Hearing Loss: Mechanisms, Assessment and Treatment

Hearing Loss: Mechanisms, Assessment and Treatment

Editor: Freya Brown

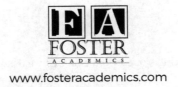

www.fosteracademics.com

www.fosteracademics.com

Cataloging-in-Publication Data

Hearing loss : mechanisms, assessment and treatment / edited by Freya Brown.
  p. cm.
Includes bibliographical references and index.
ISBN 978-1-64646-551-4
1. Deafness. 2. Deafness--Etiology. 3. Deafness--Prevention. 4. Deafness--Treatment. 5. Ear--Diseases.
6. Hearing disorders. I. Brown, Freya.
RF290 .H43 2023
617.8--dc23

Foster Academics,
118-35 Queens Blvd., Suite 400,
Forest Hills, NY 11375, USA

ISBN 978-1-64646-551-4 (Hardback)

Contents

Preface

Hearing loss refers to the partial or total loss of hearing in one or both ears, which can range from mild to profound. It is a common issue caused by illness, noise, heredity and aging. Mixed hearing loss, sensorineural hearing loss, and conductive hearing loss are the three basic types of hearing loss. There are various signs and symptoms of hearing loss including trouble understanding speech in the presence of background noise, loss of sound localization and difficulty using the telephone. The type and severity of hearing loss can be diagnosed accurately using a number of tests including auditory brainstem response (ABR), acoustic immittance and bone conduction. Some of the common treatments for hearing loss are hearing rehabilitation, medications, hearing assist devices, surgery and listening devices. This book is a valuable compilation of topics on the mechanisms, assessment and treatment of hearing loss. Its extensive content provides the readers with a thorough understanding of the subject.

This book is the end result of constructive efforts and intensive research done by experts in this field. The aim of this book is to enlighten the readers with recent information in this area of research. The information provided in this profound book would serve as a valuable reference to students and researchers in this field.

At the end, I would like to thank all the authors for devoting their precious time and providing their valuable contribution to this book. I would also like to express my gratitude to my fellow colleagues who encouraged me throughout the process.

Editor

Autophagy Contributes to the Rapamycin-Induced Improvement of Otitis Media

Daoli Xie[1†], Tong Zhao[1†], Xiaolin Zhang[2†], Lihong Kui[1], Qin Wang[1], Yuancheng Wu[1], Tihua Zheng[1], Peng Ma[3], Yan Zhang[4], Helen Molteni[5], Ruishuang Geng[1], Ying Yang[1*], Bo Li[1*] and Qing Yin Zheng[5]

[1] Hearing and Speech Rehabilitation Institute, College of Special Education, Binzhou Medical University, Yantai, China, [2] Department of Otolaryngology-Head and Neck Surgery, Binzhou Medical University Hospital, Binzhou, China, [3] Department of Genetics, School of Pharmacy, Binzhou Medical University, Yantai, China, [4] Department of Otolaryngology, Head and Neck Surgery, Second Affiliated Hospital, Xi'an Jiaotong University School of Medicine, Xi'an, China, [5] Department of Otolaryngology, Head and Neck Surgery, Case Western Reserve University, Cleveland, OH, United States

*Correspondence:
Bo Li
liboyjt@163.com
Ying Yang
yang_yingzi@163.com

†These authors have contributed equally to this work and share first authorship

Otitis media (OM) is a pervasive disease that involves hearing loss and severe complications. In our previous study, we successfully established a mouse model of human OM using *Tlr2tm1Kir* (TLR2$^{-/-}$) mice with middle ear (ME) inoculation of streptococcal peptidoglycan-polysaccharide (PGPS). In this study, we found that hearing loss and OM infections in OM mice were significantly alleviated after treatment with rapamycin (RPM), a widely used mechanistic target of RPM complex 1 (mTORC1) inhibitor and autophagy inducer. First of all, we tested the activity of mTORC1 by evaluating p-S6, Raptor, and mTOR protein expression. The data suggested that the protein expression level of p-S6, Raptor and mTOR are decreased in TLR2$^{-/-}$ mice after the injection of PGPS. Furthermore, our data showed that both the autophagosome protein LC3-II, Beclin-1, ATG7, and autophagy substrate protein p62 accumulated at higher levels in mice with OM than in OM-negative mice. The expression of lysosomal-associated proteins LAMP1, Cathepsin B, and Cathepsin D increased in the OM mice compared with OM-negative mice. Rab7 and Syntaxin 17, which is necessary for the fusion of autophagosomes with lysosomes, are reduced in the OM mice. In addition, data also described that the protein expression level of p-S6, mTOR and Raptor are lower than PGPS group after RPM treatment. The accumulation of LC3-II, Beclin-1, and ATG7 are decreased, and the expression of Rab7 and Syntaxin 17 are increased significantly after RPM treatment. Our results suggest that autophagy impairment is involved in PGPS-induced OM and that RPM improves OM at least partly by relieving autophagy impairment. Modulating autophagic activity by RPM may be a possible effective treatment strategy for OM.

Keywords: otitis media, TLR2, autophagy, PGPS, rapamycin

INTRODUCTION

OM (otitis media), one of the most common childhood infections (Rovers et al., 2004; Monasta et al., 2012), is associated with the potential burden of hearing loss and leads to excessive antibiotic consumption and severe complications (Vergison et al., 2010). The pathogenesis of OM is associated with many factors, including immune system dysfunction, genetic susceptibility, pathogen exposure, and middle ear (ME) damage (Rovers et al., 2004). ME is part of a functional system composed of the nasopharynx and eustachian tube anteriorly and the mastoid air cells posteriorly (Bluestone and Doyle, 1988). The tympanic membrane serves as the boundary between the ME and the outer ear. OM is a common inflammatory response in diseases of the auditory system (Harmes et al., 2013). Toll receptors (TLR) play a role in the innate immune response in mammals and TLR2 recognizes components from a variety of microbial pathogens (Takeda and Akira, 2015). Previously, we successfully established a mouse model of OM using *Tlr2tm1Kir* (TLR2$^{-/-}$) mice. TLR2$^{-/-}$ mice were inoculated with streptococcal peptidoglycan-polysaccharide (PGPS) into their ME by tympanic membrane puncture (Zhang et al., 2015). Our results demonstrated that compared with wild-type (WT) C57BL/6J mice, TLR2$^{-/-}$ mice inoculated with PGPS exhibited severe and long-lasting inflammation and tissue damage.

Recently, autophagy was found to be involved in immunological and inflammatory diseases. Autophagy provides a source of peptides for antigen presentation and is involved in the engulfment and degradation of intracellular pathogens, and it is also a key regulator of inflammatory cytokines (Harris et al., 2017). Autophagy plays an important role in inflammasome activation and in the release of interleukin-1 (IL-1) family cytokines, which are an essential part of innate and adaptive immune responses (Garlanda et al., 2013). Autophagy is a lysosome-dependent intracellular degradation pathway unique to eukaryotes. It is considered to have several stages: autophagy induction, autophagosome formation, the fusion of autophagosomes and lysosomes and substrate degradation (Mizushima, 2007; Glick et al., 2010). The lipidated form of microtubule-associated protein 1A/1B-light chain 3 (LC3), LC3-II, and the accumulation of the cargo receptor of autophagosomes, sequestosome 1 (SQSTM1/p62), have been used as markers for active autophagy (Tanida et al., 2004; Sou et al., 2006). In recent years, researchers have discovered that the expression of mRNA associated with autophagy, like *LC3-II* and *Beclin-1* in the ME fluid samples of patients with OM increased (Jung et al., 2020a,b), but the mechanism of autophagy involved in OM has not been clarified. Therefore, our experiment would like to verify whether autophagy is involved in OM and explore the role of autophagy in OM.

Rapamycin (RPM), an autophagy inducer, activates autophagy by repressing the mechanistic target of RPM complex 1 (mTORC1) (Sekiguchi et al., 2012). It has been used in some clinical trials, such as allograft rejection, cancer and lymphangioleiomyomatosis (Bissler et al., 2008; Li et al., 2014; Franz et al., 2016; Koenig et al., 2018; Mandrioli et al., 2018). Topical RPM appears effective and safe for treatment of tuberous sclerosis complex -related facial angiofibromas. To date, RPM has been also shown to be effective in a variety of inflammatory diseases in animal model. It relieved inflammation in experimental autoimmune encephalomyelitis in a mouse model (Li et al., 2019a,b). It also suppressed airway inflammation and inflammatory molecules in retinal inflammation (Okamoto et al., 2016; Joean et al., 2017). In

addition, it was shown to protect cartilage endplates from chronic inflammation-induced degeneration (Zuo et al., 2019). However, previous studies have not determined whether RPM treatment has an otoprotective effect in OM. We speculate that autophagy may be involved in the process of OM, and RPM may have a protective effect on OM. Therefore, we also want to find out whether RPM could relieves the OM caused by PGPS and identify the possible mechanism of this process.

We have confirmed that the ME inflammation of TLR2$^{-/-}$ mice injected with PGPS was more severe than that of WT mice through the electric otoscope image and the hematoxylin-eosin (H&E) staining firstly (**Supplementary Figures 1A,B**). In addition, we found that the protein expressions of LC3-II and p62 were increased obviously from the ME tissues injected by PGPS in TLR2$^{-/-}$ mice but not in WT mice, which suggested that the autophagy impairment may be involved in PGPS-induced OM in TLR2$^{-/-}$ mice (**Supplementary Figure 1C**). PGPS induces relatively stable OM in TLR2$^{-/-}$ mice, which provides a longer time window for drug screening and studying mechanisms of prevention and treatment. Based on the above reasons, we chose TLR2$^{-/-}$ mice as our OM model. In this study, TLR2$^{-/-}$ mice with PGPS-induced OM are called "OM mice."

In this study, we observed the therapeutic effect of RPM against PGPS-induced OM and investigated the role of autophagy in this process. Our results suggested that RPM alleviates hearing loss and inflammation in the OM mice and that normal autophagy contributes to this process. We hope that our study will help improve the clinical treatment of OM.

MATERIALS AND METHODS

Animals

Both male and female *Tlr2tm1Kir* (TLR2$^{-/-}$) mice and WT mice aged 6–8 weeks were obtained from the Jackson Laboratory (Bar Harbor, ME, United States) and housed in a pathogen-free facility. The experimental protocol was approved by the Animal Use and Care Committee of Binzhou Medical University.

Drug Treatment

Mice were treated with normal saline (NS), PGPS, NS + DMSO, or PGPS + rapamycin (RPM). Individual mice were intraperitoneally anesthetized with 4% chloral hydrate (0.01 ml/g; Biotopped Life Sciences, Beijing, China). All the mice received treatment in their right ears. The mice in the NS group received intratympanic (IT) injections of 10 μl of saline. The mice in the PGPS group received IT injections of 60 μg PGPS (100P, BD Bioscience, San Jose, CA, United States) freshly prepared in 10 μl of NS as described previously (Zhang et al., 2015). Purified (purity 99%) PGPS was extracted from the *Streptococcus pneumoniae* cell wall (Fulghum and Brown, 1998; Komori et al., 2011). RPM (Selleck, S1039, Shanghai, China) for IT injections was dissolved in 100% dimethyl sulfoxide (DMSO) to make 22 mM stock solutions and diluted with a PGPS solution immediately before injection for a final dose of either 0.35 or 0.7 μM in a 10 μl PGPS solution. 0.7 μM RPM and 0.35 μM are obtained from 22 mM stock solutions diluted with PBS. The mice in the vehicle group received IT injections of equal volumes of DMSO or NS. The mouse tympanic membranes were examined on day 3 post-injection using an otoscopic digital imaging system (MedRx VetScope System, Largo, FL, United States).

Auditory Brainstem Response and Tympanometry Procedure

The Auditory brainstem response (ABR) and tympanometry of individual experimental mice were assessed on day 3 post-injection. A computer-aided evoked potential system (IHS3.30 Intelligent Hearing Systems, Miami, FL, United States) was used for ABR measurements as described previously (Hu et al., 2016). Briefly, click, 8, 16, and 32 kHz tone burst frequencies were channeled through an earphone inserted into the right ear. The ABR threshold was identified as the lowest stimulus level at which clear and repeatable waveforms were recognized. Tympanometry measurements were performed using an MT 10 tympanometer (Interacoustics, Assens, Denmark).

Histological Analysis of the Middle Ear

The experimental mice were sacrificed on day 3 post-injection, and their right auditory bullae (including both the middle and inner ear) were dissected and subjected to pathological examination as described previously (Zhang et al., 2015). The bullae tissues were fixed with 4% paraformaldehyde for 24 h at 4°C, decalcified with a 10% EDTA solution for 5 days, and embedded in paraffin. The paraffin sections were stained with H&E and examined under a light microscope (Leica DMI4000 B, Germany).

Immunohistochemistry

The right bullae from experimental mice were fixed in 4% paraformaldehyde and decalcified before they were embedded in paraffin. The bullae tissues were sectioned at 5–7 μm. After deparaffinization, rehydration, and antigen retrieval, the sections were immunohistochemically stained with an anti-p62 antibody (Abcam, ab56416, Cambridge, England, United Kingdom), anti-Beclin-1 antibody (Abcam, ab210498), anti-ATG7 antibody (Proteintech, 10088-2-AP), anti-Cathepsin B Rabbit Polyclonal Antibody (Proteintech, 12216-1-AP), anti-Cathepsin D antibody (Proteintech, 21327-1-AP), anti-Rab7 antibody (Abcam, ab137029), anti-p-S6 antibody (Ser235/236) (Cell Signaling Technology, #4858), anti-mTOR antibody (Proteintech, 20657-1-AP), and anti-Raptor antibody (Affinity, #DF7527). The sample slides were observed under a light microscope and imaged by LAS X software (Leica DM4500 B, Leica Microsystems Inc., Buffalo Grove, IL, United States).

Immunofluorescence

After deparaffinization, rehydration, and antigen retrieval, the sections were stained with an anti-LC3B antibody (Novus Biologicals, NB100-2220, Co., United States), anti-TNF-α antibody (Proteintech, 17590-1-AP), anti-LAMP1 antibody (Abcam, ab24170), anti-Syntaxin 17 antibody (Proteintech, 17815-1-AP) and DAPI (Invitrogen, Carlsbad, United States). The stained tissues were imaged using a confocal microscope (LSM 880, Zeiss, Oberkochen, Germany).

Terminal Deoxynucleotidyl Transferase-Mediated dUTP-Biotin Nick End Labeling Staining

Paraffin sections from bullae tissues obtained from the mice were stained using a TUNEL Kit (*In Situ* Cell Death Detection Kit, Fluorescein, 11684795910; Roche Diagnostics) and following the manufacturer's protocol. The samples were then viewed under a fluorescence microscope (Leica DM4500 B, Leica Microsystems Inc., Buffalo Grove, IL, United States).

Statistical Analysis

Each experiment was repeated at least three times. All the data are presented as the mean ± SEM. Data analyses were conducted using Microsoft Excel and GraphPad Prism 9 software (GraphPad, San Diego, CA, United States). Unpaired Student's t-tests were used to determine the statistical significance when comparing two groups, and one-way ANOVA was used when comparing more than two groups. The value of $P < 0.05$ was considered statistically significant.

RESULTS

PGPS Induces Severe Otitis Media

TLR2$^{-/-}$ mice were inoculated with 10 μl of 60 μg PGPS or NS solution. Images of the mouse ears under an otoscope showed that hyperemia and hydrotympanum (white arrowhead) were present in the ears of the PGPS group (**Figure 1A**). Histological examination revealed excessive inflammatory infiltrations in the tympanic cavity and severe tissue damage in the PGPS group compared with the NS group (**Figure 1B**). The inflammatory areas in the ME of PGPS-treated mice were significantly larger than those of NS-treated mice (**Figure 1D**). Tumor Necrosis Factor α (TNF-α), an inflammatory cytokine, is responsible for a diverse range of signaling events within cells, leading to necrosis or apoptosis (Idriss and Naismith, 2000). The immunofluorescence staining revealed that expression levels of TNF-α increased in the PGPS group (**Figures 1C,E**). Taken together, these data confirmed that PGPS induced severe inflammation in the mouse ME.

Next, we investigated the hearing function of the OM mice. The average ABR thresholds and tympanometry values were measured after inoculation. Representative images of ABR waveforms for click stimuli are shown in **Figure 1F**. The mean ABR thresholds in the PGPS group were significantly higher than those in the NS solution group at click, 8 kHz and 32 kHz stimulus frequencies (**Figure 1G**). The latency of ABR wave I at click stimuli (80 dB SPL) increased in PGPS-injected mice compared with NS-injected mice (**Figure 1H**). There were significant differences in tympanometry value, compliance, and pressure between the NS and PGPS groups (**Figure 1I**).

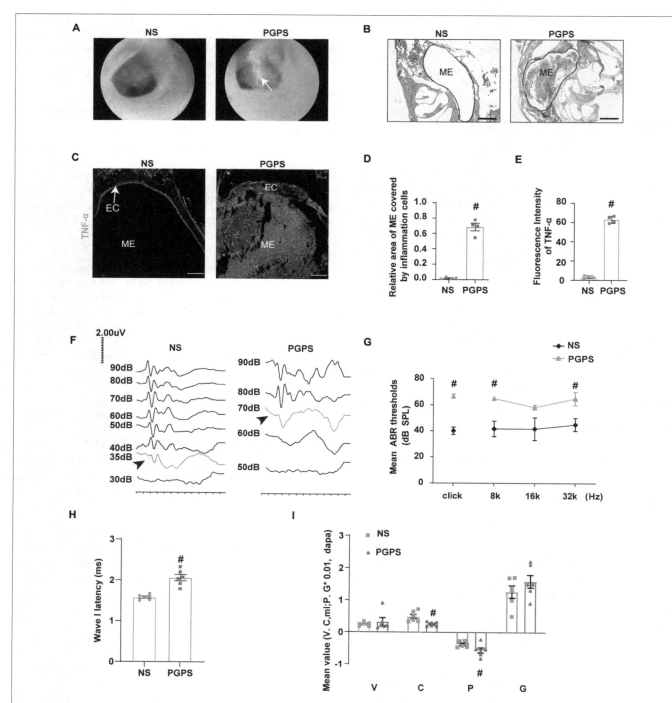

FIGURE 1 | Inoculation with PGPS induces ME inflammation and hearing loss. **(A)** Otoscopic images of ears from the NS and PGPS groups are shown. Hyperemia and hydrotympanum (white arrow) were detected in PGPS group. **(B)** H&E histology showing the structures and pathology of the ME. **(C)** Mice were inoculated with NS or PGPS for 3 days. Representative immunostaining for TNF-α expression in ME. **(D)** Quantification of the relative area of ME covered by inflammatory cells is shown in the bar graph. *n* = 4 per group **(E)** Quantification of the fluorescence intensity of TNF-α is shown in the bar graph. *n* = 4 per group **(F)** Representative images of ABR waveforms at click stimuli are shown. The red lines and arrowheads represent threshold waveforms. **(G)** Mice were inoculated with PGPS for 3 days, and the ABR thresholds were measured at the stimuli frequencies of click, 8 kHz, 16 kHz, and 32 kHz. The mean ABR thresholds in PGPS-injected mice were compared with those in NS-injected mice. The data is presented as the mean ± SEM. *n* = 10 per group **(H)** The latency of ABR wave I at click stimuli (80 dB SPL) in PGPS-injected mice compared with that in NS-injected mice is shown. Horizontal bars are mean values. *n* = 10 per group. **(I)** The tympanometry values in PGPS-injected mice are shown. The data are presented as the mean ± SEM. *n* = 10 per group. V represents the mean value of volume, C represents compliance in tympanometry parameters, G represents the gradient, and P represents the pressure. #*P* < 0.05 vs. NS group, Student's *t*-test. Scales bar, 100 μm **(B,C)**.

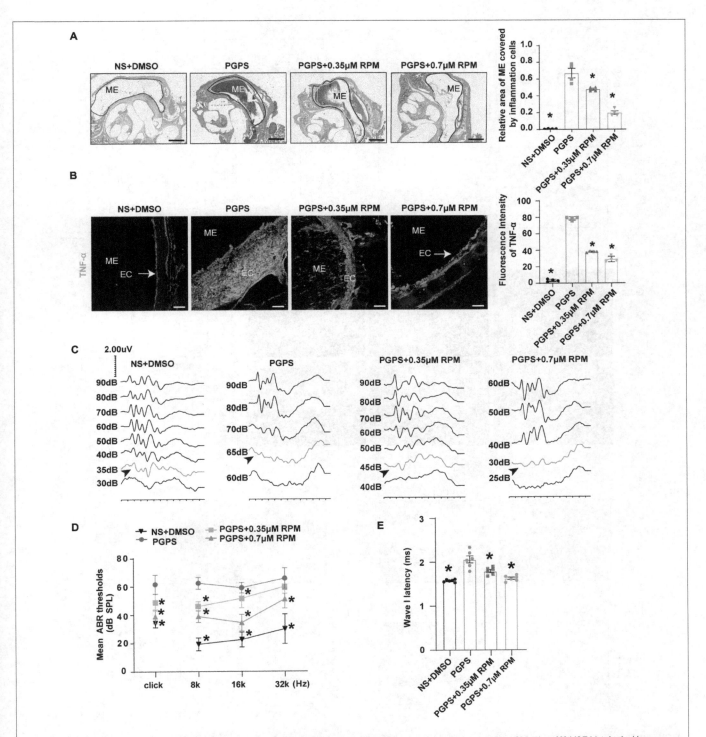

FIGURE 2 | Rapamycin treatment inhibits PGPS-induced inflammation and improves hearing function in PGPS-inoculated OM mice. **(A)** H&E histological images showing the structures and pathology of the ME. Quantification of the relative area of ME covered by inflammatory cells is shown in the bar graph. *n* = 4 per group. **(B)** Representative immunostaining for TNF-α expression in the ME. Quantification of the fluorescence intensity of TNF-α is shown in the bar graph. *n* = 4 per group. **(C)** Representative images of ABR waveforms at click stimuli are shown. The red lines and arrowheads represent threshold waveforms. **(D)** Mice were inoculated with PGPS or a combination of PGPS and either 0.35 or 0.7 μM RPM. The ABR thresholds were measured at the stimuli frequencies of click, 8, 16, and 32 kHz. The mean ABR thresholds in the NS + DMSO, PGPS + 0.35 μM RPM, and PGPS + 0.7 μM RPM groups were compared with those in the PGPS group. The data is presented as the mean ± SEM. *n* = 10 per group. **(E)** The latency of ABR wave I at click stimuli (80 dB SPL) in the NS + DMSO, PGPS + RPM combination treatment groups were compared with that in the PGPS group. Horizontal bars are mean values. *n* = 10 per group. *P < 0.05 vs. the PGPS group, one-way ANOVA, Scale bar, 100 μm **(A)**, 50 μm **(B)**.

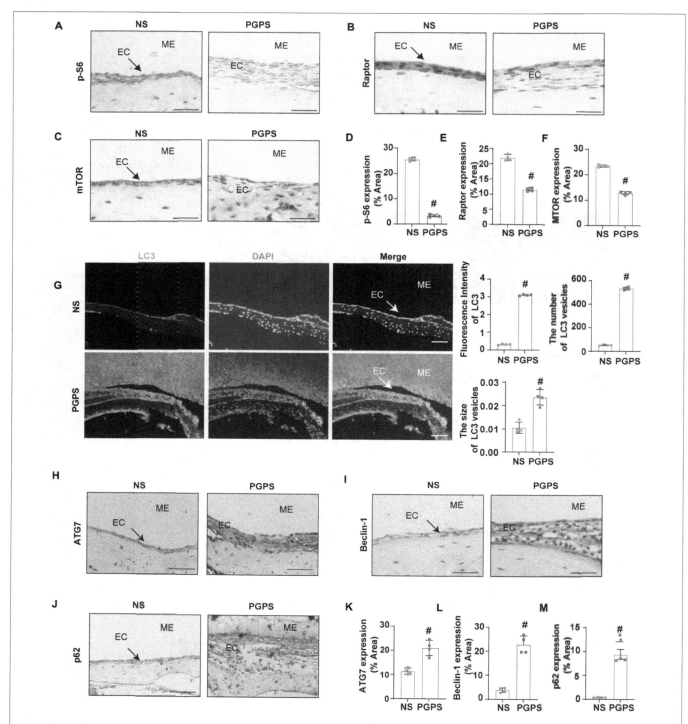

FIGURE 3 | Peptidoglycan-polysaccharide induces autophagy impairment in OM mice. Mice were inoculated with NS or PGPS for 3 days. Paraffin-embedded sections of ME tissues were immunostained with antibodies. **(A)** The representative images of p-S6 expression in ME tissues. **(B)** The representative images of Raptor expression in ME tissues. **(C)** The representative images of mTOR expression in ME tissues. **(D)** The quantification of p-S6 expression in ME tissues. **(E)** The quantification of Raptor expression in ME tissues. **(F)** The quantification of mTOR expression in ME tissues. **(G)** The representative images of LC3 expression, as well as quantitative images of the fluorescence intensity of LC3 protein expression and quantitative images of the size and number of LC3 vesicles. **(H)** The representative images of ATG7 expression in ME tissues. **(I)** The representative images of Beclin-1 expression in ME tissues. **(J)** The representative images and quantification of p62 expression in ME tissues. **(K)** The quantification of ATG7 expression in ME tissues. **(L)** The quantification of Beclin-1 expression in ME tissues. **(M)** The quantification of p-62 expression in ME tissues. $^{\#}P < 0.05$ vs. NS group, $n = 4$ per group, Student's t-test. ME represents the middle ear; EC represents epithelial cells. Scale bar = 25 μm.

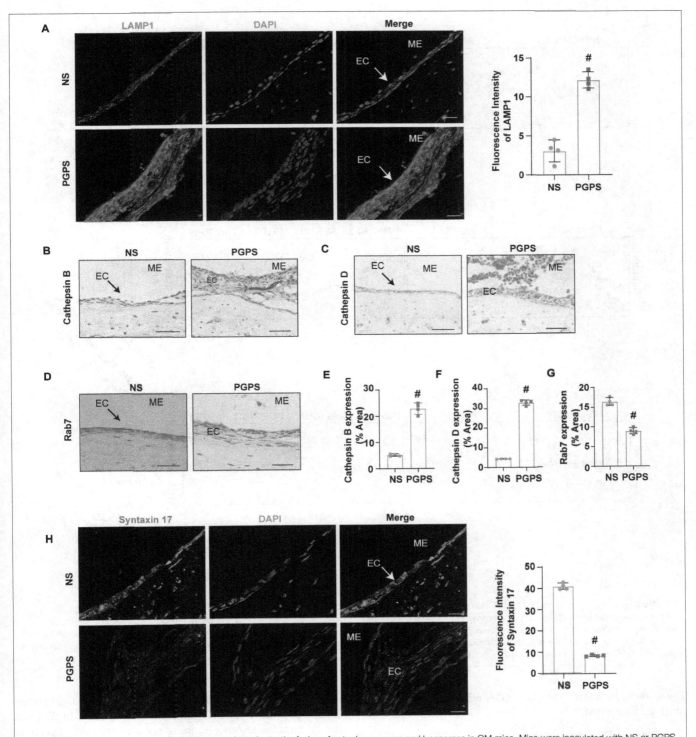

FIGURE 4 | Peptidoglycan-polysaccharide induces obstacles to the fusion of autophagosomes and lysosomes in OM mice. Mice were inoculated with NS or PGPS for 3 days. Paraffin-embedded sections of ME tissues were immunostained with antibodies. **(A)** The representative images and quantification of LAMP1 expression in ME tissues. **(B)** The representative images of Cathepsin B expression in ME tissues. **(C)** The representative images of Cathepsin D expression in ME tissues. **(D)** The representative images of Rab7 expression in ME tissues. **(E)** The quantification of Cathepsin B expression in ME tissues. **(F)** The quantification of Cathepsin D expression in ME tissues. **(G)** The quantification of Rab7 expression in ME tissues. **(H)** The representative images and quantification of Syntaxin 17 expression in ME tissues. #$P < 0.05$ vs. NS group, $n = 4$ per group, Student's t-test. ME represents the middle ear; EC represents epithelial cells. Scale bar = 25 μm.

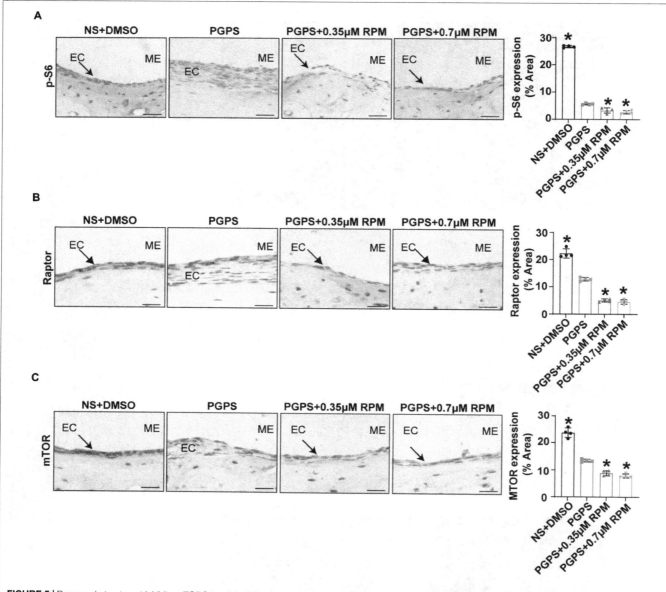

FIGURE 5 | Rapamycin treatment inhibits mTORC1 activity. Mice were inoculated with PGPS or a combination of PGPS and either 0.35 or 0.7 μM RPM. Paraffin-embedded sections of ME tissues were immunostained antibodies. **(A)** The representative images and quantification of p-S6 expression in ME tissues. **(B)** The representative images and quantification of Raptor expression in ME tissues. **(A)** The representative images and quantification of p-S6 expression in ME tissues. **(C)** The representative images and quantification of mTOR expression in ME tissues. n = 4 per group. ME represents the middle ear; EC represents epithelial cells. *P < 0.05 vs. the PGPS group, one-way ANOVA, Scale bar = 25 μm.

These data indicated that the OM mice developed severe hearing impairment.

Rapamycin Treatments Alleviate the Severity of Otitis Media Induced by PGPS

Previous studies have shown that RPM improves inflammation in organs such as the airway and retina. Thus, we investigated whether RPM has a protective effect in PGPS-induced OM mice. Histomorphological examination showed that after RPM treatment, the ME inflammation was reduced, and the

inflammation area of ME in RPM-treated mice was significantly smaller than that of PGPS-treated mice (**Figure 2A**). In addition, the immunofluorescence staining revealed that the expression of TNF-α decreased more in the RPM-treated mice than in the PGPS-treated mice (**Figure 2B**). These results showed that RPM could reduce the inflammatory infiltrates in the tympanic cavity and the expression level of TNF-α. Representative images of ABR waveforms at click stimuli are shown in **Figure 2C**. The mean ABR thresholds decreased more in the PGPS + 0.35 μM RPM group and the PGPS + 0.7 μM RPM group than in the PGPS-treated group at click, 8 and 16 kHz stimulus frequencies

(**Figure 2D**). The latency of ABR wave I at click stimuli (80 dB SPL) decreased in the PGPS + 0.7 μM RPM group compared to the PGPS-treated group (**Figure 2E**). These data suggested that RPM may ease hearing loss by attenuating PGPS-induced inflammation in OM mice.

Taking into account the complexity of RPM signaling pathways, we also injected the mice with 0.35 and 0.7 μM RPM separately. Compared with the PGPS group, the two groups of mice injected with RPM alone had normal morphology and no obvious inflammatory cells (**Supplementary Figure 2A**). The results of immunofluorescence demonstrated that the expression of TNF-α was almost invisible after the RPM injection alone (**Supplementary Figure 2B**). Compared with the PGPS group, the area of ME covered by inflammatory cells and TNF-α expression level were significantly lower in the RPM injection alone group. Compared with the NS group, there was no statistical significance. The experimental results showed that there was no obvious inflammation caused by RPM injection alone.

We also investigated the hearing function in RPM single treatment group by ABR, and the representative images of ABR waveforms at click stimuli are shown in **Supplementary Figure 2C**. Compared with the PGPS group, the average ABR thresholds of the NS group, 0.35 and 0.7 μM RPM group at click, 8, 16, and 32 kHz stimulation frequencies were lower than those in the PGPS group, and were statistically significant (**Supplementary Figure 2D**). In addition, the latency of ABR wave I in the PGPS group under the click stimulus (80 dB SPL) was longer than that of the other three groups (**Supplementary Figure 2E**). Compared with NS group, the hearing threshold and the wave I latency in RPM treatment alone group is basically no statistical significance. These data showed that after injection of RPM alone, there is almost no effect on the hearing of mice.

Autophagy Impairment Is Involved in PGPS-Induced Otitis Media

Rapamycin, an autophagy inducer, activates autophagy by repressing the mTORC1 (Sekiguchi et al., 2012). S6 ribosomal protein (S6) phosphorylation was shown to be a critical downstream component of mTOR signaling (Ruvinsky et al., 2005). mTORC1 contains mTOR, which is the catalytic subunit of the complex (Laplante and Sabatini, 2009). It also contains the large protein Raptor, which is the regulatory-associated protein of mTOR (Thoreen et al., 2009). To find out whether mTORC1 signaling is involved in PGPS-induced autophagy impairment, we examined the phosphorylation of mTORC1 substrate, S6 phosphorylation at 235/236 (p-S6) and mTORC1 components, mTOR and Raptor. PGPS treatment resulted in a significant decrease in the levels of p-S6, Raptor and mTOR compared with NS group (**Figures 3A–F**), suggesting an inhibition of mTORC1 activity. In this study, we found that the fluorescence intensity of LC3 in PGPS-treated OM mice was higher than that in NS-treated mice. Quantification of the size and number of LC3 vesicles also increased in PGPS-treated OM mice (**Figure 3G**). These results suggested that OM mice are activated at the initial stage

of autophagy, but it may also be due to the accumulation of LC3 caused by the blocked autophagy flux.

In addition, we also tested the expressions of ATG7 and Beclin-1. ATG7 is considered to be essential molecules for the induction of autophagy (Arakawa et al., 2017), and Beclin-1 initiates the nucleation step of autophagy to begin autophagic flux (Liang et al., 1999; Matsunaga et al., 2009). The results of immunohistochemistry showed that compared with the NS group, the expression of ATG7 and Beclin-1 were increased in OM mice (**Figures 3H,I,K,L**). These results suggested that after the injection of PGPS, the activity of mTORC1 was inhibited and the initial stage of autophagy was activated. We speculate that autophagy may act as an instinctive stress response to resist external stimuli by PGPS. However, p62 protein accumulation in the ME epithelial cells of OM mice was higher after PGPS treatment than after NS treatment (**Figures 3J,M**). These data indicated that PGPS could induce the initiation of autophagy, but at the same time cause impairment in the degradation of stage autophagy.

PGPS Induces Dysfunction of Autophagosome and Lysosome Fusion

The dysfunction of autophagy degradation may be due to the impairment of lysosomal function or dysfunction in the fusion stage of autophagosomes and lysosomes. Firstly, we test lysosomal function. Lysosomal activity is important for the autophagy degradation process (Tai et al., 2017). In order to investigate whether the autophagy impairment mechanism induced by PGPS is related to the dysfunction of lysosome, we examined the protein expression level of key lysosome enzymes like LAMP-1, Cathepsin B and Cathepsin D to evaluate the lysosomal function. Lysosome associated membrane protein-1 (LAMP-1) is a major protein component of the lysosomal membrane (Eskelinen, 2006). Cathepsin B, a member of the cysteine cathepsin family, involved in regulating the bioavailability of lysosomes and autophagosomes (Man and Kanneganti, 2016). Cathepsin D is one of the major lysosomal proteases indispensable for the maintenance of cellular proteostasis (Marques et al., 2020). Immunofluorescence results showed that compared with NS group, the expression of LAMP1 protein increased in the PGPS group (**Figure 4A**). The immunohistochemical results of Cathepsin B and Cathepsin D also showed a consistent increase in PGPS group (**Figures 4B,C,E,F**). These data showed that lysosome function maybe is not impaired.

Considering that lysosome function does not seem to be impaired, we examined the process of autophagosome and lysosome fusion by evaluating expression of Rab7 and Syntaxin 17 protein. Rab7 is a member of the Rab family, involved in transport to late endosomes and in the biogenesis of the perinuclear lysosome compartment (Gutierrez et al., 2004; Guerra and Bucci, 2016). It plays a critical role in the final maturation of late autophagic vacuoles (autophagosome and lysosome fusion) (Jager et al., 2004; He et al., 2019). Syntaxin 17 is also required for fusion between the autophagosome and lysosome (Itakura et al., 2012; Shen et al., 2021). Our results showed that Rab7 and Syntaxin 17 expression decreased in the PGPS group compared with the NS group (**Figures 4D,G,H**). These results suggested that PGPS may block the autophagy degradation stage mainly due to the impairment of the autophagosome and lysosome fusion stage. And PGPS may impair the fusion of autophagosomes with lysosomes by decreasing the expression of Rab7 and Syntaxin 17.

Rapamycin Treatment Enhances Autophagy in PGPS-Treated Otitis Media Mice

Immunohistochemical staining showed that after injection of PGPS + 0.35/0.7 μM RPM, p-S6, Raptor and mTOR exhibited lower protein levels than the PGPS group (**Figures 5A–C**). These results suggested that RPM may enhance autophagic initiation by inhibiting mTORC1 activity. LC3 staining in ME epithelial cells revealed lower expression of LC3 and lower numbers of LC3 vesicles in RPM-treated mice than in PGPS-treated mice, the size of LC3 vesicles did not show a significant difference (**Figure 6A**). These results suggested that there may be a certain accumulation of LC3 after injection of PGPS, and after the treatment of RPM, the autophagy flux may became smooth. Immunohistochemical staining showed that after injection of PGPS + 0.35/0.7 μM RPM, ATG7 and Beclin-1 exhibited lower protein levels than the PGPS group (**Figures 6B–C**).

In order to understand the role of RPM, we injected RPM alone in TLR2$^{-/-}$ mice. The results showed that the expression of LC3 and the number of LC3 vesicles in RPM injection group was lower than that of the PGPS group, but it was higher than that of the NS group (**Supplementary Figures 3A,B,D**). There was almost no statistical difference in the size of LC3 vesicles among the groups (**Supplementary Figures 3A,C**). These results suggested that after the injection of PGPS, the mouse ME epithelial cells activated the initiation of autophagy to resist the toxicity by PGPS. However, obstacle may occur in the autophagy degradation stage, which led to the accumulation of LC3 protein. Moreover, RPM may promote the degradation stage of autophagy.

In addition, there was less p62 protein accumulation in the RPM-treated mice than in the PGPS-treated mice (**Figure 6D**). After injection of RPM alone, the expression level of p62 was significantly lower compared with the PGPS group, and there was almost no difference compared with the NS group (**Supplementary Figure 3E**). These results indicated that degradation function may be improved after RPM treatment.

Similarly, we tested lysosome function and the fusion function of autophagosome and lysosome after RPM treatment alone. The results showed that the expression of LAMP1, Cathepsin B and Cathepsin D (**Figures 7A–C**) in the RPM-treated mice was relatively weaker than that in the PGPS group. After RPM injection alone, we found that the expression level of Cathepsin B protein was lower than that of the PGPS group, but higher than that of the NS group (**Supplementary Figure 3F**). We further speculate that the increased activity of lysosomal after PGPS injection may be a response to external stimuli by PGPS,

so the expression level of Cathepsin B is higher than that of the RPM injection group. We speculate that RPM may promote lysosome function, thus the expression level of Cathepsin B in RPM injection alone group is higher than that of NS group. In addition, the expression of Rab7 and Syntaxin 17 protein increased in the PGPS + RPM-treated mice (**Figures 8A,B**), thus RPM may promote the process of autophagosome and lysosome fusion. TUNEL staining showed that there were less apoptotic cells in the ME after RPM treatment (**Figure 9**). In addition, we did not find obvious apoptotic cells in the RPM alone group (**Supplementary Figure 4**). These data indicated that RPM may enhance the autophagic activity of OM mice by inhibiting the activity of mTORC1, increasing the fusion of autophagosomes with lysosomes and relieving ME epithelial cell apoptosis.

DISCUSSION

Otitis media, a general term for inflammatory changes in the ME cavity, is one of the most common childhood conditions (Mittal et al., 2014; Venekamp et al., 2017). The pathogenic mechanism of OM is not yet clear and excessive antibiotic treatment has also brought a heavy burden to society, so it is particularly important to explore the mechanism of OM and find suitable drug treatments (Vergison et al., 2010). In recent years, the autophagy pathway has played a certain role in inflammation, but the research on the relationship between autophagy and OM has not been in-depth. It was found that the expression of *LC3-II* was significantly increased in the inflammatory ME tissues in human (Jung et al., 2020b). Studies have shown that in the ME fluid of patients with OM, the mRNA level of autophagy initiation-related genes such as *Beclin-1*, is increased in OM patients with cholesteatom (Jung et al., 2020a). Our study aims to explore the role of autophagy in the pathogenesis of OM by TLR2$^{-/-}$ mice model, and treat OM mice by RPM, aiming to provide a theoretical basis and new treatment strategies for the treatment of clinical OM.

The mTOR is involved in the induction and initiation of autophagy (Cayo et al., 2021). We tested the expression of p-S6, Raptor and mTOR after injection of PGPS, and found that the mTORC1 activity of mice in the PGPS group was weakened. These results indicated that autophagy may be activated in the mice in the PGPS group, which seems to be consistent with the increase in the expression of proteins related to autophagy initiation like LC3, ATG7 and Beclin-1. Among them, the expressions of LC3, ATG7 and Beclin-1 in the PGPS group all showed increased compared with NS group. We speculate that autophagy may act as an instinctive stress response to resist external stimuli by PGPS. RPM + PGPS combination treatment groups showed that the protein expression of LC3, ATG7 and Beclin-1 were reduced compared with the PGPS group. Considering the complexity of the RPM pathway, we also injected RPM alone in TLR2$^{-/-}$ mice. The results suggested that the expression of LC3, ATG7, and Beclin-1 in RPM injection alone group was also lower than PGPS group, but was higher than NS group. These results indicated that the PGPS group does not seem to be impaired during the initiation of autophagy.

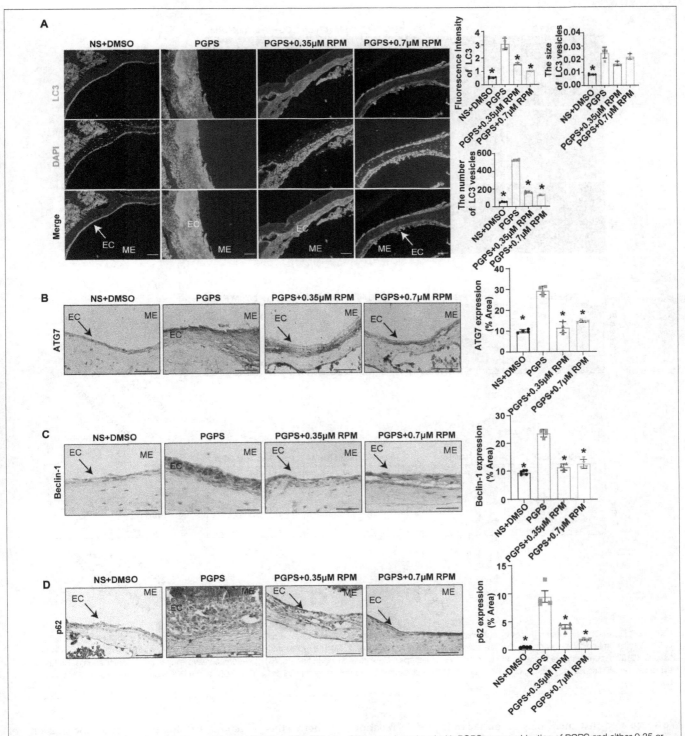

FIGURE 6 | Rapamycin treatment enhances autophagy in PGPS-treated OM mice. Mice were inoculated with PGPS or a combination of PGPS and either 0.35 or 0.7 μM RPM. Paraffin-embedded sections of ME tissues were immunostained antibodies. **(A)** The representative images of LC3 expression, as well as quantitative images of the fluorescence intensity of LC3 protein expression and quantitative images of the size and number of LC3 vesicles. $n = 4$ per group. **(B)** The representative images and quantification of ATG7 expression in ME tissues. $n = 4$ per group. **(C)** The representative images and quantification of Beclin-1 expression in ME tissues. $n = 4$ per group. **(D)** The representative images and quantification of p62 expression in ME tissues. $n = 4$ per group. ME represents the middle ear; EC represents epithelial cells. $*P < 0.05$ vs. the PGPS group, one-way ANOVA, Scale bar = 25 μm.

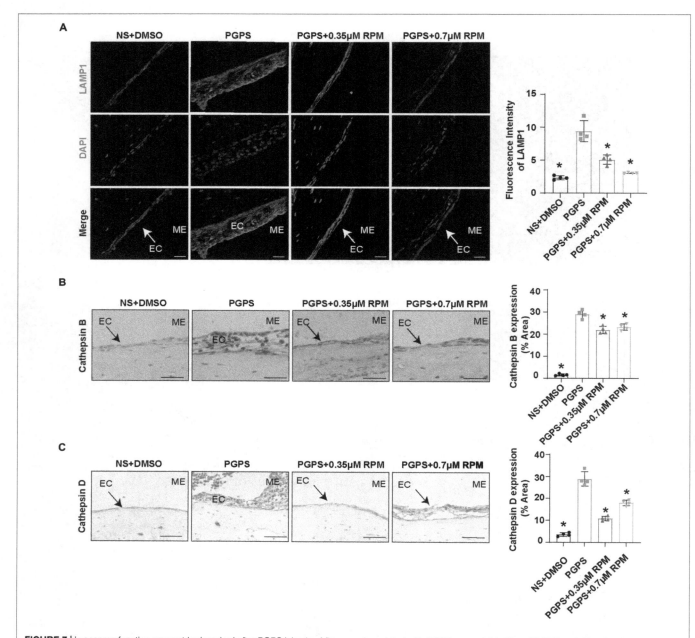

FIGURE 7 | Lysosome function may not be impaired after PGPS injection Mice were inoculated with PGPS or a combination of PGPS and either 0.35 or 0.7 μM RPM. Paraffin-embedded sections of ME tissues were immunostained antibodies. **(A)** The representative images and quantification of LAMP1 expression in ME tissues. **(B)** The representative images and quantification of Cathepsin B expression in ME tissues. **(C)** The representative images and quantification of Cathepsin D expression in ME tissues. n = 4 per group, ME represents the middle ear; EC represents epithelial cells. *P < 0.05 vs. the PGPS group, one-way ANOVA, Scale bar = 25 μm.

We speculated that there may be obstacles in the degradation stage of autophagy, resulting in accumulation of LC3 protein in PGPS group. The expression of p62 in PGPS group is more increasing than NS group, and after the injection of PGPS + RPM combination, the level of p62 decreased, which demonstrated that PGPS may induce autophagy impairment in the autophagy degradation stage and RPM may promote the degradation stage of autophagy.

Both the function of lysosome and the fusion of autophagosomes and lysosomes affect the autophagic degradation. We first evaluated the lysosomal function. Lysosome-related proteins such as LAMP1, Cathepsin B and Cathepsin D play an important role in the normal function of lysosomes (Eskelinen, 2006; Man and Kanneganti, 2016; Marques et al., 2020). In our experiment, compared with the NS group, the expression of the three proteins increased in

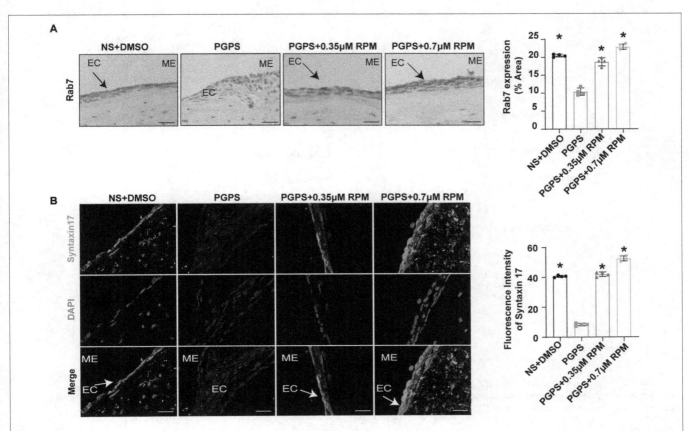

FIGURE 8 | Rapamycin treatment increases the fusion of autophagosomes and lysosomes in OM mice. Mice were inoculated with PGPS or a combination of PGPS and either 0.35 or 0.7 μM RPM. Paraffin-embedded sections of ME tissues were immunostained antibodies. **(A)** The representative images and quantification of Rab7 expression in ME tissues. **(B)** The representative images and quantification of Syntaxin 17 expression in ME tissues. $n = 4$ per group, ME represents the middle ear; EC represents epithelial cells. *$P < 0.05$ vs. the PGPS group, one-way ANOVA, Scale bar = 25 μm.

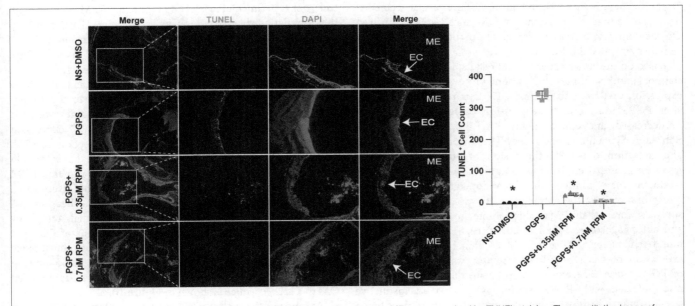

FIGURE 9 | Rapamycin treatment relieved ME epithelial cell apoptosis. Apoptotic cells in the MEs were examined by TUNEL staining. The quantitative image of apoptotic cells was shown in Figure B. The PGPS + 0.7 μM RPM group showed fewer TUNEL-positive epithelial cells than the PGPS group. ME represents the middle ear; EC represents epithelial cells. *$P < 0.05$ vs. the PGPS group, $n = 4$ per group, Scale bar = 500 μm, one-way ANOVA.

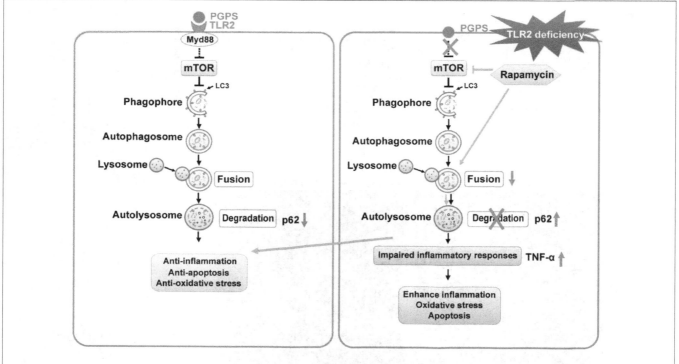

FIGURE 10 | The proposed mechanism for RPM-enhanced autophagy protects against PGPS-induced OM in TLR2$^{-/-}$ mice. TLR2 deficiency may inhibit fusion between autophagosomes and lysosomes, leading to the accumulation of p62. It may also induce inflammation and apoptosis. RPM treatment may improve the autophagic clearance ability and have a protective effect against OM injury.

the PGPS group. The expression level of the three proteins in the RPM + PGPS combination treatment group was lower than that of the PGPS group. After injection of RPM alone, the expression of Cathepsin B also decreased compared with PGPS group, but was higher than NS group. These results seemed to demonstrate that the lysosomes of OM mice are not impaired. On the contrary, increased lysosomal function may be a stress response after PGPS injection.

Based on the above experimental results, we tested the fusion stage of autophagosomes and lysosomes by evaluating the protein expression of Rab7 and Syntaxin 17. Our results showed that after PGPS injection, the expression of Rab7 and Syntaxin 17 decreased, and co-treatment with RPM, the expression of Rab7 and Syntaxin 17 increased. These results suggested that after injection of PGPS, the fusion of autophagosome and lysosome is impaired, leading to autophagy impairment. RPM treatment may stimulate the fusion of autophagosomes and lysosomes, making the autophagy pathway smoothly. Previous study also found that RPM could promote the fusion of lysosomes and autophagosomes (Choi et al., 2016). In addition, we also found that after PGPS and RPM combination treatment, the expression of p-S6, mTOR and Raptor was lower than that of PGPS alone. Therefore, we speculate that when TLR2$^{-/-}$ mice injected with PGPS, autophagy acts as an instinctive stress response to resist external stimuli. But, there may be an obstacle when autophagosomes fuse with lysosomes, which leads to obstacles in the degradation stage of autophagy and causes

protein accumulation. This may produce proteotoxic stress, and autophagy is insufficient to resist proteotoxic stress during OM. After RPM treatment, mTORC1 could be further inhibited, thereby promoting the initial stage of autophagy. At the same time, our experimental results also found that RPM may promote the degradation stage of autophagy. In summary, RPM may play a positive role in both stages, so as to exert its therapeutic effect.

In this study, we verify again that PGPS injection could cause OM in TLR2$^{-/-}$ mice, which leads to hearing loss. In addition, we demonstrated that inflammation in OM mice may be due to the impairment of autophagy pathway, mainly due to impairment in the process of autophagosome fusing to lysosomes, which is manifested by the decrease of Rab7 and Syntaxin 17 expression in the PGPS group. We also found that after injection of RPM, it could inhibit the activity of mTORC1, increase the expression level of Rab7 and Syntaxin 17 and promote autophagy flux. RPM treatment also reduce the inflammatory response of ME epithelial cells, reduce cell apoptosis, and thereby alleviate hearing loss in OM mice. Therefore, these data suggested that autophagy impairment may be involved in the development of OM and that RPM could effectively improve OM conditions, most likely by alleviating autophagy impairment. A general scheme showing that RPM-enhanced autophagy protects against PGPS-induced OM in TLR2$^{-/-}$ mice is shown in **Figure 10**.

Autophagy is a bulk degradation system that delivers cytoplasmic constituents to autolysosomes for recycling and maintaining cell homeostasis. In addition, autophagy has critical functions in cell-autonomous defense in immunity (Matsuzawa-Ishimoto et al., 2018). Many studies found autophagy impairment could mediate susceptibility to infectious and inflammatory diseases like Crohn's disease and chronic obstructive pulmonary disease (Lupfer et al., 2013; Lassen et al., 2014; Murthy et al., 2014). In this study, we found for the first time that autophagy was involved in OM and that RPM significantly alleviated autophagy impairment and improved ME inflammatory conditions.

To date, RPM has been used in some clinical trials like tuberous sclerosis complex-related facial angiofibromas (Koenig et al., 2018). It has been also shown to be effective in a variety of inflammatory diseases like autoimmune encephalomyelitis and retinal inflammation (Okamoto et al., 2016; Joean et al., 2017; Li et al., 2019a,b). In this study, we showed that RPM significantly alleviated autophagy impairment and improved ME inflammatory conditions. Some researchers also found that RPM could promote the fusion of lysosomes and autophagosomes (Choi et al., 2016; Cheng et al., 2021). Therefore, we speculate that RPM may play a positive role in the treatment of OM. Due to the complexity of RPM signaling pathways, we do not rule out the possibility that the protective effect of RPM on the OM may also involve other branches of RPM signaling in addition to autophagy. Nonetheless, our data suggest that modulating autophagy activity may be possible intervention for OM. Our study provides a theoretical basis for the clinical application of RPM in the treatment of OM. However, it has been reported that RPM has immunosuppressive side effects. Several new RPM analogs have demonstrated reduced side effects, and these new drugs may be safer and less immunosuppressive than RPM (Fu et al., 2018). Perhaps the ability of these analogs to prevent OM should be tested.

In summary, our research shows that autophagy impairment is related to OM, and impairment to the fusion of autophagosomes and lysosomes is an important factor leading to the occurrence of PGPS-induced otitis media. RPM treatment could alleviate hearing loss to a certain extent. These findings highlight the potential of specific autophagosome-to-lysosome fusion activators in reducing PGPS-induced OM. Considering that increasing autophagic clearance may be useful as a new therapeutic strategy against severe OM damage, autophagosome and lysosome fusing dysfunction may be a candidate target for therapeutic intervention. Therefore, extensive pharmaceutical studies should be performed in the near future. Future research is necessary to better explain the mechanism underlying the protective role of the normal autophagy process against the pathogenesis of OM, and then design and test potential therapeutic methods to prevent or treat OM.

AUTHOR CONTRIBUTIONS

DX, ToZ, XZ, LK, QW, and YW performed the experiments. BL and DX wrote the manuscript. ToZ and BL analyzed the data. RG, YY, PM, XZ, and YZ participated in discussion of the project. BL and QZ designed the study. YW, TiZ, HM, and QZ revised the manuscript. All authors reviewed and approved the manuscript.

ACKNOWLEDGMENTS

We would like to express the most sincere thanks to Maria Hatzoglou from Case Western Reserve University for comments and advice on the article.

REFERENCES

Arakawa, S., Honda, S., Yamaguchi, H., and Shimizu, S. (2017). Molecular mechanisms and physiological roles of Atg5/Atg7-independent alternative autophagy. *Proc. Jpn. Acad. Ser. B Phys. Biol. Sci.* 93, 378–385. doi: 10.2183/pjab.93.023

Bissler, J. J., McCormack, F. X., Young, L. R., Elwing, J. M., Chuck, G., Leonard, J. M., et al. (2008). Sirolimus for angiomyolipoma in tuberous sclerosis complex or lymphangioleiomyomatosis. *N. Engl. J. Med.* 358, 140–151.

Bluestone, C. D., and Doyle, W. J. (1988). Anatomy and physiology of eustachian tube and middle ear related to otitis media. *J. Allergy Clin. Immunol.* 81, 997–1003. doi: 10.1016/0091-6749(88)90168-6

Cayo, A., Segovia, R., Venturini, W., Moore-Carrasco, R., Valenzuela, C., and Brown, N. (2021). mTOR activity and autophagy in senescent cells, a complex partnership. *Int. J. Mol. Sci.* 22:8149. doi: 10.3390/ijms22158149

Cheng, J. T., Liu, P. F., Yang, H. C., Huang, S. J., Griffith, M., Morgan, P., et al. (2021). Tumor Susceptibility gene 101 facilitates rapamycin-induced autophagic flux in neuron cells. *Biomed. Pharmacother.* 134:111106. doi: 10.1016/j.biopha.2020.111106

Choi, J. Y., Won, N. H., Park, J. D., Jang, S., Eom, C. Y., Choi, Y., et al. (2016). From the cover: ethylmercury-induced oxidative and endoplasmic reticulum stress-mediated autophagic cell death: involvement of autophagosome-lysosome fusion arrest. *Toxicol. Sci.* 154, 27–42. doi: 10.1093/toxsci/kfw155

Eskelinen, E. L. (2006). Roles of LAMP-1 and LAMP-2 in lysosome biogenesis and autophagy. *Mol. Aspects Med.* 27, 495–502. doi: 10.1016/j.mam.2006.08.005

Franz, D. N., Belousova, E., Sparagana, S., Bebin, E. M., Frost, M. D., Kuperman, R., et al. (2016). Long-term use of everolimus in patients with tuberous sclerosis complex: final results from the EXIST-1 study. *PLoS One* 11:e0158476. doi: 10.1371/journal.pone.0158476

Fu, X., Sun, X., Zhang, L., Jin, Y., Chai, R., Yang, L., et al. (2018). Tuberous sclerosis complex-mediated mTORC1 overactivation promotes age-related hearing loss. *J. Clin. Invest.* 128, 4938–4955. doi: 10.1172/JCI98058

Fulghum, R. S., and Brown, R. R. (1998). Purified streptococcal cell wall (PG-APS) causes experimental otitis media. *Auris Nasus Larynx* 25, 5–11. doi: 10.1016/s0385-8146(97)10025-6

Garlanda, C., Dinarello, C. A., and Mantovani, A. (2013). The interleukin-1 family: back to the future. *Immunity* 39, 1003–1018. doi: 10.1016/j.immuni.2013.11.010

Glick, D., Barth, S., and Macleod, K. F. (2010). Autophagy: cellular and molecular mechanisms. *J. Pathol.* 221, 3–12. doi: 10.1002/path.2697

Guerra, F., and Bucci, C. (2016). Multiple Roles of the Small GTPase Rab7. *Cells* 5:34. doi: 10.3390/cells5030034

Gutierrez, M. G., Munafo, D. B., Beron, W., and Colombo, M. I. (2004). Rab7 is required for the normal progression of the autophagic pathway in mammalian cells. *J. Cell Sci.* 117, 2687–2697. doi: 10.1242/jcs.01114

Harmes, K. M., Blackwood, R. A., Burrows, H. L., Cooke, J. M., Harrison, R. V., and Passamani, P. P. (2013). Otitis media: diagnosis and treatment. *Am. Fam. Phys.* 88, 435–440.

Harris, J., Lang, T., Thomas, J. P. W., Sukkar, M. B., Nabar, N. R., and Kehrl, J. H. (2017). Autophagy and inflammasomes. *Mol. Immunol.* 86, 10–15.

He, K., Sun, H., Zhang, J., Zheng, R., Gu, J., Luo, M., et al. (2019). Rab7mediated autophagy regulates phenotypic transformation and behavior of smooth muscle cells via the Ras/Raf/MEK/ERK signaling pathway in human aortic dissection. *Mol. Med. Rep.* 19, 3105–3113. doi: 10.3892/mmr.2019.9955

Hu, J., Li, B., Apisa, L., Yu, H., Entenman, S., Xu, M., et al. (2016). ER stress inhibitor attenuates hearing loss and hair cell death in Cdh23(erl/erl) mutant mice. *Cell Death Dis.* 7:e2485. doi: 10.1038/cddis.2016.386

Idriss, H. T., and Naismith, J. H. (2000). TNF alpha and the TNF receptor superfamily: structure-function relationship(s). *Microsc. Res. Tech.* 50, 184–195. doi: 10.1002/1097-0029(20000801)50:3<184::AID-JEMT2>3.0.CO;2-H

Itakura, E., Kishi-Itakura, C., and Mizushima, N. (2012). The hairpin-type tail-anchored SNARE syntaxin 17 targets to autophagosomes for fusion with endosomes/lysosomes. *Cell* 151, 1256–1269. doi: 10.1016/j.cell.2012.11.001

Jager, S., Bucci, C., Tanida, I., Ueno, T., Kominami, E., Saftig, P., et al. (2004). Role for Rab7 in maturation of late autophagic vacuoles. *J. Cell Sci.* 117, 4837–4848. doi: 10.1242/jcs.01370

Joean, O., Hueber, A., Feller, F., Jirmo, A. C., Lochner, M., Dittrich, A. M., et al. (2017). Suppression of Th17-polarized airway inflammation by rapamycin. *Sci. Rep.* 7:15336. doi: 10.1038/s41598-017-15750-6

Jung, J., Jung, S. Y., Kim, M. G., Kim, Y. I., Kim, S. H., and Yeo, S. G. (2020a). Comparison of autophagy mRNA expression between chronic otitis media with and without cholesteatoma. *J. Audiol. Otol.* 24, 191–197. doi: 10.7874/jao.2020.00108

Jung, J., Park, D. C., Kim, Y. I., Lee, E. H., Park, M. J., Kim, S. H., et al. (2020b). Decreased expression of autophagy markers in culture-positive patients with chronic otitis media. *J. Int. Med. Res.* 48:300060520936174. doi: 10.1177/0300060520936174

Koenig, M. K., Bell, C. S., Hebert, A. A., Roberson, J., Samuels, J. A., Slopis, J. M., et al. (2018). Efficacy and safety of topical rapamycin in patients with facial angiofibromas secondary to tuberous sclerosis complex: the treatment randomized clinical trial. *JAMA Dermatol.* 154, 773–780. doi: 10.1001/jamadermatol.2018.0464

Komori, M., Nakamura, Y., Ping, J., Feng, L., Toyama, K., Kim, Y., et al. (2011). Pneumococcal peptidoglycan-polysaccharides regulate Toll-like receptor 2 in the mouse middle ear epithelial cells. *Pediatr. Res.* 69, 101–105. doi: 10.1203/PDR.0b013e3182055237

Laplante, M., and Sabatini, D. M. (2009). mTOR signaling at a glance. *J. Cell Sci.* 122, 3589–3594. doi: 10.1242/jcs.051011

Lassen, K. G., Kuballa, P., Conway, K. L., Patel, K. K., Becker, C. E., Peloquin, J. M., et al. (2014). Atg16L1 T300A variant decreases selective autophagy resulting in altered cytokine signaling and decreased antibacterial defense. *Proc. Natl. Acad. Sci. U.S.A.* 111, 7741–7746. doi: 10.1073/pnas.1407001111

Li, J., Kim, S. G., and Blenis, J. (2014). Rapamycin: one drug, many effects. *Cell Metab.* 19, 373–379. doi: 10.1016/j.cmet.2014.01.001

Li, Z., Nie, L., Chen, L., Sun, Y., and Guo, L. (2019a). [Rapamycin alleviates inflammation by up-regulating TGF-beta/Smad signaling in a mouse model of autoimmune encephalomyelitis]. *Nan Fang Yi Ke Da Xue Xue Bao* 39, 35–42. doi: 10.12122/j.issn.1673-4254.2019.01.06

Li, Z., Nie, L., Chen, L., Sun, Y., and Li, G. (2019b). Rapamycin relieves inflammation of experimental autoimmune encephalomyelitis by altering the balance of Treg/Th17 in a mouse model. *Neurosci. Lett.* 705, 39–45. doi: 10.1016/j.neulet.2019.04.035

Liang, X. H., Jackson, S., Seaman, M., Brown, K., Kempkes, B., Hibshoosh, H., et al. (1999). Induction of autophagy and inhibition of tumorigenesis by beclin 1. *Nature* 402, 672–676. doi: 10.1038/45257

Lupfer, C., Thomas, P. G., Anand, P. K., Vogel, P., Milasta, S., Martinez, J., et al. (2013). Receptor interacting protein kinase 2-mediated mitophagy regulates inflammasome activation during virus infection. *Nat. Immunol.* 14, 480–488. doi: 10.1038/ni.2563

Man, S. M., and Kanneganti, T. D. (2016). Regulation of lysosomal dynamics and autophagy by CTSB/cathepsin B. *Autophagy* 12, 2504–2505. doi: 10.1080/15548627.2016.1239679

Mandrioli, J., D'Amico, R., Zucchi, E., Gessani, A., Fini, N., Fasano, A., et al. (2018). Rapamycin treatment for amyotrophic lateral sclerosis: protocol for a phase II randomized, double-blind, placebo-controlled, multicenter, clinical trial (RAP-ALS trial). *Medicine (Baltimore)* 97:e11119. doi: 10.1097/MD.0000000000011119

Marques, A. R. A., Di Spiezio, A., Thiessen, N., Schmidt, L., Grotzinger, J., Lullmann-Rauch, R., et al. (2020). Enzyme replacement therapy with recombinant pro-CTSD (cathepsin D) corrects defective proteolysis and autophagy in neuronal ceroid lipofuscinosis. *Autophagy* 16, 811–825. doi: 10.1080/15548627.2019.1637200

Matsunaga, K., Saitoh, T., Tabata, K., Omori, H., Satoh, T., Kurotori, N., et al. (2009). Two Beclin 1-binding proteins, Atg14L and Rubicon, reciprocally regulate autophagy at different stages. *Nat. Cell Biol.* 11, 385–396. doi: 10.1038/ncb1846

Matsuzawa-Ishimoto, Y., Hwang, S., and Cadwell, K. (2018). Autophagy and Inflammation. *Annu. Rev. Immunol.* 36, 73–101.

Mittal, R., Kodiyan, J., Gerring, R., Mathee, K., Li, J. D., Grati, M., et al. (2014). Role of innate immunity in the pathogenesis of otitis media. *Int. J. Infect. Dis.* 29, 259–267. doi: 10.1016/j.ijid.2014.10.015

Mizushima, N. (2007). Autophagy: process and function. *Genes Dev.* 21, 2861–2873. doi: 10.1101/gad.1599207

Monasta, L., Ronfani, L., Marchetti, F., Montico, M., Vecchi Brumatti, L., Bavcar, A., et al. (2012). Burden of disease caused by otitis media: systematic review and global estimates. *PLoS One* 7:e36226. doi: 10.1371/journal.pone.0036226

Murthy, A., Li, Y., Peng, I., Reichelt, M., Katakam, A. K., Noubade, R., et al. (2014). A Crohn's disease variant in Atg16l1 enhances its degradation by caspase 3. *Nature* 506, 456–462. doi: 10.1038/nature13044

Okamoto, T., Ozawa, Y., Kamoshita, M., Osada, H., Toda, E., Kurihara, T., et al. (2016). The neuroprotective effect of rapamycin as a modulator of the mTOR-NF-kappaB axis during retinal inflammation. *PLoS One* 11:e0146517. doi: 10.1371/journal.pone.0146517

Rovers, M. M., Schilder, A. G., Zielhuis, G. A., and Rosenfeld, R. M. (2004). Otitis media. *Lancet* 363, 465–473.

Ruvinsky, I., Sharon, N., Lerer, T., Cohen, H., Stolovich-Rain, M., Nir, T., et al. (2005). Ribosomal protein S6 phosphorylation is a determinant of cell size and glucose homeostasis. *Genes Dev.* 19, 2199–2211. doi: 10.1101/gad.351605

Sekiguchi, A., Kanno, H., Ozawa, H., Yamaya, S., and Itoi, E. (2012). Rapamycin promotes autophagy and reduces neural tissue damage and locomotor impairment after spinal cord injury in mice. *J. Neurotrauma* 29, 946–956.

Shen, Q., Shi, Y., Liu, J., Su, H., Huang, J., Zhang, Y., et al. (2021). Acetylation of STX17 (syntaxin 17) controls autophagosome maturation. *Autophagy* 17, 1157–1169. doi: 10.1080/15548627.2020.1752471

Sou, Y. S., Tanida, I., Komatsu, M., Ueno, T., and Kominami, E. (2006). Phosphatidylserine in addition to phosphatidylethanolamine is an in vitro target of the mammalian Atg8 modifiers, LC3, GABARAP, and GATE-16. *J. Biol. Chem.* 281, 3017–3024. doi: 10.1074/jbc.M505888200

Tai, H., Wang, Z., Gong, H., Han, X., Zhou, J., Wang, X., et al. (2017). Autophagy impairment with lysosomal and mitochondrial dysfunction is an important characteristic of oxidative stress-induced senescence. *Autophagy* 13, 99–113. doi: 10.1080/15548627.2016.1247143

Takeda, K., and Akira, S. (2015). Toll-like receptors. *Curr. Protoc. Immunol.* 109, 14.12.1–14.12.10.

Tanida, I., Ueno, T., and Kominami, E. (2004). LC3 conjugation system in mammalian autophagy. *Int. J. Biochem. Cell Biol.* 36, 2503–2518. doi: 10.1016/j.biocel.2004.05.009

Thoreen, C. C., Kang, S. A., Chang, J. W., Liu, Q., Zhang, J., Gao, Y., et al. (2009). An ATP-competitive mammalian target of rapamycin inhibitor reveals rapamycin-resistant functions of mTORC1. *J. Biol. Chem.* 284, 8023–8032. doi: 10.1074/jbc.m900301200

Venekamp, R. P., Damoiseaux, R. A., and Schilder, A. G. (2017). Acute Otitis Media in Children. *Am Fam. Phys.* 95, 109–110.

Vergison, A., Dagan, R., Arguedas, A., Bonhoeffer, J., Cohen, R., Dhooge, I., et al. (2010). Otitis media and its consequences: beyond the earache. *Lancet Infect. Dis.* 10, 195–203. doi: 10.1016/S1473-3099(10)70012-8

Zhang, X., Zheng, T., Sang, L., Apisa, L., Zhao, H., Fu, F., et al. (2015). Otitis media induced by peptidoglycan-polysaccharide (PGPS) in TLR2-deficient (Tlr2(-/-)) mice for developing drug therapy. *Infect. Genet. Evol.* 35, 194–203. doi: 10.1016/j.meegid.2015.08.019

Zuo, R., Wang, Y., Li, J., Wu, J., Wang, W., Li, B., et al. (2019). Rapamycin induced autophagy inhibits inflammation-mediated endplate degeneration by enhancing Nrf2/Keap1 signaling of cartilage endplate stem cells. *Stem Cells* 37, 828–840. doi: 10.1002/stem.2999

2

Dual-Specificity Phosphatase 14 Regulates Zebrafish Hair Cell Formation through Activation of p38 Signaling Pathway

Guanyun Wei[1†], Xu Zhang[1,2†], Chengyun Cai[1†], Jiajing Sheng[1†], Mengting Xu[1], Cheng Wang[1], Qiuxiang Gu[1], Chao Guo[1], Fangyi Chen[3,4*], Dong Liu[1*] and Fuping Qian[1*]

[1] Key Laboratory of Neuroregeneration of MOE, Nantong Laboratory of Development and Diseases, School of Life Sciences, Co-innovation Center of Neuroregeneration, Nantong University, Nantong, China, [2] Translational Medical Research Center, Wuxi No. 2 People's Hospital, Affiliated Wuxi Clinical College of Nantong University, Wuxi, China, [3] Department of Biomedical Engineering, Southern University of Science and Technology, Shenzhen, China, [4] Department of Biology, Brain Research Center, Southern University of Science and Technology, Shenzhen, China

*Correspondence:
Fangyi Chen
chenfy@sustech.edu.cn
Dong Liu
liudongtom@gmail.com;
tom@ntu.edu.cn
Fuping Qian
qianfuping198911@163.com

† These authors have contributed equally to this work

Most cases of acquired hearing loss are due to degeneration and subsequent loss of cochlear hair cells. Whereas mammalian hair cells are not replaced when lost, in zebrafish, they constantly renew and regenerate after injury. However, the molecular mechanism among this difference remains unknown. Dual-specificity phosphatase 14 (DUSP14) is an important negative modulator of mitogen-activated protein kinase (MAPK) signaling pathways. Our study was to investigate the effects of DUSP14 on supporting cell development and hair cell regeneration and explore the potential mechanism. Our results showed that *dusp14* gene is highly expressed in zebrafish developing neuromasts and otic vesicles. Behavior analysis showed that *dusp14* deficiency resulted in hearing defects in zebrafish larvae, which were reversed by *dusp14* mRNA treatment. Moreover, knockdown of *dusp14* gene caused a significant decrease in the number of neuromasts and hair cells in both neuromast and otic vesicle, mainly due to the inhibition of the proliferation of supporting cells, which results in a decrease in the number of supporting cells and ultimately in the regeneration of hair cells. We further found significant changes in a series of MAPK pathway genes through transcriptome sequencing analysis of *dusp14*-deficient zebrafish, especially *mapk12b* gene in p38 signaling. Additionally, inhibiting p38 signaling effectively rescued all phenotypes caused by *dusp14* deficiency, including hair cell and supporting cell reduction. These results suggest that DUSP14 might be a key gene to regulate supporting cell development and hair cell regeneration and is a potential target for the treatment of hearing loss.

Keywords: DUSP14, supporting cell, hair cell, zebrafish, proliferation, regeneration

INTRODUCTION

Millions of people all over the world are subjected to different degrees of hearing loss (Morton, 1991; Sun, 2021). The main causes of hearing impairment include aging, noise, genetic mutations, and exposure to ototoxic drugs, which contributed to the sensory hair cell loss in inner ear (Furness, 2015). Most cases of acquired hearing loss are due to degeneration and subsequent loss of cochlear hair cells (Vlajkovic and Thorne, 2021). However, there are no Food and Drug Administration

(FDA)-approved drugs to protect from hearing loss, which makes urgent the task of discovering new therapeutics.

The auditory epithelium located in the cochlea is composed of sensory hair cells and non-sensory supporting cells (Kelley, 2006). Although hair cells cannot regenerate in mammalian adults, regeneration of hair cells in the inner ear and lateral line is widespread in non-mammalian vertebrates, such as chicken, amphibian, and zebrafish. Additionally, those hair cells regenerate from transdifferentiating supporting cells, which aroused the interest of many auditory scientists in understanding the inner ear hair cell and supporting cell development and regeneration, with the potential to develop biologic therapies for hearing loss (Rubel et al., 2013). Therefore, it is particularly important to understand the cellular and molecular mechanisms of such striking difference between mammalian and non-mammalian vertebrates.

Dual-specificity phosphatase (DUSP) family is a group of phosphatases, which dephosphorylate of tyrosine and/or serine or threonine residues and the resulting activity regulation of their substrates (Caunt and Keyse, 2013). DUSPs are considered to be major modulators of key signaling pathways that are dysregulated in a variety of diseases (Patterson et al., 2009a; Ríos et al., 2014; An et al., 2021). DUSPs can be divided into seven subgroups with the consideration of substrate preferences: phosphatases of regenerating liver (PRL) family, cell division cycle 14 (CDC14) phosphatases, phosphatase and tensin homologs deleted on chromosome 10 (PTEN), slingshot homolog (SSH) family of phosphatases, myotubularins, mitogen-activated protein kinase phosphatases (MKPs), and atypical DUSPs (Huang and Tan, 2012). Atypical DUSPs are mostly with low molecular weight and lack the N-terminal two CDC25 homology 2 (CH2) domain. The most atypical DUSPs are localized in the cytoplasm. It is reported that some atypical DUSPs regulate MAPK, including extracellular signal-regulated kinases (ERKs), c-Jun N-terminal kinases (JNKs), and p38 kinases, which plays an important role in cell proliferation and apoptosis (Huang and Tan, 2012).

Dual-specificity phosphatase 14, an atypical member of the DUSP family of proteins, are critical modulators in various biological processes, such as apoptosis, inflammation, proliferation, and oxidative stress. Our results showed that dusp14 gene was expressed in the inner ear and lateral line system of zebrafish, which suggest that Dusp14 may play a vital role in the regulation of hair cell fate in zebrafish.

Based on these findings, this study examined whether dusp14 gene could regulate the hair cell fate in zebrafish, especially the behavior of supporting cell. Furthermore, we aimed to evaluate whether dusp14 gene putative modulating hair cell actions would be related to modulation of the MAPK signaling pathway.

MATERIALS AND METHODS

Zebrafish Embryos

Zebrafish (*Danio rerio*) were reared and maintained at 28.5°C as Westerfield described (Westerfield, 1995). Two zebrafish lines were used in the study, including the wild-type AB line and the transgenic line *Tg(Brn3c:mGFP)*, where membrane-localized green fluorescent protein (GFP) is specifically expressed in the hair cells. Embryonic stages are defined as described (Kimmel et al., 1995). Embryos were collected after natural spawns. Embryos were moved to embryo medium containing 0.2 mM phenylthiourea at ∼20 h postfertilization (hpf) to prevent pigmentation. All animal procedures were performed according to protocols approved by the Animal Care and Use Committee of Nantong University and were consistent with the National Institutes of Health Guide for the Care and Use of Laboratory Animals.

Whole-Mount *in situ* Hybridization

The DNA fragments of zebrafish *dusp14* and *eya1* were amplified by PCR using the primers (**Supplementary Table 3**). Then, they were subcloned into the pGEM-T Easy Vector (Promega, United States), and a gene-specific digoxigenin-labeled RNA probe was transcribed *in vitro* using the DIG RNA Labeling Kit (SP6&T7) (Roche) following the manufacturer's instructions. The prefixed embryos were incubated with the probe overnight at 4°C. The alkaline phosphatase (AP)-conjugated antibody against digoxigenin (Roche) was used to detect the digoxigenin-labeled RNA probe. The AP-substrate NBT/BCIP solution (Roche) was added to the reaction system to stain the tissues specifically expressing *dusp14* gene or *eya1* gene in zebrafish.

Morpholino and CRISPR/Cas9 Microinjection

According to the manufacturer's instruction, morpholino antisense oligos (MOs; Gene Tools) were prepared at a stock concentration of 1 mM. We designed *dusp14* splice-modifying morpholino (*dusp14*-MO) to knockdown the expression of *dusp14* (**Supplementary Table 3**). MOs were diluted to 0.3 mM and injected into one-cell-stage embryos.

To generate the *dusp14* gene mutant zebrafish, as described in our previous work (Gong et al., 2017), 2–3 nL of solution containing specific single-guide RNA (sgRNA) and Cas9 mRNA was injected into one-cell-stage embryos (primers used are listed in **Supplementary Table 3**).

mRNA Synthesis and Phenotypic Rescue

dusp14 DNA fragments were synthesized by PCR using the primers, *dusp14*-*Bam*HI-F and *dusp14*-*Eco*RI-R (**Supplementary Table 3**). The DNA fragments were subcloned into the pCS2 + vector, and the recombinant plasmid was linearized using the restriction endonuclease *Not*I (New England Biolabs). The linearized product was purified as a template and transcribed into mRNA *in vitro* using the mMESSAGE mMACHINE High Yield Capped RNA Transcription kit (Ambion). Then, the synthesized *dusp14* mRNA was coinjected with *dusp14*-MO into one-cell-stage zebrafish embryos. The rate of rescued zebrafish after injection of *dusp14* mRNA was analyzed at 72 hpf.

RNA Extraction, Reverse Transcription, and Quantitative Real-Time PCR

Total RNAs of all samples were extracted using TRIzol reagent (Invitrogen, United States), and genomic DNA contamination was removed by DNase I (Promega, United States). The RNA yield was determined using NanoDrop ND-2000 (Thermo Fisher Scientific, United States), and integrity was checked on a 1% agarose gel. The cDNA was synthesized using oligo-dT primers and Superscript RT-III (Takara, JP). Quantitative real-time PCR (qRT-PCR) was performed using a Plus Real-Time PCR System (Applied Biosystems, United States). SYBR Prime ScriptTM RTPCR kit (Takara, JP) was used for mRNA qRT-PCR. Data were analyzed using the relative $2^{-\Delta\Delta CT}$ method (Livak and Schmittgen, 2001; Schmittgen and Livak, 2008). The primers for qRT-PCR are listed in **Supplementary Table 3**.

Acoustic or Vibrational Startle

Acoustic or vibrational startle protocol was based on previous studies (van den Bos et al., 2017) with appropriate modifications. Larvae (6 dpf) were transferred from petri dishes to wells filled with 1 mL of E3 medium. Both the control and *dusp14*-MO zebrafish were tested. The protocol (lights on) consisted of 10-min acclimation, followed by 9 acoustic or vibrational stimuli (DanioVision intensity setting) with a 20-s interstimulus interval (ISI). Variable of interest to show the startle response was maximum velocity (mm/s) with 1-s intervals, since the startle response is a short burst of activity best captured by this parameter. When subjects did not show a clear response to the first stimulus (values lower than 15 mm/s), they were discarded from analysis.

Acoustic Startle Reflex

The acoustic startle reflex was performed as described previously (Yang et al., 2017). The larvae (5 dpf) were put in a thin layer of culture media in a petri dish attached to mini vibrator. The response of larvae to sound stimulus (a tone burst 9 dB re. m s^{-2}, 600 Hz, for 30 ms) generated by the vibrator was recorded from above by an infrared camera over a 6-s period. The mean moving distance and peak speed were used to quantify the startle response.

Immunofluorescence Staining

For immunofluorescence staining, the embryos were anesthetized and then fixed using 4% paraformaldehyde. After washing three times with PBS-T, the embryos were incubated in the antigen retrieval solution (Beyotime Biotechnology, China, #P0088) for 15 min at 98°C. Non-specific binding was then blocked with 10% donkey serum (Solarbio, China, #SL050) in PBS-T. Next, specific primary antibodies against GFP (Abcam, #ab13970) and cleaved caspase-3 (CST, #9664), 5-bromo-2'-deoxyuridine (BrdU) (Sigma, #B5002) or SOX2 (Abcam, #ab97959) were added, and secondary antibodies were used to detect the primary antibodies.

TdT-mediated dUTP nick end labeling (TUNEL) assay was performed according to the manufacturer's instructions (Alexa Fluor 640, cat#: 40308ES20, YEASEN Biotech Co. Ltd) to detect cell death in the HCs of neuromast. In brief, the embryos were anesthetized and then fixed using 4% paraformaldehyde. After washing three times with PBST, 20 μg/mL proteinase K (Roche) was used to treat the embryos. Next, Alexa Fluor 640-12-dUTP

Labeling Mix was applied to label the apoptotic cells for at least 3 h. DAPI was applied to label the nucleus.

Images were taken with a Nikon confocal microscope A1R at 40× magnification and were analyzed by Nikon A1R NIS Elements. Exposure settings were adjusted to minimize oversaturation.

Drug Treatment

The p38 inhibitor (APExBIO, #C5248), with a working concentration at 50 ng/μL, was coinjected with *dusp14*-MO into the 1–2 cell-stage zebrafish embryos. Additionally, the injected zebrafish were raised at 28.5°C. The development status was recorded with a bright field microscope at about 72 hpf.

Statistical Analysis

All data were analyzed using GraphPad Prism 8.3.0. One-way ANOVA, unpaired Student's *t*-tests, and two-way ANOVA were used to determine statistical significance when comparing two groups. The value of $p < 0.05$ was considered as statistically significant. All data are presented as means with SEM, and all experiments were repeated at least three times.

RNA-Seq Analysis

To study gene expression changes after *dusp14* knockdown in zebrafish, we performed transcriptome sequencing. The wild-type zebrafish and *dusp14*-MO injected zebrafish of 3 days old were prepared, respectively. Three independent replicates of the samples were analyzed for each treatment. The total RNA was extracted using TRIzol reagent (Invitrogen, United States) following the manufacturer's procedure. The quantity and purity of total RNAs were checked using a Bioanalyzer 2100 and RNA 6000 Nano LabChip Kit (Agilent, CA, United States) with RIN value > 7.0. All RNA samples were submitted to GENEWIZ Science (Suzhou, China), and deep sequencings were performed on an Illumina Hiseq2500.

For RNA-seq data, the Cuffdiff was used to estimate differential expression between samples at the transcript level (Kim et al., 2013). The differentially expressed gene (DEG) was determined with *log2 fold change* > 1, *p-value* < 0.05. The R package Clusterprofer was used for Kyoto Encyclopedia of Genes and Genomes (KEGG) pathway and gene ontology (GO) annotation.

RESULTS

The *dusp14* Gene Is Expressed in the Otic Vesicles and Neuromasts in Zebrafish

First, to observe the conservation of DUSP14, we constructed an evolutionary tree of 14 species based on the amino acid sequence of DUSP14, including mouse, giant panda, domestic cat, human, big brown bat, Chinese horseshoe bat, sperm whale, sea lion, bottlenose dolphins, lizards, zebrafish, yeast, and nematodes (**Figure 1A**). The results showed that *dusp14* is an extensive

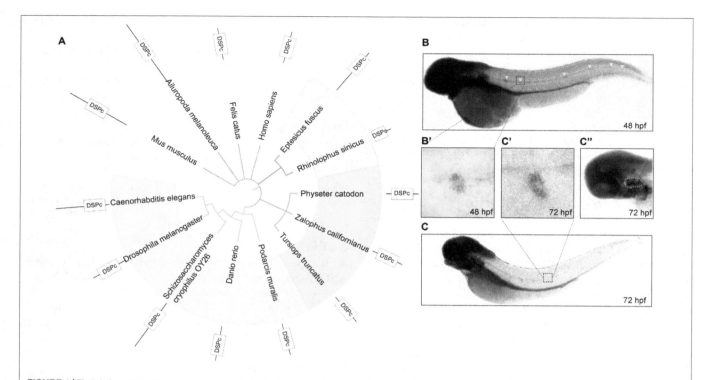

FIGURE 1 | The phylogenetic and expression analysis of zebrafish *dusp14*. **(A)** A phylogenetic tree was generated using the PhyML software base on amino acid sequences. The pictures are mouse, giant panda, domestic cat, human, big brown bat, Chinese horseshoe bat, sperm whale, sea lion, bottlenose dolphins, lizards, zebrafish, *Saccharomyces cerevisiae*, and nematodes. **(B,C)** WISH with the *dusp14* probe in wild-type zebrafish showed that the gene is expressed in the otic vesicle and lateral line at 48 hpf **(B)** and 72 hpf **(C)**. **(B',C',C")** Are the detailed information with higher magnification of the **(B,C)**, respectively.

conserved gene in many species with DUSP (dual-specificity phosphatases) conserved domain.

Next, to investigate the spatiotemporal expression of *dusp14* during the embryonic development, we performed the WISH using a *dusp14* antisense probe. As shown in **Figures 1B,B'**, *dusp14* is expressed in the neuromast at 48 hpf. At 72 h (**Figure 1C**), the *dusp14* gene expression is pronounced in the lateral line (**Figure 1C'**) and the otic vesicle (**Figure 1C"**). These results indicate that *dusp14* may play an important role in inner ear development.

Knockdown the *dusp14* Expression by Morpholino Leads to Hearing Defects in Zebrafish

To explore the effect of the *dusp14* gene on zebrafish behavioral response, we designed morpholino oligonucleotides to knockdown the expression of *dusp14*, and *dusp14*-MO was validated to effectively reduce *dusp14* expression (**Supplementary Figure 1**). Then, we performed acoustic or vibrational startle test after *dusp14*-MO injection at 5 dpf. The results showed that the response of *dusp14*-MO zebrafish to percussion stimuli becomes sluggish, whereas the injection of *dusp14* mRNA significantly rescued the phenotype (**Figures 2A,B**). In addition, there is no difference in movement rate among wide-type zebrafish, *dusp14*-MO zebrafish, and *dusp14*-mRNA and MO coinjected zebrafish during the total

test (**Figure 2C**), which suggests that the injection did not affect locomotor activities of zebrafish.

To further investigate the effects of *dusp14*-MO on hearing dysfunction, we performed the acoustic startle reflex experiment (**Figure 2D**). The results showed that the swimming trajectory (**Figure 2E**), swimming distance (**Figure 2F**), and velocity (**Figure 2G**) of *dusp14* morphants were reduced compared to the controls, which were reversed by *dusp14*-mRNA. These results indicate that *dusp14* is necessary for hearing-related behaviors.

Knockdown *dusp14* Expression by Morpholino Decreases the Number of Hair Cells and Neuromasts in Zebrafish

It is well known that hair cells in the inner ear of zebrafish are responsible for the balance perception and hearing. Therefore, to test the underlying cellular mechanisms of *dusp14* gene on ear function, we knockdown the *dusp14* expression by morpholino in the transgenic zebrafish line *Tg(Brn3c:mGFP)*, in which the GFP were specifically expressed in hair cells (**Figure 3A**). The results showed that the number of hair cells in three different crista hair cell clusters (anterior crista hair cells: AC; lateral crista hair cells: LC; posterior crista hair cells: PC) was reduced after *dusp14*-MO microinjection at 72 hpf (**Figures 3B,B'**), which was neutralized by *dusp14* mRNA treatment.

The hair cells in zebrafish are also present in the lateral line system containing the neuromasts that is important to perceive

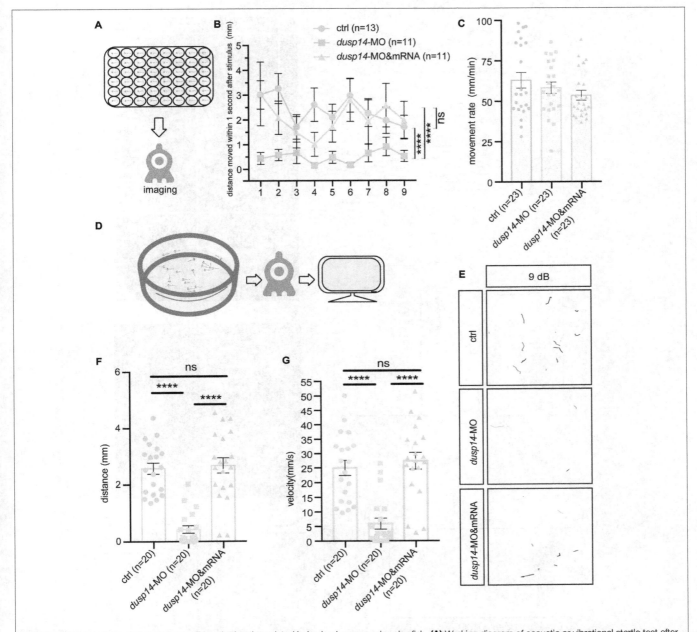

FIGURE 2 | Knockdown of *dusp14* gene affects the hearing-related behavioral response in zebrafish. **(A)** Working diagram of acoustic or vibrational startle test after *dusp14*-MO injection at 5 dpf. **(B)** The distance moved of zebrafish within 1 s after the percussion stimulation. **(C)** Statistics of the moving rate of zebrafish during the total test. **(D)** The schematic diagram shows the startle response testing equipment. **(E)** The swimming trajectory of the control, *dusp14* morphants and *dusp14*-mRNA and MO. **(F,G)** Swimming distance and peak velocity of zebrafish larvae at 5 dpf that reflected the auditory function of zebrafish larvae by examining the startle response. Values with **** above the bars are significantly different (*P* < 0.0001), ns means no significance.

changes in the surroundings. Then, we further investigate the role of *dusp14* gene on neuromast formation and found that the number of hair cell clusters in the posterior lateral line of *dusp14* morphants was significantly decreased at 72 hpf (**Figures 3C,C′**). Moreover, the number of the hair cells in the remaining neuromast L3 was also decreased (**Figures 3B,B″**). But the *dusp14* mRNA treatment interfered these changes remarkably. In addition, we used the *eya1* gene to label the

neuromast cells (Grant et al., 2005; Whitfield, 2005) in lateral line by WISH and discovered that the number of neuromasts in the posterior lateral line of *dusp14* morphants was significantly reduced (**Figures 3D,D′**). These results indicate that *dusp14* gene affects the number of hair cells in zebrafish inner ear and lateral line.

To further validate the function of *dusp14* during the hair cell development, the CRISPR/Cas9 system was utilized to knockout

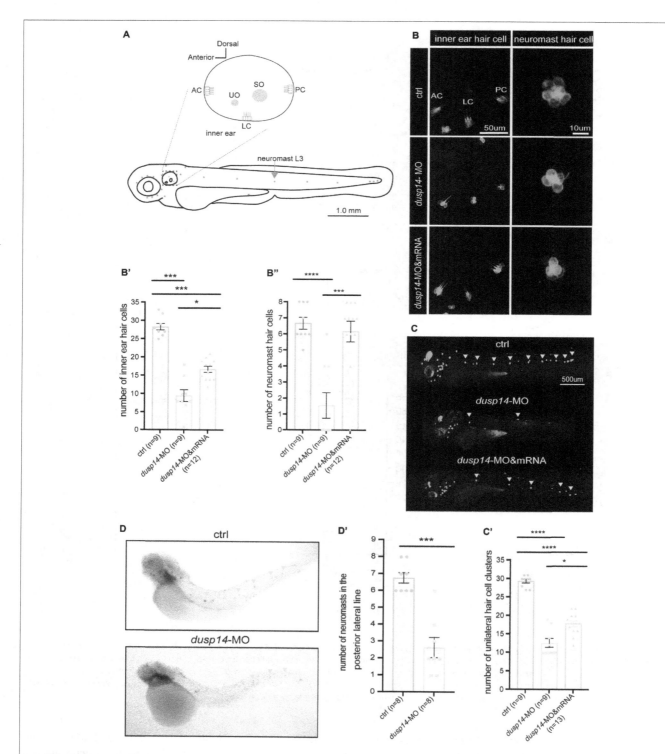

FIGURE 3 | Knockdown *dusp14* expression by morpholino decreases the number of hair cell and neuromasts in zebrafish. **(A)** Schematic diagram of zebrafish neuromast and inner ear hair cell. **(B)** Confocal imaging analysis of crista hair cells in the otic vesicle of control and *dusp14* deficiency zebrafish at 72 hpf. **(B')** The statistical analysis of the numbers of inner ear crista hair cells in the control and *dusp14* morphants at 72 hpf. **(B'')** The statistical analysis of the numbers of hair cells in the remaining neuromast L3 in the control and *dusp14* morphants at 72 hpf. **(C)** The imaging analysis of control and *dusp14* morphants at 72 hpf in fluorescent field. Scale bar = 500 μm. **(C')** Quantification of the number of unilateral hair cell clusters of control and *dusp14* morphants at 72 hpf. **(D)** *in situ* hybridization of the *eya1* gene specifically expressed in the neuromasts showed that the number of neuromasts in *dusp14*-MO zebrafish was decreased. **(D')** statistics results of D. Each bar represents the mean ± SEM. Values with *, ***, and **** above the bars are significantly different (*P* < 0.05, *P* < 0.001, and *P* < 0.0001, respectively).

dusp14 in wild-type zebrafish. As shown in **Supplementary Figure 2A**, we chose a sgRNA target site near the translation start codon in the exon1 of *dusp14* for CRISPR/Cas9-mediated mutation to abolish the protein translation. Similar to the results of the *dusp14* morphants, the number of hair cell clusters and hair cells in the posterior lateral line of the *dusp14* mutants was remarkably fewer than that of the control fish at 72 hpf, which was partially reversed by the *dusp14* mRNA injection (**Supplementary Figures 2C,C′,C″**).

Knockdown of the *dusp14* Gene Reduces the Number of Supporting Cells and Proliferation of Supporting Cells

As we know, hair cells of the inner ear and lateral line system in zebrafish regenerate from mitotic supporting cells (Williams and Holder, 2000; Kniss et al., 2016; Thomas and Raible, 2019). Since

knockdown of the *dusp14* gene caused the reduction of hair cells, we speculated that support cells, resource of hair cells, were also affected by *dusp14* morpholino injection.

To test the hypothesis, we analyzed SOX2$^+$ cells in the posterior lateral line of *dusp14* morphants by immunostaining with anti-SOX2 antibody. The results showed that SOX2$^+$ cell number was dramatically decreased after *dusp14* morpholino injection, which was substantially reserved by *dusp14* mRNA treatment (**Figures 4A,A′**). Furthermore, we performed the BrdU incorporation to measure the regeneration of supporting cells in the lateral line (**Figures 4B,B′**). Our results showed that the number of proliferating supporting cells was significantly reduced in the *dusp14* morphants. Additionally, the *dusp14* mRNA treatment partially interfered these changes. What is more, there is no difference in apoptotic signal between *dusp14* morphants and the control, which was immunostained with TUNEL and cleaved caspase 3 in zebrafish neuromasts

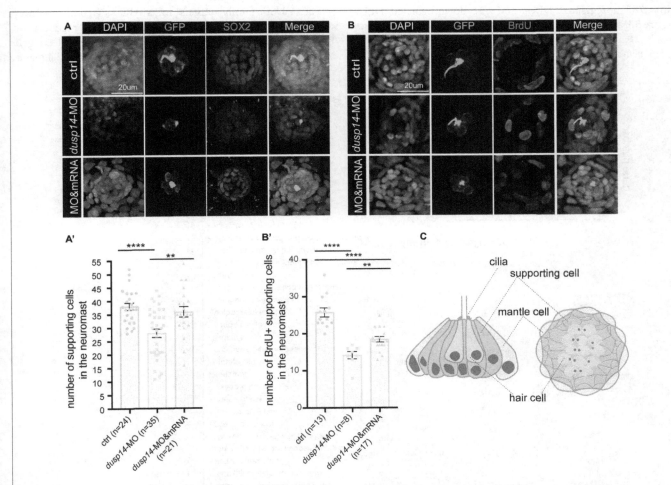

FIGURE 4 | Knockdown of the dusp14 gene reduces the number of supporting cells and proliferation of supporting cells. **(A)** The representation of SOX2 immunofluorescence images of neuromasts in the posterior lateral line of the control and *dusp14* morphants. **(A′)** Quantification of the number of supporting cells in the posterior lateral line neuromast of control and *dusp14* mutants at 72 hpf. **(B)** BrdU staining for the supporting cell in the neuromasts in the posterior lateral line of the control zebrafish and *dusp14* morphants. Scale bar = 20 μm. **(B′)** Quantification of zebrafish embryos with the BrdU$^+$ cells in the control and *dusp14* morphants. **(C)** Schematic diagram of the longitudinal structure and the plane structure of neuromast, the gray part is the mantle cell, the pink part is supporting cell, and the green represents hair cell. Experimental embryos were sampled at 72 hpf ($n > 8$). Each bar represents the mean ± SD. Values with ** and **** above the bars are significantly different ($P < 0.01$ and $P < 0.0001$, respectively).

(**Supplementary Figure 3**). Taken together, we found that *dusp14* gene may regulate the formation of hair cells and ultimately affect the hearing by modulating the proliferation of supporting cells in the zebrafish lateral line (**Figure 4C**).

Transcriptomic Sequencing Data Revealed p38 Signaling Pathways May Responsible for Regulation of *dusp14* Gene on Hearing Function

To gain a further insight into the molecular mechanism by which *dusp14* gene responsible for the regeneration of the supporting cells, we performed RNA sequencing (RNA-seq) of 72 hpf wild-type zebrafish and *dusp14*-MO zebrafish. Over 40 million valid reads per library on average were obtained after quality filtering, which was, respectively, mapped to about 90% of the zebrafish genome (**Supplementary Table 1**). The results revealed 2,418 DEGs that might be affected by the absence of *dusp14* with 1,787 upregulated DEGs and 631 downregulated DEGs (**Figure 5A** and **Supplementary Table 2**). What is more, 12 genes (*apoeb, gsta.q, pkma, meis2b, dld, prkcbb, mag, ush1ga, mkm2os.2, fbxo16, pcloa,* and *cyp26c1*) were randomly selected for qRT-PCR

analysis to confirm the quality of RNA-seq data. Notably, the expression changes of 6 among 12 genes were consistent with the results of RNA-seq data analysis (**Supplementary Figures 4A,B**), indicating the reliability of RNA-seq analysis.

Subsequently, we performed KEGG pathway enrichment analysis on the RNA-seq data. The results showed that knockdown *dusp14* gene by morpholino mainly resulted in changes in various metabolic pathways (**Supplementary Table 2**), including carbon metabolism, tryptophan metabolism, glycine metabolism, serine metabolism, tyrosine metabolism, retinol metabolism, metabolism of xenobiotics by cytochrome P450, phenylalanine metabolism, and so on. Furthermore, the most significant GO analysis enrichment terms were oxidoreductase activity, which were assigned as molecular functions. The cell membrane was the most significant GO enrichment term assigned as cellular component, and regulation of transportation was the most significant GO enrichment term assigned as a biological process (**Figure 5B**).

The DUSP family targets to MAPK signaling pathway, which modulate diverse cellular functions, such as regeneration, differentiation, and apoptosis. Therefore, we observed the gene expression changes in p38 kinases, ERKs, and JNKs signaling

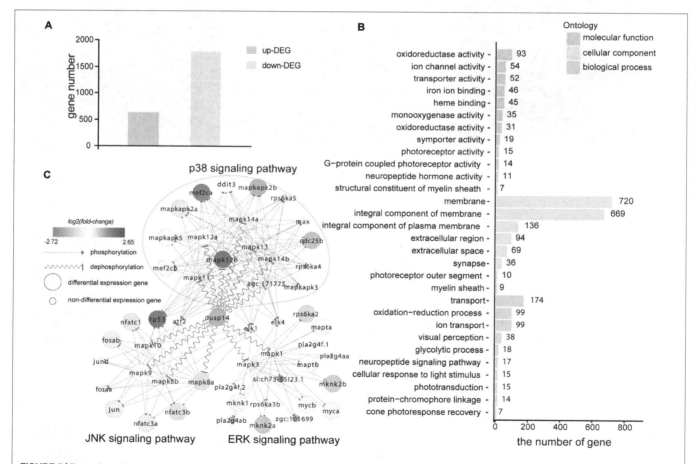

FIGURE 5 | Transcriptomic sequencing data revealed p38 signaling pathways may responsible for regulation of dusp14 gene on hearing function. **(A)** The upregulated differentially expressed genes (DEGs) and downregulated DEGs that might be affected by knockdown *dusp14* based on transcriptome data analysis. **(B)** Gene ontology (GO) annotation enrichment of DEGs. **(C)** Gene expression changes in the MAPK pathway caused by *dusp14* knockdown.

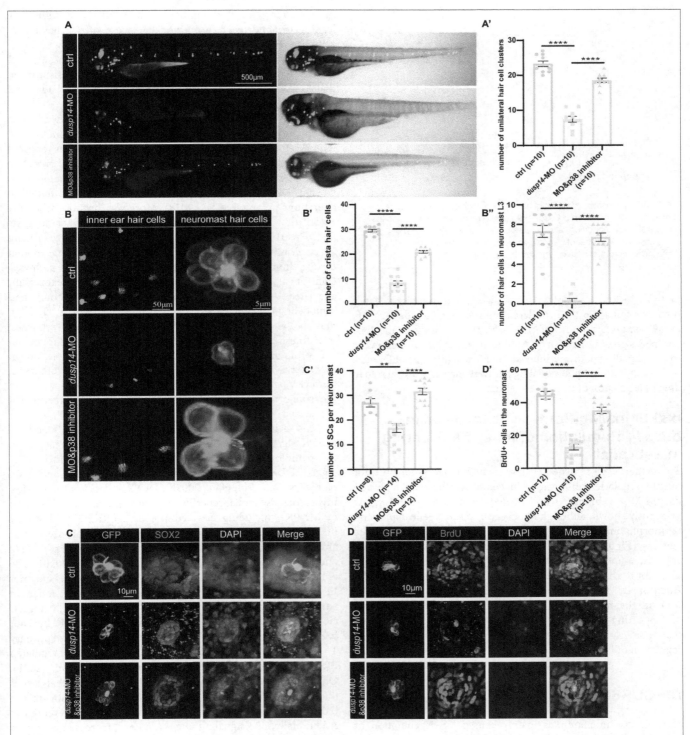

FIGURE 6 | p38 signaling pathway is involved in dusp14 regulation of inner ear hearing in zebrafish. (A) The imaging analysis of control and dusp14 mutants at 72 hpf in bright field and fluorescent field. (A') Quantification of the number of the unilateral hair cell clusters of control and dusp14 mutants at 72 hpf. (B) Confocal imaging analysis of inner ear hair cells and lateral line neuromast hair cells of control, dusp14 deficiency and dusp14-MO and p38 inhibitor coinjected zebrafish at 72 hpf. (B') The statistical analysis of the numbers of crista hair cells for panel (B). (B'') The statistical analysis of the numbers of hair cells in the remaining neuromast L3 for panel (B). (C) The representation of SOX2 immunofluorescence images of neuromasts in the posterior lateral line of the control, dusp14 morphants and dusp14-MO and p38 inhibitor coinjected zebrafish at 72 hpf. (C') Quantification of the number of supporting cells per neuromast for panel (C). (D) BrdU staining for the supporting cells in the neuromasts of the control, dusp14 morphants and dusp14-MO and p38 inhibitor coinjected zebrafish at 72 hpf. (D') Quantification of zebrafish embryos with the BrdU+ cells for panel (D). Experimental embryos were sampled at 72 hpf (n > 6). Each bar represents the mean ± SD. Values with ** and **** above the bars are significantly different (P < 0.01 and P < 0.0001, respectively).

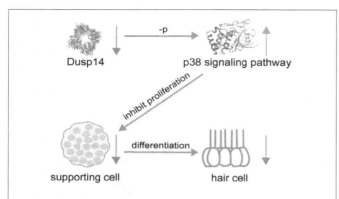

FIGURE 7 | Schematic diagram of hair cell reduction caused by *dusp14* knockdown. Knockdown of *dusp14* expression by morpholino inhibited the proliferation of supporting cells by p38 signaling pathway, resulting in a decrease in the number of hair cells and ultimately leading to abnormal hearing and balance-related behaviors in zebrafish.

pathway in RNA-seq data. As is shown in **Figure 5C**, the genes directly regulated by *dusp14* dephosphorylation include *mapk8b*, *mapk9*, *mapk12a,* and *mapk12b*, which are mainly in the JNK and p38 signaling pathways. Among them, *mapk12b* belonging to p38 signaling pathway showed the most significant difference, which suggests that p38 signaling pathway may play a vital role in *dusp14* regulation of hearing in zebrafish.

p38 Signaling Pathway Is Involved in *dusp14* Regulation of Inner Ear Hearing in Zebrafish

To further explore whether p38 signaling is responsible for *dusp14* regulation of hearing in zebrafish, the wild-type and *dusp14*-MO zebrafish were treated with p38 inhibitor. As previously shown, although knockdown *dusp14* gene expression by morpholino significantly decreased the number of hair cell clusters (**Figures 6A,A'**), the number of hair cells in inner ear cristae and neuromast L3 in the posterior lateral line, p38 inhibitor dramatically reversed these changes (**Figures 6B,B',B"**). Additionally, p38 inhibitor also blocked the effect of *dusp14*-MO on the number of supporting cell and the proliferation of supporting cells (**Figures 6C,C',D,D'**). These results indicate that p38 signaling pathway is necessary for the *dusp14* regulation of hearing.

DISCUSSION

Hearing loss in mammals mainly caused by degeneration of hair cells in the inner ear, which is an irreversible process. To date, apart from hearing aids and cochlear implants, no pharmacological therapy promoting functional recovery from hearing loss is clinically available. This study demonstrates that *dusp14*, a conserved gene between species, is highly expressed in the lateral line and otic vesicles in zebrafish. Knockdown of *dusp14* expression by morpholino inhibited the proliferation of supporting cells through p38 signaling pathway, resulting

in a decrease in the number of hair cells and ultimately leading to abnormal hearing and balance-related behaviors in zebrafish (**Figure 7**).

Dual-specificity phosphatase 14, a member of the atypical DUSPs, has been implicated in inflammation, apoptosis, cancer, diabetes, cell differentiation, and proliferation (Wada and Penninger, 2004; Turjanski et al., 2007; Lountos et al., 2009; Ríos et al., 2014). Dusp14 was characterized by yeast two hybrid systems for the first time to identify a new protein interacting with T cell costimulatory CD28 (Marti et al., 2001). It is reported that DUSP14 knockout aggravated pathological processes involved in non-alcoholic fatty liver disease development, whereas DUSP14 overexpression ameliorated these pathological alterations (Wang S. et al., 2018). Moreover, hepatic ischemia–reperfusion injury reduced Dusp14 expression, which suggests that Dusp14 is a protective factor in liver damage (Wang X. et al., 2018). Suppressing DUSP14 expression exacerbated cardiac injury through activating MAPK signaling pathways (Lin et al., 2018). Cardiac-specific Dusp14 overexpression alleviated aortic banding-induced cardiac dysfunction and remodeling (Li et al., 2016). These results indicate that DUSP14 may be a positive regulator of various cellular responses. We found that *dusp14* gene is important to supporting cell proliferating in zebrafish. Highly *dusp14* expression in the lateral line and otic vesicle in zebrafish was observed, however, whether that *dusp14* gene is specific located in the supporting cell remains unclear. The more experiments are needed.

Dusp14 is a dephosphorylate regulator that mainly acts on MAPK signaling and has different MAPK pathway targets in the pathological process of various diseases. *In vitro*, GST-tagged DUSP14 can dephosphorylate p38, ERK, and JNK pathways (Patterson et al., 2009b). DUSP14 knockout mice after myocardial ischemia–reperfusion injury induce the activation of MAPKs, including elevated p-p38, p-ERK1/2, and p-JNK in heart tissues (Lin et al., 2018). However, Dusp14 deficiency after hepatic ischemia–reperfusion injury upregulated p-JNK1/2 and p-p38, but not p-ERK1/2 (Wang X. et al., 2018). The enhanced phosphorylated p38 and JNK1/2 levels, but not ERK1/2, were also observed in Dusp14 knockout mice in aortic banding-induced hypertrophic heart tissues (Wang X. et al., 2018). The phosphorylation of ERK and JNK but not p38 increased in dominant-negative Dusp14-transduced primary T cells (Galvao et al., 2018). DUSP14 negatively regulated ERK1/2 pathway in T-cell proliferation (Sun et al., 2021). Our transcriptomic sequencing analysis showed that genes mainly regulated by *dusp14* dephosphorylation belong to the JNK and p38 signaling pathways in *dusp14*-MO zebrafish. Additionally, p38 signaling, *mapk12b* gene, increased mostly in morpholino-induced *dusp14*-deficient zebrafish. In addition, p38 inhibitor significantly inhibited the effect of *dusp14*-MO on the proliferation of supporting cells and the decrease of hair cell in zebrafish. However, further experiments are needed to confirm the regulation of *mapk12b* gene on zebrafish supporting cells. Whether JNK and ERK are involved in regulating supporting cell development and how important their roles are also needed to be further investigated.

Numerous studies in non-mammalian species since the initial discoveries have elucidated that inner ear hair cell regeneration happens by two methods: supporting cells directly transdifferentiate into hair cells, supporting cells mitosis and then one of the daughter cells transdifferentiate into hair cells (Burns and Corwin, 2013; Takeda et al., 2018). However, our understanding of the molecular mechanisms that regulates supporting cell behavior is limited. Our results indicate that DUSP14 may be an important regulator of supporting cell development. Furthermore, *DUSP14* is also reported to be involved in the hepatocyte proliferation and regeneration (Wang X. et al., 2018). In the immune system, DUSP14 negatively regulates β cell proliferation and apoptosis of cancer cells (Klinger et al., 2008).

Here, we explore the molecular mechanisms that lead to hair cell regeneration in zebrafish by exploiting their ability to regenerate hair cells. To our knowledge, this study reported the important effects of *dusp14* gene on the fate of the hair cell in zebrafish for the first time, mainly through regulating proliferation of supporting cells, providing a new insight into understand the mechanism of supporting cell development and a new potential target for the treatment of hearing loss.

AUTHOR CONTRIBUTIONS

DL and FC supervised and designed this project. GW, CC, XZ, JS, and FQ wrote the manuscript. GW, XZ, CG, and FQ analyzed the data. XZ, MX, CW, and QG performed the experiments. All authors contributed to the article and approved the submitted version.

SUPPLEMENTARY MATERIAL

Supplementary Figure 1 | The design of *Dusp14*-Mo sequence and verification of the knockdown efficiency. **(A)** The design of *dusp14* morphant sequence. **(B)** Representative images of Dusp14[+] cells of neuromasts in the posterior lateral line of the control and *dusp14* morphants. **(B′)** The statistical results of panel **(B)**. **(C)** *Left*: the result of *ef1α* RT-PCR of wild-type zebrafish and *dusp14* morphants. *Right*: the result of *dusp14* RT-PCR of wild-type zebrafish and *dusp14* morphants. **(C′)** The statistical results of panel **(C)**.

Supplementary Figure 2 | *Dusp14* knockout leads to a decrease in zebrafish hair cell. **(A)** The design of *dusp14* guide-RNA. **(B)** Mutations occurred in the target site of the *dusp14* gene in mutant zebrafish compared to the wild-type fish. **(C)** Confocal imaging analysis of the numbers of hair cell clusters and hair cells in the lateral line system of wild-type and *dusp14* mutants at 72 hpf. **(C′)** The statistical analysis of panel **(C)**. Experimental embryos were sampled at 72 hpf $n > 7$). Each bar represents the mean ± SEM. Values with *, **, ***, and **** above the bars are significantly different ($p < 0.05$, $p < 0.01$, $p < 0.001$, and $p < 0.0001$, respectively).

Supplementary Figure 3 | *Dusp14* knockdown did not induce zebrafish hair cell apoptosis. **(A)** DAPI and cleaved TUNEL staining for the L3 hair cell clusters in the posterior lateral line of the control zebrafish and *dusp14* morphants. **(B)** DAPI and cleaved caspase-3 staining for the L3 hair cell clusters in the posterior lateral line of the control zebrafish and *dusp14* morphants.

Supplementary Figure 4 | qRT-PCR of different expression gene in the control and *dusp14* morphants. **(A)** Twelve DEGs were detected in transcriptome sequencing. **(B)** The results of 12 DEGs caused by *dusp14* morphants at 72 hpf $n = 3$). Each bar represents the mean ± SEM. Values with *, **, ***, and **** above the bars are significantly different ($p < 0.05$, $p < 0.01$, $p < 0.001$, and $p < 0.0001$, respectively).

Supplementary Table 1 | Transcriptomic profiling of *dusp14*-morphant and wild-type zebrafish. The number of reads and percentage mapped to the coding genes of zebrafish genome is calculated. The 90% mapped rate presents the proportion of reads matched to the coding genes of zebrafish genome in the totally valid reads.

Supplementary Table 2 | Differentially expressed genes obtained based on transcriptome sequencing.

Supplementary Table 3 | Primer information.

REFERENCES

An, N., Bassil, K., Al Jowf, G. I., Steinbusch, H. W. M., Rothermel, M., de Nijs, L., et al. (2021). Dual-specificity phosphatases in mental and neurological disorders. *Prog. Neurobiol.* 198:101906. doi: 10.1016/j.pneurobio.2020.101906

Burns, J. C., and Corwin, J. T. (2013). A historical to present-day account of efforts to answer the question:"what puts the brakes on mammalian hair cell regeneration?". *Hear. Res.* 297, 52–67. doi: 10.1016/j.heares.2013.01.005

Caunt, C. J., and Keyse, S. M. (2013). Dual-specificity MAP kinase phosphatases (MKPs) Shaping the outcome of MAP kinase signalling. *FEBS J.* 280, 489–504. doi: 10.1111/j.1742-4658.2012.08716.x

Furness, D. N. (2015). Molecular basis of hair cell loss. *Cell Tissue Res.* 361, 387–399. doi: 10.1007/s00441-015-2113-z

Galvao, J., Iwao, K., Apara, A., Wang, Y., Ashouri, M., Shah, T. N., et al. (2018). The Krüppel-like factor gene target Dusp14 regulates axon growth and regeneration. *Invest. Ophthalmol. Vis. Sci.* 59, 2736–2747. doi: 10.1167/iovs.17-23319

Gong, J., Wang, X., Zhu, C., Dong, X., Zhang, Q., Wang, X., et al. (2017). Insm1a regulates motor neuron development in zebrafish. *Front. Mol. Neurosci.* 10:274. doi: 10.3389/fnmol.2017.00274

Grant, K. A., Raible, D. W., and Piotrowski, T. (2005). Regulation of latent sensory hair cell precursors by glia in the zebrafish lateral line. *Neuron* 45, 69–80. doi: 10.1016/j.neuron.2004.12.020

Huang, C.-Y., and Tan, T.-H. (2012). DUSPs, to MAP kinases and beyond. *Cell Biosci.* 2:24. doi: 10.1186/2045-3701-2-24

Kelley, M. W. (2006). Regulation of cell fate in the sensory epithelia of the inner ear. *Nat. Rev. Neurosci.* 7, 837–849. doi: 10.1038/nrn1987

Kim, D., Pertea, G., Trapnell, C., Pimentel, H., Kelley, R., and Salzberg, S. L. (2013). TopHat2: accurate alignment of transcriptomes in the presence of insertions, deletions and gene fusions. *Genome Biol.* 14:R36. doi: 10.1186/gb-2013-14-4-r36

Kimmel, C. B., Ballard, W. W., Kimmel, S. R., Ullmann, B., and Schilling, T. F. (1995). Stages of embryonic development of the zebrafish. *Dev. Dyn.* 203, 253–310. doi: 10.1002/aja.1002030302

Klinger, S., Poussin, C., Debril, M.-B., Dolci, W., Halban, P. A., and Thorens, B. (2008). Increasing GLP-1–induced β-cell proliferation by silencing the negative regulators of signaling cAMP response element modulator-α and DUSP14. *Diabetes* 57, 584–593. doi: 10.2337/db07-1414

Kniss, J. S., Jiang, L., and Piotrowski, T. (2016). Insights into sensory hair cell regeneration from the zebrafish lateral line. *Curr. Opin. Genet. Dev.* 40, 32–40. doi: 10.1016/j.gde.2016.05.012

Li, C.-Y., Zhou, Q., Yang, L.-C., Chen, Y.-H., Hou, J.-W., Guo, K., et al. (2016). Dual-specificity phosphatase 14 protects the heart from aortic banding-induced cardiac hypertrophy and dysfunction through inactivation of TAK1-P38MAPK/-JNK1/2 signaling pathway. *Basic Res. Cardiol.* 111:19. doi: 10.1007/s00395-016-0536-7

Lin, B., Xu, J., Feng, D.-G., Wang, F., Wang, J.-X., and Zhao, H. (2018). DUSP14 knockout accelerates cardiac ischemia reperfusion (IR) injury through activating NF-κB and MAPKs signaling pathways modulated by ROS generation. *Biochem. Biophys. Res. Commun.* 501, 24–32. doi: 10.1016/j.bbrc. 2018.04.101

Livak, K. J., and Schmittgen, T. D. (2001). Analysis of relative gene expression data using real-time quantitative PCR and the 2- ΔΔCT method. *Methods* 25, 402–408. doi: 10.1006/meth.2001.1262

Lountos, G. T., Tropea, J. E., Cherry, S., and Waugh, D. S. (2009). Overproduction, purification and structure determination of human dual-specificity phosphatase 14. *Acta Crystallogr. D Biol. Crystallogr.* 65(Pt 10), 1013–1020. doi: 10.1107/ s0907444909023762

Marti, F., Krause, A., Post, N. H., Lyddane, C., Dupont, B., Sadelain, M., et al. (2001). Negative-feedback regulation of CD28 costimulation by a novel mitogen-activated protein kinase phosphatase. MKP6. *J. Immunol.* 166, 197–206. doi: 10.4049/jimmunol.166.1.197

Morton, N. (1991). Genetic epidemiology of hearing impairment. *Ann. N. Y. Acad. Sci.* 630, 16–31. doi: 10.1111/j.1749-6632.1991.tb19572.x

Patterson, K. I., Brummer, T., O'Brien, P. M., and Daly, R. J. (2009a). Dual-specificity phosphatases: critical regulators with diverse cellular targets. *Biochem. J.* 418, 475–489. doi: 10.1042/bj20082234

Patterson, K. I., Brummer, T., O'brien, P. M., and Daly, R. J. (2009b). Dual-specificity phosphatases: critical regulators with diverse cellular targets. *Biochem. J.* 418, 475–489. doi: 10.1042/BJ20082234

Ríos, P., Nunes-Xavier, C. E., Tabernero, L., Köhn, M., and Pulido, R. (2014). Dual-specificity phosphatases as molecular targets for inhibition in human disease. *Antioxid. Redox Signal.* 20, 2251–2273. doi: 10.1089/ars.2013.5709

Rubel, E. W., Furrer, S. A., and Stone, J. S. (2013). A brief history of hair cell regeneration research and speculations on the future. *Hear. Res.* 297, 42–51. doi: 10.1016/j.heares.2012.12.014

Schmittgen, T. D., and Livak, K. J. (2008). Analyzing real-time PCR data by the comparative CT method. *Nat. Protoc.* 3, 1101–1108. doi: 10.1038/nprot.2008.73

Sun, F., Yue, T.-T., Yang, C.-L., Wang, F.-X., Luo, J.-H., Rong, S.-J., et al. (2021). The MAPK dual specific phosphatase (DUSP) proteins: a versatile wrestler in T cell functionality. *Int. Immunopharmacol.* 98:107906. doi: 10.1016/j.intimp. 2021.107906

Sun, X. (2021). Occupational noise exposure and worker's health in China. *China CDC Weekly* 3:375. doi: 10.46234/ccdcw2021.102

Takeda, H., Dondzillo, A., Randall, J. A., and Gubbels, S. P. (2018). Challenges in cell-based therapies for the treatment of hearing loss. *Trends Neurosci.* 41, 823–837. doi: 10.1016/j.tins.2018.06.008

Thomas, E. D., and Raible, D. W. (2019). Distinct progenitor populations mediate regeneration in the zebrafish lateral line. *Elife* 8:e43736. doi: 10.7554/eLife.43736

Turjanski, A. G., Vaqué, J. P., and Gutkind, J. S. (2007). MAP kinases and the control of nuclear events. *Oncogene* 26, 3240–3253. doi: 10.1038/sj.onc.1210415

van den Bos, R., Mes, W., Galligani, P., Heil, A., Zethof, J., Flik, G., et al. (2017). Further characterisation of differences between TL and AB zebrafish (*Danio rerio*): gene expression, physiology and behaviour at day 5 of the larval stage. *PLoS One* 12:e0175420.

Vlajkovic, S. M., and Thorne, P. R. (2021). *Molecular Mechanisms of Sensorineural Hearing Loss and Development of Inner Ear Therapeutics*. Basel: Multidisciplinary Digital Publishing Institute. doi: 10.3390/ijms22115647

Wada, T., and Penninger, J. M. (2004). Mitogen-activated protein kinases in apoptosis regulation. *Oncogene* 23, 2838–2849. doi: 10.1038/sj.onc.1207556

Wang, S., Yan, Z. Z., Yang, X., An, S., Zhang, K., Qi, Y., et al. (2018). Hepatocyte DUSP14 maintains metabolic homeostasis and suppresses inflammation in the liver. *Hepatology* 67, 1320–1338. doi: 10.1002/hep.29616

Wang, X., Mao, W., Fang, C., Tian, S., Zhu, X., Yang, L., et al. (2018). Dusp14 protects against hepatic ischaemia–reperfusion injury via Tak1 suppression. *J. Hepatol.* 68, 118–129.

Westerfield, M. (1995). *The Zebrafish Book: A Guide for the Laboratory Use of Zebrafish (Brachydanio rerio)*. Eugene: University of Oregon press.

Whitfield, T. T. (2005). Lateral line: precocious phenotypes and planar polarity. *Curr. Biol.* 15, R67–R70.

Williams, J. A., and Holder, N. (2000). Cell turnover in neuromasts of zebrafish larvae. *Hear. Res.* 143, 171–181. doi: 10.1016/s0378-5955(00)00039-3

Yang, Q., Sun, P., Chen, S., Li, H., and Chen, F. (2017). Behavioral methods for the functional assessment of hair cells in zebrafish. *Front. Med.* 11:178–190. doi: 10.1007/s11684-017-0507-x

3

Cingulin b is Required for Zebrafish Lateral Line Development through Regulation of Mitogen-Activated Protein Kinase and Cellular Senescence Signaling Pathways

Yitong Lu[1†], Dongmei Tang[2,3†], Zhiwei Zheng[2,3†], Xin Wang[4], Na Zuo[1], Renchun Yan[1], Cheng Wu[1], Jun Ma[1], Chuanxi Wang[1], Hongfei Xu[5], Yingzi He[2,3*], Dong Liu[4*] and Shaofeng Liu[1*]

[1] Department of Otolaryngology-Head and Neck Surgery, Yijishan Hospital of Wannan Medical College, Wuhu, China, [2] State Key Laboratory of Medical Neurobiology and MOE Frontiers Center for Brain Science, ENT Institute and Department of Otorhinolaryngology, Eye and ENT Hospital, Fudan University, Shanghai, China, [3] NHC Key Laboratory of Hearing Medicine, Fudan University, Shanghai, China, [4] Nantong Laboratory of Development and Diseases, School of Life Sciences, Co-innovation Center of Neuroregeneration, Key Laboratory of Neuroregeneration of Jiangsu and MOE, Nantong University, Nantong, China, [5] Department of Forensic Medicine, Soochow University, Suzhou, China

*Correspondence:
Yingzi He
yingzihe09611@126.com
Dong Liu
liudongtom@gmail.com;
tom@ntu.edu.cn
Shaofeng Liu
liusf_cn@163.com

† These authors have contributed equally to this work

Cingulin, a cytoplasmic element of tight junctions (TJs), is involved in maintenance of the integrity of epithelial and endothelial cells. However, the role of cingulin in the development of auditory organs remains unclear. Zebrafish is popular as a model organism for hearing research. Using the whole mount *in situ* hybridization (WISH) experiment, we detected the expression of *cingulin b* in the posterior lateral line system (PLLs) of zebrafish. We traced the early development progress of zebrafish PLLs from 36 hpf to 72 hpf, and found that inhibition of *cingulin b* by target morpholinos resulted in severe developmental obstruction, including decreased number of neuromasts, reduced proliferative cells in the primordium, and repressed hair cell differentiation in the neuromasts. To examine the potential mechanism of *cingulin b* in the development of zebrafish PLL neuromasts, we performed RNA-seq analysis to compare the differently expressed genes (DEGs) between *cingulin b* knockdown samples and the controls. The KEGG enrichment analysis revealed that MAPK signaling pathway and cellular senescence were the key pathways with most DEGs in *cingulin b*-MO morphants compared to the Control-MO embryos. Furthermore, quantitative RT-PCR analysis confirmed the findings by RNA-seq that the transcript levels of cell cycle negative regulators such as *tp53* and *cdkn1a*, were remarkably upregulated after inhibition of *cingulin b*. Our results therefore indicated an important role of *cingulin b* in the development of auditory organs, and MAPK signaling pathway was inhibited while cellular senescence pathway was activated after downregulation of *cingulin b*. We bring forward new insights of cingulin by exploring its function in auditory system.

Keywords: cingulin b, zebrafish, development, MAPK signaling pathway, cellular senescence

Abbreviations: DEGs, differently expressed genes; HCs, hair cells; hpf, hours post-fertilization; JNK, Jun N-terminal kinase; MAPK, Mitogen-activated protein kinase; PLL, posterior lateral line; qRT-PCR, quantitative real-time PCR; TJ, tight junctions; WISH, whole mount *in situ* hybridization; GFP, green fluorescent protein.

INTRODUCTION

Tight junctions (TJs), mainly composed of claudins, occludin, ZO proteins, cingulin and paracingulin, are widely localized at the apicolateral borders of cells, and play important roles in maintaining the integrity, permeability and polarity of cells (González-Mariscal et al., 2014; Citi, 2019). Cingulin is localized in the cytoplasmic region of TJs, comprised of a head, a rod and a tail domain (Cordenonsi et al., 1999). Cingulin connects to actin and microtubule cytoskeleton in the head domain, and interacts with Rho family GTPases in the coiled-coil rod region (Cordenonsi et al., 1999; D'atri et al., 2002; Ohnishi et al., 2004; Van Itallie et al., 2009; Yano et al., 2013). Cingulin is mainly involved in regulating the paracellular and blood-brain barrier, for example, edema is more severe in the specific cingulin knock-out mouse model compared to the controls (Hawkins and Davis, 2005; Zhuravleva et al., 2020). In addition, cingulin is found expressed in the organ of Corti, and its distribution is rearranged after high-intensity noise exposure (Raphael and Altschuler, 1991). In a kanamycin damaged guinea pig model, cingulin together with adherens junctions such as E-cadherin and beta-catenin are found reorganized in two distinct planes, and they would preserve the integrity of tissues during scar formation and hair cell degeneration, indicating a barrier function of cingulin in the organ of Corti (Leonova and Raphael, 1997). Cingulin is also expressed in key regions of mouse cochlea, such as spiral ligament, stria vascularis, spiral limbus, and tectorial membrane (Batissoco et al., 2018). However, the role of cingulin in the development of auditory system is unknown.

Zebrafish have a high genetic similarity with the genome of human, and many critical genes required for the development of eyes, ear, brain, heart and other organs are highly conserved between zebrafish and humans, which makes zebrafish an excellent model for studying the human disease (Dooley and Zon, 2000; Howe et al., 2013; Kalueff et al., 2014). Besides, the characteristics of short reproductive cycle, strong reproductive ability, and transparent embryos increase the popularity of zebrafish as an animal model compared to mice (Mandrekar and Thakur, 2009; He et al., 2017). The mature neuromast of zebrafish PLL is consisted of the central hair cells (HCs) and the surrounding supporting cells (SCs), which share many structural and functional similarities with the inner ear cochlea of mammals (Nicolson, 2005), making zebrafish lateral line system a significant model for studying hair cell development, survival and regeneration (Driever et al., 1994; Pyati et al., 2007; Brignull et al., 2009).

In this study, we chose zebrafish as the animal model to explore the potential role of cingulin in the development of lateral line system of zebrafish. In zebrafish, *cingulin b* is orthologous to human cingulin. We firstly designed anti-sense morpholinos to downregulate the expression of *cingulin b*, and the efficacy of *cingulin b*-MO was confirmed by ISH staining and qPCR analysis of *cingulin b*. We observed reduced number of neuromasts, decreased cell proliferation, and repressed HC differentiation in the PLL system of zebrafish after knocking down *cingulin b* compared to the control group. The RNA-seq analysis revealed that MAPK signaling pathway and cellular senescence genes were involved in the development of zebrafish PLL after inhibition of *cingulin b*. Our findings uncover a potential role of cingulin in the development of zebrafish mechanosensory organs.

MATERIALS AND METHODS

Animal Operations

All zebrafish, including the wild type AB line and the transgenic *Tg (cldnb: lynGFP)* and *Tg (brn3c: mGFP)^{s356t}* lines were bred in 28.5°C constant temperature incubator in embryo medium according to the standard formula (Kimmel et al., 1995). The stage of embryonic development was marked as hours- or days- after fertilization (hpf or dpf) (Kimmel et al., 1995). In order to avoid pigmentation, the embryos should be further immersed in 1-phenyl-2-thiourea (PTU) (Sigma-Aldrich) in the culture medium from 10 hpf (Tang et al., 2019). The operations on zebrafish were discussed and permitted by the Animal Conservation and Utilization Committee of Fudan University in Shanghai.

Morpholino Injection and mRNA Rescue Test

Cingulin b-MO, sequenced in 5'-TCCTGTCCGCAGAGAGGG AACTCAT-3', was injected at a dose of 2 ng or 3 ng at one or two cell stage of embryos to reduce the expression of *cingulin b*. The other siblings were considered as controls by injection with a sequence of 5'-CCTCTTACCTCAGT TACAATTTATA-3', namely control-MO (Control-MO). For the messenger RNA (mRNA) rescue experiment, a mixture of *cingulin b*-MO and *cingulin b* mRNA (Forward primer: 5'-AT GAGTTCCCTCTCTGCGGA-3'; Reverse primer: 5'-TCAACAG CTGGTGGTCTGAA-3') was injected at the same stage with other groups.

Whole Mount *in situ* Hybridization in Zebrafish

WISH experiment was operated as previously disclosed (He et al., 2014; Thisse and Thisse, 2014). To examine the expression pattern of *cingulin b* in zebrafish, we collected embryos at various stages including 3.7, 14, and 48 hpf. To verify the efficacy of *cingulin b*-MO in the lateral line system of zebrafish, we collected embryos at 48 hpf. After a series of gradient solutions for dehydration, the collected embryos were stored in pure methanol (100% concentration) at −20°C. Before hybridization, the embryos would be gradient rehydrated first, and then digested with 20 μg/ml protease K. The probe was added and hybridized at 65°C constant temperature overnight. After thorough washes with the SSC-series at 65°C, the embryos were blocked in 2x BBR at room temperature for at least 1 h. Anti- digoxigenin (Dig)-AP Fab fragment (Roche) was added and incubated with specimens overnight at 4°C. Primers for synthesizing the objective genes were listed in **Supplementary Table 1**. Color reaction was implemented with BM purple AP substrate (Roche) in the dark at 37°C, and stopped with NTMT. The embryos after three times rinses were then re-fixed in 4% PFA and treated

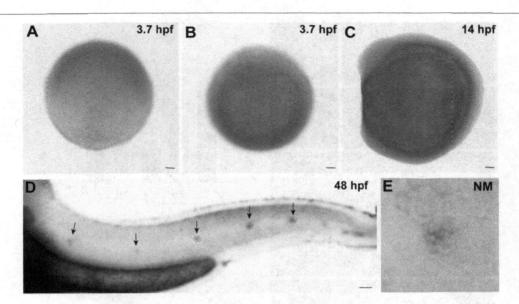

FIGURE 1 | Expression of *cingulin b* is detected during the early development of zebrafish. **(A,B)** *In situ* hybridization staining of *cingulin b* at 3.7 hpf (*n* = 13) from the lateral view **(A)** and the top view **(B)**. **(C)** *Cingulin b* is expressed in the whole somite at 14 hpf from the lateral view (*n* = 14). **(D–E)** The expression of *cingulin b* is focused on the neuromasts of the posterior lateral line system at 48 hpf (*n* = 11). Scale bars mark 50 μm in panel **(A–D)**. The black arrows in D indicate neuromasts, and the white dotted lines labeled neuromast in D is magnified in panel **(E)**.

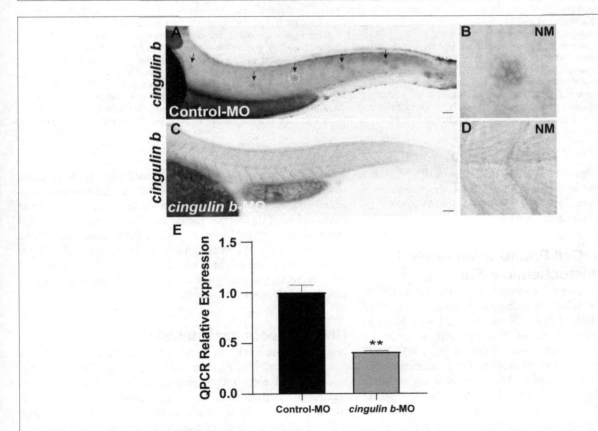

FIGURE 2 | The efficacy of *cingulin b*-MO. **(A–D)** The expression of *cingulin b* is significantly reduced in the *cingulin b*-MO morphants **(C)**, *n* = 8 compared to that in the Control-MO embryos **(A)** *n* = 5. **(E)** Quantitative analysis on the level of *cingulin b* between Control-MO and *cingulin b*-MO groups (*n* = 8 in each group). Data are shown in mean ± SEM, **$p < 0.01$. Scale bars in panel **(A,C)** mark 50 μm. The black arrows in panel **(A)** indicate the neuromasts, and the white dotted lines labeled neuromasts in panel **(A,C)** are magnified in panel **(B,D)**, respectively.

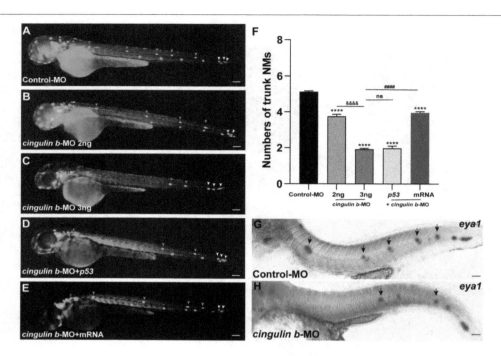

FIGURE 3 | Inhibition of *cingulin b* affects the normal deposition of neuromasts in zebrafish. **(A–E)** In transgenic *cldnb:lynGFP* embryos, the neuromasts of PLL are labeled with green fluorescence. At 48 hpf, the deposition of neuromasts in zebrafish is shown in the control group **(A)**, *cingulin b* knockdown group **(B,C)**, *cingulin b*-MO + *p53* group **(D)**, and *cingulin b*-MO + *cingulin b* mRNA group **(E)**, respectively. **(F)** The number of PLL neuromasts in controls (*n* = 235), *cingulin b* knockdown (2 ng or 3 ng) group (*n* = 86 and 264, respectively), *cingulin b*-MO (3 ng) + *p53* group (*n* = 81), and *cingulin b*-MO (3 ng) + mRNA embryos (*n* = 180) at 48 hpf. The number of neuromasts decreased dose-dependently after knockdown of *cingulin b* **(A–C,F)**. The decrease in the number of neuromasts is also confirmed when co-injecting with *cingulin b*-MO and *p53* **(C,D,F)**. Combined injection of *cingulin b*-MO and *cingulin b* mRNA can partially rescue the decrease in the number of neuromasts caused by *cingulin b*-MO **(E,F)**. Red arrowheads mark the neuromasts in the trunk, and white arrowheads mark the terminal neuromasts of the PLL system **(A–E)**. Scale bars represent 100 μm. Data are shown in mean ± SEM. *Stands by the comparison with the control group: ***p < 0.0001. #Stands by the comparison between *cingulin b*-MO group and *cingulin b*-MO + *cingulin b* mRNA group: ####p < 0.0001. &Stands by the comparison between 2 ng *cingulin b*-MO group and 3 ng *cingulin b*-MO group: &&&&p < 0.0001. ns means no significance. **(G,H)** The number of *eya1* labeled neuromasts is markedly reduced after knocking down of *cingulin b* **(G)** *n* = 21 compared to the Control-MOs **(H)** *n* = 14. The black arrows in G and H indicate the neuromasts. Scale bars in panel **(G,H)** mark 50 μm.

with different gradients of glycerol/PBS. The final specimens were stored in 100% glycerol and photographed by fluorescence stereoscopic microscope. All images were prepared by Photoshop and Illustrator software (2018, Adobe).

BrdU Labeled Cell Proliferation Analysis and Immunohistochemical Staining

Bromodeoxyuridine (BrdU) co-incubation was conducted to label the proliferative cells. The dechorionated embryos at 34 hpf were incubated in 10 mM BrdU (Sigma-Aldrich) for 2 hours to show the cell proliferation in the PLL primordium, while the dechorionated larvae at 2 dpf were incubated in 10 mM BrdU (Sigma-Aldrich) for 24 hours to examine the proliferative cells in PLL neuromasts of zebrafish. The corresponding embryos or larvae were collected, anesthetized in 0.02%MS-222 (Sigma-Aldrich), and fixed in 4% PFA at 4°C overnight. After washing with PBT-2 for 3 times, the collected embryos were soaked in 2 N HCl at 37°C for 30 min. After incubation with the primary anti-BrdU monoclonal antibody (1:200 dilution; Santa Cruz Biotechnology) for 1 h at 37°C following 4°C overnight, the samples were washed for several times and then incubated

with the secondary Cy3 polyclonal antibody (1:300 dilution; Jackson) for 1 h at 37°C. DAPI (1:800 dilution; Invitrogen) was added and incubated with the embryos or larvae for 20 min at room temperature to label the nuclei. The fluorescence-labeled embryos were imaged by Leica confocal fluorescence microscope (TCS SP8; Leica). The images obtained were further rotated, cut, and adjusted in the brightness by Photoshop (2018, Adobe) and then the images were aligned and added with fonts or labels by Illustrator software (2018, Adobe).

RNA-Sequencing Analysis

Before specimen collection, the zebrafish embryos at 48 hpf accepted depletion of chorion and the yolk sac. The total RNA was extracted with TRIzol reagent (Thermo Fisher Science) and reversely transcribed into cDNA using the first strand of transcriptional cDNA synthesis kit (Roche). An Illumina HiSeq X Ten platform was used for library sequencing. Raw reads were firstly filtered out the data in low-quality, and the remaining high quality raw data were used for downstream analyses. We used the Spliced Transcripts Alignment to a Reference (STAR) software as the reference genome library. Differential expression analysis was conducted with the DESeq (2012) R package, and p-value <0.05 indicated significant difference. R package was performed for KEGG pathway enrichment analysis of DEGs on the basis of hypergeometric distribution. KEGG pathway database were the reference for further functional and pathway enrichment analysis.

Quantitative Real-Time PCR

In order to fully quantity the mRNA level of target genes, a quantitative real-time PCR (qRT-PCR) system (LightCycler®480) was operated on 48 hpf larvae in the Control-MO group and the *cingulin b*-MO group, using the PrimeScript RT reagent Kit (RR047A, Takara Biomedical Technology) and the SYBR PreMix Ex Taq Kit (RR820A, Takara Biomedical Technology). $^{\Delta\Delta}$Ct method was chosen for results analysis. The primer sequences used in the study were described in **Supplementary Table 2**. Each qPCR assay was repeated in triplicate, and GAPDH was used as the internal reference genes.

Statistical Analysis

All statistics were performed with GraphPad Prism software (version, 8.0c). Comparison between two groups was conducted with double-tailed Student t test, while comparisons among multiple groups were carried out by One-way ANOVA. Statistics were recorded as mean ± SEM (standard error of mean), and

the difference was considered to be of significant difference with p-value less than 0.05.

RESULTS

Expression of *Cingulin b* in Zebrafish

In order to detect whether *cingulin b* is expressed in zebrafish, we collected embryos at various stages and conducted WISH analysis for *cingulin b* staining. As shown in **Figure 1**, *cingulin b* was detected expressed in the oblong stage at 3.7 hpf (**Figures 1A,B**), the 10-somite stage at 14 hpf (**Figure 1C**), and the deposited PLL neuromasts at 48 hpf (**Figure 1D**), mainly in the central HC area (**Figure 1E**). To confirm the expression of *cingulin b* in the early development of zebrafish, we also conducted the sense control probe for *cingulin b* at 48 hpf, however, we didn't detect any expression of *cingulin b* in the lateral line system of zebrafish compared to that using antisense mRNA probe for *cingulin b* (**Supplementary Figure 1**).

Cingulin b Is Required for Normal Deposition of Neuromasts in Posterior Lateral Line System of Zebrafish

To explore the role of *cingulin b* in the development of zebrafish, we injected specific morpholino (MO) targeting *cingulin b* at

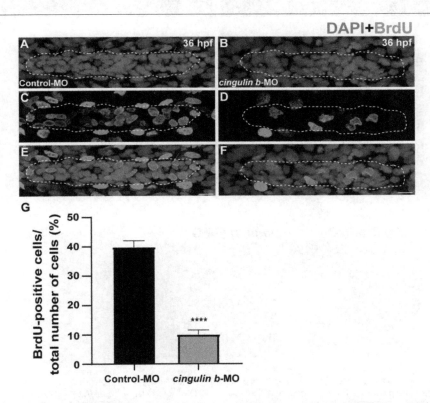

FIGURE 4 | The proliferative cells in the PLL primordium are severely decreased while downregulation of *cingulin b*. **(A–F)** Representative images of BrdU positive proliferating cells and DAPI labeled nuclei in the controls **(A,C,E)** and *cingulin b*-deficient embryos **(B,D,F)** at 36 hpf. Red arrows indicate the rosette-shaped cell clusters in the primordium **(A)**. Scale bars mark the 10 μm scale. **(G)** The quantitative analysis of BrdU index in control ($n = 16$) and *cingulin b*-MO embryos ($n = 18$). Data are shown in mean ± SEM. ****$p < 0.0001$.

one or two cell stage of embryos for knockdown of *cingulin b*. The control group was injected with Control-MO to eliminate the effect of injection operation. The efficacy of *cingulin b*-MO-injection was examined by *in situ* staining of *cingulin b* and qRT-PCR analysis, that we found significantly down-regulated expression of *cingulin b* in the PLL neuromasts in the *cingulin b*-MO morphants compared to the controls (**Figures 2A–D**), and the quantitative level of *cingulin b* was remarkably decreased after *cingulin b*-MO injection compared to the embryos injected with

Control-MO (**Figure 2E**). We also examined the embryos as a whole in the Control-MO and *cingulin b*-MO groups, and we did not find any obvious malformation in the entire zebrafish after injection with *cingulin b*-MO (**Supplementary Figure 2**).

The *Tg (cldnb: lynGFP)* zebrafish were used in this study to directly observe the morphology of neuromasts (**Figure 3A**). We counted the number of neuromasts at 48 hpf, a time point when the PLL primordium stops migration and finishes deposition (Kimmel et al., 1995; Nechiporuk and Raible, 2008).

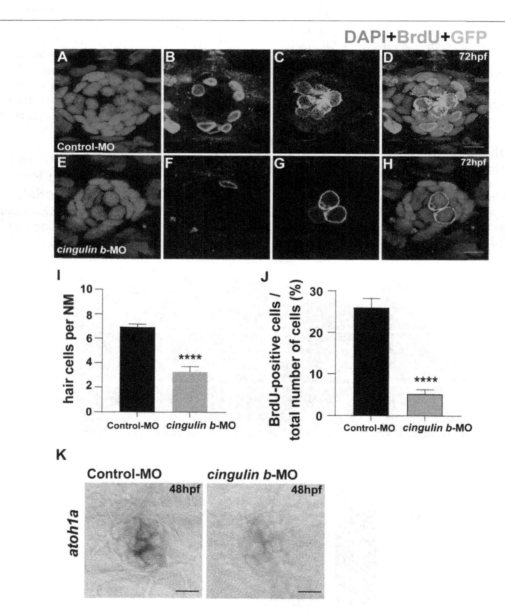

FIGURE 5 | Knockdown of *cingulin b* reduces the number of HCs and cell proliferation in the neuromasts of zebrafish at 72 hpf. **(A–H)** The immunochemical staining of PLL neuromasts in the Control-MO group (*n* = 19) and *cingulin b*-MO group (*n* = 15). DAPI (green) labels nuclei **(A,E)** and BrdU (red) labels proliferative cells in the neuromast **(B,F)**. In transgenic *Tg (brn3c: mGFP)^s356t* lines, the membrane of HCs in PLL neuromasts are labeled with green fluorescence (GFP) **(C,G)**. **(I)** The average number of hair cells per neuromast is significantly reduced after inhibition of *cingulin b*. **(J)** BrdU index in the neuromasts is also severely downregulated in the *cingulin b*-MO injected embryos compared to the controls. Scale bars mark 10 μm **(A–H)**. Data are shown in mean ± SEM, and ****p < 0.0001. **(K)** The differentiation of HCs indicated by *atoh1* ISH staining is inhibited after injection with *cingulin b*-MO. Scale bars in panel **(K)** mark 30 μm.

The average number of neuromasts in the trunk was notably decreased in the *cingulin b*-MO-injected morphants compared to that in the Control-MO-injected embryos (**Figures 3A–C,F**). The average number of neuromasts was even lower in 3 ng *cingulin b*-MO group than that in 2 ng *cingulin b*-MO group (**Figures 3B–C,F**), showing a dose-dependent manner, thus, we chose 3 ng dose for the following experiments. To avoid the non-specific effect of morpholino technology, we co-injected *p53* with *cingulin b*-MO, and surprisingly the average number of neuromasts in the trunk in *cingulin b*-MO + *p53* group was equivalent to that in *cingulin b*-MO-only group (**Figures 3C–D,F**). In addition, we also carried out rescue experiment, that combined injection with *cingulin b* mRNA and morpholino could partially restore the reduced number of neuromasts in the trunk (**Figures 3E,F**). The findings suggested that loss of *cingulin b* would affect the normal deposition of PLL neuromasts during the embryonic development of zebrafish. These findings were further validated by the expression of *eya1*, a marker for the neuromast in the lateral line of zebrafish (Kozlowski et al., 2005), that the number of neuromasts in the trunk was severely reduced in the *cingulin b*-MO morphants compared to that in the Control-MO embryos (**Figures 3G,H**). Taken together, our

findings indicated that *cingulin b* was required in the lateral line system of zebrafish.

Knockdown of *Cingulin b* Inhibits Cell Proliferation and Hair Cell Differentiation in the Lateral Line System of Zebrafish

During the development of zebrafish lateral line, the collective cells migrate and form rosette-like structure in the trailing region (Aman and Piotrowski, 2008). The deposition of neuromasts occurs after assembly of the last rosette (Nechiporuk and Raible, 2008). Here, we found that cell proliferation in the primordium was destroyed during the embryonic development of zebrafish by BrdU staining after knocking down the gene expression of *cingulin b* (**Figures 4A–F**). BrdU index was defined as the number of BrdU-positive cells divided by the number of total cells labeled by DAPI in this article, which was used to evaluate cell proliferation ability. In 36 dpf, the BrdU index in the primordium of *cingulin b*-MO morphants decreased significantly, that the BrdU index was 10.04% ± 0.02 ($n = 17$) compared to 39.74% ± 0.02 in the Control-MO group (**Figure 4G**).

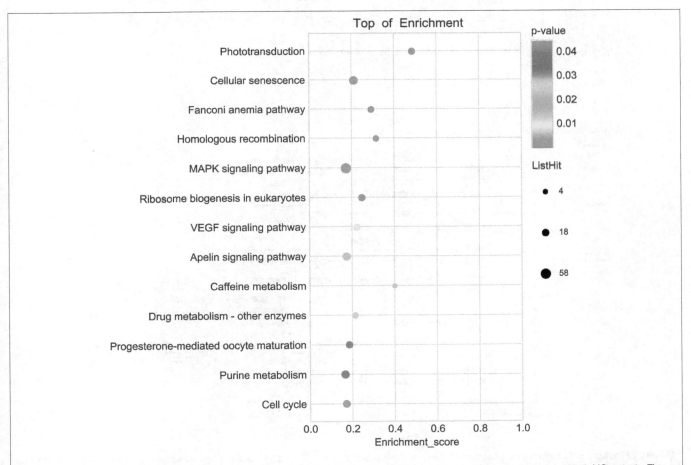

FIGURE 6 | KEGG enrichment analysis screens out top 13 pathways which are highly differentiated expressed between controls and *cingulin b*-MO mutants. The analysis is conducted from three independent experiments in different groups (n = 30 embryos in each group), and p value <0.05 is considered as remarkable difference.

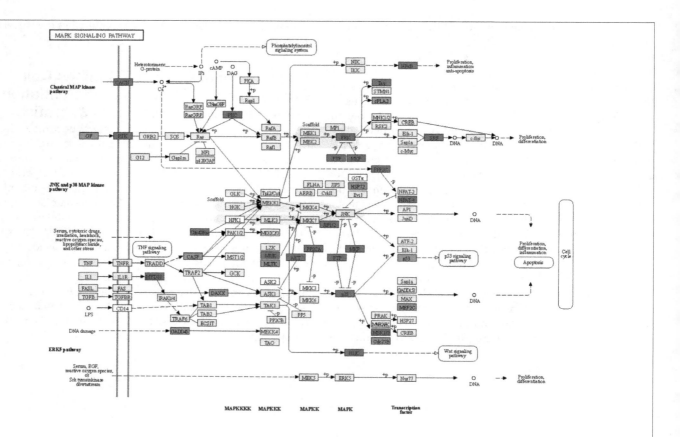

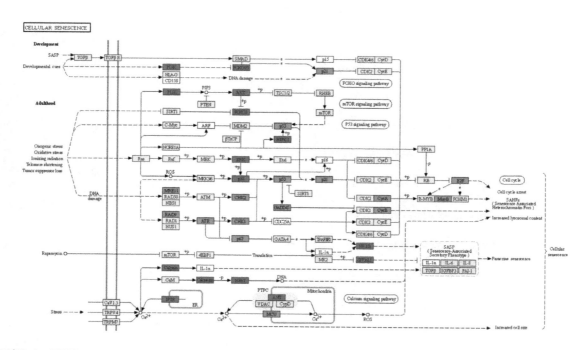

FIGURE 7 | The key KEGG pathways: MAPK signaling pathway and cellular senescence signaling pathway. The red nodes represent upregulated DEGs in *cingulin b*-MO mutants, the green marked node represents downregulated DEGs in *cingulin b*-MO mutants, and the blue marked node represents overlapping targets between Control-MO and *cingulin b*-MO embryos. The analysis is conducted from three independent experiments in different groups, and each group has 30 embryos.

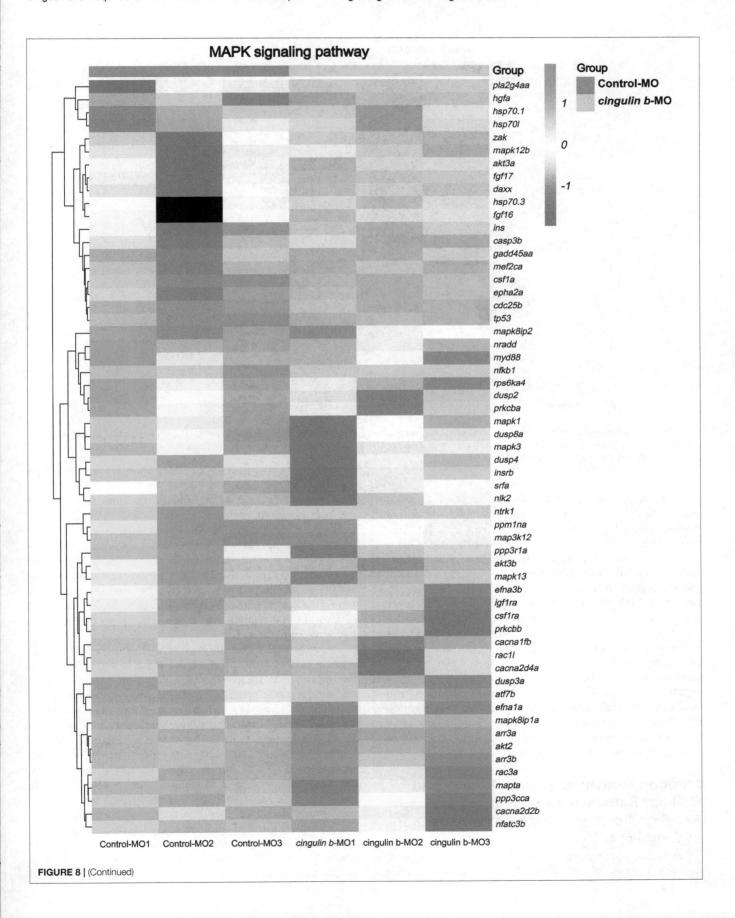

FIGURE 8 | (Continued)

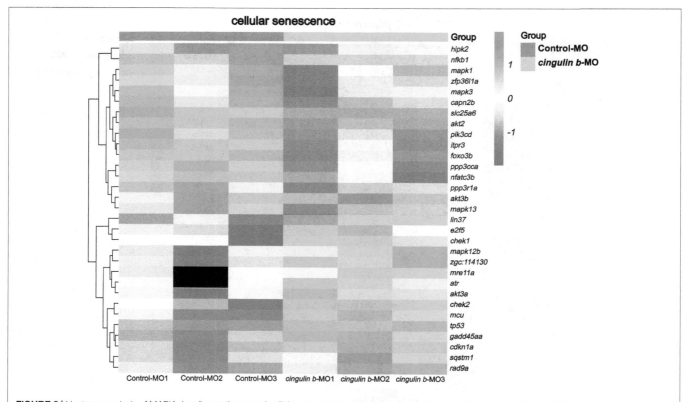

FIGURE 8 | Heatmap analysis of MAPK signaling pathway and cellular senescence signaling pathway in comparison between Control-MO embryos and *cingulin b*-MO morphants. The red indicates upregulated DEGs and the blue indicates downregulated DEGs. The analysis is conducted from three independent experiments in different groups, and each group has 30 embryos.

To investigate the sustained effect of *cingulin b* in zebrafish embryonic development, we stained the proliferative cells with BrdU (**Figures 5B,F**) and collected embryos at 3 dpf. The *Tg (brn3c: mGFP)^{s356t}* zebrafish were used here because of the HCs in neuromasts were labeled with GFP (**Figures 5C,G**). The total cells in neuromast were labeled with DAPI (**Figures 5A,E**). The merged images were shown in **Figures 5D,H**. The number of neuromast HCs in the trunk in *cingulin b*-MO experimental group decreased significantly compared to that of Control-MO group (**Figure 5I**). The BrdU index was also decreased severely in the *cingulin b*-MO group compared to that in the Control-MO group (**Figure 5J**). We also performed ISH staining of *atohla*, a maeker of HC, and found the expression of *atoh1a* was significantly decressed after knocking down of *cigulin b* compared to the control group (**Figure 5K**). Altogether, the data showed that knocking down *cingulin b* inhibited cell proliferation during primordia migration and neuromasts deposition in the early development process of zebrafish PLL system.

Mitogen-Activated Protein Kinase and Cellular Senescence Signaling Pathway Are Significantly Affected After Inhibition of *Cingulin b*

To explore the potential mechanism of *cingulin b* in regulating the development of zebrafish PLL system, we conducted

RNA sequencing analysis to compare the difference between the control group and the *cingulin b*-MO mutants. KEGG analysis figured out the 13 top enriched pathways, of which MAPK signaling pathway and cellular senescence were the most two significant pathways evaluated by *p* value and gene counts (**Figure 6**). The key KEGG pathways, namely MAPK signaling pathway and cellular senescence pathway were listed in **Figure 7**. Also, the location of DEGs in *cingulin b*-MO siblings and overlapping genes of enriched pathways were revealed.

Heatmap analysis of DEGs of MAPK pathway and cellular senescence was screened in **Figure 8** for Control-MO group vs. *cingulin b*-MO experimental group, respectively. RT-PCR analysis for some genes from MAPK and cellular senescence signaling pathways was conducted to verify our findings in RNA-sequencing data. The primer sequences were as listed in **Supplementary Table 2**. As shown in **Figure 9**, a total 9 genes in MAPK signaling pathways, 4 genes in cellular senescence pathway, and 9 genes overlapped in the two signaling pathways were examined. The mRNA levels of *mapk1*, *mapk3*, *akt2*, *akt3b*, *atf7b*, *ppp3cca*, and *ppp3r1a* were significantly decreased after knockdown of *cingulin b*, while the expression levels of *tp53*, *mef2ca*, *mapk12b*, and *gadd45aa* were significantly increased in *cingulin b*-MO group. The results of qRT-PCR were in consistency with those found in KEGG analysis, indicating that MAPK signaling was inhibited

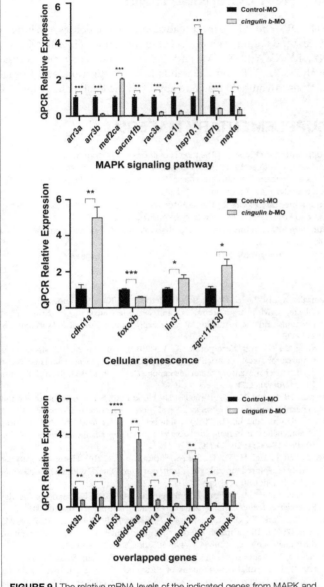

FIGURE 9 | The relative mRNA levels of the indicated genes from MAPK and cellular senescence signaling pathways were normalized to the GAPDH level as determined by qRT-PCR. The results are recorded as mean ± SEM from three independent experiments (n = 8 embryos in each group). *p < 0.05, **p < 0.01, ***p < 0.001, and ****p < 0.0001.

whereas cellular senescence was activated by repression of *cingulin b*.

DISCUSSION

Cingulin is found interacting with connexin-26, a GJB2 encoding gene pivotal in hearing (Kelsell et al., 1997; Najmabadi et al., 2002), through the protein-protein interaction analysis (Batissoco et al., 2018). Besides, cingulin and connexin-26 are also found co-immuno-precipitated in the mouse organ of Cotri and stria vascularis (Batissoco et al., 2018). However,

the role of cingulin in the cochlear development has not been identified. Previous studies have demonstrated that the PLL system of zebrafish is a good animal model for the research of mechanosensory organ development for the reason that the HCs in PLL neuromasts share similar structure and function with the mammalian inner ear HCs (He et al., 2017; Tang et al., 2019; Tang et al., 2021). In this study, we detected obvious expression of *cingulin b* in the PLL neuromasts of zebrafish. However, the number of PLL neuromasts was significantly decreased after knockdown of *cingulin b* by antisense MO injection, and we also found severe repression of cell proliferation and hair cell differentiation in the PLL primordium and neuromasts. Additionally, the RNA sequence analysis revealed that MAPK signaling was downregulated while cellular senescence signaling was upregulated in the *cingulin b*-MO embryos compared to the Control-MO injection embryos. Furthermore, we also confirmed the findings by heatmap differential analysis through qRT-PCR experiment. Our findings demonstrated that *cingulin b* was required for the normal development of zebrafish posterior lateral line by regulating the MAPK and cellular senescence signaling pathways.

Mitogen-activated protein kinase (MAPK) has been reported to be related to the formation of primordium in the posterior lateral line system of zebrafish (Harding and Nechiporuk, 2012). MAPK signaling pathway has three subfamilies, namely classical ERK pathway, Jun N-terminal kinase (JNK) pathway, and p38 pathway (Zhang and Liu, 2002). Activation of *ERK1/2* enhances cell proliferation (Lavoie et al., 2020), induces the expression of Cyclin D1 (Chen et al., 2020), and regulates the G1/S progression of cell cycle (Jirmanova et al., 2002). JNK and p38 pathways are often activated by stresses from environment or toxic agents, and usually exert antagonistic effects on cell proliferation and cell survival (Wagner and Nebreda, 2009). As previously reported, *p38* is considered as a negative regulator of cell cycle procession through downregulating cyclins and upregulating inhibitors of cyclin-dependent kinase (CDKIs) (Thornton and Rincon, 2009). In our previous study, we find that JNK inhibitor SP600125 suppresses the development of zebrafish lateral line by induction of *p21* and *p53* (Cai et al., 2016), which links the JNK pathway with tumor suppressor *p53*. Another study also demonstrates that JNK is the negative modulation of *p53* (Das et al., 2007). In the present study, *mapk1* and *mapk3* were significantly downregulated while *tp53* and *gadd45aa* were remarkably upregulated after knockdown of *cingulin b* in comparison with the Control-MO-injected controls, which were in consistency with the previous reporters.

Cellular senescence is a permanent cell cycle arrest after different damages, such as aging, oncogenes, oxidative agents, chemotherapeutic drugs, or epigenetic modulators (Hernandez-Segura et al., 2018). Senescent cells have variable phenotypes but share some common hallmarks in the mechanism, of which CDKIs are widely involved in the progression of cellular senescence, and the main components driving cell cycle arrest in senescence are *cdkn1a* (*p21*), *cdkn2a* (*p16*), and *cdkn2b* (*p15*) (Hernandez-Segura et al., 2018). Cellular senescence is found relevant to the development and tissue regeneration of zebrafish (Da Silva-Alvarez et al., 2020a,b). In this study, we observed strong elevation in the expression of *tp53*, *cdkn1a*, and *gadd45aa* in the morphants injected with *cingulin b*-MO compared to the control embryos, suggesting the activation of cellular senescence after inhibition of *cingulin b*.

CONCLUSION

We demonstrate that *cingulin b* is required in the development of zebrafish lateral line system, and MAPK signaling pathway and cellular senescence are regulated by morpholino knockdown of *cingulin b*. To our knowledge, it's the first time that the function of *cingulin b* is explored in the mechanosensory organs of zebrafish, but further studies are needed to detect direct evidence between auditory organ development and cingulin, the proteins of tight junctions.

AUTHOR CONTRIBUTIONS

YH, DL, and SL: conceptualization, methodology, writing— review and editing, and project administration. YL, DT, ZZ, XW, NZ, RY, CeW, HX, JM, and CuW: methodology and formal analysis. YL, DT, and ZZ: validation, investigation, and formal analysis. All authors read and approved the final manuscript.

SUPPLEMENTARY MATERIAL

Supplementary Figure 1 | The representative S (sense control) and AS (antisense mRNA probe) images of *cingulin b* in the PLL of zebrafish at 48 hpf. Black arrowheads indicate neuromasts. Scale bars represent 50 μm, *n* = 10 in S group, and *n* = 7 in AS group.

Supplementary Figure 2 | The representative images of embryos as a whole as followed in the Control-MO and *cingulin b*-MO groups.

Supplementary Table 1 | Primers for the synthesis of objective genes in WISH experiment.

Supplementary Table 2 | Primers for Real-Time PCR experiment.

REFERENCES

Aman, A., and Piotrowski, T. (2008). Wnt/beta-catenin and Fgf signaling control collective cell migration by restricting chemokine receptor expression. *Dev. Cell* 15, 749–761. doi: 10.1016/j.devcel.2008.10.002

Batissoco, A. C., Salazar-Silva, R., Oiticica, J., Bento, R. F., Mingroni-Netto, R. C., and Haddad, L. A. (2018). A Cell Junctional Protein Network Associated with Connexin-26. *Int. J. Mol. Sci.* 2018:19. doi: 10.3390/ijms19092535

Brignull, H. R., Raible, D. W., and Stone, J. S. (2009). Feathers and fins: non-mammalian models for hair cell regeneration. *Brain Res.* 1277, 12–23. doi: 10.1016/j.brainres.2009.02.028

Cai, C., Lin, J., Sun, S., and He, Y. (2016). JNK Inhibition Inhibits Lateral Line Neuromast Hair Cell Development. *Front. Cell Neurosci.* 10:19. doi: 10.3389/fncel.2016.00019

Chen, C. A., Chang, J. M., Yang, Y. L., Chang, E. E., and Chen, H. C. (2020). Macrophage migration inhibitory factor regulates integrin-β1 and cyclin D1 expression *via* ERK pathway in podocytes. *Biomed. Pharmacother.* 124:109892. doi: 10.1016/j.biopha.2020.109892

Citi, S. (2019). The mechanobiology of tight junctions. *Biophys. Rev.* 11, 783–793. doi: 10.1007/s12551-019-00582-7

Cordenonsi, M., D'atri, F., Hammar, E., Parry, D. A., Kendrick-Jones, J., Shore, D., et al. (1999). Cingulin contains globular and coiled-coil domains and interacts with ZO-1, ZO-2, ZO-3, and myosin. *J. Cell Biol.* 147, 1569–1582. doi: 10.1083/jcb.147.7.1569

Da Silva-Alvarez, S., Guerra-Varela, J., Sobrido-Camean, D., Quelle, A., Barreiro-Iglesias, A., Sanchez, L., et al. (2020a). Cell senescence contributes to tissue regeneration in zebrafish. *Aging Cell* 19:e13052. doi: 10.1111/acel.13052

Da Silva-Alvarez, S., Guerra-Varela, J., Sobrido-Camean, D., Quelle, A., Barreiro-Iglesias, A., Sanchez, L., et al. (2020b). Developmentally-programmed cellular senescence is conserved and widespread in zebrafish. *Aging* 12, 17895–17901. doi: 10.18632/aging.103968

Das, M., Jiang, F., Sluss, H. K., Zhang, C., Shokat, K. M., Flavell, R. A., et al. (2007). Suppression of p53-dependent senescence by the JNK signal transduction pathway. *Proc. Natl. Acad. Sci. U S A* 104, 15759–15764. doi: 10.1073/pnas.0707782104

D'atri, F., Nadalutti, F., and Citi, S. (2002). Evidence for a functional interaction between cingulin and ZO-1 in cultured cells. *J. Biol. Chem.* 277, 27757–27764. doi: 10.1074/jbc.M203717200

Dooley, K., and Zon, L. I. (2000). Zebrafish: a model system for the study of human disease. *Curr. Opin. Genet. Dev.* 10, 252–256. doi: 10.1016/s0959-437x(00)00074-5

Driever, W., Stemple, D., Schier, A., and Solnica-Krezel, L. (1994). Zebrafish: genetic tools for studying vertebrate development. *Trends Genet.* 10, 152–159. doi: 10.1016/0168-9525(94)90091-4

González-Mariscal, L., Domínguez-Calderón, A., Raya-Sandino, A., Ortega-Olvera, J. M., Vargas-Sierra, O., and Martínez-Revollar, G. (2014). Tight junctions and the regulation of gene expression. *Semin. Cell Dev. Biol.* 36, 213–223.

Harding, M. J., and Nechiporuk, A. V. (2012). Fgfr-Ras-MAPK signaling is required for apical constriction *via* apical positioning of Rho-associated kinase during mechanosensory organ formation. *Development* 139, 3130–3135. doi: 10.1242/dev.082271

Hawkins, B. T., and Davis, T. P. (2005). The blood-brain barrier/neurovascular unit in health and disease. *Pharmacol. Rev.* 57, 173–185. doi: 10.1124/pr.57.2.4

He, Y., Bao, B., and Li, H. (2017). Using zebrafish as a model to study the role of epigenetics in hearing loss. *Expert Opin. Drug Discov.* 12, 967–975. doi: 10.1080/17460441.2017.1340270

He, Y., Wu, J., Mei, H., Yu, H., Sun, S., Shou, J., et al. (2014). Histone deacetylase activity is required for embryonic posterior lateral line development. *Cell Prolif* 47, 91–104. doi: 10.1111/cpr.12081

Hernandez-Segura, A., Nehme, J., and Demaria, M. (2018). Hallmarks of Cellular Senescence. *Trends Cell Biol.* 28, 436–453. doi: 10.1016/j.tcb.2018.02.001

Howe, K., Clark, M. D., Torroja, C. F., Torrance, J., Berthelot, C., Muffato, M., et al. (2013). The zebrafish reference genome sequence and its relationship to the human genome. *Nature* 496, 498–503. doi: 10.1038/nature12111

Jirmanova, L., Afanassieff, M., Gobert-Gosse, S., Markossian, S., and Savatier, P. (2002). Differential contributions of ERK and PI3-kinase to the regulation of cyclin D1 expression and to the control of the G1/S transition in mouse embryonic stem cells. *Oncogene* 21, 5515–5528. doi: 10.1038/sj.onc.1205728

Kalueff, A. V., Stewart, A. M., and Gerlai, R. (2014). Zebrafish as an emerging model for studying complex brain disorders. *Trends Pharmacol. Sci.* 35, 63–75. doi: 10.1016/j.tips.2013.12.002

Kelsell, D. P., Dunlop, J., Stevens, H. P., Lench, N. J., Liang, J. N., Parry, G., et al. (1997). Connexin 26 mutations in hereditary non-syndromic sensorineural deafness. *Nature* 387, 80–83. doi: 10.1038/387080a0

Kimmel, C. B., Ballard, W. W., Kimmel, S. R., Ullmann, B., and Schilling, T. F. (1995). Stages of embryonic development of the zebrafish. *Dev. Dyn.* 203, 253–310. doi: 10.1002/aja.1002030302

Kozlowski, D. J., Whitfield, T. T., Hukriede, N. A., Lam, W. K., and Weinberg, E. S. (2005). The zebrafish dog-eared mutation disrupts eya1, a gene required for cell survival and differentiation in the inner ear and lateral line. *Dev. Biol.* 277, 27–41. doi: 10.1016/j.ydbio.2004.08.033

Lavoie, H., Gagnon, J., and Therrien, M. (2020). ERK signalling: a master regulator of cell behaviour, life and fate. *Nat. Rev. Mol. Cell Biol.* 21, 607–632. doi: 10.1038/s41580-020-0255-7

Leonova, E. V., and Raphael, Y. (1997). Organization of cell junctions and cytoskeleton in the reticular lamina in normal and ototoxically damaged organ of Corti. *Hear Res.* 113, 14–28. doi: 10.1016/s0378-5955(97)00130-5

Mandrekar, N., and Thakur, N. L. (2009). Significance of the zebrafish model in the discovery of bioactive molecules from nature. *Biotechnol. Lett.* 31, 171–179. doi: 10.1007/s10529-008-9868-1

Najmabadi, H., Cucci, R. A., Sahebjam, S., Kouchakian, N., Farhadi, M., Kahrizi, K., et al. (2002). GJB2 mutations in Iranians with autosomal recessive non-syndromic sensorineural hearing loss. *Hum. Mutat.* 19:572. doi: 10.1002/humu.9033

Nechiporuk, A., and Raible, D. W. (2008). FGF-dependent mechanosensory organ patterning in zebrafish. *Science* 320, 1774–1777. doi: 10.1126/science.1156547

Nicolson, T. (2005). The genetics of hearing and balance in zebrafish. *Annu. Rev. Genet.* 39, 9–22. doi: 10.1146/annurev.genet.39.073003.105049

Ohnishi, H., Nakahara, T., Furuse, K., Sasaki, H., Tsukita, S., and Furuse, M. (2004). JACOP, a novel plaque protein localizing at the apical junctional complex with sequence similarity to cingulin. *J. Biol. Chem.* 279, 46014–46022. doi: 10.1074/jbc.M402616200

Pyati, U. J., Look, A. T., and Hammerschmidt, M. (2007). Zebrafish as a powerful vertebrate model system for *in vivo* studies of cell death. *Semin. Cancer Biol.* 17, 154–165. doi: 10.1016/j.semcancer.2006.11.007

Raphael, Y., and Altschuler, R. A. (1991). Reorganization of cytoskeletal and junctional proteins during cochlear hair cell degeneration. *Cell Motil. Cytoskeleton.* 18, 215–227. doi: 10.1002/cm.970180307

Tang, D., He, Y., Li, W., and Li, H. (2019). Wnt/β-catenin interacts with the FGF pathway to promote proliferation and regenerative cell proliferation in the zebrafish lateral line neuromast. *Exp. Mol. Med.* 51, 1–16. doi: 10.1038/s12276-019-0247-x

Tang, D., Lu, Y., Zuo, N., Yan, R., Wu, C., Wu, L., et al. (2021). The H3K27 demethylase controls the lateral line embryogenesis of zebrafish. *Cell Biol. Toxicol.* 2021:9669. doi: 10.1007/s10565-021-09669-y

Thisse, B., and Thisse, C. (2014). In situ hybridization on whole-mount zebrafish embryos and young larvae. *Methods Mol. Biol.* 1211, 53–67. doi: 10.1007/978-1-4939-1459-3_5

Thornton, T. M., and Rincon, M. (2009). Non-classical p38 map kinase functions: cell cycle checkpoints and survival. *Int. J. Biol. Sci.* 5, 44–51. doi: 10.7150/ijbs.5.44

Van Itallie, C. M., Fanning, A. S., Bridges, A., and Anderson, J. M. (2009). ZO-1 stabilizes the tight junction solute barrier through coupling to the perijunctional cytoskeleton. *Mol. Biol. Cell* 20, 3930–3940. doi: 10.1091/mbc.e09-04-0320

Wagner, E. F., and Nebreda, A. R. (2009). Signal integration by JNK and p38 MAPK pathways in cancer development. *Nat. Rev. Cancer* 9, 537–549. doi: 10.1038/nrc2694

Yano, T., Matsui, T., Tamura, A., Uji, M., and Tsukita, S. (2013). The association of microtubules with tight junctions is promoted by cingulin phosphorylation by AMPK. *J. Cell Biol.* 203, 605–614. doi: 10.1083/jcb.201304194

Zhang, W., and Liu, H. T. (2002). MAPK signal pathways in the regulation of cell proliferation in mammalian cells. *Cell Res.* 12, 9–18. doi: 10.1038/sj.cr.7290105

Zhuravleva, K., Goertz, O., Wölkart, G., Guillemot, L., Petzelbauer, P., Lehnhardt, M., et al. (2020). The tight junction protein cingulin regulates the vascular response to burn injury in a mouse model. *Microvasc. Res.* 132:104067. doi: 10.1016/j.mvr.2020.104067

4

Cognitive Function in Acquired Bilateral Vestibulopathy: A Cross-Sectional Study on Cognition, Hearing and Vestibular Loss

Bieke Dobbels[1,2]*, Griet Mertens[1,2], Annick Gilles[1,2], Annes Claes[1,2], Julie Moyaert[2],
Raymond van de Berg[3,4], Paul Van de Heyning[1,2], Olivier Vanderveken[1,2] and
Vincent Van Rompaey[1,2]

[1] Faculty of Medicine and Health Sciences, University of Antwerp, Antwerp, Belgium, [2] Department of Otorhinolaryngology and Head and Neck Surgery, Antwerp University Hospital, Edegem, Belgium, [3] Division of Balance Disorders, Department of Otorhinolaryngology and Head and Neck Surgery, Maastricht University Medical Center, Maastricht, Netherlands, [4] Faculty of Physics, Tomsk State University, Tomsk, Russia

*Correspondence:
Bieke Dobbels
bieke.dobbels@uza.be;
biekedobbels@gmail.com

Background: Several studies have demonstrated cognitive deficits in patients with bilateral vestibulopathy (BVP). So far, little attention has been paid to the hearing status of vestibular patients when evaluating their cognition. Given the well-established link between sensorineural hearing loss (SNHL) and cognitive decline and the high prevalence of SNHL in BVP patients, it is therefore uncertain if the cognitive deficits in BVP patients are solely due to their vestibular loss or might be, partially, explained by a concomitant SNHL.

Objective: To evaluate the link between cognition, hearing, and vestibular loss in BVP patients.

Design: Prospective cross-sectional analysis of cognitive performance in patients with BVP and control participants without vestibular loss. Both groups included subjects with a variety of hearing (dys)function. Cognition was assessed by means of the Repeatable Battery for the Assessment of Neuropsychological Status for Hearing Impaired Individuals (RBANS-H).

Results: Sixty-four BVP patients were evaluated and compared with 83 control participants. For each subscale and the totale RBANS-H scale a multiple linear regression model was fitted with the following variables: vestibular loss, hearing loss, age, gender, and education. Hearing loss seemed to be associated with worse outcome on the total RBANS-H scale and subscales immediate memory and language. Vestibular loss, on the other hand, was linked to worse performance on the attention subscale of the RBANS-H. Furthermore, we did not observe a correlation between saccular function and cognition.

Conclusion: This study has found general cognitive deficits in a large sample size of BVP patients. Multiple linear regression models revealed that both vestibular and hearing dysfunction were associated with different subscales of the cognitive test battery, the RBANS-H. Whereas hearing loss was associated with worse performance on total RBANS-H score, immediate memory and language, vestibular loss was observed to negatively affect attention performance.

Keywords: bilateral vestibulopathy, hearing loss, sensorineural, COCH protein, human, causality, cognition

INTRODUCTION

The vestibular apparatus, which includes the three semicircular canals and two otolith organs, is known to be crucial in maintaining balance and gaze stabilization. However, a growing body of literature recognizes that the role of the vestibular system goes far beyond these primitive reflexes. Over the past decades, numerous animal studies have repeatedly demonstrated spatial cognitive deficits in rodents with vestibular lesions (Wallace et al., 2002; Zheng et al., 2007, 2009a,b, 2012a,b, 2013; Baek et al., 2010). These findings have prompted researchers to evaluate whether human patients with vestibular lesions also suffer from cognitive dysfunction. Because of their bilateral loss of peripheral vestibular input, patients with bilateral vestibulopathy (BVP) are of specific interest to investigate the cognitive repercussions of vestibular loss. Numerous studies have demonstrated spatial cognitive deficits in BVP patients (Brandt et al., 2005; Grabherr et al., 2011; Kremmyda et al., 2016; Popp et al., 2017; Xie et al., 2017; Wei et al., 2018). Besides spatial cognitive impairment, more recent studies also show evidence of general cognitive deficits in BVP patients (Bessot et al., 2012; Popp et al., 2017; Wei et al., 2018). For instance, Popp et al. showed a statistically significant impairment of executive function, visuospatial abilities, attention and short-term memory in BVP patients (Popp et al., 2017). These findings are supported by the recent findings of Wei and colleagues, who examines executive function and attention in patients with Alzheimer's disease (AD) and mild cognitive impairment (MCI). In this study, subjects with bilateral absent saccular function performed significantly worse compared to peers with normal saccular function on the Trial Making Test-B (Wei et al., 2018).

The growing evidence of cognitive impairment in BVP patients has led to speculation on a causal relationship between peripheral vestibular loss and dementia (Previc, 2013; Harun et al., 2016). A recent cross-sectional study has found an increased prevalence of AD in individuals with bilateral absent saccular function (Harun et al., 2016). Up to now, convincing evidence to recognize vestibular loss as an independent risk-factor for dementia is lacking.

The pathomechanism that underpins the cognitive deficits in subjects with vestibular loss is not fully understood. Substantial research suggest that the extensive vestibular-cortical network forms the basis of this relationship (Smith and Zheng, 2013; Hitier et al., 2014; Smith, 2017). The vestibular system, more than any other sensory system, has widespread projections to many cortical areas, including those involved in autonomic functions, sleep, emotions, and cognition. As such, the spatial cognitive impairment in BVP patients seems to be related to an atrophy of the hippocampal formation, i.e., the hippocampus and parahippocampus, which is known to play a key role in spatial memory and navigation (Zheng et al., 2013; Hitier et al., 2014; Smith, 2017). Studies comparing brain volumes on MRI imaging using voxel-based morphometry, indeed revealed smaller hippocampal formation volumes in BVP patients compared with matched controls (Brandt et al., 2005; Gottlich et al., 2016; Kremmyda et al., 2016). Likewise, patients with Menière's disease were observed to have hippocampal atrophy compared to healthy controls. Moreover, their hippocampal volume was significantly correlated with the severity of vestibular loss ($p < 0.05$) and hearing dysfunction ($p < 0.001$) (Seo et al., 2016).

However, probably related to the wide cortical vestibular network, vestibular patients are prone to also develop anxiety, depression, and sleep disturbances (van de Berg et al., 2015; Kremmyda et al., 2016; Smith, 2017; Lucieer et al., 2018; Smith et al., 2018). In addition, some of peripheral vestibular diseases are frequently associated with sensorineural hearing loss (SNHL), e.g., Menière's disease, BVP, ototoxicity, … Both psychiatric comorbidities and hearing loss are known to negatively influence cognition themselves (Livingston et al., 2017). Multiple cohort (Lin et al., 2013; Gurgel et al., 2014) and cross-sectional studies (Lin, 2011; Lin et al., 2011; Quaranta et al., 2014; Loughrey et al., 2018) have demonstrated that SNHL is an independent risk factor for cognitive decline and even dementia. Therefore, the question is raised whether the observed cognitive deficits in vestibular patients are a result of these other comorbidities or whether they can be independently attributed to vestibular loss (Smith, 2017; Dobbels et al., 2018; Smith et al., 2018).

Recently, Smith and colleagues demonstrated short-term memory deficits in patients with a variety of vestibular syndromes, independently of psychiatric disorders, fatigue and sleep disturbances (Smith et al., 2018).

Yet, studies investigating cognition in vestibular patients thereby taking their hearing status into account, are limited. For example, Semenov and colleagues demonstrated cognitive deficits in 757 subjects with vestibular dysfunction, independently of SNHL. However, study participants did not receive laboratory vestibular testing to reassure peripheral vestibular loss. Moreover, only a subset of patients received auditory assessment (Semenov et al., 2016). A recent systematic review pointed out that none of the studies investigating cognition in BVP patients, diagnosed by means of calorics, rotatory chair test, and/or (video) head impulse test as suggested by the BVP diagnostic criteria of the Bárány Society, corrected for SNHL. Nonetheless, prevalence of SNHL in BVP patients range from 31 to 44% (Zingler et al., 2007; Lucieer et al., 2016).

Therefore, it is uncertain whether the cognitive impairment demonstrated in BVP patients could be solely attributed to the loss of vestibular input as suggested in previous studies. These cognitive deficits in BVP patients might be partially caused by a concomitant hearing loss.

In the light of the above uncertainty, this study specifically aims to evaluate the link between cognition, vestibular and hearing dysfunction in BVP patients with established vestibular loss by laboratory vestibular testing. Therefore, the general cognitive performance of BVP patients was compared to controls without vestibular loss and a variety of hearing (dys)function. To assess cognitive function, an instrument specifically designed to exclude any potential bias from hearing loss was used: the Repeatable Battery for the Assessment of Neuropsychological Status for Hearing Impaired Individuals (RBANS-H). This test battery assesses immediate and delayed memory, attention, language and visuospatial abilities.

MATERIALS AND METHODS

Study Design

This was a single-center, prospective, cross-sectional study recruiting from October 2017 until August 2018 at the Antwerp University Hospital. BVP patients were assessed during two separate visits of approximately 1.5–2 h by two ICH-GCP-accredited clinical researchers. Cognitive assessment was always performed at the start of each visit – by means of the Repeatable Battery for the Assessment of Neuropsychological Status for Hearing Impaired Individuals (RBANS-H) – in order to avoid loss of attention due to fatigue.

Study Participants
BVP Patients

Patients with a previous tentative diagnosis of BVP were recruited from the patient's database at the Otorhinolaryngology, Head and Neck surgery department at the Antwerp University Hospital, Belgium. All patients who accepted enrolment in this study, received new neuro-otological testing on site. The evaluation of the lower frequencies function of the lateral semi-circular canals was performed by electronystagmography (ENG) with bithermal caloric tests and rotatory chair test (Nystagliner Toennies, Germany). At our clinic, rotatory chair tests are performed using sinusoidal rotation (0.05 Hz) with a peak velocity of 60°/sec. Further detailed methodology and normative data had been previously described (Van der Stappen et al., 2000). In the first 35 patients, caloric irrigation was performed with water. Due to change in local patient safety guidelines, caloric insufflation in the other patients had to be performed with air: warm (47°C) and cold (26°C) air for 30 s. High-frequency function of all six semicircular canals was measured by the video head impulse test (vHIT). Angular head velocity was determined by three mini-gyroscopes, eye velocity by means of an infrared camera recording the right eye, all incorporated in commercially

available vHIT goggles (Otometrics, Taastrup, Denmark). Vestibulo-ocular reflex (VOR) gain was defined as the ratio of the area under the eye velocity curve to the head velocity curve from the impulse onset until the head velocity was again 0 (Macdougall et al., 2013). According to the recently established Bárány society criteria (Strupp et al., 2017), BVP diagnosis can be made based upon a bilaterally reduced function of the lateral semi-circular canals. Additionally, we evaluated saccular function by performing c-VEMP testing. Details on the procedure have been published previously (Colebatch et al., 1994; Vanspauwen et al., 2011). In brief, a patient's saccular function is quantified by the response of the ipsilateral sternocleidomastoid muscle to air-conducted 500 Hz tone bursts delivered monoaurally via insert phones. Recordings were made with an auditory evoked potential system equipped with electromyographic software (Neuro-Audio, Difra, Belgium), with self-adhesives electrodes (Blue sensor, Ambu, Denmark). The presence of a typically biphasic shape, with a positive peak after 13 ms (p13) and a negative peak after 23 ms (n23), was evaluated. When no p13n23 wave was seen above 100 dB acoustic clicks, a patient was considered to have an absent cVEMP response.

Inclusion criteria for BVP patients were:

(1) Bilaterally reduced vestibular function, as defined by the Bárány Society Criteria for BVP (Strupp et al., 2017):

- horizontal angular VOR gain < 0.6 measured by the vHIT, and/or
- reduced caloric response (sum of bithermal, 30 and 44°, maximum peak slow phase velocity (SPV) on each side < 6°/sec), and/or
- reduced horizontal angular VOR gain < 0.1 upon sinusoidal stimulation on a rotatory chair

(2) Disease duration of BVP > 6 months, in order to exclude acute pathology with possible remaining vertigo spells. Moreover, in the case of a vestibular neuritis recovery can occur in the first 6 months.
(3) Subjects might suffer from a post-lingual hearing loss.

Control Participants (CPs)

Control participants were recruited on the one hand, for subjects with hearing loss, from the hospital patient's database and on the other hand, for subjects without expected hearing loss, by means of the population registries at the local city councils in southern Antwerp (Belgium), by advertisements in the hospital and by approaching friends, family, and colleagues. Only subjects with no history of vertigo and scores < 5 on the Dizziness Handicap Inventory (DHI) were considered for enrolment in the study. After a screening phase, in which medical history was questioned and the DHI administered, hearing performance was examined. If participants suffered from SNHL, rotatory chair test with electronystagmographic registration of the vestibulo-ocular reflex was performed to exclude severe vestibular dysfunction. Only subjects with a gain > 0.3 were enrolled as controls in the study. This cut-off value was chosen in compliance with the current criteria for presbyvestibulopathy, which are in development by the Bárány Society (Agrawal et al., 2018). In these criteria, a gain lower than 0.3 upon sinusoidal stimulation on a rotatory chair is considered pathological.

For both BVP patients and CP the following additional inclusion criteria were applied: (1) Age ≥ 18 years; (2) Fluency in Dutch; (3) No history of neurological diseases (e.g., dementia, Parkinson's disease, cerebrovascular accident, etc.); (4) Absence of clinical signs indicating dementia or MCI.

Education of all participants was classified as primary school, lower secondary school, upper secondary school and college/university.

Cognitive Assessment

The assessment of cognition was based on a validated neuropsychological test battery, designed by Randolph: the Repeatable Battery for the Assessment of Neuropsychological Status (RBANS) (Randolph et al., 1998; Randolph, 2012). Advantages of this test battery include the comprehensive insight on general cognitive performance, the relatively short administering time (30–40 min), good sensitivity, the established test–retest reliability and its age-corrected normative data (Duff et al., 2005; Randolph, 2012).

In the RBANS-H, modifications are made to create a test battery suitable for hearing impaired subjects (Claes et al., 2016). In addition to the RBANS, in which all instructions are given orally, written instructions through PowerPoint presentation are provided (Claes et al., 2016). Regarding the inclusion of participants with SNHL, the additional written instructions are necessary to test our study population. With only oral instructions, patients with SNHL are at a possible disadvantage of not hearing correctly the instructions and thus obtain lower scores compared with normal hearing peers.

Similar to the RBANS, the RBANS-H is a complete cognitive test battery consisting of 12 subtests evaluating five cognitive domains: immediate memory, delayed memory, attention, language and visuospatial abilities (**Table 1**).

As considered of special interest, the tasks evaluating visuospatial cognition will be discussed briefly. In the task 'Figure Copy,' participants are shown a complex geometric figure on a screen. While remaining visually available, participants are asked to copy the figure on a paper with special attention to the correctness of each element and its relative location to the rest of the figure. In the second subtest, Line orientation, 13 identical lines radiating out from a single point and forming half of a circular pattern, are shown. Below this pattern of numbered lines (1–13), two

identical lines that match two of the lines from the original pattern are displayed. The participant is asked to give the numbers of the lines in the original pattern to which the two lines correspond.

All subtests are scored separately to generate the index score of the corresponding cognitive domain, and total score RBANS-H score. All index and total scores can be converted to age-appropriate scores with a normal distribution with a mean of 100 and a standard deviation of 15.

Hearing Assessment

To correct cognitive outcome measures for the hearing status of the enrolled participants, a speech audiometry in noise was performed. In order to correspond as much as possible to their daily life hearing performance, participants were asked to use their habitual hearing aids if they had any. Assessment was conducted in free field in an audiometric soundproof booth using the Leuven Intelligibility Sentences Test (LIST) (van Wieringen and Wouters, 2008). This speech material consists of several lists of 10 sentences. An adaptive procedure was used to determine the speech reception threshold (SRT). The level of the speech-weighted noise was fixed at 65 dB SPL and the intensity level of the sentences varied in steps of 2 dB adaptively in a one-down, one-up procedure according to participant's response. The SRT was ascertained based on the level of the last six sentences of two lists, including an imaginary 11th sentence. A lower SRT indicates better speech in noise perception and thus better hearing function. The average SRT in an normal hearing population is -7.8 ± 1.17 dB speech-to-noise ratio (van Wieringen and Wouters, 2008).

Data Collection and Statistics

Data were stored in OpenClinica LLC (Waltham, MA, United States), an online database for electronic data registration and data management developed for clinical research. Data were stored with a password secured access to the online database. We used IBMS SPSS Statistics 24 (IBM; Armonk, NY, United States) for the statistical analyses. Demographic data were analyzed with t-test (continuous data) and chi-squared test (categorical data), or the appropriate non-parametric tests. To adjust for confounders in the comparison of cognitive performance between BVP patients and CP, a multiple linear regression model was fitted. The RBANS-H score, either the total scale or the subscales, was entered as dependent variable. Group, SNHL (SRT in noise), age, gender, and education were entered as covariates in all models. These models evaluate whether BVP patients have worse cognitive function than CP when correcting for hearing dysfunction and other confounders. The same models can test if the effect of SNHL on the RBANS-H (sub)scores is significant, when adjusting for vestibular loss and other confounders. Multicollinearity was checked by means of variance inflation factors. Normality of the residuals were checked with QQ-plots. Homoscedasticity, independence of error and linearity assumptions were controlled by means of residuals plots.

Finally, a linear regression model was fitted to assess the link between saccular function and cognition in the BVP group.

TABLE 1 | The five cognitive domains and 12 subtests of the RBANS.

Immediate memory	Delayed memory	Visuospatial	Language	Attention
List learning	List recall	Figure copy	Picture naming	Digit span
Story memory	List recognition	Line orientation	Semantic fluency	Coding
	Story recall			
	Figure recall			

TABLE 2 | Demographic characteristics and hearing status of study population.

	BVP patients	Control participants	
	n = 64	*n* = 83	
Age (mean, SD)	59 (14.3)	68.4 (10.5)	$p < 0.05$
Sex (*n*, %)			$p = 0.4$
Male	38 (59)	43 (52)	
Female	26 (41)	40 (48)	
Education (*n*, %)			$p = 0.1$
Less than primary school	1 (1.8)	0	
Primary school	2 (3.6)	12 (14.5)	
Lower secondary school	11 (19.6)	10 (12)	
Upper secondary school	20 (35.7)	23 (27.7)	
College/University	22 (39.3)	38 (45.8)	
Hearing performance			
Speech reception threshold in noise (mean, SD in dB)	+0.65 (± 6.5)	−0.27 (± 7.4)	$p = 0.4$
Conventional hearing aid (n)	12	12	
Other hearing aid: CI, BAHA (n)	19	1	

BVP, bilateral vestibulopathy; CI, cochlear implant; BAHA, bone anchored hearing aid.

Both, the amplitude of the p13n23 wave and the cVEMP response (unilateral absent, bilateral absent, or bilateral present response) were entered as dependent variable. Again, these two models were adjusted for SNHL (SRT in noise), age, sex, and education.

RESULTS

Study Population

The database consisted of 234 patients with a tentative diagnosis of bilateral vestibulopathy. Of these patients, 127 patients declined to participate in the study, 34 patients did not meet the Bárány Society criteria for BVP based on their vestibular test results, three patients did not speak Dutch and two patients died before the start of the study.

Finally, sixty-four BVP patients with a mean age of 59 ± 14.3 years met the study inclusion criteria; 59% of them were male. Eighty-three CP with a mean age of 68.4 ± 10.5 years, were enrolled in the study; 52% of them were male (**Table 2**). There was no statistically significant difference between BVP patients and CP concerning sex, education level and hearing performance (SRT in noise). CP were significantly older than BVP patients.

To be enrolled as BVP patient, the Bárány Society criteria needed to be fulfilled (Strupp et al., 2017). Forty percent of BVP patients met all Bárány society criteria: a bilateral reduced response on caloric testing, rotatory chair test and vHIT. In 30% of BVP patients two out of three Bárány society criteria were fulfilled, and in the remaining 30% of the BVP patients there was only found a vestibular hypofunction in one of the three vestibular tests (**Figure 1**).

An underlying cause of vestibular loss could not be identified in 33.9% of BVP patients. With a prevalence of nearly 20%,

a mutation in the COCH gene causing DFNA9, was the most frequent underlying non-idiopathic etiology in our BVP cohort. In 16% of BVP patients, an infectious cause was found (e.g., meningitis, neuritis, Lyme disease). Ménière's disease and head trauma accounted for respectively 6 and 11% of BVP causes. In four BVP patients an ototoxic cause was suspected (3 aminoglycosides antibiotics and 1 chemotherapy, not further specified) (**Figure 2**).

Among the BVP patients, the mean SRT during speech in noise was +0.65 (± 6.5) dB SNR and ranged from −7 to +20 dB SNR. This was not significantly different from control participants (mean SRT during speech in noise −0.27 (± 7.4); range −7 to +20 dB SNR).

The Effect of Vestibular Loss and Hearing Loss on Cognitive Performance

All 64 BVP patients completed the RBANS-H except from five participants: four refused any cognitive assessment; one participant witnessed the RBANS-H test procedure in his father and was thus excluded because of a potential practice effect. Thus, in total 59 BVP patients were included for statistical analysis concerning RBANS-H results. We did not observe a statistically significant difference on total RBANS-H score or any RBANS-H subscales between BVP patients diagnosed by caloric irrigation with water, compared with those diagnosed by insufflation with air.

Results of the RBANS-H total score and index-scores are presented in **Figure 3**. Overall, BVP patients performed worse on the RBANS-H (mean total score in BVP patients 95.6 ± 17.2 versus 98.7 ± 13.1 in CP). Mean performance on Immediate Memory, Attention, Language, and Visuospatial was worse in BVP patients (see **Table 3**). Delayed Memory seemed to be slightly better in BVP patients compared to CP.

To evaluate the presence of a statistically significant association between vestibular loss, SNHL and cognition, a multiple linear regression model was conducted for each outcome measure (total RBANS-H scale and every subscale) (**Table 3**). All models were adjusted for SNHL (SRT in noise), age, sex, and education. As previously mentioned, the same model evaluates whether there is a statistically significant effect of group (BVP versus CP) and SNHL on the cognitive outcome measure. Model coefficients were designed in such way that a negative model coefficient always indicated poorer cognition in the BVP group. Similarly, a negative coefficient pointed at a negative impact of SNHL (higher SRT) on cognitive performance.

Regarding the link between vestibular loss and cognition, only a statistically significant difference was found between BVP patients and CP on the subscale Attention (mean score of 89.1 ± 18 in BVP patients, versus mean score of 94.2 ± 16.1 in CP, $p = 0.045$, β = −5.9). In contrast, hearing dysfunction, in both BVP and CP,was statistically significant associated with worse cognitive performance on the Total scale of the RBANS-H and on the subscales Immediate Memory and Language. More specifically, one dB lower SRT in noise was associated with a 0.4 lower Total scale ($p = 0.027$), a 0.6 lower Immediate

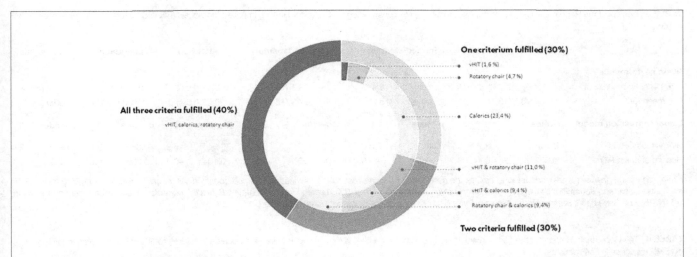

FIGURE 1 | According to the Barany Criteria, bilateral vestibular loss is defined by a hypofunction measured by means of caloric irrigation, rotatory chair test, or vHIT. In this figure, the percentages of BVP who fulfilled all these criteria or less are presented.

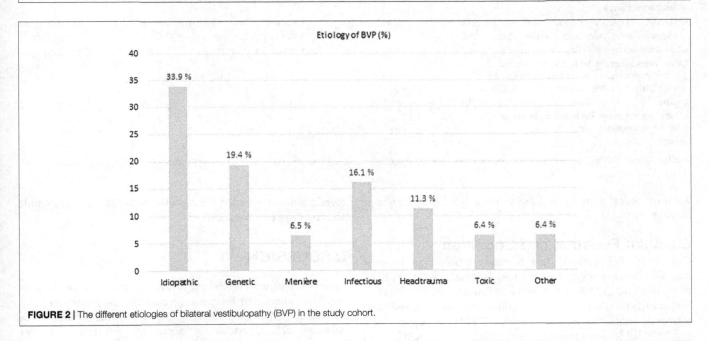

FIGURE 2 | The different etiologies of bilateral vestibulopathy (BVP) in the study cohort.

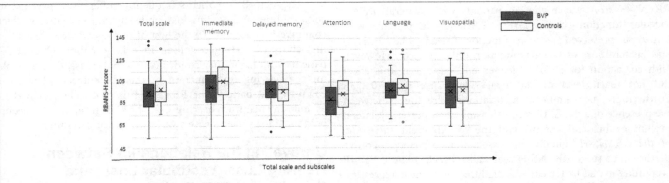

FIGURE 3 | Cognitive outcome measures. Boxplots of the RBANS-H total and index scores are shown for the CP group (control participants) and BVP group (bilateral vestibulopathy).

TABLE 3 | Results of the Repeatable Battery for the Assessment of Neuropsychological Status for Hearing Impaired Individuals (RBANS-H) total and index scores in BVP patients and CP.

	Total RBANS-H scale		Immediate memory		Delayed memory		Attention		Language		Visuospatial	
Mean performance												
BVP patients: mean (SD)	95.6 (17.2)		100.4 (18.4)		99.1 (14.2)		89.1 (18.0)		97.7 (11.6)		96.3 (16.3)	
CP: mean (SD)	98.7 (13.1)		105.7 (15.9)		97.9 (12.4)		94.2 (16.1)		101.3 (12.1)		96.9 (14.2)	
Linear regression model	*p*-value	β	*p*-value	β	*p*-value	β	*p*-value	β	*p*-value	β	*p*-value	β
BVP versus CP	0.142	−3.7	0.07	−5.0	0.73	0.8	0.045	−5.9	0.083	−3.6	0.396	−2.4
Hearing status (SRT)	0.027	−0.4	0.009	−0.5	0.115	−0.3	0.104	−0.4	0.002	−0.5	0.492	0.1

Linear regression analyses were conducted to assess the association between vestibular loss, hearing loss and cognition. All models adjusted for hearing loss (SRT in noise), age, sex, and education. Statistical significant p-values are shown in gray. BVP, bilateral vestibulopathy; CP, healthy controls; SRT, speech reception threshold; RBANS-H, The Repeatable Battery for the Assessment of Neuropsychological Status for Hearing Impaired Individuals.

TABLE 4 | The Repeatable Battery for the Assessment of Neuropsychological Status for Hearing Impaired Individuals (RBANS-H) total and index scores regarding c-VEMP response in BVP patients.

	Total scale	Immediate memory	Delayed memory	Attention	Language	Visuospatial
Mean performance						
Bilateral absent c-VEMP response: mean (SD)	90.4 (15.6)	96.0 (18.3)	96.9 (15.5)	85.7 (16.8)	94.2 (11.0)	91.2 (17.1)
Unilateral present c-VEMP response: mean (SD)	95.8 (17.5)	96.5 (16.3)	100.0 (9.4)	90.2 (21.5)	100.0 (13.5)	96.5 (11.0)
Bilateral present c-VEMP response: mean (SD)	116.0 (9.8)	124.5 (13.7)	110.3 (11.6)	101.5 (7.1)	107.8 (7.6)	112.8 (11.0)
Linear regression model in 3 VEMP groups *(bilateral absent response/unilateral present response/bilateral present response)*						
p-value	0.4	0.06	0.8	0.5	0.4	0.1
Linear regression model with amplitude of c-VEMP of the better ear						
p-value	0.6	0.3	1	0.8	0.5	0.6

c-VEMP, cervical vestibular evoked myogenic potentials. All linear regression models adjusted for hearing (speech reception threshold in noise), age, sex, and education.

Memory index score (*p* = 0.009) and a 0.5 lower Language score (*p* = 0.002).

Saccular Function and Cognition

Only four BVP patients had a bilateral preserved saccular function. Twenty-seven patients had bilateral absent c-VEMP responses, and in 13 BVP patients a unilateral c-VEMP response was measured. Due to practical considerations or insufficient sternocleidomastoid muscle tension, c-VEMP responses could not be reliably measured in the remaining 20 patients. *Total RBANS-H score* was higher in patients with bilateral present saccular function (mean: 116 ± 9.8) than in patients with unilateral preserved saccular function (mean: 95.8 ± 17.5) and bilateral loss of saccular function (90.4 ± 15.6). However, with correction for SNHL, age, sex and education, this effect did not reach level of statistical significance (*p* = 0.253). Furthermore, no significant associations were found between the presence of a c-VEMP response (unilateral present, bilateral present or bilateral absent) and the five different *sub scales of the RBANS-H*. Finally, an association between cognitive performance (total RBANS-H scale, all subscales) and c-VEMP amplitude in the better ear was explored in a linear regression model for each outcome, all correcting for SNHL, age, gender and education (**Table 4**). Neither on the RBANS-H total scale, nor on any of the index scores, a significant

correlation was revealed between the p13-n23 wave amplitude and cognitive performance.

DISCUSSION

Despite the extensive research demonstrating cognitive impairment in animal and human subjects suffering from vestibular lesions, it remains a matter of debate to which extent these cognitive deficits are solely dependent on their vestibular loss. As such, BVP patients frequently suffer from psychiatric comorbidities and hearing loss, both known to negatively affect cognitive functioning. To the best of our knowledge, this is the first study evaluating cognition in a large cohort of 64 BVP patients with laboratory confirmed vestibular loss, that controls for the hearing (dys)function of the test subjects. The used cognitive test battery, the RBANS-H, is especially designed to exclude any bias from hearing loss. The BVP group and CP group both included subjects with a variety of hearing dysfunction.

Unraveling the Relationship Between Hearing Loss, Vestibular Loss, and Cognition in BVP Patients

In general, BVP patients were observed to perform worse on the total RBANS-H scale and the following subscales: immediate memory, attention, language, and visuospatial. By means of a multiple linear regression model fitted for each outcome measure, it was evaluated if the worse outcome in BVP patients was significantly linked to vestibular loss (group) or hearing loss (SRT in noise), thereby additionally adjusting for age, gender and education. Hearing loss, in both BVP patients and CP, was observed to be associated with a worse score on the total RBANS-H scale and on the subscales immediate memory and language. More specifically, 5 dB higher SRT resulted on average in two points lower on the total RBANS-H scale, three points lower on immediate memory and 2.5 points lower on language. These effects can be considered rather small (Randolph, 2012). On the other hand, vestibular loss seemed to be associated with a worse performance on the attention tasks of the RBANS-H. BVP patients scored on average 6 points less on the attention sub score.

In other words, these results confirm the previously observed cognitive deficits in BVP patients. However, it seems that not only the vestibular loss of BVP patients, but also their hearing loss, contributes to their impaired cognition. Particularly, attention seemed to be associated with vestibular (dys)function in this study. Interestingly, next to spatial cognitive deficits, attentional deficits have indeed been observed most frequently in previous BVP cohort studies (Dobbels et al., 2018). However, also memory deficits have been previously described in BVP patients (Popp et al., 2017). Our results suggest that these deficits might be more correlated to the hearing loss of BVP patients than to their vestibular loss. Language function, which is in this study negatively influenced by hearing loss, has never been assessed before in BVP patients.

Spatial Cognition in BVP Patients

Because numerous studies have observed spatial cognitive deficits in animals and humans with vestibular loss, it is of potential interest that our results could not confirm this finding in a relatively large sample size of BVP patients. Even without correction for hearing loss, no significant difference in Visuospatial performance was found between CP and BVP patients. This rather contradictory result might rely on the kind of tasks used to assess visuospatial abilities. Previous literature seem to be more focused on spatial memory and navigation than constructional cognition (e.g., copying a figure) (Jandl et al., 2015; Kremmyda et al., 2016; Brandt and Dieterich, 2017; Popp et al., 2017). It is reasonable that the figure coping and line orientation task are not sensitive enough to detect spatial cognitive deficits in BVP patients. Moreover, a big animal literature repeatedly linked spatial cognition to the vestibular system. Several of these studies attempted to control for the bias of SNHL by removing the tympanic membrane of the sham control animals. Although this is only considered a partial auditory control, researchers repeatedly found that rodents without vestibular lesions but with a removed tympanic membrane outperformed rodents with vestibular lesions on a variety of spatial cognitive tasks (Zheng et al., 2007, 2009a,b, 2012b; Baek et al., 2010; Smith and Zheng, 2013).

In human BVP patients, the virtual Morris water task have been shown to be sensitive enough to detect spatial

cognitive deficits in (small sample sizes of) BVP patients (Brandt et al., 2005; Kremmyda et al., 2016). Further research should be undertaken to investigate if spatial memory and navigation is impaired in BVP patients, regardless of their hearing status., for example by using the virtual Morris water task (Hamilton et al., 2009).

Hearing Loss in BVP Patients

Compared with literature, the prevalence of SNHL in our BVP cohort was relatively high: 85% BVP patients with abnormal hearing in at least one ear. This might lead to a more substantial effect of hearing loss on cognition in our BVP patients compared to other BVP study groups. Therefore, these results need to be interpreted with caution and must be reproduced by future research. A possible explanation for the high occurrence of hearing loss in our BVP cohort, might be the high prevalence of genetic causes of BVP, i.e., COCH mutations. This is an autosomal dominant disorder, causing progressive otovestibular decline starting at the 3rd to 5th life decade. As the burden of a genetic disease might not be underestimated, it is not excluded that cognitive evolution behaves differently in DFNA9 patients compared with BVP patients caused by other pathologies. According to a recent literature review, cognition has never been explored in DFNA9 patients (De Belder et al., 2017).

Nonetheless, our findings underpin the importance of adjusting for hearing when reporting on cognition in a vestibular patient group. On the one hand, it is necessary to correct for hearing when investigating cognition in patients with vestibular disorders. Since positive effects of hearing aids on cognition have been reported in literature (Amieva et al., 2015), we chose to adjust for hearing in a best aided situation with the SRT in noise. When relying on hearing in an unaided situation, the effect of hearing might be overestimated as it does not represent the daily life situation of a patient. On the other hand, the instrument of cognitive assessment needs to be adapted for hearing-impaired participants. Otherwise, hearing loss might negatively affect the cognitive outcomes, as the to-be-repeated or to-be-remembered items may not be well-perceived by the participant (Dupuis et al., 2015).

Given the negative association between vestibular loss and attention and the close anatomical link between the cochlea and the vestibular system, future research investigating cognition in patients with severe hearing loss should take, vice versa, the vestibular function of the study group into account.

Otolith Function and Cognition

To the best of our knowledge, previous research investigating cognition in BVP patients has not corrected for hearing (Glasauer et al., 1994, 2002; Brandt et al., 2005; Grabherr et al., 2011; Bessot et al., 2012; Jandl et al., 2015; Kremmyda et al., 2016; Popp et al., 2017). In these studies a diagnosis of BVP was based on bilateral hypofunction of the lateral semicircular canal, which is equivalent to the Bárány society criteria applied in this study. As the Bárány society criteria were only recently established, cut-off values to determine vestibular hypofunction vary across the latter studies (Dobbels et al., 2018). Interestingly, few studies found an association of saccular function with cognition (Bigelow and Agrawal, 2015; Xie et al., 2017; Wei et al., 2018). Otolith function, measured by ocular or cervical vestibular evoked myogenic potentials, is not incorporated in the Bárány society criteria for BVP. Importantly, one of the studies investigating saccular function and cognition adjusted for hearing (Bigelow et al., 2015). In this study, patients with absent c-VEMP response were excluded. After correction for hearing loss, a significant link between c-VEMP amplitude in the better ear with cognition remained. Therefore, we additionally investigated a link between saccular function and cognition in our BVP cohort. First, the association between a present or absent c-VEMP and cognitive performance was explored. Second, the amplitude of the c-VEMP response in the better ear was used as value for saccular function in the analysis. However, in contrast with the study of Bigelow and colleagues, we did not detect a significant correlation between saccular function on cognition. This might be mediated by the differences between both study protocols. In our study, we only analyzed saccular function in the BVP cohort and not in CP. Literature about the contribution of the saccule to cognitive function is sparse. Future research investigating this link might be of particular interest.

Limitations

Due to the establishment of new patient safety guidelines at the Antwerp University Hospital, the electronystagmography procedure was changed from caloric irrigation with water to air insufflation. In total, 35 BVP patients received caloric irrigation with water. As higher responses are obtained for water irrigation compared to air insufflation, the former group of 35 BVP patients might suffer from a more profound vestibular loss the latter group with air irrigation (Maes et al., 2007). Surprisingly, the former group patients performed better on all subscales and on total RBANS-H scores, although not at a statistically significant level. Furthermore, the group of CP was significantly older than the BVP group. This seemed an inevitable consequence of matching CP and BVP on their hearing status. SNHL prevalence is relatively high in young BVP patients, whereas young controls with SNHL but without vestibular loss, confirmed by rotatory chair testing, are sparse. Yet, all subscales and the total RBANS-H scale are age-corrected. Furthermore, the disadvantage of the significantly older control group was tried to minimize by entering age as a covariate in all statistical models. Nonetheless, the older CP group makes it more difficult to reveal significant cognitive deficits in the BVP group.

Finally, this the first study using the RBANS(-H) to assess cognition in vestibular patients. The RBANS-H was chosen because it is a comprehensive test evaluating nearly all cognitive subdomains, thereby providing age-corrected sub- and total scores. Furthermore, Claes and colleagues demonstrated its suitability to test cognition in patients with severe SNHL (Claes et al., 2016, 2018a,b). The RBANS is more sensitive compared to cognitive screening tests such as the Montreal Cognitive Assessment (MoCA) (Claes et al., 2016). Nonetheless, as the RBANS-H has not been compared to other test batteries in vestibular patients, its sensitivity to detect cognitive dysfunction in this population is unknown.

CONCLUSION

The current study was designed to evaluate the relationship between cognition, hearing, and vestibular loss in BVP patients. Cognitive performance was compared between BVP patients and subjects without vestibular loss, by using the RBANS-H, a cognitive task adapted for hearing-impaired subjects. In both groups subjects with a variety of hearing (dys)function were included. On the one hand a significant negative association was observed between hearing loss and total RBANS-H score, immediate memory and language. On the other hand, vestibular loss was associated with worse performance on the attention subscale of the RBANS-H.

AUTHOR CONTRIBUTIONS

BD conceived and designed the study, acquired, analyzed, and interpreted the data, and wrote the manuscript with input from all authors. GM and AG conceived and designed the study, analyzed and interpreted the data, and critically revised the manuscript for important intellectual content. JM acquired and stored the data. AC contributed to normative data cognitive assessment. RVdB critically revised the manuscript for important intellectual content. PVH and VVR conceived and designed the study, analyzed and interpreted the data, critically revised the manuscript for important intellectual content, and supervised the study. OV critically revised the manuscript for important intellectual content and supervised the study.

ACKNOWLEDGMENTS

All authors would like to acknowledge Olivier Peetermans, Bram Boon, Stijn Matthysen, Jonas de Belder, Nick Janssen, Jonas Janssens, and Timoti Dom for their contributions to the data storage of the study.

REFERENCES

Agrawal, Y., Van de Berg, R., Wuyts, F., Walther, L., Magnusson, M., Oh, E., et al. (2018). Presbyvestibulopathy: diagnostic criteria. *J. Vestib. Res.* Available

at: http://www.jvr-web.org/images/Presbyvestibulopathy-Diagnostic-Criteria-090618ab-MS01.pdf [Epub ahead of print].
Amieva, H., Ouvrard, C., Giulioli, C., Meillon, C., Rullier, L., and Dartigues, J. F. (2015). Self-reported hearing loss, hearing aids, and cognitive decline in elderly

adults: a 25-year study. *J. Am. Geriatr. Soc.* 63, 2099–2104. doi: 10.1111/jgs. 13649

Baek, J. H., Zheng, Y., Darlington, C. L., and Smith, P. F. (2010). Evidence that spatial memory deficits following bilateral vestibular deafferentation in rats are probably permanent. *Neurobiol. Learn. Mem.* 94, 402–413. doi: 10.1016/j.nlm. 2010.08.007

Bessot, N., Denise, P., Toupet, M., Van Nechel, C., and Chavoix, C. (2012). Interference between walking and a cognitive task is increased in patients with bilateral vestibular loss. *Gait Posture* 36, 319–321. doi: 10.1016/j.gaitpost.2012. 02.021

Bigelow, R. T., and Agrawal, Y. (2015). Vestibular involvement in cognition: visuospatial ability, attention, executive function, and memory. *J. Vestib. Res.* 25, 73–89. doi: 10.3233/VES-150544

Bigelow, R. T., Semenov, Y. R., Trevino, C., Ferrucci, L., Resnick, S. M., Simonsick, E. M., et al. (2015). Association between visuospatial ability and vestibular function in the baltimore longitudinal study of aging. *J. Am. Geriatr. Soc.* 63, 1837–1844. doi: 10.1111/jgs.13609

Brandt, T., and Dieterich, M. (2017). The dizzy patient: dont forget disorders of the central vestibular system. *Nat. Rev. Neurol.* 13, 352–362. doi: 10.1038/nrneurol. 2017.58

Brandt, T., Schautzer, F., Hamilton, D. A., Bruning, R., Markowitsch, H. J., Kalla, R., et al. (2005). Vestibular loss causes hippocampal atrophy and impaired spatial memory in humans. *Brain* 128, 2732–2741. doi: 10.1093/brain/awh617

Claes, A. J., Mertens, G., Gilles, A., Hofkens-Van den Brandt, A., Fransen, E., Van Rompaey, V., et al. (2016). The repeatable battery for the assessment of neuropsychological status for hearing impaired individuals (rbans-h) before and after cochlear implantation: a protocol for a prospective, longitudinal cohort study. *Front. Neurosci.* 10:512. doi: 10.3389/fnins.2016.00512

Claes, A. J., Van de Heyning, P., Gilles, A., Hofkens-Van den Brandt, A., Van Rompaey, V., Mertens, G., et al. (2018a). Impaired cognitive functioning in cochlear implant recipients over the age of 55 years: a cross-sectional study using the repeatable battery for the assessment of neuropsychological status for hearing-impaired individuals (RBANS-H). *Front. Neurosci.* 12:580. doi: 10. 3389/fnins.2018.00580

Claes, A. J., Van de Heyning, P., Gilles, A., Van Rompaey, V., and Mertens, G. (2018b). Cognitive performance of severely hearing-impaired older adults before and after cochlear implantation: preliminary results of a prospective, longitudinal cohort study using the RBANS-H. *Otol. Neurotol.* 39, e765–e773. doi: 10.1097/MAO.000000000000 1936

Colebatch, J. G., Halmagyi, G. M., and Skuse, N. F. (1994). Myogenic potentials generated by a click-evoked vestibulocollic reflex. *J. Neurol. Neurosurg. Psychiatry* 57, 190–197. doi: 10.1136/jnnp.57.2.190

De Belder, J., Matthysen, S., Claes, A. J., Mertens, G., Van de Heyning, P., and Van Rompaey, V. (2017). Does otovestibular loss in the autosomal dominant disorder dfna9 have an impact of on cognition? A systematic review. *Front. Neurosci.* 11:735. doi: 10.3389/fnins.2017. 00735

Dobbels, B., Peetermans, O., Boon, B., Mertens, G., Van de Heyning, P., and Van Rompaey, V. (2018). Impact of bilateral vestibulopathy on spatial and nonspatial cognition: a systematic review. *Ear Hear.* doi: 10.1097/AUD. 0000000000000679 [Epub ahead of print].

Duff, K., Beglinger, L. J., Schoenberg, M. R., Patton, D. E., Mold, J., Scott, J. G., et al. (2005). Test-retest stability and practice effects of the RBANS in a community dwelling elderly sample. *J. Clin. Exp. Neuropsychol.* 27, 565–575. doi: 10.1080/ 13803390490918363

Dupuis, K., Pichora-Fuller, M. K., Chasteen, A. L., Marchuk, V., Singh, G., and Smith, S. L. (2015). Effects of hearing and vision impairments on the montreal cognitive assessment. *Neuropsychol. Dev. Cogn. B Aging Neuropsychol. Cogn.* 22, 413–437. doi: 10.1080/13825585.2014.968004

Glasauer, S., Amorim, M. A., Viaud-Delmon, I., and Berthoz, A. (2002). Differential effects of labyrinthine dysfunction on distance and direction during blindfolded walking of a triangular path. *Exp. Brain Res.* 145, 489–497. doi: 10.1007/s00221-002-1146-1

Glasauer, S., Amorim, M. A., Vitte, E., and Berthoz, A. (1994). Goal-directed linear locomotion in normal and labyrinthine-defective subjects. *Exp. Brain Res.* 98, 323–335. doi: 10.1007/BF00228420

Gottlich, M., Jandl, N. M., Sprenger, A., Wojak, J. F., Munte, T. F., Kramer, U. M., et al. (2016). Hippocampal gray matter volume in bilateral vestibular failure. *Hum. Brain Mapp.* 37, 1998–2006. doi: 10.1002/hbm.23152

Grabherr, L., Cuffel, C., Guyot, J. P., and Mast, F. W. (2011). Mental transformation abilities in patients with unilateral and bilateral vestibular loss. *Exp. Brain Res.* 209, 205–214. doi: 10.1007/s00221-011-2535-0

Gurgel, R. K., Ward, P. D., Schwartz, S., Norton, M. C., Foster, N. L., and Tschanz, J. T. (2014). Relationship of hearing loss and dementia: a prospective, population-based study. *Otol. Neurotol.* 35, 775–781. doi: 10.1097/MAO. 0000000000000313

Hamilton, D. A., Johnson, T. E., Redhead, E. S., and Verney, S. P. (2009). Control of rodent and human spatial navigation by room and apparatus cues. *Behav. Process.* 81, 154–169. doi: 10.1016/j.beproc.2008.12.003

Harun, A., Oh, E. S., Bigelow, R. T., Studenski, S., and Agrawal, Y. (2016). Vestibular impairment in dementia. *Otol. Neurotol.* 37, 1137–1142. doi: 10. 1097/MAO.0000000000001157

Hitier, M., Besnard, S., and Smith, P. F. (2014). Vestibular pathways involved in cognition. *Front. Integr. Neurosci.* 8:59. doi: 10.3389/fnint.2014. 00059

Jandl, N. M., Sprenger, A., Wojak, J. F., Gottlich, M., Munte, T. F., Kramer, U. M., et al. (2015). Dissociable cerebellar activity during spatial navigation and visual memory in bilateral vestibular failure. *Neuroscience* 305, 257–267. doi: 10.1016/j.neuroscience.2015.07.089

Kremmyda, O., Hufner, K., Flanagin, V. L., Hamilton, D. A., Linn, J., Strupp, M., et al. (2016). Beyond dizziness: virtual navigation, spatial anxiety and hippocampal volume in bilateral vestibulopathy. *Front. Hum. Neurosci.* 10:139. doi: 10.3389/fnhum.2016.00139

Lin, F. R. (2011). Hearing loss and cognition among older adults in the United States. *J. Gerontol. A. Biol. Sci. Med. Sci.* 66, 1131–1136. doi: 10.1093/ gerona/glr115

Lin, F. R., Ferrucci, L., Metter, E. J., An, Y., Zonderman, A. B., and Resnick, S. M. (2011). Hearing loss and cognition in the baltimore longitudinal study of aging. *Neuropsychology* 25, 763–770. doi: 10.1037/a0024238

Lin, F. R., Yaffe, K., Xia, J., Xue, Q. L., Harris, T. B., Purchase-Helzner, E., et al. (2013). Hearing loss and cognitive decline in older adults. *JAMA Intern. Med.* 173, 293–299. doi: 10.1001/jamainternmed.2013.1868

Livingston, G., Sommerlad, A., Orgeta, V., Costafreda, S. G., Huntley, J., Ames, D., et al. (2017). Dementia prevention, intervention, and care. *Lancet* 390, 2673–2734. doi: 10.1016/S0140-6736(17)31363-6

Loughrey, D. G., Kelly, M. E., Kelley, G. A., Brennan, S., and Lawlor, B. A. (2018). Association of Age-related hearing loss with cognitive function, cognitive impairment, and dementia: a systematic review and meta-analysis. *JAMA Otolaryngol. Head Neck Surg.* 144, 115–126. doi: 10.1001/jamaoto.2017.2513

Lucieer, F., Duijn, S., Van Rompaey, V., Perez Fornos, A., Guinand, N., Guyot, J. P., et al. (2018). Full spectrum of reported symptoms of bilateral vestibulopathy needs further investigation-a systematic review. *Front. Neurol.* 9:352. doi: 10. 3389/fneur.2018.00352

Lucieer, F., Vonk, P., Guinand, N., Stokroos, R., Kingma, H., and van de Berg, R. (2016). Bilateral vestibular hypofunction: insights in etiologies, clinical subtypes, and diagnostics. *Front. Neurol.* 7:26. doi: 10.3389/fneur.2016.00026

Macdougall, H. G., McGarvie, L. A., Halmagyi, G. M., Curthoys, I. S., and Weber, K. P. (2013). The video head impulse test (vHIT) detects vertical semicircular canal dysfunction. *PLoS One* 8:e61488. doi: 10.1371/journal.pone.0061488

Maes, L., Dhooge, I., De Vel, E., DHaenens, W., Bockstael, A., and Vinck, B. M. (2007). Water irrigation versus air insufflation: a comparison of two caloric test protocols. *Int. J. Audiol.* 46, 263–269. doi: 10.1080/14992020601178147

Popp, P., Wulff, M., Finke, K., Ruhl, M., Brandt, T., and Dieterich, M. (2017). Cognitive deficits in patients with a chronic vestibular failure. *J. Neurol.* 264, 554–563. doi: 10.1007/s00415-016-8386-7

Previc, F. H. (2013). Vestibular loss as a contributor to alzheimers disease. *Med. Hypotheses* 80, 360–367. doi: 10.1016/j.mehy.2012.12.023

Quaranta, N., Coppola, F., Casulli, M., Barulli, M. R., Panza, F., Tortelli, R., et al. (2014). The prevalence of peripheral and central hearing impairment and its relation to cognition in older adults. *Audiol. Neurootol.* 19(Suppl. 1), 10–14. doi: 10.1159/000371597

Randolph, C. (2012). *RBANS Update: Repeatable Battery for the Assessment of Neuropsychological Status. Second.* London: Pearson, 182.

Randolph, C., Tierney, M. C., Mohr, E., and Chase, T. N. (1998). The repeatable battery for the assessment of neuropsychological status (RBANS): preliminary clinical validity. *J. Clin. Exp. Neuropsychol.* 20, 310–319. doi: 10.1076/jcen.20.3. 310.823

Semenov, Y. R., Bigelow, R. T., Xue, Q. L., du Lac, S., and Agrawal, Y. (2016). Association between vestibular and cognitive function in U.S. adults: data from the national health and nutrition examination survey. *J. Gerontol. A Biol. Sci. Med. Sci.* 71, 243–250. doi: 10.1093/gerona/glv069

Seo, Y. J., Kim, J., and Kim, S. H. (2016). The change of hippocampal volume and its relevance with inner ear function in menieres disease patients. *Auris Nasus Larynx* 43, 620–625. doi: 10.1016/j.anl.2016.01.006

Smith, L., Wilkinson, D., Bodani, M., Bicknell, R., and Surenthiran, S. S. (2018). Short-term memory impairment in vestibular patients can arise independently of psychiatric impairment, fatigue, and sleeplessness. *J. Neuropsychol.* doi: 10.1111/jnp.12157 [Epub ahead of print].

Smith, P. F. (2017). The vestibular system and cognition. *Curr. Opin. Neurol.* 30, 84–89. doi: 10.1097/WCO.0000000000000403

Smith, P. F., and Zheng, Y. (2013). From ear to uncertainty: vestibular contributions to cognitive function. *Front. Integr. Neurosci.* 7:84. doi: 10.3389/fnint.2013.00084

Strupp, M., Kim, J. S., Murofushi, T., Straumann, D., Jen, J. C., Rosengren, S. M., et al. (2017). Bilateral vestibulopathy: diagnostic criteria. consensus document of the classification committee of the bárány society. *J. Vestib. Res.* 27, 177–189. doi: 10.3233/VES-170619

van de Berg, R., van Tilburg, M., and Kingma, H. (2015). Bilateral vestibular hypofunction: challenges in establishing the diagnosis in adults. *ORL J. Otorhinolaryngol. Relat. Spec.* 77, 197–218. doi: 10.1159/000433549

Van der Stappen, A., Wuyts, F. L., and Van de Heyning, P. H. (2000). Computerized electronystagmography: normative data revisited. *Acta Otolaryngol.* 120, 724–730. doi: 10.1080/000164800750000243

van Wieringen, A., and Wouters, J. (2008). LIST and LINT: sentences and numbers for quantifying speech understanding in severely impaired listeners for flanders and the Netherlands. *Int. J. Audiol.* 47, 348–355. doi: 10.1080/14992020801895144

Vanspauwen, R., Weerts, A., Hendrickx, M., Buytaert, K. I., Blaivie, C., Jorens, P. G., et al. (2011). No effects of anti-motion sickness drugs on vestibular evoked myogenic potentials outcome parameters. *Otol. Neurotol.* 32, 497–503. doi: 10.1097/MAO.0b013e31820d94d0

Wallace, D. G., Hines, D. J., Pellis, S. M., and Whishaw, I. Q. (2002). Vestibular information is required for dead reckoning in the rat. *J. Neurosci.* 22, 10009–10017. doi: 10.1523/JNEUROSCI.22-22-10009.2002

Wei, E. X., Oh, E. S., Harun, A., Ehrenburg, M., and Agrawal, Y. (2018). Vestibular loss predicts poorer spatial cognition in patients with alzheimers disease. *J. Alzheimers Dis.* 61, 995–1003. doi: 10.3233/JAD-170751

Xie, Y., Bigelow, R. T., Frankenthaler, S. F., Studenski, S. A., Moffat, S. D., and Agrawal, Y. (2017). Vestibular loss in older adults is associated with impaired spatial navigation: data from the triangle completion task. *Front. Neurol.* 8:173. doi: 10.3389/fneur.2017.00173

Zheng, Y., Balabhadrapatruni, S., Baek, J. H., Chung, P., Gliddon, C., Zhang, M., et al. (2012a). The effects of bilateral vestibular loss on hippocampal volume, neuronal number, and cell proliferation in rats. *Front. Neurol.* 3:20. doi: 10.3389/fneur.2012.00020

Zheng, Y., Cheung, I., and Smith, P. F. (2012b). Performance in anxiety and spatial memory tests following bilateral vestibular loss in the rat and effects of anxiolytic and anxiogenic drugs. *Behav. Brain Res.* 235, 21–29. doi: 10.1016/j.bbr.2012.07.025

Zheng, Y., Balabhadrapatruni, S., Masumura, C., Munro, O., Darlington, C. L., and Smith, P. F. (2009a). Bilateral vestibular deafferentation causes deficits in a 5-choice serial reaction time task in rats. *Behav. Brain Res.* 203, 113–117. doi: 10.1016/j.bbr.2009.04.027

Zheng, Y., Goddard, M., Darlington, C. L., and Smith, P. F. (2009b). Long-term deficits on a foraging task after bilateral vestibular deafferentation in rats. *Hippocampus* 19, 480–486. doi: 10.1002/hipo.20533

Zheng, Y., Goddard, M., Darlington, C. L., and Smith, P. F. (2007). Bilateral vestibular deafferentation impairs performance in a spatial forced alternation task in rats. *Hippocampus* 17, 253–256. doi: 10.1002/hipo.20266

Zheng, Y., Wilson, G., Stiles, L., and Smith, P. F. (2013). Glutamate receptor subunit and calmodulin kinase II expression, with and without T maze training, in the rat hippocampus following bilateral vestibular deafferentation. *PLoS One* 8:e54527. doi: 10.1371/journal.pone.0054527

Zingler, V. C., Cnyrim, C., Jahn, K., Weintz, E., Fernbacher, J., Frenzel, C., et al. (2007). Causative factors and epidemiology of bilateral vestibulopathy in 255 patients. *Ann. Neurol.* 61, 524–532. doi: 10.1002/ana.21105

5

Mechanism and Prevention of Spiral Ganglion Neuron Degeneration in the Cochlea

Li Zhang[1], Sen Chen[1] and Yu Sun[1,2]*

[1] Department of Otorhinolaryngology, Union Hospital, Tongji Medical College, Huazhong University of Science and Technology, Wuhan, China, [2] Institute of Otorhinolaryngology, Tongji Medical College, Huazhong University of Science and Technology, Wuhan, China

Correspondence:
Yu Sun
sunyu@hust.edu.cn

Sensorineural hearing loss (SNHL) is one of the most prevalent sensory deficits in humans, and approximately 360 million people worldwide are affected. The current treatment option for severe to profound hearing loss is cochlear implantation (CI), but its treatment efficacy is related to the survival of spiral ganglion neurons (SGNs). SGNs are the primary sensory neurons, transmitting complex acoustic information from hair cells to second-order sensory neurons in the cochlear nucleus. In mammals, SGNs have very limited regeneration ability, and SGN loss causes irreversible hearing loss. In most cases of SNHL, SGN damage is the dominant pathogenesis, and it could be caused by noise exposure, ototoxic drugs, hereditary defects, presbycusis, etc. Tremendous efforts have been made to identify novel treatments to prevent or reverse the damage to SGNs, including gene therapy and stem cell therapy. This review summarizes the major causes and the corresponding mechanisms of SGN loss and the current protection strategies, especially gene therapy and stem cell therapy, to promote the development of new therapeutic methods.

Keywords: spiral ganglion neuron, sensorineural hearing loss, gene therapy, stem cell therapy, cochlea

INTRODUCTION

Hearing loss is one of the major health problems worldwide, affecting over 5% of the population of the world or approximately 466 million people[1]. Children with hearing loss have difficulties in language and cognitive development, thus affecting their school performance, ability to integrate into mainstream job markets, and overall quality of life (Wake et al., 2004; Borton et al., 2010). Hearing loss in the elderly may increase the risk of dementia and Alzheimer's disease (Lin et al., 2011). Based on the affected cochlear sites, hearing loss is generally categorized into conductive and sensorineural hearing loss (SNHL). SNHL is usually caused by irreversible damage to cells along the auditory pathway, including spiral ganglion neurons (SGNs). The major causes of SGN loss include harmful extrinsic (noise, ototoxic drugs, etc.) and intrinsic causes (genetic factors, aging, etc.). The mature sensorineural tissues of the cochlea in mammals, including hair cells (HCs) and SGNs, have very limited repair capacity and do not regenerate, so this damage is usually permanent.

The somata of SGNs reside in Rosenthal's spiral canal. Each cell body of SGNs gives rise to a peripheral process that extends toward the organ of Corti and a central process that connects

[1]https://www.who.int/news-room/fact-sheets/detail/deafness-and-hearing-loss

together to form the auditory nerve emitting into the brain, thus establishing a point-to-point communication between the cochlear HCs and the cochlear nucleus. Human SGNs are divided into two types: type I and type II afferent neurons. Ninety-five percent of the neuron population in the spiral ganglion consists of type I afferent neurons, which are myelinated and connect inner hair cells (IHC) with the cochlear nuclei of the brainstem (Eybalin, 1993). Each dendrite of type I afferent neurons innervates only one IHC, while each IHC receives contacts from 10 to 20 dendrites from type I afferent neurons (Eybalin, 1993). Type II afferent neurons account for only 5–10% of the neuron population (Spoendlin, 1972; Ruggero et al., 1982) and they are pseudounipolar and non-myelinated neurons (Berglund and Ryugo, 1986, 1991). Each type II afferent neuron innervates approximately 15 to 20 outer hair cells (OHCs), which are from the same row, while each OHC receives only one contact from one type II afferent neuron.

Until recently, the only treatments for SNHL have been hearing aids and cochlear implants, both of which are highly unnatural compared with normal sound stimulation, and they perform poorly in noisy environments. Cochlear implants are the standard therapy for severe to profound hearing loss, and their performance is variable, which is likely related to the number of residual SGNs (Seyyedi et al., 2014). No clinical therapies existed to rescue the dying SGNs or regenerate these cells once lost. Fortunately, great progress has been made in new biological therapies, such as gene therapy and stem cell therapy, providing promising perspectives for the future restoration of hearing in deaf people. This review summarizes the major causes and the related mechanisms leading to the degeneration of SGNs and discusses recent therapeutic strategies in gene therapy and stem cell therapy research to reverse SGN damage.

MAJOR CAUSES AND CORRESPONDING MECHANISMS OF SPIRAL GANGLION NEURONS LOSS

Noise Exposure

Exposure to excessive levels of sound leads to a temporary threshold shift (TTS) that can fully recover to normal or a permanent threshold shift (PTS) that fails to return to pre-exposure levels. The loss of afferent ribbon synapses and the degeneration of SGNs can be triggered by noise exposure (Fernandez et al., 2015). After mild noise exposure with TTS, swelling of afferent endings and the primary degeneration of SGNs were observed in a mouse model (Puel et al., 1998; Kujawa and Liberman, 2009). During the early stage of noise exposure, the quantity and quality of the ribbon synapses significantly deceased without total recovery even after several days when the hearing was fully recovered (Shi et al., 2015). This form of damage is thought to contribute to hearing difficulties in noisy environments, tinnitus, and other auditory dysfunctions (Kujawa and Liberman, 2009). However, high-intensity exposure (>100 dB sound pressure level, SPL) or repeated overstimulation leads to PTSs (Spoendlin, 1985). After overexposure, hair cell

damage can be visible within minutes, while the death of SGNs is delayed by months to years (Johnsson, 1974).

Excitotoxicity is a complex process triggered by the overactivation of glutamate receptors that results in degenerative neuronal cell death (Lai et al., 2014). Type I SGNs are activated by glutamate, and excessive release of the excitatory neurotransmitter (glutamate) from IHC could lead to the death of SGNs. Excitotoxicity is thought to play an essential role in noise-induced hearing loss. SGN afferent synapse swelling after noise exposure is likely due to glutamate toxicity (Robertson, 1983; Puel et al., 1998). Excessive glutamate release after noise overstimulation leads to the overactivation of glutamate receptors on the postsynaptic membrane of SGNs. Such overactivation leads to an influx of cations such as Na^+ and Ca^{2+}. Then, Cl^- and water molecules passively cross the plasma membrane, leading to edema and even death of the SGNs (Pujol and Puel, 1999; Wang et al., 2002). Administration of exogenous glutamate receptor agonists, including AMPA and kainite, to the cochlea could mimic this process (Ruel et al., 2000; Le Prell et al., 2004), while swelling of the afferent synapse could be prevented by treatment with a glutamate antagonist (Puel et al., 1998). These results suggest a contribution of excitotoxicity to SGN damage induced by noise exposure. In addition, an influx of Ca^{2+} into the afferent nerves of the cochlea leads to calcium-dependent caspase-mediated apoptosis by the intrinsic (mitochondria-mediated) pathway (Puel et al., 1998; Pujol and Puel, 1999; Ruel et al., 2007).

Toxic Drugs

Certain therapeutic agents could cause functional impairment and cellular degeneration of SGNs. More than 130 drugs have been found to be ototoxic (Liu et al., 2011, 2012; Lanvers-Kaminsky et al., 2017). Two important classes are aminoglycoside antibiotics (Jeong et al., 2010; Wang et al., 2021) and platinum-based antineoplastic agents (Tsukasaki et al., 2000; Liu et al., 2019b, 2021), which could cause permanent hearing loss. Cisplatin, the most commonly used platinum-based antineoplastic agent and the most ototoxic drug in frequent use in the clinic (Muggia et al., 2015), results in OHC loss in a basal to apical gradient and SGN and cell loss in the stria vascularis (Schacht et al., 2012). Degeneration of SGNs caused by toxic drugs is frequently observed secondary to hair cell loss. However, Wang et al. (2003) found that the neurotoxic effects after carboplatin treatment occurred approximately 1 day before the IHCs were injured. A unique case showed that the benefit of cochlear implantation (CI) was lost due to the use of cisplatin (Harris et al., 2011). These results indicate that SGNs are the primary injury sites after treatment with platinum-based antineoplastic agents, and they are not limited to hair cell loss. However, the mechanisms of SGN damage induced by cisplatin have not been fully explained. One of these mechanisms is thought to be mediated through ROS generation, subsequently inducing calcium influx and apoptosis (Kawai et al., 2006; Mohan et al., 2014). Cisplatin also activates apoptosis by increasing the release of cytochrome c (Garcia-Berrocal et al., 2007; Jeong et al., 2007). The expression of JNK, phospho-JNK, c-Jun, and phospho-c-Jun are also increased (Jeong et al., 2010), indicating that activation of the c-Jun N-terminal kinase signaling pathway is involved in SGN apoptosis in response to oxidative stress. Liu et al. (2019b) found that Wnt signaling activated TIGAR, protecting SGNs against cisplatin-induced damage through the suppression of oxidative stress and apoptosis. Autophagic flux was found to be activated by PRDX1 *via* the PTEN/AKT signaling pathway in SGNs after cisplatin damage, attenuating ROS accumulation to mediate protective effects (Liu et al., 2021).

Infections

Infection with some viruses or bacteria, such as cytomegalovirus (CMV) and *Streptococcus pneumoniae*, leads to SNHL due to the degeneration of SGNs. CMV is the leading cause of congenital virus infection, and it affects around 0.5–1% of all live births worldwide, with approximately 10% of infected infants developing hearing loss (Lombardi et al., 2010; Plosa et al., 2012). A histopathological study of the human temporal bone showed that the total number of SGNs was significantly reduced in ears with congenital infectious diseases compared to normal ears (Miura et al., 2002). However, the mechanisms of the pathogenesis are still unclear. Mouse models of CMV-induced profound SNHL have shown that SGNs are preferentially infected by CMV and that the number of SGNs dramatically decreases (Juanjuan et al., 2011; Schachtele et al., 2011; Bradford et al., 2015; Ikuta et al., 2015). These results indicate that a reduction in the number of SGNs may be the major cause of congenital CMV infection-induced SNHL. Increased numbers of macrophages and CD3 + mononuclear cells were detected in the SGNs of infected mice with hearing loss (Schachtele et al., 2011; Bradford et al., 2015). High levels of ROS were found to be involved in CMV-induced profound SNHL (Schachtele et al., 2011; Zhuang et al., 2018). Multiple proinflammatory molecules, including tumor necrosis factor-α, interleukin-6, CCL8, CXCL9, and CXCL10 were increased in CMV infection-induced SNHL (Teissier et al., 2011; Gabrielli et al., 2013; Melnick and Jaskoll, 2013; Bradford et al., 2015). Li et al. (2016) demonstrated that SGN apoptosis has an important relationship with SNHL induced by CMV infection. In addition to CMV, *Streptococcus pneumonia* and *Mycobacterium tuberculosis* infection-induced SNHL also led to a markedly decreased density of SGNs (Klein et al., 2003; Kuan et al., 2007; Perny et al., 2016).

Genetic Factors

Genetic factors play a crucial role in SNHL, including congenital and later-onset hearing loss. More than 150 genes have been identified to be directly associated with SNHL. Among the genes identified are those encoding transcription factors (*POU3F4*), ion channels (*KCNQ1* and *KCNE1*), extracellular matrix components (*COCH*), cytoskeletal proteins (several unconventional myosins), and proteins of unknown function (*DFNA5*). Mutations in these genes result in either primary and/or secondary SGN damage. Primary SGN degeneration is more likely to be observed with mutations of genes that play an important role in neuronal survival and the regulation of synaptic transmission, such as *POU3F4*, *SLC17A8*, and *PJVK* (Ruel et al., 2008; Brooks et al., 2020; Cheng et al., 2020). Mutations in *POU3F4/Pou3f4*, the encoding of a transcription factor, and POU-domain protein cause deafness in humans and mice (Kandpal et al., 1996;

Minowa et al., 1999). *Pou3f4*$^{-/-}$ mice showed disrupted radial bundle fasciculation and synapse formation (Coate et al., 2012) and degeneration of SGNs (Coate et al., 2012; Brooks et al., 2020). The hair cells and supporting cells in the *Pou3f4*$^{-/-}$ mice appeared normal, indicating that the degeneration of SGNs is primary in this mouse model. Secondary SGN degeneration often occurs due to mutations in genes affecting hair cells or supporting cells. Mutations in the *GJB2* gene, expressed in supporting cells, are the most common cause of hereditary hearing loss. Conditional Cx26-null mice exhibit secondary SGN degeneration resulting from the degeneration of hair cells and supporting cells (Wang et al., 2009; Takada et al., 2014). Degeneration of SGNs was observed in mice with mutations in other deafness genes, such as *KCNQ1* and *KCNE1* (Vetter et al., 1996; Eugene et al., 2009). In addition, hundreds of genes, including mitochondrial genes and antioxidant defense-related genes, are thought to predispose people to noise-induced, drug-induced and age-related hearing loss by aggravating SGN damage (Wang and Puel, 2018).

Aging

Age-related hearing loss (ARHL) is the third most prevalent chronic medical condition affecting the elderly (Lethbridge-Cejku et al., 2004), and it is characterized by difficulties in speech discrimination and sound detection and localization, particularly in the presence of background noise. It is symmetric, progressive, and sensorineural, and it begins in the high-frequency region and spreads toward the low-frequency regions as age advances. SGNs are frequently lost during aging secondary to the loss of HCs (Schacht and Hawkins, 2005) as hair cells and supporting cells provide neurotrophic support, including neurotrophin-3 (NT3), brain-derived neurotrophic factor (BDNF), and glial cell line-derived neurotrophic factor (GDNF) for SGN survival (Ernfors et al., 1995; Fritzsch et al., 1997; Takeno et al., 1998). However, SGN degeneration without HC loss is common among mammals during aging. The loss of SGNs is probably independent of the age-related loss of HCs. Primary and secondary degeneration of SGNs may coincide in the same cochlea (Hequembourg and Liberman, 2001). It may be impossible to separate the primary and secondary degeneration of SGNs during the early degeneration stages of aging. Oxidative metabolism is involved in age-related SGN loss. Significant age-related loss of SGN fibers has been observed prior to HC in mice lacking copper/zinc superoxide dismutase, the first-line defense against oxidative damage caused by ROS (Keithley et al., 2005). Mitochondria play a key role in ROS generation. It has been shown that age-related loss of SGNs in mice with mitochondrial dysfunction is more severe than in control mice (Niu et al., 2007; Yamasoba et al., 2007). In addition to ROS generation, mitochondria may also promote ARHL *via* apoptosis and calcium signaling pathways.

Signaling pathways that impact the aging of the whole organism could influence age-related SGN loss, as age is the most important predictor of SGN survival. Two key molecular pathways, the insulin/insulin-like growth factor-1 (IGF-1) pathway and the lipophilic/steroid hormone pathway, are closely related to the survival of SGNs. Caloric restriction

(CR) can effectively modulate the IGF-1 pathway to prevent age-related neuronal loss of the enteric nervous system (Cowen, 2002; Thrasivoulou et al., 2006). CR was found to delay auditor brainstem response (ABR) threshold shifts during aging and ameliorate SGN degeneration in mice (Park et al., 1990; Willott et al., 1995; Someya et al., 2007; Yamasoba et al., 2007). Glucocorticoids, lipophilic/steroid hormones, have been shown to have detrimental effects on neuronal function during aging (Sapolsky et al., 1986; Miller and O'Callaghan, 2005; Landfield et al., 2007). In mice lacking the β2 subunit of the nicotinic acetylcholine receptor, SGN loss was accelerated (Bao et al., 2005) and serum corticosterone (a major glucocorticoid) increased (Zoli et al., 1999) during ageing. Acceleration of age-related SGN loss was also found in mice lacking NF-κB (Lang et al., 2006) whose translocation in SGNs appears to be controlled by glucocorticoids (Tahera et al., 2006).

PROTECTION AND REGENERATION OF SPIRAL GANGLION NEURONS

Currently, there are no clinical therapies to prevent SGN degeneration or to regenerate these cells once lost. Numerous efforts have been made to explore potential therapies that could ameliorate the degeneration of SGNs. It is not surprising that agents that could interfere with the progression of SGN degeneration are promising candidates for SNHL. These pharmacological therapies include mitochondrial metabolic regulators, autophagy modulators, antioxidants or inhibitors of kinases, and apoptosis. However, there are no known drugs specifically approved by the FDA to prevent SGN degeneration or promote SGN repair. Although osmotic pumps containing neurotrophic factors (NTs) have been used to treat deaf animal models and have shown promising results, concerns about infection and the duration of efficacy restrict their widespread clinical application (Ma et al., 2019). More recent studies have focused on gene therapy and stem cell therapy, which could possibly provide long-term treatment efficacy (Liu et al., 2019a).

Gene Therapy

Gene therapy is a method that introduces a target foreign gene or gene regulatory element into target cells to replace or fix defective genes (Mulligan, 1993). Factors including vector types, administration routes, administration time, etc., have a vital role in the treatment effect. Currently, transfer vectors include viral and non-viral vectors. The most commonly used and most promising vectors in cochlear gene therapy are adenovirus (Ad)-based and vector adeno-associated virus (AAV)-based vectors, as both have effective transduction of many cochlear cell types (Kesser and Lalwani, 2009; Ruan et al., 2010). The capacity of Ad vectors is large (26–45 kb), which greatly expands the number of target genes, while AAV vectors have limited capacity (4–5 kb). AAV vectors are not associated with any known human disease, making them unique among viral vectors. In addition to choosing a proper vector, a safe and efficient administration route is required for inner ear gene therapies. The most commonly used routes for introducing delivery vectors into the inner ear

of neonatal and adult animals are through the scala media, scala tympani, and the semicircular canal (Kilpatrick et al., 2011; Gassner et al., 2012; Chien et al., 2015). Some studies also delivered viral vectors in utero (Bedrosian et al., 2006; Gubbels et al., 2008). Gene therapy goals for SGNs include preventing the degeneration of SGNs and promoting the regeneration of SGNs. The most studied gene therapies in animal models to protect the SGN are NTs, such as BDNF and NT3 (Wan et al., 2014; Budenz et al., 2015; Pfingst et al., 2017). Neurotrophins regulate neuronal differentiation and survival during cochlear development (Fritzsch et al., 1999; Farinas et al., 2001; Rubel and Fritzsch, 2002; Yang et al., 2011). BDNF and NT3, mainly provided by supporting cells of the organ of Corti, have important roles in the development and maintenance of SGNs (Schecterson and Bothwell, 1994; Fritzsch et al., 1999; Stankovic et al., 2004). Loss of BDNF and NT3 support leads to the gradual degeneration of SGNs (Fritzsch et al., 1999; Alam et al., 2007).

Exogenous NT (BDNF, GDNF, NT3, CNTF, and others) administration into the cochlea can prevent precipitous SGN loss (Gillespie et al., 2003) and also promote long-term survival of SGNs (Shepherd et al., 2008; Agterberg et al., 2009; Leake et al., 2011), especially when combined with electrical stimulation (Shepherd et al., 2005; Leake et al., 2013). Several studies in deaf animal models, including guinea pigs, mice (Fukui et al., 2012), rats (Wu et al., 2011) and cats, have reported improved SGN survival with virally mediated NT expression compared to controls after acoustic trauma (**Table 1**). Staecker et al. (1998) reported that an HSV-1 vector containing BDNF could almost completely rescue the damaged SGNs caused by neomycin despite the destruction of all HCs. Another study demonstrated that enhanced SGN survival was observed for up to 4 weeks in aminoglycoside/diuretic-induced deafened guinea pigs with the administration of Ad-mediated transfection of GDNF compared to the controls (Yagi et al., 2000). Ad-mediated gene transfer of BDNF and NT3 also prevented SGN degeneration after aminoglycoside-induced deafness in guinea pigs (Wise et al., 2010). HSV1-mediated NT3 expression protected SGNs from degeneration caused by cisplatin-induced ototoxicity in aged mice (Bowers et al., 2002). In addition to SGN protection, gene therapy with NTs could also improve the survival and resprouting of the radial nerve fibers of SGNs (Shibata et al., 2010; Wise et al., 2010; Atkinson et al., 2012, 2014; Fukui et al., 2012; Chen et al., 2018).

Noise-induced synapse loss could be prevented with inner ear gene therapy with NTs. SGN degeneration and hearing loss in rats exposed to blast waves were prevented by gene therapy with Ad-mediated human beta-nerve growth factor gene transfer (Wu et al., 2011). Synapse damage caused by noise exposure could be prevented by Ntf3 overexpression via gene therapy (Wan et al., 2014). AAV-mediated NT3 overexpression prevented and repaired noise-induced synaptopathy (Chen et al., 2018; Hashimoto et al., 2019). Pfingst et al. (2017) also demonstrated that AAV-mediated NT3 gene therapy could prevent SGN degeneration in deafened, implanted guinea pigs.

A proper administration approach is important for SGN gene therapy. Wise et al. (2010) demonstrated that injection of vectors into the scala media resulted in more localized gene

TABLE 1 | Studies of gene therapy for SGNs rescue in deafened animals.

Animal	Damage model	Administration route	Viral vectors	Morphological protection	References
CBA/6J mice	Neomycin	scala tympani	HSV1-*BDNF*	significantly improved SGNs survival	Staecker et al., 1998
Guinea pig	Kanamycin + ethacrynic acid	scala tympani	Ad5-*GDNF*	significantly enhanced SGNs survival	Yagi et al., 2000
Guinea pig	Kanamycin + ethacrynic acid	Scala media	AAV-*BDNF*	significantly enhanced SGNs survival	Lalwani et al., 2002
CBA/CaJ aging mice	cisplatin	scala tympani	HSV1-*NT3*	significantly improved SGNs survival	Bowers et al., 2002
Guinea pig	Kanamycin + ethacrynic acid	scala tympani	Ad-*BDNF* Ad-*CNTF*	*BDNF* alone and the combined *BDNF* and *CNTF* treatment significantly enhanced SGN survival. *CNTF* did not enhance the protective effect of *BDNF*.	Nakaizumi et al., 2004
Guinea pig	Kanamycin + ethacrynic acid	scala tympani	Ad-*BDNF*	significantly preserved SGNs in the basal turns	Rejali et al., 2007
Guinea pig	Neomycin	scala tympani	Ad-*BDNF*	higher SGNs survival and lower CI thresholds	Chikar et al., 2008
Rat	Kanamycin	scala tympani	AAV1-*GDNF*	Significantly reduced SGNs damage and improved auditory function	Liu et al., 2008
Guinea pig	Kanamycin + furosemide	scala tympani scala media	Ad5-*BDNF* Ad5-*NT3*	significant preservation of SGNs and radial nerve fiber survival	Wise et al., 2010
Rat	Noise exposure	scala tympani	Ad-*hNGFβ*	Significant greater number of SGNs and smaller ABR threshold shift	Wu et al., 2011
Guinea pig	Kanamycin + furosemide	scala media	Ad5-*BDNF* or Ad5-*NT3*	Significant SGNs protection in the entire basal turn for the 1 week deaf group, in the lower basal turn for the 4 week deaf group and no protection for the 8 week deaf group	Wise et al., 2011
Mutant mice	*Pou4f3* mutant	scala media	Ad-*BDNF*	Enhanced preservation of SGNs and pronounced sprouting of nerve fiber	Fukui et al., 2012
Guinea pigs	Kanamycin + furosemide	scala media	Ad5-*BDNF* Ad5-*NT3*	Sustain protection of SGNs and directed peripheral fiber regrowth (4–11 weeks)	Atkinson et al., 2012
Guinea pigs	Kanamycin + furosemide	scala tympani	Plasmid-*BDNF*	Regeneration of SGNs neurites	Pinyon et al., 2014
Guinea pigs	Kanamycin + furosemide	scala media	Ad5-*BDNF* Ad5-*NT3*	Long term protection of SGNs (6 months)	Atkinson et al., 2014
Guinea pigs	Neomycin or Kanamycin + furosemide	scala tympani	AAV-*BDNF* AAV-*NT3*	A transient elevation in NT levels can sustain the cochlear neural substrate in the long term; BDNF was more effective than NT3 in preserving SGNs	Budenz et al., 2015
Guinea pigs	Neomycin	scala tympani	AAV2-*NT3*	Long term protection of SGNs (5–14 months)	Pfingst et al., 2017
Guinea pigs	Noise exposure	scala tympani	AAV8-*NT3*	Significant SGNs synaptic protection	Chen et al., 2018
Cat	Neomycin	scala tympani	AAV2-*hBDNF* AAV5-*GDNF*	Improved SGNs and radial nerve fiber survival	Leake et al., 2019

SGNs, spiral ganglion neurons; HSV1, Herpes simplex virus type 1; Ad, adenovirus; AAV, adeno-associated virus; BDNF, brain-derived neurotrophic factor; GDNF, glial cell line-derived neurotrophic factor; NT3, neurotrophin-3; CNTF, ciliary neurotrophic factor.

expression, greater neuron survival, and more localized fiber responses than scala tympani injection. This result indicates that vector injection into the scala media may be a better method for gene therapy of SGNs. Another important factor to consider with gene therapy is the acute treatment window. Andrew et al. showed that the efficacy of SGNs protection of viral-mediated NT expression diminished with an increasing duration of deafness, which indicates that there is a treatment window of gene therapy (Wise et al., 2011). Interestingly, Budenz et al. (2015) reported that BDNF was more effective in preventing SGN degeneration after deafness, while NT3 had a greater effect in eliciting the regrowth of radial nerve fibers. These results suggest that combining the overexpression of *BDNF* and *NT3* may have a better effect on SGN protection.

Although great progress has been made in gene therapy for protecting SGNs, there are some problems that need to be solved. NT overexpression has been reported to have detrimental effects on hearing. A recent study showed that overexpression of *Ntf3* in normal guinea pig cochleae led to disruption of synapses in the cochlea and hearing loss (Lee et al., 2016). Another study also found that overexpression of human *GDNF* in normal mice caused severe neurological symptoms and hearing loss (Akil et al., 2019). These findings indicate that extremely high levels of transgene NT expression should be avoided. Another obstacle for gene therapy application is that the gene therapy effect gradually disappears due to degeneration of the transduced cell (Atkinson et al., 2014). A long-term study on NT gene therapy showed that the efficacy of one-time injection could only last for up to 11 weeks (Atkinson et al., 2012). At 3 months after gene therapy with *BDNF* or *NT3*, peripheral auditory fibers still showed considerable regrowth in the basilar membrane area compared to the controls, although the neurotrophin levels were not significantly elevated in the cochlear fluids (Budenz et al., 2015). Finally, an important limitation blocking the

TABLE 2 | Studies of stem cell in animal models for SGN regeneration.

Animals	Damages	Type of cells	Delivery site of transplantation	Morphology change	Hearing outcome	References
Mouse	Cisplatin	mNSCs	Modiolus	Robust survival of transplant-derived cells in the modiolus of the cochlea, but the majority of grafted NSCs differentiated into glial cells	Not mentioned	Tamura et al., 2004
Guinea pig	Kanamycin and ethacrynic acid	mESCs	Modiolus	Transplanted cell was found in cochlea and project neurites toward peripheral and central nervous systems.	Significant improvement in the ABR thresholds	Okano et al., 2005
Guinea pig	Neomycin	mESCs	Scala tympani	Transplanted cells were found close both to the sensory epithelium, and the SGNs with peripheral dendritic processes projecting to the organ of Corti. Co-transplantation with mDRGs increased SGNs survival.	Not mentioned	Hu et al., 2005a
Rat	NA	mDRGs	Scala tympani	A significant difference was identified in the number of DRG neurons between the NGF and non-NGF groups. Extensive neurite projections from DRGs were found penetrating the osseous modiolus toward the spiral ganglion.	Not mentioned	Hu et al., 2005b
Guinea pig	Neomycin	mNSCs	Scala tympani	Transplanted cells expressed the neuronal marker and were found close to the sensory epithelium and adjacent to the SGNs and their peripheral processes.	Not mentioned	Hu et al., 2005c
Guinea pig	Kanamycin and frusemide	mESCs	Scala tympani	Small numbers of MESCs were detected in the scala tympani for up to 4 weeks and a proportion of these cells retained expression of neurofilament protein.	Not mentioned	Coleman et al., 2006
Gerbil	Ouabain	mESCs	cochlear nerve trunk	SGNs and neuronal processes near the sensory epithelium increased	Not mentioned	Corrales et al., 2006
Gerbil	Ouabain	BM-MSCs	Scala tympani or Modiolus	Transplanted cells were able to survive in the modiolus.	Not mentioned	Matsuoka et al., 2007
Mice and guinea pig	Noise	NSC	Scala tympani	Transplanted cells showed characteristic of both neuron tissues and the cells of the organ of Corti. SGNs increased.	Not mentioned	Parker et al., 2007
Gerbil	Ouabain	mESCs	Perilymph or endolymph	ESCs introduced into perilymph most differentiated into glia-like cells. ESCs transplanted into endolymph survived poorly.	Not mentioned	Lang et al., 2008
Guinea pig	Kanamycin and ethacrynic acid	mESCs	Scala tympani	50–75% of transplanted cells express markers of early neurons, and a majority of these cells had a glutamatergic phenotype.	Not mentioned	Reyes et al., 2008
Mouse	NA	miPSCs	Scala tympani	Neurons derived from iPS cells projected neurites toward cochlear hair cells.	Not mentioned	Nishimura et al., 2009
Rat	β-bungarotoxin	mESCs	Modiolus or internal auditory meatus	Transplanted cells were found in the scala tympani, the modiolus, the auditory never trunk. BDNF increased cell survival and neuronal differentiation.	Not mentioned	Ganat et al., 2012
Rat	Noise Neomycin	hBM-MSCs	Intravenous administration	Delivered hMSCs were largely entrapped in the lungs; Recruitment of hMSCs was limited to the spiral ganglion area	No improvement	Choi B. Y. et al., 2012
Guinea pig	Neomycin and Ouabain	hUC-MSCs	Intravenous administration	Increase in spiral ganglion and hair cells	Significant improvement in the ABR thresholds	Choi M. Y. et al., 2012
Gerbil	Ouabain	hESCs	Modiolus	Forming an ectopic spiral ganglion	improvement in the ABR thresholds	Chen et al., 2012
Rat	Ouabain	oe-NSCs	Cochlear lateral wall	NSCs migrated into RC with a high efficiency and differentiated into neurons in a degenerated SGN	Not mentioned	Zhang et al., 2013
Rat	Ouabain	mNSCs	Scala tympani	Transplanted mNSCs were more likely to differentiate into neurons in SGN-degenerated cochleae than in control cochleae	Not mentioned	He et al., 2014

(Continued)

TABLE 2 | (Continued)

Animals	Damages	Type of cells	Delivery site of transplantation	Morphology change	Hearing outcome	References
Guinea pig	Neomycin	hMSCs	Scala tympani	Significant SGN increase	Not mentioned	Jang et al., 2015
Congenital deaf albino pig	Hereditary	hUC-MSCs	subarachnoid cavity	UMSC cells were detected in SGNs, basal membrane and Stria Vescularis	Detectible wave change of ABR	Ma et al., 2016
Guinea pig	Neomycin and Ouabain	hPD-MSCs	Intravenous administration	Significant SGN increase	improvement in the ABR and DOPAE thresholds	Kil et al., 2016
Rat	Noise	oe-NSCs	retroauricular approach	Oe-NSC survived and migrated around the SGNs in RC	Hearing loss was restored	Xu et al., 2016
Mouse	Neomycin	miPSCs	Scala tympani	miPSC could differentiate into hair cell-like cells and spiral ganglion-like cells	No improvement	Chen et al., 2017
Guinea pig	NA	hiPSCs	Scala tympani	The survival of transplant-derived neurons was achieved when inflammatory responses were appropriately controlled	Not mentioned	Ishikawa et al., 2017
Guinea pig	Ouabain	hESCs	Internal auditory meatus	Transplanted cells survival was poor	Partially recovered of ABR	Hackelberg et al., 2017
Mouse	NA	miPSCs	Scala tympani	Transplanted cells were observed in the cochlear perilymph, endolymph, and modiolus, and some cells expressed neural cell markers.	No improvement	Zhu et al., 2018
Guinea pig	Kanamycin and furosemide	hMSCs	Scala tympani	In deafened animals, the alginate-MSC coating of the CI significantly prevented SGN from degeneration, but the injection of alginate-MSCs only did not.	No improvement	Scheper et al., 2019a
DTR mice	DT	hESCs	Scala tympani	Transplanted hESC-derived ONP spheroids survived and neuronally differentiated into otic neuronal lineages and also extended neurites toward the bony wall of the cochlea	Not mentioned	Chang et al., 2020

SGNs, spiral ganglion neurons; RC, Rosenthal's canal; NA, Not Applied; mNSCs, mouse neural stem cells; mDRGs, mouse embryonic dorsal root ganglion cells; NGF, nerve growth factor; hMB-MSCs, Human mesenchymal stem cells from bone marrow; hESCs, human embryonic stem cells; rESCs, rat embryonic stem cells; mESCs, murine embryonic stem cells; hUC-MSCs, human umbilical cord mesenchymal stem cells; hPD-MSCs, human placenta mesenchymal stem cells; miPSCs, mouse induced pluripotent stem cells; oe-NSCs, olfactory epithelium neural stem cells; hPSCs, human pluripotent stem cells.

transition into clinical practice is the lack of diagnostic tools to detect synaptopathy.

Stem Cell Therapy

Cell therapy refers to the use of live cells to repair damaged cells or to replace lost cells. Stem cells and differentiated cells can be used for these purposes (Parker, 2011). Stem cells, including embryonic stem cells (ESCs), adult stem cells (ASCs), and induced pluripotent stem cells (iPSCs), are involved in the regeneration of SGNs. There are two strategies for stem cell-based therapy: to stimulate resident stem cells within the organ of Corti to differentiate into SGNs and to supply exogenous stem cells (stem cell transplantation) into the inner ear. Theoretically, the first approach is supposed to be the best strategy for repairing or replacing damaged SGNs. Unfortunately, there is an insufficient number of resident stem cells in the adult cochlea, and they are not capable of restoring hearing.

Consequently, recent studies (**Table 2**) have focused on the second approach (Maharajan et al., 2021). Stem cell therapy includes stem cell differentiation into target cells *in vitro* and differentiated cell transplantation into the cochlea. Gunewardene et al. (2012) proposed the stepwise differentiation of ESCs and iPSCs into otic or neuronal precursors. In our opinion, the major challenge in stem cell therapy is cell transplantation, as

the environment in the cochlea is hostile to the survival of foreign stem cells. Strategies to introduce exogenous neural stem cells into the cochlea include administration *via* the perilymph and endolymph (Lang et al., 2008) into the modiolus or the cochlear nerve (Corrales et al., 2006; Ogita et al., 2009) and into the lateral wall (Zhang et al., 2013). Although transplantation into the modiolus has shown a higher cell survival rate and increased populations of exogenous cells in Rosenthal's canal compared to transplantation into the perilymph and endolymph (Matsuoka et al., 2007; Lang et al., 2008), the transplantation process may cause hearing damage (Corrales et al., 2006; Ogita et al., 2009). The transplantation of stem cells into the sidewall of the cochlea achieved efficient results and temporary relief of auditory impairment (Zhang et al., 2013). This method may be a better choice for transplantation. Lee et al. (2017) preconditioned the scala media to reduce the potassium concentration before transplantation, thus increasing the survival of transplanted cells. However, some stem cells lose their pluripotency and differentiation ability.

Embryonic stem cells (ESCs) are pluripotent stem cells and have limitless potential to proliferate and differentiate. Studies have demonstrated that human ESCs (hESCs) are able to differentiate into otic neuronal progenitors (ONPs) and SGN-like cells. Newly differentiated SGN-like cells have genotypic and phenotypic SGN-specific features, and their neurites extend toward the cochlear nucleus (Matsuoka et al., 2017). Hyakumura et al. (2019) recently found that human pluripotent stem cells (hPSCs) could be derived from sensory neuronal cells, which formed synaptic connections with hair cells and cochlear nuclei in organotypic coculture. ESC-derived mouse neural progenitor cells were transplanted *via* a round window membrane into ouabain-deafened gerbils, and they successfully engrafted into the modiolus and formed ectopic ganglia with differentiated neuronal-type cells that projected to sensory cells in the organ of Corti (Corrales et al., 2006). Chen et al. (2012) demonstrated that transplantation of neural progenitors into adult ouabain-deafened animals rescued the auditory function of the deafened animals. Although hESCs have high proliferative capacity, ethical concerns, immunological rejection, difficulty in procurement, and tumorigenic potential limit their utilization.

ASCs are thought to be a promising resource for SGN regeneration from both ethical and patient compatibility perspectives. Some cell markers of stem cells in the olfactory epithelium are the same as some cells in the auditory epithelium, and they have good regenerative capacity in adults, making them a good source of SGNs (Graziadei and Graziadei, 1979; Roisen et al., 2001). Olfactory stem cells can survive and migrate to Rosenthal's canal after transplantation (Zhang et al., 2013; Xu et al., 2016), ameliorating noise-induced hearing impairment (Xu et al., 2016). Bone marrow stromal stem cells (Naito et al., 2004) and a purified subpopulation of glial cells expressing Sox2 isolated from the auditory nerve also showed efficient cell migration and differentiation ability (Lang et al., 2015). However, ASCs showed far less differentiation ability than ESCs, which limited their application.

In recent years, much attention has been given to iPSCs with the development of reprogramming technology. iPSCs are adult differentiated cells that are genetically reprogrammed to form pluripotent stem cells. iPSCs can easily be obtained from the somatic cells of the patient. Thus, there is no concern about immunological rejection and fewer ethical problems. A research group demonstrated that hiPSC-derived neurons could form presynaptic connections with HCs in the *in vitro* coculture system (Gunewardene et al., 2016). iPSCs also have some disadvantages, such as a low proliferation rate, the tendency to differentiate into the original somatic tissue, and tumorigenicity (Nishimura et al., 2012). One main concern in regards to their tumorigenicity is the use of viral vectors during reprogramming. A recent study described a specific stepwise neural induction method for hiPSCs to eliminate undifferentiated cells from transplants, allowing the use of only terminally differentiated neurons, thus reducing the probability of tumorigenicity. First, a neural induction method was established on Matrigel-coated plates. Then, hiPSCs were differentiated into neurons on a 3D collagen matrix, and the neuron subtypes were examined. Finally, the cultured neurons were transplanted into the guinea pig cochlea (Ishikawa et al., 2017). Boddy et al. (2020) found that human-induced pluripotent cell lines are capable of differentiating into otic cell types, including hair cells and neuronal lineages, using the non-integration approach. This technology lacks genetic integration problems, making it highly attractive in the field of regenerative medicine.

CONCLUSION AND FUTURE PROSPECTS

Different approaches are being developed for the treatment of deafness. Great progress has been made in gene therapy and stem cell therapy over the last decade. There are some problems that need to be solved, including viral safety and long-term treatment effects. Ad and AAV are widely used in cochlear gene therapy, and their safety has been confirmed in animal models. Additional research should be conducted to assess the safety and efficiency of treating humans. The treatment efficacy gradually decreases over time, so a second or even regular repeated treatments may be a solution. With regard to stem cell therapy, iPSC technology is thought to be promising. As a transplant source, autologous neurons from patient-derived iPSCs are ideal for the replacement of neurons in the injured cochlea. However, some challenges need to be overcome before application to humans, such as tumorigenesis and controlled growth of transplanted cells. Future therapies to rescue auditory function must consider multiple targets.

Combining several therapeutic strategies, for instance, stem cell delivery, gene therapy and cochlear implants, may achieve better performance. The treatment effect of cochlear implants relies at least partially on the number of surviving SGNs (Yagi et al., 2000). It is not surprising that gene therapy or stem cell therapy combined with cochlear implants could enhance the performance of cochlear implants, as gene therapy and stem cell therapy could prevent SGN degeneration. Guinea pigs treated with Ad-*BDNF* had a lower CI threshold and higher survival of SGNs, indicating that the combination of Ad-*BDNF* inoculation and electrical stimulation improved the functional measures of cochlear implant performance (Chikar et al., 2008). Scheper et al. (2019a) also showed that the alginate-MSC coating of CI significantly prevented SGN degeneration. A study demonstrated that coculture with Wnt1-expressing Schwann cells enhanced the neuronal differentiation of transplanted neural stem cells (He et al., 2014). This result reminds us that cotransplantation modified cells expressing specific cytokines along with stem cells may help us overcome the barrier of a low transplant survival rate. Genetically modified hMSCs overexpressing BDNF protect neurons significantly better from degeneration than native MSCs (Scheper et al., 2019b), which indicates that genetic modification prior to stem cell transplantation may provide a better effect. Efforts should continue toward the development of gene therapy and stem cell therapy for treating deafness.

AUTHOR CONTRIBUTIONS

YS conceived and designed the manuscript. SC and LZ wrote the manuscript. All authors contributed to the article and approved the submitted version.

REFERENCES

Agterberg, M. J., Versnel, H., van Dijk, L. M., de Groot, J. C., and Klis, S. F. (2009). Enhanced survival of spiral ganglion cells after cessation of treatment with brain-derived neurotrophic factor in deafened guinea pigs. *J. Assoc. Res. Otolaryngol.* 10, 355–367. doi: 10.1007/s10162-009-0170-2

Akil, O., Blits, B., Lustig, L. R., and Leake, P. A. (2019). Virally mediated overexpression of glial-derived neurotrophic factor elicits age- and dose-dependent neuronal toxicity and hearing loss. *Hum. Gene Ther.* 30, 88–105. doi: 10.1089/hum.2018.028

Alam, S. A., Robinson, B. K., Huang, J., and Green, S. H. (2007). Prosurvival and proapoptotic intracellular signaling in rat spiral ganglion neurons *in vivo* after the loss of hair cells. *J. Comp. Neurol.* 503, 832–852. doi: 10.1002/cne.21430

Atkinson, P. J., Wise, A. K., Flynn, B. O., Nayagam, B. A., and Richardson, R. T. (2014). Viability of long-term gene therapy in the cochlea. *Sci. Rep.* 4:4733. doi: 10.1038/srep04733

Atkinson, P. J., Wise, A. K., Flynn, B. O., Nayagam, B. A., Hume, C. R., O'Leary, S. J., et al. (2012). Neurotrophin gene therapy for sustained neural preservation after deafness. *PLoS One* 7:e52338. doi: 10.1371/journal.pone.0052338

Bao, J., Lei, D., Du, Y., Ohlemiller, K. K., Beaudet, A. L., and Role, L. W. (2005). Requirement of nicotinic acetylcholine receptor subunit beta2 in the maintenance of spiral ganglion neurons during aging. *J. Neurosci.* 25, 3041–3045. doi: 10.1523/JNEUROSCI.5277-04.2005

Bedrosian, J. C., Gratton, M. A., Brigande, J. V., Tang, W., Landau, J., and Bennett, J. (2006). *In vivo* delivery of recombinant viruses to the fetal murine cochlea: transduction characteristics and long-term effects on auditory function. *Mol. Ther.* 14, 328–335. doi: 10.1016/j.ymthe.2006.04.003

Berglund, A. M., and Ryugo, D. K. (1986). A monoclonal antibody labels type II neurons of the spiral ganglion. *Brain Res.* 383, 327–332. doi: 10.1016/0006-8993(86)90034-x

Berglund, A. M., and Ryugo, D. K. (1991). Neurofilament antibodies and spiral ganglion neurons of the mammalian cochlea. *J. Comp. Neurol.* 306, 393–408. doi: 10.1002/cne.903060304

Boddy, S. L., Romero-Guevara, R., Ji, A. R., Unger, C., Corns, L., Marcotti, W., et al. (2020). Generation of otic lineages from integration-free human-induced pluripotent stem cells reprogrammed by mRNAs. *Stem Cells Int.* 2020:3692937. doi: 10.1155/2020/3692937

Borton, S. A., Mauze, E., and Lieu, J. E. (2010). Quality of life in children with unilateral hearing loss: a pilot study. *Am. J. Audiol.* 19, 61–72. doi: 10.1044/1059-0889(2010/07-0043)

Bowers, W. J., Chen, X., Guo, H., Frisina, D. R., Federoff, H. J., and Frisina, R. D. (2002). Neurotrophin-3 transduction attenuates cisplatin spiral ganglion neuron ototoxicity in the cochlea. *Mol. Ther.* 6, 12–18. doi: 10.1006/mthe.2002.0627

Bradford, R. D., Yoo, Y. G., Golemac, M., Pugel, E. P., Jonjic, S., and Britt, W. J. (2015). Murine CMV-induced hearing loss is associated with inner ear inflammation and loss of spiral ganglia neurons. *PLoS Pathog.* 11:e1004774. doi: 10.1371/journal.ppat.1004774

Brooks, P. M., Rose, K. P., MacRae, M. L., Rangoussis, K. M., Gurjar, M., Hertzano, R., et al. (2020). Pou3f4-expressing otic mesenchyme cells promote spiral ganglion neuron survival in the postnatal mouse cochlea. *J. Comp. Neurol.* 528, 1967–1985. doi: 10.1002/cne.24867

Budenz, C. L., Wong, H. T., Swiderski, D. L., Shibata, S. B., Pfingst, B. E., and Raphael, Y. (2015). Differential effects of AAV.BDNF and AAV.Ntf3 in the deafened adult guinea pig ear. *Sci. Rep.* 5:8619. doi: 10.1038/srep08619

Chang, H. T., Heuer, R. A., Oleksijew, A. M., Coots, K. S., Roque, C. B., Nella, K. T., et al. (2020). An engineered three-dimensional stem cell niche in the inner ear by applying a nanofibrillar cellulose hydrogel with a sustained-release neurotrophic factor delivery system. *Acta Biomater.* 108, 111–127. doi: 10.1016/j.actbio.2020.03.007

Chen, H., Xing, Y., Xia, L., Chen, Z., Yin, S., and Wang, J. (2018). AAV-mediated NT-3 overexpression protects cochleae against noise-induced synaptopathy. *Gene Ther.* 25, 251–259. doi: 10.1038/s41434-018-0012-0

Chen, J., Guan, L., Zhu, H., Xiong, S., Zeng, L., and Jiang, H. (2017). Transplantation of mouse-induced pluripotent stem cells into the cochlea for the treatment of sensorineural hearing loss. *Acta Otolaryngol.* 137, 1136–1142. doi: 10.1080/00016489.2017.1342045

Chen, W., Jongkamonwiwat, N., Abbas, L., Eshtan, S. J., Johnson, S. L., Kuhn, S., et al. (2012). Restoration of auditory evoked responses by human ES-cell-derived otic progenitors. *Nature* 490, 278–282. doi: 10.1038/nature11415

Cheng, Y. F., Tsai, Y. H., Huang, C. Y., Lee, Y. S., Chang, P. C., Lu, Y. C., et al. (2020). Generation and pathological characterization of a transgenic mouse model carrying a missense PJVK mutation. *Biochem. Biophys. Res. Commun.* 532, 675–681. doi: 10.1016/j.bbrc.2020.07.101

Chien, W. W., McDougald, D. S., Roy, S., Fitzgerald, T. S., and Cunningham, L. L. (2015). Cochlear gene transfer mediated by adeno-associated virus: comparison of two surgical approaches. *Laryngoscope* 125, 2557–2564. doi: 10.1002/lary.25317

Chikar, J. A., Colesa, D. J., Swiderski, D. L., Di Polo, A., Raphael, Y., and Pfingst, B. E. (2008). Over-expression of BDNF by adenovirus with concurrent electrical stimulation improves cochlear implant thresholds and survival of auditory neurons. *Hear. Res.* 245, 24–34. doi: 10.1016/j.heares.2008.08.005

Choi, B. Y., Song, J. J., Chang, S. O., Kim, S. U., and Oh, S. H. (2012). Intravenous administration of human mesenchymal stem cells after noise- or drug-induced hearing loss in rats. *Acta Otolaryngol.* 132(Suppl. 1), S94–S102. doi: 10.3109/00016489.2012.660731

Choi, M. Y., Yeo, S. W., and Park, K. H. (2012). Hearing restoration in a deaf animal model with intravenous transplantation of mesenchymal stem cells derived from human umbilical cord blood. *Biochem. Biophys. Res. Commun.* 427, 629–636. doi: 10.1016/j.bbrc.2012.09.111

Coate, T. M., Raft, S., Zhao, X., Ryan, A. K., Crenshaw, E. B. III, and Kelley, M. W. (2012). Otic mesenchyme cells regulate spiral ganglion axon fasciculation through a Pou3f4/EphA4 signaling pathway. *Neuron* 73, 49–63. doi: 10.1016/j.neuron.2011.10.029

Coleman, B., Hardman, J., Coco, A., Epp, S., de Silva, M., Crook, J., et al. (2006). Fate of embryonic stem cells transplanted into the deafened mammalian cochlea. *Cell Transplant.* 15, 369–380. doi: 10.3727/000000006783981819

Corrales, C. E., Pan, L., Li, H., Liberman, M. C., Heller, S., and Edge, A. S. (2006). Engraftment and differentiation of embryonic stem cell-derived neural progenitor cells in the cochlear nerve trunk: growth of processes into the organ of Corti. *J. Neurobiol.* 66, 1489–1500. doi: 10.1002/neu.20310

Cowen, T. (2002). Selective vulnerability in adult and ageing mammalian neurons. *Auton. Neurosci.* 96, 20–24. doi: 10.1016/s1566-0702(01)00376-9

Ernfors, P., Van De Water, T., Loring, J., and Jaenisch, R. (1995). Complementary roles of BDNF and NT-3 in vestibular and auditory development. *Neuron* 14, 1153–1164. doi: 10.1016/0896-6273(95)90263-5

Eugene, D., Deforges, S., Vibert, N., and Vidal, P. P. (2009). Vestibular critical period, maturation of central vestibular neurons, and locomotor control. *Ann. N. Y. Acad. Sci.* 1164, 180–187. doi: 10.1111/j.1749-6632.2008.03727.x

Eybalin, M. (1993). Neurotransmitters and neuromodulators of the mammalian cochlea. *Physiol. Rev.* 73, 309–373. doi: 10.1152/physrev.1993.73.2.309

Farinas, I., Jones, K. R., Tessarollo, L., Vigers, A. J., Huang, E., Kirstein, M., et al. (2001). Spatial shaping of cochlear innervation by temporally regulated neurotrophin expression. *J. Neurosci.* 21, 6170–6180.

Fernandez, K. A., Jeffers, P. W., Lall, K., Liberman, M. C., and Kujawa, S. G. (2015). Aging after noise exposure: acceleration of cochlear synaptopathy in "recovered" ears. *J. Neurosci.* 35, 7509–7520. doi: 10.1523/JNEUROSCI.5138-14.2015

Fritzsch, B. I, Silos-Santiago, I., Bianchi, L. M., and Farinas, I. I. (1997). Effects of neurotrophin and neurotrophin receptor disruption on the afferent inner ear innervation. *Semin. Cell Dev. Biol.* 8, 277–284.

Fritzsch, B., Pirvola, U., and Ylikoski, J. (1999). Making and breaking the innervation of the ear: neurotrophic support during ear development and its clinical implications. *Cell Tissue Res.* 295, 369–382. doi: 10.1007/s004410051244

Fukui, H., Wong, H. T., Beyer, L. A., Case, B. G., Swiderski, D. L., Di Polo, A., et al. (2012). BDNF gene therapy induces auditory nerve survival and fiber sprouting in deaf Pou4f3 mutant mice. *Sci. Rep.* 2:838. doi: 10.1038/srep00838

Gabrielli, L., Bonasoni, M. P., Santini, D., Piccirilli, G., Chiereghin, A., Guerra, B., et al. (2013). Human fetal inner ear involvement in congenital cytomegalovirus infection. *Acta Neuropathol. Commun.* 1:63. doi: 10.1186/2051-5960-1-63

Ganat, Y. M., Calder, E. L., Kriks, S., Nelander, J., Tu, E. Y., Jia, F., et al. (2012). Identification of embryonic stem cell-derived midbrain dopaminergic neurons for engraftment. *J. Clin. Invest.* 122, 2928–2939. doi: 10.1172/JCI58767

Garcia-Berrocal, J. R., Nevado, J., Ramirez-Camacho, R., Sanz, R., Gonzalez-Garcia, J. A., Sanchez-Rodriguez, C., et al. (2007). The anticancer drug cisplatin induces an intrinsic apoptotic pathway inside the inner ear. *Br. J. Pharmacol.* 152, 1012–1020. doi: 10.1038/sj.bjp.0707405

Gassner, D., Durham, D., Pfannenstiel, S. C., Brough, D. E., and Staecker, H. (2012). Canalostomy as a surgical approach for cochlear gene therapy in the rat. *Anat. Rec. (Hoboken)* 295, 1830–1836. doi: 10.1002/ar.22593

Gillespie, L. N., Clark, G. M., Bartlett, P. F., and Marzella, P. L. (2003). BDNF-induced survival of auditory neurons *in vivo*: cessation of treatment leads to accelerated loss of survival effects. *J. Neurosci. Res.* 71, 785–790. doi: 10.1002/jnr.10542

Graziadei, P. P., and Graziadei, G. A. (1979). Neurogenesis and neuron regeneration in the olfactory system of mammals. I. Morphological aspects of differentiation and structural organization of the olfactory sensory neurons. *J. Neurocytol.* 8, 1–18. doi: 10.1007/BF01206454

Gubbels, S. P., Woessner, D. W., Mitchell, J. C., Ricci, A. J., and Brigande, J. V. (2008). Functional auditory hair cells produced in the mammalian cochlea by in utero gene transfer. *Nature* 455, 537–541. doi: 10.1038/nature07265

Gunewardene, N., Crombie, D., Dottori, M., and Nayagam, B. A. (2016). Innervation of cochlear hair cells by human induced pluripotent stem cell-derived neurons *in vitro*. *Stem Cells Int.* 2016:1781202. doi: 10.1155/2016/1781202

Gunewardene, N., Dottori, M., and Nayagam, B. A. (2012). The convergence of cochlear implantation with induced pluripotent stem cell therapy. *Stem Cell Rev. Rep.* 8, 741–754. doi: 10.1007/s12015-011-9320-0

Hackelberg, S., Tuck, S. J., He, L., Rastogi, A., White, C., Liu, L., et al. (2017). Nanofibrous scaffolds for the guidance of stem cell-derived neurons for auditory nerve regeneration. *PLoS One* 12:e0180427. doi: 10.1371/journal.pone.0180427

Harris, M. S., Gilbert, J. L., Lormore, K. A., Musunuru, S. A., and Fritsch, M. H. (2011). Cisplatin ototoxicity affecting cochlear implant benefit. *Otol. Neurotol.* 32, 969–972. doi: 10.1097/MAO.0b013e3182255893

Hashimoto, K., Hickman, T. T., Suzuki, J., Ji, L., Kohrman, D. C., Corfas, G., et al. (2019). Protection from noise-induced cochlear synaptopathy by virally mediated overexpression of NT3. *Sci. Rep.* 9:15362. doi: 10.1038/s41598-019-51724-6

He, Y., Zhang, P. Z., Sun, D., Mi, W. J., Zhang, X. Y., Cui, Y., et al. (2014). Wnt1 from cochlear schwann cells enhances neuronal differentiation of transplanted neural stem cells in a rat spiral ganglion neuron degeneration model. *Cell Transplant.* 23, 747–760. doi: 10.3727/096368913X669761

Hequembourg, S., and Liberman, M. C. (2001). Spiral ligament pathology: a major aspect of age-related cochlear degeneration in C57BL/6 mice. *J. Assoc. Res. Otolaryngol.* 2, 118–129. doi: 10.1007/s101620010075

Hu, Z., Andang, M., Ni, D., and Ulfendahl, M. (2005a). Neural cograft stimulates the survival and differentiation of embryonic stem cells in the adult mammalian auditory system. *Brain Res.* 1051, 137–144. doi: 10.1016/j.brainres.2005.06.016

Hu, Z., Ulfendahl, M., and Olivius, N. P. (2005b). NGF stimulates extensive neurite outgrowth from implanted dorsal root ganglion neurons following transplantation into the adult rat inner ear. *Neurobiol. Dis.* 18, 184–192. doi: 10.1016/j.nbd.2004.09.010

Hu, Z., Wei, D., Johansson, C. B., Holmstrom, N., Duan, M., Frisen, J., et al. (2005c). Survival and neural differentiation of adult neural stem cells transplanted into the mature inner ear. *Exp. Cell Res.* 302, 40–47. doi: 10.1016/j.yexcr.2004.08.023

Hyakumura, T., McDougall, S., Finch, S., Needham, K., Dottori, M., and Nayagam, B. A. (2019). Organotypic cocultures of human pluripotent stem cell derived-neurons with mammalian inner ear hair cells and cochlear nucleus slices. *Stem Cells Int.* 2019:8419493. doi: 10.1155/2019/8419493

Ikuta, K., Ogawa, H., Hashimoto, H., Okano, W., Tani, A., Sato, E., et al. (2015). Restricted infection of murine cytomegalovirus (MCMV) in neonatal mice with MCMV-induced sensorineural hearing loss. *J. Clin. Virol.* 69, 138–145. doi: 10.1016/j.jcv.2015.06.083

Ishikawa, M., Ohnishi, H., Skerleva, D., Sakamoto, T., Yamamoto, N., Hotta, A., et al. (2017). Transplantation of neurons derived from human iPS cells cultured on collagen matrix into guinea-pig cochleae. *J. Tissue Eng. Regen. Med.* 11, 1766–1778. doi: 10.1002/term.2072

Jang, S., Cho, H. H., Kim, S. H., Lee, K. H., Jun, J. Y., Park, J. S., et al. (2015). Neural-induced human mesenchymal stem cells promote cochlear cell regeneration in deaf Guinea pigs. *Clin. Exp. Otorhinolaryngol.* 8, 83–91. doi: 10.3342/ceo.2015.8.2.83

Jeong, H. J., Kim, S. J., Moon, P. D., Kim, N. H., Kim, J. S., Park, R. K., et al. (2007). Antiapoptotic mechanism of cannabinoid receptor 2 agonist on cisplatin-induced apoptosis in the HEI-OC1 auditory cell line. *J. Neurosci. Res.* 85, 896–905. doi: 10.1002/jnr.21168

Jeong, S. W., Kim, L. S., Hur, D., Bae, W. Y., Kim, J. R., and Lee, J. H. (2010). Gentamicin-induced spiral ganglion cell death: apoptosis mediated by ROS and the JNK signaling pathway. *Acta Otolaryngol.* 130, 670–678. doi: 10.3109/00016480903428200

Johnsson, L. G. (1974). Sequence of degeneration of Corti's organ and its first-order neurons. *Ann. Otol. Rhinol. Laryngol.* 83, 294–303. doi: 10.1177/000348947408300303

Juanjuan, C., Yan, F., Li, C., Haizhi, L., Ling, W., Xinrong, W., et al. (2011). Murine model for congenital CMV infection and hearing impairment. *Virol. J.* 8:70. doi: 10.1186/1743-422X-8-70

Kandpal, G., Jacob, A. N., and Kandpal, R. P. (1996). Transcribed sequences encoded in the region involved in contiguous deletion syndrome that comprises X-linked stapes fixation and deafness. *Somat. Cell Mol. Genet.* 22, 511–517. doi: 10.1007/BF02369442

Kawai, Y., Nakao, T., Kunimura, N., Kohda, Y., and Gemba, M. (2006). Relationship of intracellular calcium and oxygen radicals to Cisplatin-related renal cell injury. *J. Pharmacol. Sci.* 100, 65–72. doi: 10.1254/jphs.fp0050661

Keithley, E. M., Canto, C., Zheng, Q. Y., Wang, X., Fischel-Ghodsian, N., and Johnson, K. R. (2005). Cu/Zn superoxide dismutase and age-related hearing loss. *Hear. Res.* 209, 76–85. doi: 10.1016/j.heares.2005.06.009

Kesser, B. W., and Lalwani, A. K. (2009). Gene therapy and stem cell transplantation: strategies for hearing restoration. *Adv. Otorhinolaryngol.* 66, 64–86. doi: 10.1159/000218208

Kil, K., Choi, M. Y., Kong, J. S., Kim, W. J., and Park, K. H. (2016). Regenerative efficacy of mesenchymal stromal cells from human placenta in sensorineural hearing loss. *Int. J. Pediatr. Otorhinolaryngol.* 91, 72–81. doi: 10.1016/j.ijporl.2016.10.010

Kilpatrick, L. A., Li, Q., Yang, J., Goddard, J. C., Fekete, D. M., and Lang, H. (2011). Adeno-associated virus-mediated gene delivery into the scala media of the normal and deafened adult mouse ear. *Gene Ther.* 18, 569–578. doi: 10.1038/gt.2010.175

Klein, M., Koedel, U., Pfister, H. W., and Kastenbauer, S. (2003). Morphological correlates of acute and permanent hearing loss during experimental pneumococcal meningitis. *Brain Pathol.* 13, 123–132. doi: 10.1111/j.1750-3639.2003.tb00012.x

Kuan, C. C., Kaga, K., and Tsuzuku, T. (2007). Tuberculous meningitis-induced unilateral sensorineural hearing loss: a temporal bone study. *Acta Otolaryngol.* 127, 553–557. doi: 10.1080/00016480600951418

Kujawa, S. G., and Liberman, M. C. (2009). Adding insult to injury: cochlear nerve degeneration after "temporary" noise-induced hearing loss. *J. Neurosci.* 29, 14077–14085. doi: 10.1523/JNEUROSCI.2845-09.2009

Lai, T. W., Zhang, S., and Wang, Y. T. (2014). Excitotoxicity and stroke: identifying novel targets for neuroprotection. *Prog. Neurobiol.* 115, 157–188. doi: 10.1016/j.pneurobio.2013.11.006

Lalwani, A. K., Han, J. J., Castelein, C. M., Carvalho, G. J., and Mhatre, A. N. (2002). *In vitro* and *in vivo* assessment of the ability of adeno-associated virus-brain-derived neurotrophic factor to enhance spiral ganglion cell survival following ototoxic insult. *Laryngoscope* 112, 1325–1334. doi: 10.1097/00005537-200208000-00001

Landfield, P. W., Blalock, E. M., Chen, K. C., and Porter, N. M. (2007). A new glucocorticoid hypothesis of brain aging: implications for Alzheimer's disease. *Curr. Alzheimer Res.* 4, 205–212. doi: 10.2174/156720507780362083

Lang, H., Schulte, B. A., Goddard, J. C., Hedrick, M., Schulte, J. B., Wei, L., et al. (2008). Transplantation of mouse embryonic stem cells into the cochlea of an auditory-neuropathy animal model: effects of timing after injury. *J. Assoc. Res. Otolaryngol.* 9, 225–240. doi: 10.1007/s10162-008-0119-x

Lang, H., Schulte, B. A., Zhou, D., Smythe, N., Spicer, S. S., and Schmiedt, R. A. (2006). Nuclear factor kappaB deficiency is associated with auditory nerve degeneration and increased noise-induced hearing loss. *J. Neurosci.* 26, 3541–3550. doi: 10.1523/JNEUROSCI.2488-05.2006

Lang, H., Xing, Y., Brown, L. N., Samuvel, D. J., Panganiban, C. H., Havens, L. T., et al. (2015). Neural stem/progenitor cell properties of glial cells in the adult mouse auditory nerve. *Sci. Rep.* 5:13383. doi: 10.1038/srep13383

Lanvers-Kaminsky, C., Zehnhoff-Dinnesen, A. A., Parfitt, R., and Ciarimboli, G. (2017). Drug-induced ototoxicity: mechanisms, Pharmacogenetics, and protective strategies. Clin. Pharmacol. Ther. 101, 491–500. doi: 10.1002/cpt.603

Le Prell, C. G., Yagi, M., Kawamoto, K., Beyer, L. A., Atkin, G., Raphael, Y., et al. (2004). Chronic excitotoxicity in the guinea pig cochlea induces temporary functional deficits without disrupting otoacoustic emissions. J. Acoust. Soc. Am. 116, 1044–1056. doi: 10.1121/1.1772395

Leake, P. A., Hradek, G. T., Hetherington, A. M., and Stakhovskaya, O. (2011). Brain-derived neurotrophic factor promotes cochlear spiral ganglion cell survival and function in deafened, developing cats. J. Comp. Neurol. 519, 1526–1545. doi: 10.1002/cne.22582

Leake, P. A., Rebscher, S. J., Dore, C., and Akil, O. (2019). AAV-Mediated neurotrophin gene therapy promotes improved survival of cochlear spiral ganglion neurons in neonatally deafened cats: comparison of AAV2-hBDNF and AAV5-hGDNF. J. Assoc. Res. Otolaryngol. 20, 341–361. doi: 10.1007/s10162-019-00723-5

Leake, P. A., Stakhovskaya, O., Hetherington, A., Rebscher, S. J., and Bonham, B. (2013). Effects of brain-derived neurotrophic factor (BDNF) and electrical stimulation on survival and function of cochlear spiral ganglion neurons in deafened, developing cats. J. Assoc. Res. Otolaryngol. 14, 187–211. doi: 10.1007/s10162-013-0372-5

Lee, M. Y., Hackelberg, S., Green, K. L., Lunghamer, K. G., Kurioka, T., Loomis, B. R., et al. (2017). Survival of human embryonic stem cells implanted in the guinea pig auditory epithelium. Sci. Rep. 7:46058. doi: 10.1038/srep46058

Lee, M. Y., Kurioka, T., Nelson, M. M., Prieskorn, D. M., Swiderski, D. L., Takada, Y., et al. (2016). Viral-mediated Ntf3 overexpression disrupts innervation and hearing in nondeafened guinea pig cochleae. Mol. Ther. Methods Clin. Dev. 3:16052. doi: 10.1038/mtm.2016.52

Lethbridge-Cejku, M., Schiller, J. S., and Bernadel, L. (2004). Summary health statistics for U.S. adults: national health interview survey, 2002. Vital Health Stat. 10, 1–151.

Li, X., Shi, X., Wang, C., Niu, H., Zeng, L., and Qiao, Y. (2016). Cochlear spiral ganglion neuron apoptosis in neonatal mice with murine cytomegalovirus-induced sensorineural hearing loss. J. Am. Acad. Audiol. 27, 345–353. doi: 10.3766/jaaa.15061

Lin, F. R., Metter, E. J., O'Brien, R. J., Resnick, S. M., Zonderman, A. B., and Ferrucci, L. (2011). Hearing loss and incident dementia. Arch. Neurol. 68, 214–220.

Liu, W., Fan, Z., Han, Y., Lu, S., Zhang, D., Bai, X., et al. (2011). Curcumin attenuates peroxynitrite-induced neurotoxicity in spiral ganglion neurons. Neurotoxicology 32, 150–157. doi: 10.1016/j.neuro.2010.09.003

Liu, W., Fan, Z., Han, Y., Zhang, D., Li, J., and Wang, H. (2012). Intranuclear localization of apoptosis-inducing factor and endonuclease G involves in peroxynitrite-induced apoptosis of spiral ganglion neurons. Neurol. Res. 34, 915–922. doi: 10.1179/1743132812Y.0000000098

Liu, W., Xu, X., Fan, Z., Sun, G., Han, Y., Zhang, D., et al. (2019b). Wnt signaling activates TP53-induced glycolysis and apoptosis regulator and protects against Cisplatin-induced spiral ganglion neuron damage in the mouse cochlea. Antioxid. Redox Signal. 30, 1389–1410. doi: 10.1089/ars.2017.7288

Liu, W., Wang, X., Wang, M., and Wang, H. (2019a). Protection of spiral ganglion neurons and prevention of auditory neuropathy. Adv. Exp. Med. Biol. 1130, 93–107. doi: 10.1007/978-981-13-6123-4_6

Liu, W., Xu, L., Wang, X., Zhang, D., Sun, G., Wang, M., et al. (2021). PRDX1 activates autophagy via the PTEN-AKT signaling pathway to protect against cisplatin-induced spiral ganglion neuron damage. Autophagy 1–23. doi: 10.1080/15548627.2021.1905466

Liu, Y., Okada, T., Shimazaki, K., Sheykholeslami, K., Nomoto, T., Muramatsu, S. I., et al. (2008). Protection against aminoglycoside-induced ototoxicity by regulated AAV vector-mediated GDNF gene transfer into the cochlea. Mol. Ther. 16, 474–480.

Lombardi, G., Garofoli, F., and Stronati, M. (2010). Congenital cytomegalovirus infection: treatment, sequelae and follow-up. J. Matern. Fetal Neonatal Med. 23(Suppl. 3), 45–48. doi: 10.3109/14767058.2010.506753

Ma, Y., Guo, W., Yi, H., Ren, L., Zhao, L., Zhang, Y., et al. (2016). Transplantation of human umbilical cord mesenchymal stem cells in cochlea to repair sensorineural hearing. Am. J. Transl. Res. 8, 5235–5245.

Ma, Y., Wise, A. K., Shepherd, R. K., and Richardson, R. T. (2019). New molecular therapies for the treatment of hearing loss. Pharmacol. Ther. 200, 190–209. doi: 10.1016/j.pharmthera.2019.05.003

Maharajan, N., Cho, G. W., and Jang, C. H. (2021). Therapeutic application of mesenchymal stem cells for cochlear regeneration. In Vivo 35, 13–22. doi: 10.21873/invivo.12227

Matsuoka, A. J., Kondo, T., Miyamoto, R. T., and Hashino, E. (2007). Enhanced survival of bone-marrow-derived pluripotent stem cells in an animal model of auditory neuropathy. Laryngoscope 117, 1629–1635. doi: 10.1097/MLG.0b013e31806bf282

Matsuoka, A. J., Morrissey, Z. D., Zhang, C., Homma, K., Belmadani, A., Miller, C. A., et al. (2017). Directed differentiation of human embryonic stem cells toward placode-derived spiral ganglion-like sensory neurons. Stem Cells Transl. Med. 6, 923–936. doi: 10.1002/sctm.16-0032

Melnick, M., and Jaskoll, T. (2013). An in vitro mouse model of congenital cytomegalovirus-induced pathogenesis of the inner ear cochlea. Birth Defects Res. A Clin. Mol. Teratol. 97, 69–78. doi: 10.1002/bdra.23105

Miller, D. B., and O'Callaghan, J. P. (2005). Aging, stress and the hippocampus. Ageing Res. Rev. 4, 123–140. doi: 10.1016/j.arr.2005.03.002

Minowa, O., Ikeda, K., Sugitani, Y., Oshima, T., Nakai, S., Katori, Y., et al. (1999). Altered cochlear fibrocytes in a mouse model of DFN3 nonsyndromic deafness. Science 285, 1408–1411. doi: 10.1126/science.285.5432.1408

Miura, M., Sando, I., Hirsch, B. E., and Orita, Y. (2002). Analysis of spiral ganglion cell populations in children with normal and pathological ears. Ann. Otol. Rhinol. Laryngol. 111, 1059–1065. doi: 10.1177/000348940211101201

Mohan, S., Smyth, B. J., Namin, A., Phillips, G., and Gratton, M. A. (2014). Targeted amelioration of cisplatin-induced ototoxicity in guinea pigs. Otolaryngol. Head Neck Surg. 151, 836–839. doi: 10.1177/0194599814544877

Muggia, F. M., Bonetti, A., Hoeschele, J. D., Rozencweig, M., and Howell, S. B. (2015). Platinum antitumor complexes: 50 years since barnett rosenberg's discovery. J. Clin. Oncol. 33, 4219–4226. doi: 10.1200/JCO.2015.60.7481

Mulligan, R. C. (1993). The basic science of gene therapy. Science 260, 926–932.

Naito, Y., Nakamura, T., Nakagawa, T., Iguchi, F., Endo, T., Fujino, K., et al. (2004). Transplantation of bone marrow stromal cells into the cochlea of chinchillas. Neuroreport 15, 1–4. doi: 10.1097/00001756-200401190-00001

Nakaizumi, T., Kawamoto, K., Minoda, R., and Raphael, Y. (2004). Adenovirus-mediated expression of brain-derived neurotrophic factor protects spiral ganglion neurons from ototoxic damage. Audiol. Neurootol. 9, 135–143. doi: 10.1159/000077264

Nishimura, K., Nakagawa, T., Ono, K., Ogita, H., Sakamoto, T., Yamamoto, N., et al. (2009). Transplantation of mouse induced pluripotent stem cells into the cochlea. Neuroreport 20, 1250–1254.

Nishimura, K., Nakagawa, T., Sakamoto, T., and Ito, J. (2012). Fates of murine pluripotent stem cell-derived neural progenitors following transplantation into mouse cochleae. Cell Transplant. 21, 763–771. doi: 10.3727/096368911X623907

Niu, X., Trifunovic, A., Larsson, N. G., and Canlon, B. (2007). Somatic mtDNA mutations cause progressive hearing loss in the mouse. Exp. Cell Res. 313, 3924–3934. doi: 10.1016/j.yexcr.2007.05.029

Ogita, H., Nakagawa, T., Lee, K. Y., Inaoka, T., Okano, T., Kikkawa, Y. S., et al. (2009). Surgical invasiveness of cell transplantation into the guinea pig cochlear modiolus. ORL J. Otorhinolaryngol. Relat. Spec. 71, 32–39. doi: 10.1159/000165915

Okano, T., Nakagawa, T., Endo, T., Kim, T. S., Kita, T., Tamura, T., et al. (2005). Engraftment of embryonic stem cell-derived neurons into the cochlear modiolus. Neuroreport 16, 1919–1922. doi: 10.1097/01.wnr.0000187628.38010.5b

Park, J. C., Cook, K. C., and Verde, E. A. (1990). Dietary restriction slows the abnormally rapid loss of spiral ganglion neurons in C57BL/6 mice. Hear. Res. 48, 275–279. doi: 10.1016/0378-5955(90)90067-y

Parker, M. A. (2011). Biotechnology in the treatment of sensorineural hearing loss: foundations and future of hair cell regeneration. J. Speech Lang. Hear. Res. 54, 1709–1731. doi: 10.1044/1092-4388(2011/10-0149)

Parker, M. A., Corliss, D. A., Gray, B., Anderson, J. K., Bobbin, R. P., Snyder, E. Y., et al. (2007). Neural stem cells injected into the sound-damaged cochlea migrate throughout the cochlea and express markers of hair cells, supporting cells, and spiral ganglion cells. Hear. Res. 232, 29–43. doi: 10.1016/j.heares.2007.06.007

Perny, M., Roccio, M., Grandgirard, D., Solyga, M., Senn, P., and Leib, S. L. (2016). The severity of infection determines the localization of damage and extent of sensorineural hearing loss in experimental pneumococcal meningitis. *J. Neurosci.* 36, 7740–7749. doi: 10.1523/JNEUROSCI.0554-16.2016

Pfingst, B. E., Colesa, D. J., Swiderski, D. L., Hughes, A. P., Strahl, S. B., Sinan, M., et al. (2017). Neurotrophin gene therapy in deafened ears with cochlear implants: long-term effects on nerve survival and functional measures. *J. Assoc. Res. Otolaryngol.* 18, 731–750. doi: 10.1007/s10162-017-0633-9

Pinyon, J. L., Tadros, S. F., Froud, K. E., Wong, Y. A. C., Tompson, I. T., Crawford, E. N., et al. (2014). Close-field electroporation gene delivery using the cochlear implant electrode array enhances the bionic ear. *Sci. Transl. Med.* 6:233ra54.

Plosa, E. J., Esbenshade, J. C., Fuller, M. P., and Weitkamp, J. H. (2012). Cytomegalovirus infection. *Pediatr. Rev.* 33, 156–163; quiz 63.

Puel, J. L., Ruel, J., Gervais d'Aldin, C., and Pujol, R. (1998). Excitotoxicity and repair of cochlear synapses after noise-trauma induced hearing loss. *Neuroreport* 9, 2109–2114. doi: 10.1097/00001756-199806220-00037

Pujol, R., and Puel, J. L. (1999). Excitotoxicity, synaptic repair, and functional recovery in the mammalian cochlea: a review of recent findings. *Ann. N. Y. Acad. Sci.* 884, 249–254. doi: 10.1111/j.1749-6632.1999.tb08646.x

Rejali, D., Lee, V. A., Abrashkin, K. A., Humayun, N., Swiderski, D. L., and Raphael, Y. (2007). Cochlear implants and ex vivo BDNF gene therapy protect spiral ganglion neurons. *Hear. Res.* 228, 180–187. doi: 10.1016/j.heares.2007. 02.010

Reyes, J. H., O'Shea, K. S., Wys, N. L., Velkey, J. M., Prieskorn, D. M., Wesolowski, K., et al. (2008). Glutamatergic neuronal differentiation of mouse embryonic stem cells after transient expression of neurogenin 1 and treatment with BDNF and GDNF: *in vitro* and *in vivo* studies. *J. Neurosci.* 28, 12622–12631. doi: 10.1523/JNEUROSCI.0563-08.2008

Robertson, D. (1983). Functional significance of dendritic swelling after loud sounds in the guinea pig cochlea. *Hear. Res.* 9, 263–278. doi: 10.1016/0378-5955(83)90031-x

Roisen, F. J., Klueber, K. M., Lu, C. L., Hatcher, L. M., Dozier, A., Shields, C. B., et al. (2001). Adult human olfactory stem cells. *Brain Res.* 890, 11–22.

Ruan, Q., Chen, D., Wang, Z., Chi, F., He, J., Wang, J., et al. (2010). Effects of Kir2.1 gene transfection in cochlear hair cells and application of neurotrophic factors on survival and neurite growth of co-cultured cochlear spiral ganglion neurons. *Mol. Cell. Neurosci.* 43, 326–339. doi: 10.1016/j.mcn.2009.12.006

Rubel, E. W., and Fritzsch, B. (2002). Auditory system development: primary auditory neurons and their targets. *Annu. Rev. Neurosci.* 25, 51–101. doi: 10. 1146/annurev.neuro.25.112701.142849

Ruel, J., Bobbin, R. P., Vidal, D., Pujol, R., and Puel, J. L. (2000). The selective AMPA receptor antagonist GYKI 53784 blocks action potential generation and excitotoxicity in the guinea pig cochlea. *Neuropharmacology* 39, 1959–1973. doi: 10.1016/s0028-3908(00)00069-1

Ruel, J., Emery, S., Nouvian, R., Bersot, T., Amilhon, B., Van Rybroek, J. M., et al. (2008). Impairment of SLC17A8 encoding vesicular glutamate transporter-3, VGLUT3, underlies nonsyndromic deafness DFNA25 and inner hair cell dysfunction in null mice. *Am. J. Hum. Genet.* 83, 278–292. doi: 10.1016/j.ajhg. 2008.07.008

Ruel, J., Wang, J., Rebillard, G., Eybalin, M., Lloyd, R., Pujol, R., et al. (2007). Physiology, pharmacology and plasticity at the inner hair cell synaptic complex. *Hear. Res.* 227, 19–27. doi: 10.1016/j.heares.2006.08.017

Ruggero, M. A., Santi, P. A., and Rich, N. C. (1982). Type II cochlear ganglion cells in the chinchilla. *Hear. Res.* 8, 339–356. doi: 10.1016/0378-5955(82)90023-5

Sapolsky, R. M., Krey, L. C., and McEwen, B. S. (1986). The neuroendocrinology of stress and aging: the glucocorticoid cascade hypothesis. *Endocr. Rev.* 7, 284–301. doi: 10.1210/edrv-7-3-284

Schacht, J., and Hawkins, J. E. (2005). Sketches of otohistory. Part 9: presby[a]cusis. *Audiol. Neurootol.* 10, 243–247. doi: 10.1159/000086524

Schacht, J., Talaska, A. E., and Rybak, L. P. (2012). Cisplatin and aminoglycoside antibiotics: hearing loss and its prevention. *Anat. Rec. (Hoboken)* 295, 1837–1850. doi: 10.1002/ar.22578

Schachtele, S. J., Mutnal, M. B., Schleiss, M. R., and Lokensgard, J. R. (2011). Cytomegalovirus-induced sensorineural hearing loss with persistent cochlear inflammation in neonatal mice. *J. Neurovirol.* 17, 201–211. doi: 10.1007/s13365-011-0024-7

Schecterson, L. C., and Bothwell, M. (1994). Neurotrophin and neurotrophin receptor mRNA expression in developing inner ear. *Hear. Res.* 73, 92–100. doi: 10.1016/0378-5955(94)90286-0

Scheper, V., Hoffmann, A., Gepp, M. M., Schulz, A., Hamm, A., Pannier, C., et al. (2019a). Stem cell based drug delivery for protection of auditory neurons in a guinea pig model of cochlear implantation. *Front. Cell. Neurosci.* 13:177. doi: 10.3389/fncel.2019.00177

Scheper, V., Schwieger, J., Hamm, A., Lenarz, T., and Hoffmann, A. (2019b). BDNF-overexpressing human mesenchymal stem cells mediate increased neuronal protection in vitro. *J. Neurosci. Res.* 97, 1414–1429. doi: 10.1002/jnr. 24488

Seyyedi, M., Viana, L. M., and Nadol, J. B. Jr. (2014). Within-subject comparison of word recognition and spiral ganglion cell count in bilateral cochlear implant recipients. *Otol. Neurotol.* 35, 1446–1450. doi: 10.1097/MAO. 0000000000000443

Shepherd, R. K., Coco, A., and Epp, S. B. (2008). Neurotrophins and electrical stimulation for protection and repair of spiral ganglion neurons following sensorineural hearing loss. *Hear. Res.* 242, 100–109. doi: 10.1016/j.heares.2007. 12.005

Shepherd, R. K., Coco, A., Epp, S. B., and Crook, J. M. (2005). Chronic depolarization enhances the trophic effects of brain-derived neurotrophic factor in rescuing auditory neurons following a sensorineural hearing loss. *J. Comp. Neurol.* 486, 145–158. doi: 10.1002/cne.20564

Shi, L., Liu, K., Wang, H., Zhang, Y., Hong, Z., Wang, M., et al. (2015). Noise induced reversible changes of cochlear ribbon synapses contribute to temporary hearing loss in mice. *Acta Otolaryngol.* 135, 1093–1102. doi: 10.3109/00016489. 2015.1061699

Shibata, S. B., Cortez, S. R., Beyer, L. A., Wiler, J. A., Di Polo, A., Pfingst, B. E., et al. (2010). Transgenic BDNF induces nerve fiber regrowth into the auditory epithelium in deaf cochleae. *Exp. Neurol.* 223, 464–472. doi: 10.1016/j. expneurol.2010.01.011

Someya, S., Yamasoba, T., Weindruch, R., Prolla, T. A., and Tanokura, M. (2007). Caloric restriction suppresses apoptotic cell death in the mammalian cochlea and leads to prevention of presbycusis. *Neurobiol. Aging* 28, 1613–1622. doi: 10.1016/j.neurobiolaging.2006.06.024

Spoendlin, H. (1972). Innervation densities of the cochlea. *Acta Otolaryngol.* 73, 235–248.

Spoendlin, H. (1985). Histopathology of noise deafness. *J. Otolaryngol.* 14, 282–286.

Staecker, H., Gabaizadeh, R., Federoff, H., and Van De Water, T. R. (1998). Brain-derived neurotrophic factor gene therapy prevents spiral ganglion degeneration after hair cell loss. *Otolaryngol. Head Neck Surg.* 119, 7–13. doi: 10.1016/S0194-5998(98)70194-9

Stankovic, K., Rio, C., Xia, A., Sugawara, M., Adams, J. C., Liberman, M. C., et al. (2004). Survival of adult spiral ganglion neurons requires erbB receptor signaling in the inner ear. *J. Neurosci.* 24, 8651–8661. doi: 10.1523/JNEUROSCI. 0733-04.2004

Tahera, Y., Meltser, I., Johansson, P., Bian, Z., Stierna, P., Hansson, A. C., et al. (2006). NF-kappaB mediated glucocorticoid response in the inner ear after acoustic trauma. *J. Neurosci. Res.* 83, 1066–1076. doi: 10.1002/jnr. 20795

Takada, Y., Beyer, L. A., Swiderski, D. L., O'Neal, A. L., Prieskorn, D. M., Shivatzki, S., et al. (2014). Connexin 26 null mice exhibit spiral ganglion degeneration that can be blocked by BDNF gene therapy. *Hear. Res.* 309, 124–135. doi: 10.1016/j.heares.2013.11.009

Takeno, S., Wake, M., Mount, R. J., and Harrison, R. V. (1998). Degeneration of spiral ganglion cells in the chinchilla after inner hair cell loss induced by carboplatin. *Audiol. Neurootol.* 3, 281–290. doi: 10.1159/000013800

Tamura, T., Nakagawa, T., Iguchi, F., Tateya, I., Endo, T., Kim, T. S., et al. (2004). Transplantation of neural stem cells into the modiolus of mouse cochleae injured by cisplatin. *Acta Otolaryngol. Suppl.* 124, 65–68. doi: 10.1080/ 03655230310016780

Teissier, N., Delezoide, A. L., Mas, A. E., Khung-Savatovsky, S., Bessieres, B., Nardelli, J., et al. (2011). Inner ear lesions in congenital cytomegalovirus infection of human fetuses. *Acta Neuropathol.* 122, 763–774. doi: 10.1007/ s00401-011-0895-y

Thrasivoulou, C., Soubeyre, V., Ridha, H., Giuliani, D., Giaroni, C., Michael, G. J., et al. (2006). Reactive oxygen species, dietary restriction and neurotrophic factors in age-related loss of myenteric neurons. *Aging Cell* 5, 247–257. doi: 10.1111/j.1474-9726.2006.00214.x

Tsukasaki, N., Whitworth, C. A., and Rybak, L. P. (2000). Acute changes in cochlear potentials due to cisplatin. *Hear. Res.* 149, 189–198. doi: 10.1016/s0378-5955(00)00182-9

Vetter, D. E., Mann, J. R., Wangemann, P., Liu, J., McLaughlin, K. J., Lesage, F., et al. (1996). Inner ear defects induced by null mutation of the isk gene. *Neuron* 17, 1251–1264. doi: 10.1016/s0896-6273(00)80255-x

Wake, M., Hughes, E. K., Poulakis, Z., Collins, C., and Rickards, F. W. (2004). Outcomes of children with mild-profound congenital hearing loss at 7 to 8 years: a population study. *Ear Hear.* 25, 1–8. doi: 10.1097/01.AUD.0000111262.12219.2F

Wan, G., Gomez-Casati, M. E., Gigliello, A. R., Liberman, M. C., and Corfas, G. (2014). Neurotrophin-3 regulates ribbon synapse density in the cochlea and induces synapse regeneration after acoustic trauma. *Elife* 3:e03564. doi: 10.7554/eLife.03564

Wang, J., and Puel, J. L. (2018). Toward cochlear therapies. *Physiol. Rev.* 98, 2477–2522.

Wang, J., Ding, D., and Salvi, R. J. (2003). Carboplatin-induced early cochlear lesion in chinchillas. *Hear. Res.* 181, 65–72. doi: 10.1016/s0378-5955(03)00176-x

Wang, M., Han, Y., Wang, X., Liang, S., Bo, C., Zhang, Z., et al. (2021). Characterization of EGR-1 expression in the auditory cortex following kanamycin-induced hearing loss in mice. *J. Mol. Neurosci.* 71, 2260–2274. doi: 10.1007/s12031-021-01791-0

Wang, Y., Chang, Q., Tang, W., Sun, Y., Zhou, B., Li, H., et al. (2009). Targeted connexin26 ablation arrests postnatal development of the organ of Corti. *Biochem. Biophys. Res. Commun.* 385, 33–37. doi: 10.1016/j.bbrc.2009.05.023

Wang, Y., Hirose, K., and Liberman, M. C. (2002). Dynamics of noise-induced cellular injury and repair in the mouse cochlea. *J. Assoc. Res. Otolaryngol.* 3, 248–268. doi: 10.1007/s101620020028

Willott, J. F., Erway, L. C., Archer, J. R., and Harrison, D. E. (1995). Genetics of age-related hearing loss in mice. II. Strain differences and effects of caloric restriction on cochlear pathology and evoked response thresholds. *Hear. Res.* 88, 143–155. doi: 10.1016/0378-5955(95)00107-f

Wise, A. K., Hume, C. R., Flynn, B. O., Jeelall, Y. S., Suhr, C. L., Sgro, B. E., et al. (2010). Effects of localized neurotrophin gene expression on spiral ganglion neuron resprouting in the deafened cochlea. *Mol. Ther.* 18, 1111–1122. doi: 10.1038/mt.2010.28

Wise, A. K., Tu, T., Atkinson, P. J., Flynn, B. O., Sgro, B. E., Hume, C., et al. (2011). The effect of deafness duration on neurotrophin gene therapy for spiral ganglion neuron protection. *Hear. Res.* 278, 69–76. doi: 10.1016/j.heares.2011.04.010

Wu, J., Liu, B., Fan, J., Zhu, Q., and Wu, J. (2011). Study of protective effect on rat cochlear spiral ganglion after blast exposure by adenovirus-mediated human beta-nerve growth factor gene. *Am. J. Otolaryngol.* 32, 8–12. doi: 10.1016/j.amjoto.2009.08.012

Xu, Y. P., Shan, X. D., Liu, Y. Y., Pu, Y., Wang, C. Y., Tao, Q. L., et al. (2016). Olfactory epithelium neural stem cell implantation restores noise-induced hearing loss in rats. *Neurosci. Lett.* 616, 19–25. doi: 10.1016/j.neulet.2016.01.016

Yagi, M., Kanzaki, S., Kawamoto, K., Shin, B., Shah, P. P., Magal, E., et al. (2000). Spiral ganglion neurons are protected from degeneration by GDNF gene therapy. *J. Assoc. Res. Otolaryngol.* 1, 315–325. doi: 10.1007/s101620010011

Yamasoba, T., Someya, S., Yamada, C., Weindruch, R., Prolla, T. A., and Tanokura, M. (2007). Role of mitochondrial dysfunction and mitochondrial DNA mutations in age-related hearing loss. *Hear. Res.* 226, 185–193. doi: 10.1016/j.heares.2006.06.004

Yang, T., Kersigo, J., Jahan, I., Pan, N., and Fritzsch, B. (2011). The molecular basis of making spiral ganglion neurons and connecting them to hair cells of the organ of Corti. *Hear. Res.* 278, 21–33. doi: 10.1016/j.heares.2011.03.002

Zhang, P. Z., He, Y., Jiang, X. W., Chen, F. Q., Chen, Y., Shi, L., et al. (2013). Stem cell transplantation *via* the cochlear lateral wall for replacement of degenerated spiral ganglion neurons. *Hear. Res.* 298, 1–9.

Zhu, H., Chen, J., Guan, L., Xiong, S., and Jiang, H. (2018). The transplantation of induced pluripotent stem cells into the cochleae of mature mice. *Int. J. Clin. Exp. Pathol.* 11, 4423–4430.

Zhuang, W., Wang, C., Shi, X., Qiu, S., Zhang, S., Xu, B., et al. (2018). MCMV triggers ROS/NLRP3-associated inflammasome activation in the inner ear of mice and cultured spiral ganglion neurons, contributing to sensorineural hearing loss. *Int. J. Mol. Med.* 41, 3448–3456. doi: 10.3892/ijmm.2018.3539

Zoli, M., Picciotto, M. R., Ferrari, R., Cocchi, D., and Changeux, J. P. (1999). Increased neurodegeneration during ageing in mice lacking high-affinity nicotine receptors. *EMBO J.* 18, 1235–1244. doi: 10.1093/emboj/18.5.1235

6

Functional Age-Related Changes within the Human Auditory System Studied by Audiometric Examination

Oliver Profant [1,2]*, Milan Jilek [1], Zbynek Bures [1,3], Vaclav Vencovsky [1], Diana Kucharova [1,4], Veronika Svobodova [1,4], Jiri Korynta [5] and Josef Syka [1]

[1]Department of Auditory Neuroscience, Institute of Experimental Medicine of the Czech Academy of Sciences, Prague, Czechia, [2]Department of Otorhinolaryngology of Faculty Hospital Královské Vinohrady and 3rd Faculty of Medicine, Charles University, Prague, Czechia, [3]Department of Technical Studies, College of Polytechnics, Jihlava, Czechia, [4]Department of Otorhinolaryngology and Head and Neck Surgery, 1st Faculty of Medicine, Charles University in Prague, University Hospital Motol, Prague, Czechia, [5]Eye Clinic Liberec, Liberec, Czechia

*Correspondence:
Oliver Profant
oliver.profant@iem.cas.cz
orcid.org/0000-0002-7738-1791

Age related hearing loss (presbycusis) is one of the most common sensory deficits in the aging population. The main subjective ailment in the elderly is the deterioration of speech understanding, especially in a noisy environment, which cannot solely be explained by increased hearing thresholds. The examination methods used in presbycusis are primarily focused on the peripheral pathologies (e.g., hearing sensitivity measured by hearing thresholds), with only a limited capacity to detect the central lesion. In our study, auditory tests focused on central auditory abilities were used in addition to classical examination tests, with the aim to compare auditory abilities between an elderly group (elderly, mean age 70.4 years) and young controls (young, mean age 24.4 years) with clinically normal auditory thresholds, and to clarify the interactions between peripheral and central auditory impairments. Despite the fact that the elderly were selected to show natural age-related deterioration of hearing (auditory thresholds did not exceed 20 dB HL for main speech frequencies) and with clinically normal speech reception thresholds (SRTs), the detailed examination of their auditory functions revealed deteriorated processing of temporal parameters [gap detection threshold (GDT), interaural time difference (ITD) detection] which was partially responsible for the altered perception of distorted speech (speech in babble noise, gated speech). An analysis of interactions between peripheral and central auditory abilities, showed a stronger influence of peripheral function than temporal processing ability on speech perception in silence in the elderly with normal cognitive function. However, in a more natural

Abbreviations: ABR, auditory brainstem responses; DP, distortion product OAE; "elderly," elderly group; GDT, gap detection threshold; HFA, high frequency audiometry; ILD, interaural level difference; ITD, interaural time difference; MoCA, Montreal cognitive assessment; OAE, otoacoustic emissions; PTAV, pure tone average; SIN, speech in noise; SNHL, sensorineural hearing loss; SRT, speech reception threshold; TE, transient evoked OAE; "young", young controls.

environment mimicked by the addition of background noise, the role of temporal processing increased rapidly.

Keywords: presbycusis, central hearing loss, temporal processing, laterogram, cognition

HIGHLIGHTS

- Specific auditory tests reveal the central component of presbycusis.
- Temporal processing deteriorates in the elderly with normal hearing thresholds.
- Speech processing is altered in the elderly without clear cognitive pathology.

INTRODUCTION

The deterioration of hearing with age is a physiological process that starts to become evident after 30 years of age and reaches substantial levels above the age of 60, when it is called presbycusis (Gates and Cooper, 1991). Presbycusis is typically diagnosed in clinical practice by the elevation of hearing thresholds at frequencies above 2 kHz, however the most typical subjective symptom is a deteriorated speech perception under strenuous conditions (background noise; Pronk et al., 2013).

One view on presbycusis is the hypofunction of the auditory periphery. Schuknecht and Gacek (1993) described four types of presbycusis; sensory, metabolic, neural and mechanical, and correlated them with the type of auditory thresholds. Gates et al. (1990) also described four different shapes of auditory thresholds related to presbycusis: sharply sloping, gradually sloping, flat and notched; the proportion of which in the population differs not only according to increasing age but also according to gender.

Another approach to understanding presbycusis was focused on its possible central components as described by the Committee on Hearing, Bioacoustics, and Biomechanics, Commission on Behavioral and Social Sciences and Education, National Research Council (CHABA, 1998). CHABA (1998) and later Humes (1996) and Humes et al. (2012) also took into account speech related difficulties in the elderly, and proposed two additional presbycusis hypotheses: central auditory and cognitive hypotheses. The central auditory hypothesis is based on the additional pathology within the supracochlear parts of the auditory system, which can either result from peripheral pathology or can emerge independently of peripheral pathology. The cognitive hypothesis focuses on the overall effect of aging that leads to cognitive impairment and decreased speech processing (Pichora-Fuller and Singh, 2006; Jayakody et al., 2018). Recently, Füllgrabe and Moore (2014) suggested that the decline in speech perception in older people is partly caused by cognitive and perceptual changes, which is separate from age-related changes in audiometric sensitivity. The most dominant cognitive declines are auditory memory deficits, attention deficits and an executive function that can be correlated with the elevation of auditory thresholds (Pearman et al., 2000; Lin et al., 2011). Willott (1996) in his classical review (1996), differentiated between the central effects of biological aging (connected with the deleterious effects of histopathology and/or pathophysiology of neurons and neural circuits within the central auditory system) and the central effects of peripheral pathology (based on the deleterious effects of the age-related alterations of cochlear neural input to the central auditory system).

One of the most common central pathologies in presbycusis is the inability to detect the temporal features of sound (Grose and Mamo, 2010) which is most likely due to the hypofunction of the inhibitory system responsible for the coding of the rapid sound changes (Suta et al., 2011) or potential neuronal fiber degeneration. Although correlations between the functional/behavioral age-related functional decline and a hearing decline were observed in animal experiments (for review see Syka, 2010), in humans the data is inconclusive. The results of recent clinical studies with presbycusis indicated morphological and biochemical changes in the auditory cortex and auditory pathway (Profant et al., 2013, 2014). Functional changes (Profant et al., 2015; Giroud et al., 2018) in patients with presbycusis show increased activation of the right auditory cortex with aging, which is also supported by the loss of left ear dominance in the periphery (Tadros et al., 2005). However, the degree of hearing loss seemed to have only a minor effect on the changes in the central auditory system (Ouda et al., 2015). Therefore it is unclear whether these changes are due to age related hearing loss, age related cognitive decline or if they solely represent the effect of aging *per se*.

In this study we investigated the auditory functions in elderly participants with clinically normal hearing ability, as detected by auditory thresholds and speech reception threshold (SRT; although these participants exhibited a very mild degree of pathology due to natural aging, their auditory thresholds and SRT did not exceed the clinical normality as defined by WHO), and compared them with young controls. The goal was to improve characterization of age related hearing changes and its specific parameters at different levels of the auditory system in a group of elderly participants with normal hearing by a range of detailed auditory tests. Our battery of tests included examination of the processing of temporal auditory information, its relation to the processing of distorted speech and the possible interactions with cognitive abilities. In clinical practice, elderly patients quite commonly emerge with normal or close to normal hearing thresholds and complain of hearing difficulties related to speech processing, especially in background noise. These deficits cannot be explained by increased hearing thresholds and suggest a central component of the hearing pathology. We hypothesize that even healthy elderly subjects with minimal peripheral pathology and normal cognitive function will display some degree of supracochlear dysfunction, especially in their ability to process temporal parameters of sound.

MATERIALS AND METHODS

Fifty-six participants were examined in this study; 28 elderly participants (elderly; 13 women and 15 men) between the ages of 64–79 (mean age 70.4) and 28 young participants (10 men and 18 women) between 17 and 29 (mean age 24.36) were used as controls (young). The elderly participants included in this study had to meet the following criteria: age above 64 years, no subjective hearing loss, auditory thresholds not exceeding 25 dB on speech frequencies. All of the examined participants declined any previous otologic surgery: vestibular lesion, tinnitus, chronic exposure to loud noise, severe head trauma, lesion of the facial nerve, disorder of the cervical spine or had self-reported a central nervous system disorder. None of the participants were musical professionals, but several in the elderly group played musical instruments sporadically. An otoscopic examination, with removal of the cerumen and confirmation of an intact tympanic membrane, was performed on all of the participants. The examination procedures were approved by the Ethics Committee of the University Hospital Motol, in Prague. All participants signed written informed consent.

Measurement and Stimulation

All acoustic stimuli, except for pure tone audiometry, laterogram and otoacoustic emission (OAE), were presented so that the same signal was delivered simultaneously to both ears. Apart from the measurement of OAEs, acoustic signals were delivered *via* Sennheiser HDA 200 high-frequency audiometric headphones connected to a Madsen Orbiter 922 clinical audiometer. In the case of pure-tone audiometry, the tonal stimuli were generated by the audiometer. In the remaining tests, the signals were either played from a CD or generated by an external generator and routed to the audiometer. The measurements that related to temporal processing employed a custom-made gating device inserted between the signal generator or CD player and the audiometer.

The gating device provided click generation, white noise generation, precise gating of the input signal (used in the gap detection task and the gated speech task), and also a mutual temporal shift of the two auditory channels (used in the laterogram task). The gating device is equipped with two separate audio channels controlled by a PIC18F4550 controller and operated *via* USB from a standard PC using custom-made software. Each channel is provided with an attenuator (1 dB step) and variable rise/fall gating with a variable time shift between channels. The parameters can either be set manually or dedicated software modules can be used for the specific measurement tasks (e.g., the laterogram, see below).

The audio equipment was calibrated using the Brüel and Kjær 2231 sound level meter and Brüel and Kjær 4153 Artificial Ear equipped with Brüel and Kjær 4134 pressure microphone. The pure tones were calibrated according to ISO 389-5, ISO 389-8. Clicks were measured as peak-to-peak equivalent SPL according to IEC 60645-3. The speech level was measured as C-weighted equivalent SPL according to IEC 60645-2. The OAEs were measured using the Otodynamics ILO 292 analyzer and calibrated using the 2 ccm cavity (coupler) supplied by the manufacturer.

Pure Tone Audiometry

Pure tone audiometry was measured over an extended frequency range from 125 Hz to 16 kHz (specifically, at 0.125, 0.25, 0.5, 0.71, 1, 1.6, 2, 3.15, 4, 6.3, 8, 10, 12.5, and 16 kHz). Hearing thresholds were measured separately for each ear with a resolution of 2 dB. No significant differences between the left and right audiograms were found (see "Results" section), therefore the thresholds of both ears were analyzed together. Pure tone average (PTAV) was calculated as an average hearing loss at 0.5, 1, and 2 kHz. Hearing loss was also expressed in % according to Fowler correction (Fowler and Sabine, 1942) that uses an average value related to the degree of hearing loss at 0.5, 1, 2 and 4 kHz (the weighted value for each frequency and level of hearing loss is estimated on the basis of the importance of each frequency within the auditory field for speech perception). To express the hearing thresholds over the entire frequency range in a single number, a weighted average of the hearing threshold levels was calculated. Weighting coefficients were estimated with respect to speech recognition capability (highest weight at 2 kHz) with high frequency preference, such as a counterbalance to PTAV, which does not even take into account frequencies above 2 kHz. Coefficients were set with an average equal to 1 [example: if hearing loss is equal for all frequencies, e.g., 10 dB HL, then the result is that value (i.e., 10 dB HL)]. Coefficients for frequencies between 1 and 8 kHz were greater than 1, for frequencies outside of this range were less than 1 and coefficients for frequencies below 500 Hz were even lower. For a typical audiogram of an elderly participant, which has a loss of about 10 dB up to 2 kHz, a slight decrease up to higher frequencies and a sharp drop above 6 kHz (high frequency slope), the result is about 24 dB. The goal to use pure tone audiometry, was to gain more detailed information about the volunteers hearing within the extended frequency range in comparison with standard clinical practice (testing up to 8 kHz).

Speech Audiometry

For speech audiometry in silence, a standard CD recording of Czech word audiometry, according to (Seeman, 1960), was used. One set of ten words was presented at each intensity and the recognition score (percentage of understood words) was determined. The measurement started at 60 dB SPL; should the recognition score at this intensity be lower than 70%, the intensity was increased to 80 dB SPL. Subsequently the sound level was decreased with 10 dB steps until near-zero intelligibility was reached. The threshold was stated as the intensity where the recognition score equaled 50%. Speech audiometry is a basic clinical test. The goal was to use clinical information from the test and compare its contribution with the results of more detailed speech tests.

Speech in Noise Audiometry

For the speech audiometry in noise, a standard CD recording of Czech sentence audiometry, according to (Dlouhá et al., 2013), was used. The speech level was kept at 65 dB SPL, while the background babble noise level was increased from 64 to 76 dB in 2 dB steps. Ten sentences were presented for each noise level and the recognition score (percentage of sentences understood) was recorded. A correctly understood complete sentence was counted as 1; a partially understood sentence was counted as half. A psychometric function was constructed by plotting the recognition score as the function of the noise level; the noise level at which the psychometric function crossed 50% was taken as the result. Speech audiometry in noise provides improved information on speech processing compared to basic speech audiometry, and mimics the life situations that cause hearing problems in the elderly.

Periodically Gated Speech (Chopper)

Short sentences (unused sentences from the set created for the speech audiometry in noise) were periodically gated (cycle duration 200 ms) with a given duty cycle (approx. 30% to 70%); the percentage represents the proportion of the total cycle duration containing the speech signal, the remaining segment of the cycle was muted. The signal was ramped using a raised cosine ramp with 15 ms duration. Gated sentences were generated using a CD player and a custom-made gating device. Ten sentences were presented for each value of duty cycle and the recognition score (percentage of sentences understood) was recorded. The measurement proceeded from small duty cycles (usually 20%) to larger duty cycles in 10% steps until the recognition score reached nearly 100%. It should be noted that the ascending order of duty cycles provides different results than the descending order, hence it was important to strictly adhere to the procedure. This is due to the fact that the person learns during the test. In the case of an ascending order, when the person at first does not understand, his/her chance to learn is restricted. A correctly understood complete sentence was counted as 1; a partially understood sentence was counted as half. The recognition score was plotted as the function of the duty cycle, and the duty cycle corresponding to the 50% recognition score was taken as the result. Chopper is the most complicated speech test in our battery of tests and focuses on central speech processing and its integration with cognitive abilities (specifically working memory, auditory memory and attention deficits).

Binaural Time-Intensity Interchange Ratio (Laterogram)

This measurement is employed to evaluate the ability to perceive interaural time (ITD) and interaural level differences (ILD) that the auditory system uses for space perception: when a sound source is deviated from the medial plane, the sound at the contralateral ear has a lower intensity than in the ipsilateral ear due to an acoustic shade of the head, and it arrives with a certain delay due to the longer path. Participants were exposed to stimuli with a different interaural time and intensity difference. The stimuli consisted of trains of 10 clicks (100 μs duration; 100 ms repetition rate; SPL = 100 dB, measured as peak-to-peak

equivalent SPL). Each click pair had a certain ITD (−500 μs to 500 μs, 50 μs step) and ILD (−15 dB to 15 dB, 1 dB step) between the left and right ear. The time-intensity trading ratio allows us to compensate one parameter (simulating lateralization to one side) by another parameter (simulating lateralization to the other side), resulting in the perception of the signal in the middle position. Other combinations lead to a lateralized perception. The participants had to indicate their subjective perception of sound source lateralization (left; right; center). The laterogram test was developed to evaluate the integration of bilateral auditory information, providing the possibility to separately evaluate its temporal and intensity aspects. Based on the physiological processing of the auditory signal, it enables the evaluation of the processing of acoustical signals at the subcortical levels.

Detection Threshold of Gap in Noise (Gap)

For the gap detection measurement, trains of three successive pauses in a continuous white noise at 70 dB SPL (150 ms intervals between gaps) were presented randomly in time. The subject had to indicate by pressing a button whenever he/she perceived the gaps. Starting at 10 ms, the gap duration was varied (2 ms up, 1 ms down) until the approximate detection threshold was obtained. Close to the approximated threshold, a fine threshold was subsequently determined by varying the gap duration with 0.1 ms steps in a zig-zag manner. The resulting value of the threshold was the gap duration for which the subject's detection scores equaled 50%, i.e., the duration at which the subject correctly responded in 50% of trials. Gap is widely used as the test for evaluating temporal processing abilities. Based on the results of animal experiments it is believed that it takes place in the auditory cortex. The comparison of gap (cortex) and ITD (subcortical level—most probably inferior colliculus) results enables the differentiation between the two levels of auditory temporal processing.

Detection Threshold of Clicks

The auditory thresholds were also measured for clicks, with the aim to exclude frequency specificity and to take into account the processing of extremely short stimulus durations. The detection threshold of short clicks, depending on their level, was measured analogously to the measurement of detection thresholds of pure tones. Trains of three rectangular pulses (100 μs duration, 100 ms inter-pulse interval) were presented to both ears. The intensity of the click trains was varied until the detection threshold was obtained. The initial intensity was estimated at approximately 20 dB above the expected threshold. The intensity of the click trains was varied until the detection threshold was obtained. The level of the click in dB was defined as a peak-to-peak equivalent value. The click threshold was used to minimize the effect of the frequency specific hearing pathology (high frequency hearing loss in elderly) on the cochlea.

Detection of Short Tones

The hearing thresholds for tone at 1 kHz were measured as the function of tone duration. The procedure for obtaining the threshold was analogous to the measurement of the pure-tone hearing threshold however, for detection of short tones the signal was presented to both ears and the resolution was improved to

1 dB. The hearing threshold for tone durations of 70, 30, 20, 10, and 5 ms were measured. The short tones examination was used with the aim to exclude the high frequency hearing loss (there were no pathologies at the level of 1 kHz in the elderly group) and its integration with temporal processing (threshold for different duration). Stimulus duration coding is another temporal feature that, based on the data from animal experiments, occurs at the level of cochlea and cochlear nerve.

OAE Measurement

The distortion product OAE (DPOAE) and the transiently evoked OAE (TEOAE) with and without contralateral white noise of 70 dB SPL were recorded in both ears. The difference between the response with and without the noise was considered as the suppression. The stimulus for the TEOAEs was the conventional, broadband nonlinear click (0.5–6.0 kHz), with stimulus gain adjusted to 81 dB peak. The stimuli for eliciting DPOAEs at $2f_1$-f_2 were two primary tones ($f_2/f_1 = 1.22$ with $L_1 = 70$ and $L_2 = 70$ dB SPL). Both TEOAE and DPOAE provide information about the function of the outer hair cell population. The addition of contralateral suppression allows the evaluation of the function of the efferent auditory pathway.

MoCA

Montreal Cognitive Assessment (MoCA; Nasreddine et al., 2005) was used for the assessment of cognitive abilities of examinees. Three versions of Czech variant (Reban, 2006) were used with a maximum score of 30, and the borderline for cognitive impairment set at 26 (Rektorová, 2011).

Data Analysis

Laterogram Analysis

For the analysis of the laterogram, the responses were plotted in a 3D space (ITD × ILD × response value) and evaluated by means of non-linear surface fitting. Lateralization responses were assigned numerical values (-1 = left, 0 = center, 1 = right) to create a real function of two variables, ITD and ILD. This function was interpolated using a 2D smoothing cubic spline interpolation, to obtain a smooth and high-resolution approximation of the subject's lateralization responses over the whole range of ITDs and ILDs (see **Figure 1**). First, to determine the subject's ability to trade off between ITD and ILD, the interpolated surface was cut with a horizontal plane at zero (i.e., at the "center" response, see **Figure 1**). The obtained curve was fitted with a third order polynomial and the coefficient of the linear term, determining the slope near the origin, was evaluated. Second, to separate the contribution of ITD and ILD parameters alone, the interpolated surface was cut with two vertical planes, one at ILD = 0, the other at ITD = 0. The resulting curves were subsequently fitted using a sigmoidal Boltzmann-like function to obtain a parameterized approximation of a psychometric function. The sensitivity to ITD or ILD was evaluated as the slope (first order derivative) of the fit in the mid-point. The sensitivity to ITD and ILD may be interpreted as an index of temporal and intensity resolution of the auditory system.

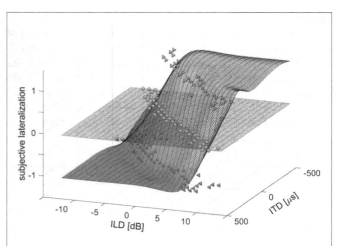

FIGURE 1 | Example of a laterogram plot in 3D space [interaural time difference (ITD) × interaural level difference (ILD) × response value] evaluated by means of non-linear surface fitting.

The Analysis of Detection of Short Tones

The analysis of short tone detection utilized the fact that the thresholds increase with shorter durations; the shape and steepness of this dependence was quantified using an exponential fit. The worsening of the threshold relative to the threshold for the 70 ms tone was plotted as the function of the tone duration, obtaining a decreasing curve converging to zero. The function was fitted with a single exponential curve in the form of $A\exp(-kt)$ and both parameters A and k were taken as the results. This approach allowed us to quantify the steepness of the dependence between the tone duration and its detection threshold independently of the absolute detection thresholds.

Statistical Analysis

Normality of distributions of the data sets was tested using the Lilliefors test prior to subsequent analyses. Some data sets were found to have a distribution significantly deviating from the normality. For this reason, two-sided Wilcoxon rank sum tests were computed for comparisons of the medians of two data sets. For easier interpretation of the results however, the data are presented as mean ± SEM rather than medians. The possible relationships between the selected parameters were tested using Spearman's correlation coefficient. In all cases, the alpha level was set to 0.05. Statistical analyses were performed using Matlab software (Mathworks, Inc., Natick, MA, USA).

RESULTS

Hearing Thresholds

To exclude the possibility of biased results due to asymmetry of hearing thresholds, the differences between the left and right hearing thresholds at individual frequencies in all participants were calculated. The difference was not significant (0.11 ± 0.29 dB HL, $p = 0.25$, Wilcoxon sign rank test). The auditory thresholds of the elderly volunteers were elevated compared to the young, particularly above ca. 2 kHz (**Figure 2**). When PTAV was used to express the hearing function

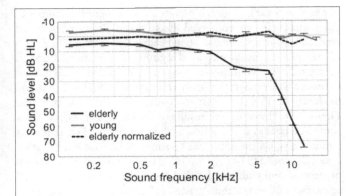

FIGURE 2 | Average audiograms of elderly and young, with the broken line expressing the normalized values of elderly according to correction from Jilek et al. (2014) suggesting physiologic auditory thresholds in our elderly group.

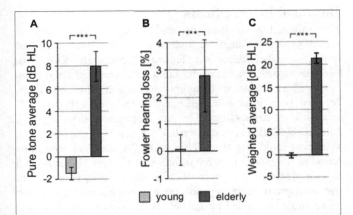

FIGURE 3 | All graphs show the comparison of different threshold-related values used in audiometry, showing significant differences between young and elderly. **(A)** Comparison of pure tone average (PTAV; 0.5, 1, 2 kHz). **(B)** Comparison of hearing loss according to Fowler correction. **(C)** Comparison of weighted averaged thresholds computed over the whole frequency range (***$p < 0.001$).

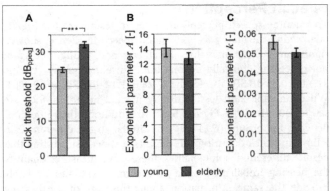

FIGURE 4 | All graphs show the comparison of different threshold-related values. **(A)** Comparison of click threshold. Comparison of parameters of exponential fits of thresholds for 1 kHz tones depending on their duration expressed as exponential parameter A **(B)** and exponential parameter k **(C**; ***$p < 0.001$).

(**Figure 3A**), the differences between young and elderly values were statistically significant (7.97 ± 1.06 vs. −1.46 ± 0.43 in dB HL; $p < 0.0001$, Wilcoxon rank sum test), however from a clinical point of view such a difference is considered non-significant. Similar differences were present when expressed using Fowler weighting coefficients (2.78 ± 0.6 vs. 0.07 ± 0.05 in %; $p < 0.0001$, Wilcoxon rank sum test; **Figure 3B**). The most profound differences in expressing hearing thresholds as a single number were present when a weighted coefficient for each measured frequency up to 16 kHz was used (23.44 ± 1.43 vs. −0.13 ± 0.55 in dB HL; $p < 0.0001$, Wilcoxon rank sum test; **Figure 3C**).

The auditory thresholds were also measured for clicks (with the aim to exclude frequency specificity and take into account the processing of extreme short stimulus durations; **Figure 4A**) and short tones at 1 kHz (**Figure 4B**). These types of stimuli might also reveal a possible auditory neuropathy (Zeng et al., 2005). Although the mean click threshold values in both groups (young: 24.89 ± 0.81 dB$_{ppeq}$; elderly: 32.17 ± 0.85 dB$_{ppeq}$) were

higher compared to mean PTAV due to different measuring techniques and units (PTAV is expressed in dB HL, click level as dB peak-to-peak equivalent), the age-related elevation of hearing thresholds measured using clicks is similar as in the case of PTAV (click: 7.29 dB vs. PTAV: 9.43 dB), indicating that both quantities convey similar information about the state of hearing. Therefore, despite its simplicity, the PTAV correlated strongly with the weighted average of hearing loss across the whole frequency range ($\rho = 0.71$, $p < 0.0001$, Spearman correlation), with the Fowler's coefficient ($\rho = 0.75$, $p < 0.0001$, Spearman correlation), and with the thresholds for click ($\rho = 0.69$, $p < 0.0001$, Spearman correlation). Therefore it seems that in the case of the normal aging process, the PTAV conveys very similar information as the other measures of hearing thresholds. For this reason, we chose the PTAV for further joint analyses. In the case of 1 kHz threshold dependent on the tone duration, the difference between the groups was not significant for any of the exponential parameters (parameter A, young: 14.12 ± 1.16 vs. elderly: 12.72 ± 0.77; parameter k, young: 0.055 ± 0.0035 vs. elderly: 0.050 ± 0.0022; $p > 0.2$ in all cases, Wilcoxon rank sum tests), suggesting minimal age related pathology (**Figures 4B,C**).

Otoacoustic Emissions

The function of the outer hair cells was examined by recording TEOAE and DPOAE. Overall, the presence of measurable TE was 100% in young vs. 76% in elderly and in the case of DP was again 100% in young vs. 92% in elderly. Both types of OAE showed significant differences in their respective amplitudes, with lower values in elderly (TEOAE, young: 11.63 ± 1.13 dB vs. elderly: 3.58 ± 1.51 dB SPL, $p < 0.001$, Wilcoxon rank sum test; DPOAE, young: 12.26 ± 0.7 dB SPL vs. elderly: 3.1 ± 0.91 dB SPL, $p < 0.0001$, Wilcoxon rank sum test). The contralateral suppression of OAEs showed the effectiveness of the efferent auditory pathway. In both groups the decrease of amplitude caused by the contralateral stimulation, was similar for TE (young: 1.68 ± 0.19 dB SPL vs. elderly: 1.91 ± 0.27 dB SPL, $p = 0.78$, Wilcoxon rank sum test) and also for DP (young: 0.87 ± 0.24 dB SPL vs. elderly: 0.42 ± 0.23 dB SPL, $p = 0.06$, Wilcoxon rank sum test).

Speech Perception

To examine speech perception, different tests were used. SRT, quantifying the ability to understand speech in silence, showed significantly different values in elderly and young, yet again not exceeding clinically normal limits in either group (young: 21.14 ± 0.45 dB SPL vs. elderly: 27.28 ± 1.12 dB SPL; $p < 0.0001$, Wilcoxon rank sum test; clinically normal limits for SRT are set at 30 dB SPL; **Figure 5A**). In addition, the difference between the groups (6.14 dB) was similar to the differences in PTAV and click detection threshold (see above), suggesting that despite different absolute values, these three measures quantify the hearing impairment in a very similar way and probably provide the same information about the state of the hearing system. In the speech in babble noise test (SIN), the level of background babble noise resulting in a 50% recognition score was 73.74 ± 0.52 dB SPL in young, compared to 70.68 ± 0.32 dB SPL in elderly ($p < 0.0001$, Wilcoxon rank sum test; **Figure 5B**).

For further testing of speech perception and cognitive abilities of our participants, we employed the so-called chopper test based on the ability to understand periodically gated speech. The results of chopper test again displayed significant differences between young and elderly; the lowest proportion of speech signal needed to reach a 50% recognition score was in young $28.71 \pm 1.00\%$ and in elderly $40.85 \pm 1.28\%$ ($p < 0.0001$, Wilcoxon rank sum test; **Figure 5C**). However, the results of the chopper measurements should be treated with caution as they are yet to be validated. As a more complex indicator, the Gardner-Robertson classification scale (Gardner and Robertson, 1988) was used to integrate speech perception and auditory threshold with the aim to use a clinical assessment of serviceable (grade 1, 2)/non-serviceable (grade 3, 4 and 5) hearing, showing only grade 1 (PTAV $\geq$ 30 dB HL and $\geq70\%$ speech discrimination score at dB SPL stimulus) in both groups.

Binaural Interactions

The interaction of intensity and temporal parameters of sound within the bilateral auditory pathways was examined by the so-called laterogram. **Figure 6** depicts an example of one laterogram measurement, along with averaged laterogram curves. The collected data revealed significant differences between both groups in their ability to trade between ITD and ILD as demonstrated by the laterogram slope (young: 0.044 ± 0.002 dB/ms vs. elderly: 0.033 ± 0.003 dB/ms; $p < 0.001$, Wilcoxon rank sum test; **Figures 6B, 7A**). A shallower slope found in the elderly group indicates that a larger ITD is needed to compensate for a given ILD in the elderly. However, as the laterogram slope depends on two parameters, this result alone could be caused by age-related changes in the detection of both ITD and/or ILD. For this reason, we also analyzed the subjective sound source lateralization for the ITD and ILD separately. We found that while the ILD-induced lateralization was similar in both groups (ILD lateralization slope, young: 0.203 ± 0.012 vs. elderly: 0.196 ± 0.015; $p > 0.55$, Wilcoxon rank sum test; see **Figure 7C**), the ITD-induced lateralization

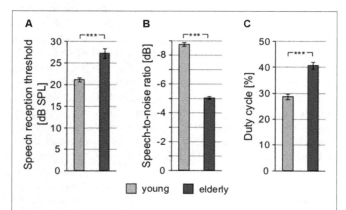

FIGURE 5 | Speech perception tests show significant differences between young and elderly. **(A)** Speech reception thresholds (SRTs). **(B)** Speech-to-noise ratio at which participants reach 50% recognition score (negative SNR values mean higher noise level). **(C)** Proportion of signal in the gated speech needed for 50% recognition score (***$p < 0.001$).

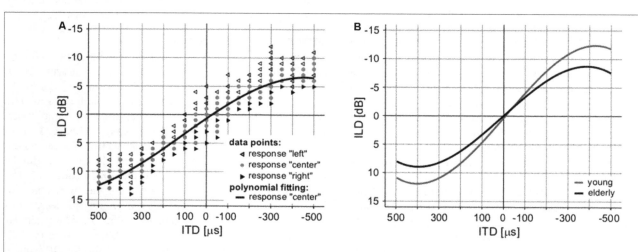

FIGURE 6 | An example of a laterogram of one subject. **(A)** Averaged laterograms of young controls and elderly group **(B)** showing a shallower slope of the trading function in the elderly.

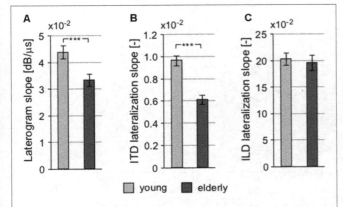

FIGURE 7 | Several parameters of the laterogram suggest significant differences in extracting binaural auditory information at subcortical levels. **(A)** Slope of the laterogram compares the ability to trade between ITD and ILD and is significantly shallower in the elderly. This is probably due to the reduced ability to process the temporal differences between the auditory inputs indicated by the different ITD lateralization slope **(B)** without any pathology in the processing of the intensity parameter, the ILD lateralization slope **(C)**; ***$p < 0.001$).

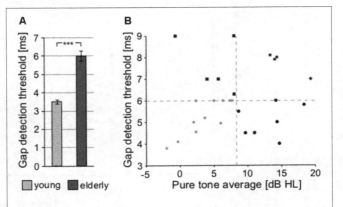

FIGURE 8 | **(A)** Processing of the temporal parameter of sound (gap in noise detection threshold) at cortical level (***$p < 0.001$). **(B)** Relationship between the gap detection threshold (GDT) and PTAV values for individual participants of the elderly group, providing an option for the further characterization of presbycusis subpopulations.

was significantly smaller in the elderly (ITD lateralization slope, young: 0.0097 ± 0.0005 vs. elderly: 0.0062 ± 0.0004; $p < 0.0001$, Wilcoxon rank sum test; **Figure 7B**). Hence the different laterogram slope was mainly due to lower sensitivity to the temporal parameter of the signal. Similar as in the case of chopper, data from laterogram measurements should be treated with caution as they are yet to be validated.

Temporal Parameters

To further investigate the processing of the temporal parameters of the sound, a gap detection threshold (GDT) test was used (**Figure 8A**). Significant differences between both groups were observed (young: 3.504 ± 0.114 ms vs. elderly: 6.007 ± 0.278 ms; $p < 0.0001$, Wilcoxon rank sum test), confirming the finding that the elderly participants exhibit poorer temporal processing, as already observed with the ITD-based lateralization. Gap detection is processed at the level of the temporal cortex (Rybalko et al., 2010; Mitsudo et al., 2014) and thus it was chosen for further analyses as a fundamental measure of the central auditory processing, along with the PTAV, as a fundamental index of peripheral processing. When the GDT and PTAV are plotted together in a 2D space (**Figure 8B**), it is clear that they are only unsubstantially related ($r = 0.14$, $p = 0.41$, Spearman correlation) and that besides people with both parameters, either good or bad, there also exist participants with physiological peripheral processing and deteriorated central processing (top-left corner) or participants with physiological central processing and deteriorated peripheral processing (bottom-right corner). The combined analysis of PTAV and GDT appears to be a promising method for a more detailed characterization of presbycustic subpopulations.

Cognitive Abilities

The cognitive abilities of volunteers from both groups were assessed by a MoCA questionnaire. The average scores were

28.79 ± 0.29 in young and 27.06 ± 0.44 in elderly ($p < 0.01$, Wilcoxon rank sum test), the lowest score in the young was 26 and in elderly was 23 (three participants scored lower then 26 within the elderly).

Correlation of Peripheral and Central Auditory and Cognitive Parameters

To examine the possible relationships between various parameters of interest, joint analyses of selected parameters were performed in the elderly group. First, we focused on the correlation of hearing thresholds with parameters of the function of central auditory system. Considering the temporal parameters, the PTAV (as well as the other peripheral measures) was not correlated with either of them (ITD lateralization slope: $\rho = -0.29$, $p > 0.05$; GDT: $\rho = 0.27$, $p > 0.05$; Spearman correlation). However, the speech comprehension measures, especially the SRT, were all correlated with the PTAV (SRT: $\rho = 0.75$, $p < 0.0001$; SIN: $\rho = -0.58$, $p < 0.01$; gated speech: $\rho = 0.53$, $p < 0.01$; Spearman correlation). Hence it appears that the hearing threshold is a strong predictor of speech comprehension ability. The GDT was found to be weakly correlated with the ITD lateralization slope ($\rho = -0.37, p = 0.05$, Spearman correlation), the correlation is nevertheless at the edge of statistical significance and therefore these two temporal measures could most likely be taken as independent. The GDT was also not correlated with the speech recognition threshold ($\rho = 0.32$, $p > 0.05$, Spearman correlation). On the other hand, the GDT significantly correlated with the ability to understand distorted speech, especially the speech in babble noise (SIN: $\rho = 0.51$, $p < 0.01$; gated speech: $\rho = 0.41$, $p < 0.05$; Spearman correlation; **Figures 9A,B**).

From the non-auditory parameters, we focused on the MoCA index and age. Interestingly, the MoCA index was not related to speech comprehension ability (in all three cases $\rho < 0.35$, $p > 0.05$, Spearman correlation). It was also not correlated with GDT ($\rho = -0.15$, $p > 0.05$, Spearman correlation), ITD slope ($\rho = 0.27$, $p > 0.05$, Spearman correlation), and age ($\rho = -0.32$,

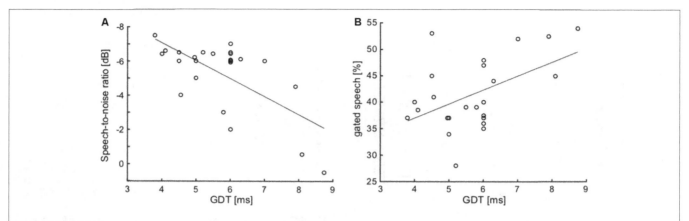

FIGURE 9 | Correlations of GDT with SIN **(A)** and with gated speech **(B)** suggest the importance of the temporal processing factor for speech understanding in a complex listening environment.

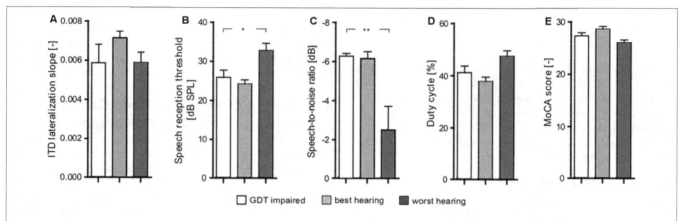

FIGURE 10 | Comparison of three groups of elderly subjects (GDT impaired, best hearing, worst hearing) based on their peripheral (PTAV) and central (GDT) functions inspired by **Figure 8B**, shows significant differences between worst hearing and both other groups in SIN ($p < 0.01$; **C**) and SRT ($p < 0.05$) parameters **(B)** and close to statistical significance [Cliff's d was medium-to-large ($d = 0.62$)] in gated speech **(D)**. In none of the other parameters [ITD lateralization slope **(A)** Montreal Cognitive Assessment (MoCA) **(E)**] was a significant difference present. Comparison of best hearing and GDT impaired did not show any significant differences (*$p < 0.05$, **$p < 0.01$).

$p > 0.05$, Spearman correlation). However, the MoCA depended on PTAV—the larger the hearing loss, the lower the MoCA index ($\rho = -0.57$, $p < 0.01$, Spearman correlation). In the case of age within the elderly group, only the ITD slope changes significantly ($\rho = -0.53$, $p < 0.01$, Spearman correlation); all the other tested parameters (PTAV, SRT, SIN, gated speech, GDT) do not depend on age within the elderly (in all cases $\rho < 0.25$, $p > 0.05$, Spearman correlation). Considering that these parameters all differ between the elderly and young, it can be assumed that age-related changes do occur, but either more slowly than can be displayed by the variability of age within the elderly, or that the progress of changes with age is not linear or gradual.

The correlation takes into account all the measured data points. Inspired by the plot shown in **Figure 8B**, it was interesting that the group of participants have deficits in central processing, despite having relatively good periphery. In the plot, these participants appear in the top-left quadrant. Specifically, we

extracted the elderly participants who have PTAV lower or equal than median, and GDT higher or equal than median (GDT impaired). We subsequently compared these participants with participants from the top-right quadrant (similar GDT, but worse hearing thresholds-worst hearing), and bottom-left quadrant (similar thresholds, but better GDT-best hearing).

The examined parameters were ITD slope, SRT, SIN, gated speech, and MoCA (**Figure 10**). Interestingly, the GDT impaired participants exhibited no significant differences ($p > 0.05$ in all cases, Wilcoxon rank sum tests) of the tested parameters in comparison with the group of the worst hearing participants (bottom-left quadrant). When compared with the worst hearing participants (top-right quadrant), these GDT impaired participants have better SRT (GDT impaired: 25.9 ± 1.9 dB SPL vs. worst hearing: 32.75 ± 1.8 dB SPL, $p < 0.05$; Wilcoxon rank sum test; **Figure 10B**) and SIN (GDT impaired: -6.27 ± 0.14 dB vs. worst hearing: -2.51 ± 1.2 dB, $p < 0.01$; Wilcoxon rank sum test; **Figure 10C**). GDT impaired participants also tend to have a better ability to understand the gated speech (GDT impaired: 41.21 ± 2.5% vs. worst hearing: 47.42 ± 2.1%, $p = 0.07$; Wilcoxon rank sum test; **Figure 10D**). Despite the fact that the difference did not reach statistical significance due to the low number of observations, the effect size expressed as Cliff's d was medium-to-large ($d = 0.62$) and therefore the difference might potentially be important. The other parameters were not significantly different ($p > 0.05$, Wilcoxon rank sum tests) (**Figures 10A,E**). Overall, it appears that despite that GDT is in general correlated with the speech comprehension abilities, the hearing thresholds are more important for speech understanding, at least in our group of participants.

DISCUSSION

In the current study we have investigated the auditory function in elderly volunteers with clinically normal hearing thresholds with the aim to identify possible central auditory dysfunctions and explore its interactions with peripheral impairments. Regular auditory tests [high frequency audiometry (HFA), speech audiometry, OAE] were complemented by additional audiometric tests (gated speech—chopper, binaural time-intensity tradeoff—laterogram, GDT, detection of clicks and short tones) and by cognitive screening (MoCA). Although the auditory thresholds of our elderly (up to 6 kHz) only show a very mild elevation due to normal aging with only minimal clinical signs of hearing pathology, our data show otherwise. Even in the elderly population without subjective hearing pathology and with only minor elevation of auditory thresholds, supracochlear structures of the auditory system show deteriorated functions. The results of the laterogram, and specifically ITD sensitivity, express altered integration of the binaural information, especially with respect of the temporal parameter. GDTs provide information about the ability of central processing of the temporal parameters of sound, which is altered independently of the function of the inner ear. Speech audiometry in babble noise and chopper, integrate the auditory information with cognitive processing and both tests show a clear deterioration with age, while the MoCA results are within the physiologic range with the exception of three borderline participants.

Pure tone audiogram represents the "gold standard" of audiometric examinations, providing basic information about the hearing ability of the subject. Under standard conditions, hearing thresholds are measured up to 8 kHz and the elevation of auditory thresholds above 25 dB HL are considered by the majority of clinicians, and also according to WHO, to be mild hearing loss. In our elderly participants, hearing thresholds up to 8 kHz showed clinically normal values, according to ISO 7029. High frequency pure tone audiometry (HFA) examines hearing thresholds up to 16 (in our case) or 20 kHz. Our elderly participants demonstrated significant deterioration of hearing above 8 kHz, which is in agreement with Matthews et al. (1997), therefore it is necessary to use HFA in specific conditions [for example: tinnitus, sensorineural hearing loss (SNHL), etc.; Wiley et al., 1998; Vielsmeier et al., 2015]. Although our study did not

focus on the shape of hearing thresholds as described by Gates et al. (1990), all of the elderly participants showed a shallow sloping type. The difference in the auditory thresholds between both groups is numerically expressed by PTAV and Fowler's percentage of hearing loss. Although the differences of these measures between elderly and young are statistically significant, both values are considered clinically normal. Furthermore, as shown by correlation analysis, the PTAV and Fowler's coefficient are mutually dependent.

The examination of click hearing thresholds also provides a comparison of auditory thresholds, but without the frequency dependency. It also takes into account the short duration of clicks. Considering the click duration and the altered ability to track temporal changes, we expected a greater impairment of the click thresholds with aging compared to pure tone thresholds, nonetheless our results show otherwise. Although clicks are regularly used as a stimulus for brainstem audiometry, in the case of subjective audiometry the click hearing thresholds do not seem to provide any additional information to PTAV.

The analysis of the effect of stimulus duration on the auditory threshold (in our case 1 kHz tone) allows the examination of temporal processing within the inner ear and also possibly the synchrony of the auditory nerve activity (Zeng et al., 2005). The sensitivity to the stimulus duration is essential for both the individual properties of sound within the sound sequence, and for the rate characteristics of the sequence as a whole (Fitzgibbons and Gordon-Salant, 2011). As previously reported, a shorter duration of the stimulus leads to an increase of threshold (Abel, 1972), however, hearing loss does not seem to have a significant effect on duration discrimination (Fitzgibbons and Gordon-Salant, 1994) as the temporal discrimination has previously been shown as independent from the hearing threshold elevation (Grose et al., 2006; Fitzgibbons and Gordon-Salant, 2011). The deteriorated ability of duration discrimination seems to occur even in middle aged men (Grose et al., 2006). On the other hand, Fitzgibbons and Gordon-Salant (1995) showed that stimulus duration discrimination also depends on the context, suggesting that simple tone discrimination is not a good predictor for discrimination, even of the same sound presented within a more complex sequential pattern. In the case of 1 kHz tone, the hearing threshold in our elderly seems to be unaffected by aging, therefore the factor of intensity should not play a significant role in the processing of 1 kHz signal. In our study, we quantified the steepness of the dependence between the tone duration and its detection threshold using the parameters of the exponential fit. Since none of the parameters differ between young and elderly, temporal integration at the level of the inner ear appears unaffected by aging. This information is important since one of the most influential effects of aging is the decreased ability to detect fast changing (temporal) auditory cues (Grose and Mamo, 2010; Ozmeral et al., 2016a). However, comparing our results in a gap detection task and in its "inverse," the short tone detection task, it seems that processing of the temporal aspects of sound is different in the case of detection of pauses or valleys in the stimulus envelope and in the case of the detection of amplitude peaks.

One of the explanations of impaired temporal processing that could also advocate for near normal audiograms is cochlear synaptopathy. Cochlear synaptopathy, in humans, sometimes also referred to as a hidden hearing loss, is a pathology described by Kujawa and Liberman (2009). Although initially described as a result of noise induced hearing loss, it has also recently been confirmed in aging animals as an effect of presbycusis (Sergeyenko et al., 2013). Impaired temporal processing in cochlear synaptopathy is probably due specifically to its effect on low spontaneous rate auditory nerve fibers, which would also explain the minimal elevation of auditory threshold (Liberman and Kujawa, 2017). Although the cited data seem promising, the phenomenon has not been proved to be completely transferable to humans, and the presence of cochlear synaptopathy in humans remains inconclusive (for review see Hickox et al., 2017). In our study, the peripheral auditory impairment represented by increased PTAV does not correlate with the changes of auditory temporal processing represented by ITD and GDT, which further supports the idea of independence between possible peripheral temporal processing impairment (as described in relation to cochlear synaptopathy) and more centrally located temporal processing impairments.

OAE examination provides information about the functionality of outer hair cells. As expected, in the elderly the amplitudes are lower for both types of evoked responses (TE and DP), which is a sign of hypofunction of the outer hair cell populations common in aging (Helleman et al., 2010). Lower amplitudes are accompanied by a lower number of functional outer hair cell populations (Mazelová et al., 2003; Ueberfuhr et al., 2016). The outer hair cell hypofunction in the elderly causes a deterioration of the auditory input that leads to a diminished neural signal reaching the central auditory structures. The decrease of DPOAEs amplitudes of contralateral suppression due to aging is also present in our study, although these changes were not statistically significant. This mild effect of aging on contralateral suppression suggests a relatively weak alteration of the efferent auditory system in our elderly. However, several authors have clearly demonstrated the substantial effect of aging on contralateral suppression (Kim et al., 2002; Jacobson et al., 2003). Interestingly this decrease already starts in middle age (Kim et al., 2002). The impaired function of the outer hair cells could be compensated by the proper function of the efferent auditory system. Although the exact function of the efferent auditory system remains unclear, several reports describe its positive effect on the improved extraction of auditory cues from a complex acoustic background, that could lead to an improved auditory stream segregation (Sussman et al., 2007; Füllgrabe and Moore, 2014; Pannese et al., 2015). Evidently, the deteriorated function of the efferent auditory system may contribute significantly to the problems of people with expressed presbycusis, in the identification of speech in a noisy environment.

Altered speech processing is common in the elderly. Our elderly show a normal ability to understand speech in silence (SRT), which is in agreement with the auditory threshold examination. However, the difference between young and elderly becomes apparent in SIN and seems even more profound in the understanding of temporally degraded speech, where the elderly participants need a significantly larger proportion of speech signal to understand the sentence than the young. Speech signal carries several types of information: phonetic, phonemic and syllabic and lexicosyntactics (Greenber, 1996). Although an altered auditory system could lead to the deterioration of word recognition, for example in speech (sentences) processing, the lost information (phonetic) can be compensated by use of the context (phonemic; Pichora-Fuller and Singh, 2006; Sheldon et al., 2008). However, such compensation increases the requirements on the working memory (Bopp and Verhaeghen, 2009) that might lead to an overall slowing down of the cognitive processing, especially if conditions worsen (for example in the chopper test).

One of the explanations for altered comprehension of SIN and gated speech in the elderly is their worsened ability to extract fine temporal structure information (Moore, 2016), and to track fast temporal changes (Fogerty et al., 2015). Another important factor for speech processing is sensitivity to segment duration that is significant for the better identification of stress or accent patterns (Pickett, 1999). In our case, the correlation between GDT and SIN and chopper, but absent correlation between GDT and SRT supports the idea that temporal parameters become increasingly important for speech understanding in a complex environment. Similar findings were also observed in tinnitus patients with normal hearing thresholds (Bureš et al., under review; Moon et al., 2015) that showed a beneficiary effect of sensitivity to temporal modulation on SIN in comparison to volunteers without tinnitus. Bureš et al. (under review) also showed stronger correlations between ITD and speech recognition in tinnitus patients. In this case the tinnitus plays the role of a distractor (similar speech perception in silence compared to SIN) that most likely leads to more efficient utilization of the temporal information by tinnitus patients. The detection of a gap in noise is a simple test of the temporal processing in the central auditory system, as demonstrated in experimental animals by Rybalko et al. (2010) and Suta et al. (2011) that deteriorates with age. The auditory cortex is involved in the processing of GDT since its dysfunction in rats results in prolongation of the GDT values (Syka, 2002). Age-related prolongation of GDT has also been demonstrated in humans (Mazelová et al., 2003). GDTs can be elevated, even in the elderly with normal hearing (Strouse et al., 1998). However, a certain proportion of the elderly may have GDTs similar to young subjects (Snell, 1997). In experimental animals, age-related alterations in the neuronal processing of gaps in noise were demonstrated in the inferior colliculus (Walton et al., 1998). Williamson et al. (2015) used gaps in noise auditory brainstem response (ABR) tests in a mice model of presbycusis and showed that age related changes of temporal processing already start in middle-aged animals. Age-related GDT differences become more apparent if more complex stimuli are used, such as if the gap is located near the stimulus offset or onset (He et al., 1999), or when the components bordering the gaps shift their spectral contents (Fitzgibbons and Gordon-Salant, 1994). One of the possible explanations of the deteriorated ability to track fast temporal changes is the alteration of the inhibitory mechanisms (Schatteman et al., 2008;

Anderson et al., 2012). Such changes have been documented, especially in animal models of aging, as a reduction in the number of inhibitory interneurons, with lower levels of the inhibitory neurotransmitter GABA at the level of AC, as well as in the IC (Caspary et al., 2005; Ouda et al., 2015; Popelář et al., 2013), and in the case of glycine as low as in the cochlear nucleus (Frisina and Walton, 2006).

Our chopper results correspond with the results of previously used time compressed speech tests that also contain reduced linguistic and semantic cues (Gordon-Salant and Fitzgibbons, 1993), specifically naturally fast speech (Gordon-Salant et al., 2014), which alters speed processing and working memory abilities (Wingfield et al., 2006). Chopper and time-compressed speech are similar in the way that they both contain fewer contextual cues and therefore are more demanding on cognitive processing resources. Unfortunately, it is not possible to completely separate the influence of the cognitive and auditory abilities in our experimental paradigm. Although the results of MoCA screen for normal cognitive function in the elderly with the exception of three borderline participants (Nasreddine et al., 2005), the deteriorated speech signal is much more difficult to compensate by the cognitive system. Akeroyd (2008) showed that none of the commonly used cognitive tests correlate with speech in noise perception performance, supporting the idea that for auditory processing, different cognitive abilities are necessary than those examined by general cognitive tests. Decreased temporal processing also alters the integration of complex processing that uses cognitive resources and working memory (Frisina and Frisina, 1997; Grady, 2008), which could explain the lower chopper scores and normal results of the MoCA tests. Previously, an increase of working memory load has been identified as an important factor in the age related speech processing decline, especially in the case of sentences with low context cues (Wingfield, 1996). Another factor that influences the cognitive processing of speech, is the processing rate as mentioned in the case of time-compressed speech, however in the majority of individuals, a decrease of speech rate does not improve speech understanding (Gordon-Salant and Fitzgibbons, 1997). An important role that age-related changes in cognition play in the auditory ability was recently reported by Grassi and Borella (2013).

In a detailed analysis of the relationship between cognitive tasks and hearing, Füllgrabe and Moore (2014) described age related differences in the majority of cognitive tests in the young and elderly with normal hearing thresholds. Specifically, selective attention, attention switching and working memory test results were affected by aging. The results of cognitive tests were significantly correlated with altered speech processing in noise and also with temporal processing. In our study the MoCA results did not correlate with either the speech parameters or with the temporal processing parameters, suggesting that MoCA is probably not optimally suited for evaluation of the cognitive abilities related to hearing function. The effects of age and hearing loss on the processing of auditory temporal fine structure (TFS) was recently summarized by Moore (2016), taking into account that in many studies the effects of hearing loss and age have been confounded. In monaural processing,

both hearing loss and aging negatively influence the output from the cochlea, represented by the TFS whereas the slowly varying envelope (ENV) is hardly affected. In the binaural version of speech stimulation, the TFS, which is important for sound localization and binaural masking level difference, is also negatively influenced by hearing loss and aging, with aging being more influential. The binaural processing of ENV also deteriorates with aging. It is difficult to compare our data with the results of psychoacoustic tests used by Füllgrabe and Moore (2014) and Moore (2016), yet even our data strongly support the view that aging is connected in humans with the deterioration of the processing of temporal aspects of the acoustical signal. For example, our data clearly show that in monaural stimulation, deterioration of the GDT frequently occurs, whereas in binaural stimulation, elderly subjects suffer from deterioration of ITD.

For some time, ABRs were used for the examination of the auditory pathway from the level of cochlear nuclei to the inferior colliculus. In our previous study (Profant et al., 2017), we showed that in spite of normal ABR results, the function of the auditory pathway might be impaired. Laterogram compares the ability to trade between the time and intensity differences of the acoustic signal coming from both ears. The ability to integrate the signal from both ears is crucial in speech processing in background noise, and in auditory stream segregation. Similarly to the decline of the peripheral and central auditory functions, orientation in acoustic space (a natural outcome of the bilateral hearing) is also altered by hearing impairment (Noble et al., 1994) and aging (Abel et al., 2000). From a clinical point of view, on the grounds of the auditory thresholds and speech perception, both groups show a normal auditory function, however there is a significant difference in the ability to extract the binaural temporal information with only minor changes in the intensity difference detection. Based on the anatomy of the auditory pathway, the integration of the acoustic cues in bilateral hearing and taking into account the normal integration of temporal information within the inner ear (duration vs. detection threshold of 1 kHz stimuli, click detection thresholds), the impaired ITD sensitivity suggests that the temporal processing impairment is probably already present at the level of auditory brainstem and inferior colliculus. The different localization of the processing of ITD vs. GDT is also supported by their very low correlation. From this perspective, the ITD detection test may be used as a complement for the gap detection test to examine the temporal processing ability at the different levels of the auditory pathway. However, it has to be taken into account that a hearing loss above 4 kHz (typical sign of presbycusis) affects ITD to a greater extent than a low frequency hearing loss (Abel and Hay, 1996). Our findings of age related decline in ITD and only minimal changes in ILD are in agreement with previous reports (Babkoff et al., 2002; Ross et al., 2007). However, when taking into account the ability to separate speech and background noise based on the different spatial localization of sources, the age related difference in ITD processing does not seem to have an effect (Füllgrabe and Moore, 2014). This is very likely due to the ability to utilize additional cues such as monaural spectral cues and ILD

(Singh et al., 2008; Füllgrabe and Moore, 2014). Although the ITD as a temporal processing ability seems to play a major role in spatial orientation, another aspect affecting the temporal interaural interactions is the neural synchrony parameter, which is also negatively affected by age (Ozmeral et al., 2016b). For the binaural interactions and specifically spatial coding, the neural synchrony at the level of medial superior olive is important and is negatively affected by insufficient inhibitory inputs due to aging (Pecka et al., 2008).

One of the aims of our project was to better characterize SNHL. According to the reported data it seems that even in a homogenous population of elderly with clinically normal hearing (deterioration of auditory thresholds is in agreement with their age "hearing age"), clear differences are present. There is variability at the level of the inner ear, auditory pathway and also at the level of auditory cortex and in interactions with the cognitive network. For the purpose of improved identification of SNHL, we correlated a basic inner ear parameter—PTAV—with a basic central hearing parameter—GDT. The auditory periphery/center correlation proposes at least four possible subgroups: the real "golden ears" with almost perfect function of the auditory periphery and center, groups with either good periphery and declined central auditory function or declined peripheral auditory function and good central function, and a fourth group with both functions deteriorated. Another finding is that in our elderly the relatively minor degree of purely central pathology represented by higher GDT (GDT impaired subgroup of elderly) has only limited influence on speech processing, especially in comparison with the effect of peripheral function represented by PTAV. Additional comprehensive examination is needed, especially in the elderly with a more profound hearing deterioration, to further stress this classification and potentially add more presbycustic subpopulations. Our approach might complete the missing pieces in several theories of presbycusis as proposed by CHABA (1998).

Our data present a new insight (specifically the chopper and laterogram tests) into auditory processing in humans with a potential impact on the diagnosis of SNHL. This is especially in contrast with the classic clinical approach to the diagnosis of hearing loss that uses only limited examination. As presented above, none of our elderly participants had an auditory function that would be considered by clinical standards as pathological, however our detailed tests show otherwise. We believe that in specific diagnosis such as presbycusis or potentially tinnitus, a more thorough examination is necessary. We aim to use our battery of tests to further classify the different subtypes of presbycusis that might eventually lead to a different approach of how to rehabilitate hearing impairment. Nonetheless, at this point there is no clear clinical recommendation for the use of a novel part of the test battery since more data is needed for

validation. Among the clinically available tests in specific cases when a patient's subjective feeling does not correlate with the results of basic audiometric examination, HFA, SIN and the effect of contralateral suppression on OAE should be complemented.

Although our results provide a new insight into the pathophysiology of the age related changes in the auditory system, it is necessary to point out that the novel tests (specifically laterogram, chopper and short tone audiogram) have not been validated yet. However, based on the results of these tests and their correlation with the standardized auditory and cognitive measurements, convergent validity approach can be implemented. Nonetheless, in the near future, we plan to produce validated results of these tests for each age group (in 10 year intervals) that would provide reference data and allow a more general use of these tests.

CONCLUSION

Presbycusis is a complex disorder affecting different parts of the auditory system. Although the elevation of hearing thresholds is its most common expression indicating inner ear (peripheral) pathology, several other central auditory features are affected as well. The presented data demonstrate the deterioration of the interaural auditory processing (laterogram), specifically of temporal information (ITD), decreased ability of auditory cortex to identify fast signal changes (GDT) and an overall decline of the integration of auditory and cognitive abilities (speech in noise, chopper). The analysis of the interactions of peripheral and central auditory abilities showed a stronger influence of peripheral function (expressed as hearing thresholds) than temporal processing ability on speech perception in silence, however in a more natural environment such as with the addition of noise to speech, the role of temporal processing increases rapidly. Our data reveal several pathologies causing presbycusis and suggest that they are to some extent independent of each other and, in particular, that hearing threshold elevation does not predict the state of the supracochlear auditory function.

AUTHOR CONTRIBUTIONS

OP: manuscript preparation, examination, auditory tests creation, statistical analysis, work load ca 25%. MJ: examination, software preparation, auditory tests creation, work load ca 15%. ZB: software preparation, auditory tests creation, statistical analysis, manuscript preparation, work load ca 15%. VV: examination, software preparation, work load ca 10%. DK and VS: examination, database administration, work load ca 10%. JK: software preparation, work load ca 5%. JS: manuscript preparation, auditory test creation, project overview, work load 10%.

REFERENCES

Abel, S. M. (1972). Duration discrimination of noise and tone bursts. *J. Acoust. Soc. Am.* 51, 1219–1223. doi: 10.1121/1.1912963

Abel, S. M., Giguère, C., Consoli, A., and Papsin, B. C. (2000). The effect of aging on horizontal plane sound localization. *J. Acoust. Soc. Am.* 108, 743–752. doi: 10.1121/1.429607

Abel, S. M., and Hay, V. H. (1996). Sound localization. The interaction of aging, hearing loss and hearing protection. *Scand. Audiol.* 25, 3–12. doi: 10.3109/01050399609047549

Akeroyd, M. A. (2008). Are individual differences in speech reception related to individual differences in cognitive ability? A survey of twenty experimental studies with normal and hearing-impaired adults. *Int. J. Audiol.* 47, S53–S71. doi: 10.1080/14992020802301142

Anderson, S., Parbery-Clark, A., White-Schwoch, T., and Kraus, N. (2012). Aging affects neural precision of speech encoding. *J. Neurosci.* 32, 14156–14164. doi: 10.1523/JNEUROSCI.2176-12.2012

Babkoff, H., Muchnik, C., Ben-David, N., Furst, M., Even-Zohar, S., and Hildesheimer, M. (2002). Mapping lateralization of click trains in younger and older populations. *Hear. Res.* 165, 117–127. doi: 10.1016/s0378-5955(02)00292-7

Bopp, K. L., and Verhaeghen, P. (2009). Working memory and aging: separating the effects of content and context. *Psychol. Aging* 24, 968–980. doi: 10.1037/a0017731

Caspary, D. M., Schatteman, T. A., and Hughes, L. F. (2005). Age-related changes in the inhibitory response properties of dorsal cochlear nucleus output neurons: role of inhibitory inputs. *J. Neurosci.* 25, 10952–10959. doi: 10.1523/JNEUROSCI.2451-05.2005

CHABA. (1998). Speech understanding and aging. working group on speech understanding and aging. committee on hearing, bioacoustics and biomechanics, commission on behavioral and social sciences and education, national research council. *J. Acoust. Soc. Am.* 83, 859–895.

Dlouhá, O., Vokřál, J., and Cerny, L. (2013). Test of sentence intelligibility in babble noise in persons with normal hearing. *Otorhinolaryngol. Foniatrie* 61, 240–244.

Fitzgibbons, P. J., and Gordon-Salant, S. (1994). Age effects on measures of auditory duration discrimination. *J. Speech Hear. Res.* 37, 662–670. doi: 10.1044/jshr.3703.662

Fitzgibbons, P. J., and Gordon-Salant, S. (1995). Age effects on duration discrimination with simple and complex stimuli. *J. Acoust. Soc. Am.* 98, 3140–3145. doi: 10.1121/1.413803

Fitzgibbons, P. J., and Gordon-Salant, S. (2011). Age effects in discrimination of repeating sequence intervals. *J. Acoust. Soc. Am.* 129, 1490–1500. doi: 10.1121/1.3533728

Fogerty, D., Ahlstrom, J. B., Bologna, W. J., and Dubno, J. R. (2015). Sentence intelligibility during segmental interruption and masking by speech-modulated noise: effects of age and hearing loss. *J. Acoust. Soc. Am.* 137, 3487–3501. doi: 10.1121/1.4921603

Fowler, E. P., and Sabine, P. E. (1942). Tentative standard procedure for evaluating the percentage of useful hearing loss in medicolegal cases. *JAMA* 119, 1108–1109.

Frisina, D. R., and Frisina, R. D. (1997). Speech recognition in noise and presbycusis: relations to possible neural mechanisms. *Hear. Res.* 106, 95–104. doi: 10.1016/s0378-5955(97)00006-3

Frisina, R. D., and Walton, J. P. (2006). Age-related structural and functional changes in the cochlear nucleus. *Hear. Res.* 216–223. doi: 10.1016/j.heares.2006.02.003

Füllgrabe, C., and Moore, B. C. J. (2014). Effects of age and hearing loss on stream segregation based on interaural time differences. *J. Acoust. Soc. Am.* 136, EL185–EL191. doi: 10.1121/1.4890201

Gardner, G., and Robertson, J. H. (1988). Hearing preservation in unilateral acoustic neuroma surgery. *Ann. Otol. Rhinol. Laryngol.* 97, 55–66. doi: 10.1177/000348948809700110

Gates, G. A., and Cooper, J. C. (1991). Incidence of hearing decline in the elderly. *Acta. Otolaryngol.* 111, 240–248. doi: 10.3109/00016489109137382

Gates, G. A., Cooper, J. C., Kannel, W. B., and Miller, N. J. (1990). Hearing in the elderly: the Framingham cohort, 1983-1985. Part I. Basic audiometric test results. *Ear Hear.* 11, 247–256.

Giroud, N., Hirsiger, S., Muri, R., Kegel, A., Dillier, N., and Meyer, M. (2018). Neuroanatomical and resting state EEG power correlates of central hearing loss in older adults. *Brain Struct. Funct.* 223, 145–163. doi: 10.1007/s00429-017-1477-0

Gordon-Salant, S., and Fitzgibbons, P. J. (1993). Temporal factors and speech recognition performance in young and elderly listeners. *J. Speech Hear. Res.* 36, 1276–1285. doi: 10.1044/jshr.3606.1276

Gordon-Salant, S., and Fitzgibbons, P. J. (1997). Selected cognitive factors and speech recognition performance among young and elderly listeners. *J. Speech Lang. Hear. Res. JSLHR* 40, 423–431. doi: 10.1044/jslhr.4002.423

Gordon-Salant, S., Zion, D. J., and Espy-Wilson, C. (2014). Recognition of time-compressed speech does not predict recognition of natural fast-rate speech by older listeners. *J. Acoust. Soc. Am.* 136, EL268–274. doi: 10.1121/1.4895014

Grady, C. L. (2008). Cognitive neuroscience of aging. *Ann. N Y Acad. Sci.* 1124, 127–144. doi: 10.1196/annals.1440.009

Grassi, M., and Borella, E. (2013). The role of auditory abilities in basic mechanisms of cognition in older adults. *Front. Aging Neurosci.* 5:59. doi: 10.3389/fnagi.2013.00059

Greenber, S. (1996). "Auditory processing of speech," in *Principles of Experimental Phonetics*, ed. N. Lass (St. Louis: Mosby), 364–407.

Grose, J. H., Hall, J. W., and Buss, E. (2006). Temporal processing deficits in the pre-senescent auditory system. *J. Acoust. Soc. Am.* 119, 2305–2315.

Grose, J. H., and Mamo, S. K. (2010). Processing of temporal fine structure as a function of age. *Ear Hear.* 31, 755–760. doi: 10.1097/AUD.0b013e3181e627e7

He, N. J., Horwitz, A. R., Dubno, J. R., and Mills, J. H. (1999). Psychometric functions for gap detection in noise measured from young and aged subjects. *J. Acoust. Soc. Am.* 106, 966–978. doi: 10.1121/1.427109

Helleman, H. W., Jansen, E. J. M., and Dreschler, W. A. (2010). Otoacoustic emissions in a hearing conservation program: general applicability in longitudinal monitoring and the relation to changes in pure-tone thresholds. *Int. J. Audiol.* 49, 410–419. doi: 10.3109/14992020903527616

Hickox, A. E., Larsen, E., Heinz, M. G., Shinobu, L., and Whitton, J. P. (2017). Translational issues in cochlear synaptopathy. *Hear. Res.* 349, 164–171. doi: 10.3410/f.727192264.793532887

Humes, L. E. (1996). Speech understanding in the elderly. *J. Am. Acad. Audiol.* 7, 161–167.

Humes, L. E., Dubno, J. R., Gordon-Salant, S., Lister, J. J., Cacace, A. T., Cruickshanks, K. J., et al. (2012). Central presbycusis: a review and evaluation of the evidence. *J. Am. Acad. Audiol.* 23, 635–666. doi: 10.3766/jaaa.23.8.5

Jacobson, M., Kim, S., Romney, J., Zhu, X., and Frisina, R. D. (2003). Contralateral suppression of distortion-product otoacoustic emissions declines with age: a comparison of findings in CBA mice with human listeners. *Laryngoscope* 113, 1707–1713. doi: 10.1097/00005537-200310000-00009

Jayakody, D. M. P., Friedland, P. L., Martins, R. N., and Sohrabi, H. R. (2018). Impact of aging on the auditory system and related cognitive functions: a narrative review. *Front. Neurosci.* 12:125. doi: 10.3389/fnins.2018.00125

Jilek, M., Šuta, D., and Syka, J. (2014). Reference hearing thresholds in an extended frequency range as a function of age. *J. Acoust. Soc. Am.* 136, 1821–1830. doi: 10.1121/1.4894719

Kim, S., Frisina, D. R., and Frisina, R. D. (2002). Effects of age on contralateral suppression of distortion product otoacoustic emissions in human listeners with normal hearing. *Audiol. Neurootol.* 7, 348–357. doi: 10.1159/000066159

Kujawa, S. G., and Liberman, M. C. (2009). Adding insult to injury: cochlear nerve degeneration after "temporary" noise-induced hearing loss. *J. Neurosci. Off. J. Soc. Neurosci.* 29, 14077–14085. doi: 10.1523/JNEUROSCI.2845-09.2009

Liberman, M. C., and Kujawa, S. G. (2017). Cochlear synaptopathy in acquired sensorineural hearing loss: Manifestations and mechanisms. *Hear. Res.* 349, 138–147. doi: 10.1016/j.heares.2017.01.003

Lin, F. R., Ferrucci, L., Metter, E. J., An, Y., Zonderman, A. B., and Resnick, S. M. (2011). Hearing loss and cognition in the Baltimore Longitudinal Study of Aging. *Neuropsychology* 25, 763–770. doi: 10.1037/a0024238

Matthews, L. J., Lee, F. S., Mills, J. H., and Dubno, J. R. (1997). Extended high-frequency thresholds in older adults. *J. Speech Lang. Hear. Res.* 40, 208–214. doi: 10.1044/jslhr.4001.208

Mazelová, J., Popelar, J., and Syka, J. (2003). Auditory function in presbycusis: peripheral vs. central changes. *Exp. Gerontol.* 38, 87–94. doi: 10.1016/s0531-5565(02)00155-9

Mitsudo, T., Hironaga, N., and Mori, S. (2014). Cortical activity associated with the detection of temporal gaps in tones: a magnetoencephalography study. *Front. Hum. Neurosci.* 8:763. doi: 10.3389/fnhum.2014.00763

Moon, I. J., Won, J. H., Kang, H. W., Kim, D. H., An, Y.-H., and Shim, H. J. (2015). Influence of tinnitus on auditory spectral and temporal resolution and speech perception in tinnitus patients. *J. Neurosci.* 35, 14260–14269. doi: 10.1523/JNEUROSCI.5091-14.2015

Moore, B. C. J. (2016). Effects of age and hearing loss on the processing of auditory temporal fine structure. *Adv. Exp. Med. Biol.* 894, 1–8. doi: 10.1007/978-3-319-25474-6_1

Nasreddine, Z. S., Phillips, N. A., Bédirian, V., Charbonneau, S., Whitehead, V., Collin, I., et al. (2005). The montreal cognitive assessment, MoCA: a brief screening tool for mild cognitive impairment. *J. Am. Geriatr. Soc.* 53, 695–699. doi: 10.1111/j.1532-5415.2005.53221.x

Noble, W., Byrne, D., and Lepage, B. (1994). Effects on sound localization of configuration and type of hearing impairment. *J. Acoust. Soc. Am.* 95, 992–1005. doi: 10.1121/1.408404

Ouda, L., Burianova, J., and Syka, J. (2015). Age-related changes in calbindin and calretinin immunoreactivity in the central auditory system of the rat. *Exp. Gerontol.* 47, 497–506. doi: 10.1016/j.exger.2012.04.003

Ozmeral, E. J., Eddins, A. C., Frisina, D. R., and Eddins, D. A. (2016a). Large cross-sectional study of presbycusis reveals rapid progressive decline in auditory temporal acuity. *Neurobiol. Aging* 43, 72–78. doi: 10.1016/j.neurobiolaging.2015.12.024

Ozmeral, E. J., Eddins, D. A., and Eddins, A. C. (2016b). Reduced temporal processing in older, normal-hearing listeners evident from electrophysiological responses to shifts in interaural time difference. *J. Neurophysiol.* 116, 2720–2729. doi: 10.1152/jn.00560.2016

Pannese, A., Grandjean, D., and Frühholz, S. (2015). Subcortical processing in auditory communication. *Hear. Res.* 328, 67–77. doi: 10.1016/j.heares.2015.07.003

Pearman, A., Friedman, L., Brooks, J. O., and Yesavage, J. A. (2000). Hearing impairment and serial word recall in older adults. *Exp. Aging Res.* 26, 383–391. doi: 10.1080/036107300750015769

Pecka, M., Brand, A., Behrend, O., and Grothe, B. (2008). Interaural time difference processing in the mammalian medial superior olive: the role of glycinergic inhibition. *J. Neurosci.* 28, 6914–6925. doi: 10.1523/jneurosci.1660-08.2008

Pichora-Fuller, M. K., and Singh, G. (2006). Effects of age on auditory and cognitive processing: implications for hearing aid fitting and audiologic rehabilitation. *Trends Amplif.* 10, 29–59. doi: 10.1177/108471380601000103

Pickett, J. M. (1999). *The Acoustics of Speech Communication: Fundamentals, Speech Perception Theory and Technology.* Boston: Allyn and Bacon.

Popelář, J., Rybalko, N., Burianová, J., Schwaller, B., and Syka, J. (2013). The effect of parvalbumin deficiency on the acoustic startle response and prepulse inhibition in mice. *Neurosci. Lett.* 553, 216–220. doi: 10.1016/j.neulet.2013.08.042

Profant, O., Balogová, Z., Dezortová, M., Wagnerová, D., Hájek, M., and Syka, J. (2013). Metabolic changes in the auditory cortex in presbycusis demonstrated by MR spectroscopy. *Exp. Gerontol.* 48, 795–800. doi: 10.1016/j.exger.2013.04.012

Profant, O., Roth, J., Bureš, Z., Balogová, Z., Lišková, I., Betka, J., et al. (2017). Auditory dysfunction in patients with Huntington's disease. *Clin. Neurophysiol.* 128, 1946–1953. doi: 10.1016/j.clinph.2017.07.403

Profant, O., Škoch, A., Balogová, Z., Tintěra, J., Hlinka, J., and Syka, J. (2014). Diffusion tensor imaging and MR morphometry of the central auditory pathway and auditory cortex in aging. *Neuroscience* 260, 87–97. doi: 10.1016/j.neuroscience.2013.12.010

Profant, O., Tintěra, J., Balogová, Z., Ibrahim, I., Jilek, M., and Syka, J. (2015). Functional changes in the human auditory cortex in ageing. *PLoS One* 10:e0116692. doi: 10.1371/journal.pone.0116692

Pronk, M., Deeg, D. J., Festen, J. M., Twisk, J. W., Smits, C., Comijs, H. C., et al. (2013). Decline in older persons' ability to recognize speech in noise: the influence of demographic, health-related, environmental, and cognitive factors. *Ear Hear.* 34, 722–732. doi: 10.1097/AUD.0b013e3182994eee

Reban, J. (2006). Montrealský kognitivni test /MoCA/: přínos k diagnostice predemencí. *Čes Ger Revue* 4, 224–229.

Rektorová, I. (2011). Screeningové škály pro hodnocení demence. *Neurol. Praxi* 12, 37–45.

Ross, B., Fujioka, T., Tremblay, K. L., and Picton, T. W. (2007). Aging in binaural hearing begins in mid-life: evidence from cortical auditory-evoked responses to changes in interaural phase. *J. Neurosci.* 27, 11172–11178. doi: 10.1523/jneurosci.1813-07.2007

Rybalko, N., Suta, D., Popelár, J., and Syka, J. (2010). Inactivation of the left auditory cortex impairs temporal discrimination in the rat. *Behav. Brain Res.* 209, 123–130. doi: 10.1016/j.bbr.2010.01.028

Schatteman, T. A., Hughes, L. F., and Caspary, D. M. (2008). Aged-related loss of temporal processing: altered responses to amplitude modulated tones in rat dorsal cochlear nucleus. *Neuroscience* 154, 329–337. doi: 10.1016/j.neuroscience.2008.02.025

Schuknecht, H. F., and Gacek, M. R. (1993). Cochlear pathology in presbycusis. *Ann. Otol. Rhinol. Laryngol.* 102, 1–16. doi: 10.1177/00034894931020s101

Seeman, M., (1960). *Czech Speech Audiometry.* Prague: SZN.

Sergeyenko, Y., Lall, K., Liberman, M. C., and Kujawa, S. G. (2013). Age-related cochlear synaptopathy: an early-onset contributor to auditory functional decline. *J. Neurosci.* 33, 13686–13694. doi: 10.1523/jneurosci.1783-13.2013

Sheldon, S., Pichora-Fuller, M. K., and Schneider, B. A. (2008). Priming and sentence context support listening to noise-vocoded speech by younger and older adults. *J. Acoust. Soc. Am.* 123, 489–499. doi: 10.1121/1.2783762

Singh, G., Pichora-Fuller, M. K., and Schneider, B. A. (2008). The effect of age on auditory spatial attention in conditions of real and simulated spatial separation. *J. Acoust. Soc. Am.* 124, 1294–1305. doi: 10.1121/1.2949399

Snell, K. B. (1997). Age-related changes in temporal gap detection. *J. Acoust. Soc. Am.* 101, 2214–2220. doi: 10.1121/1.418205

Strouse, A., Ashmead, D. H., Ohde, R. N., and Grantham, D. W. (1998). Temporal processing in the aging auditory system. *J. Acoust. Soc. Am.* 104, 2385–2399. doi: 10.1121/1.423748

Sussman, E. S., Horváth, J., Winkler, I., and Orr, M. (2007). The role of attention in the formation of auditory streams. *Percept. Psychophys.* 69, 136–152. doi: 10.3758/bf03194460

Suta, D., Rybalko, N., Pelánová, J., Popelář, J., and Syka, J. (2011). Age-related changes in auditory temporal processing in the rat. *Exp. Gerontol.* 46, 739–746. doi: 10.1016/j.exger.2011.05.004

Syka, J. (2002). Plastic changes in the central auditory system after hearing loss, restoration of function, and during learning. *Physiol. Rev.* 82, 601–636. doi: 10.1152/physrev.00002.2002

Syka, J. (2010). The fischer 344 rat as a model of presbycusis. *Hear. Res.* 264, 70–78. doi: 10.1016/j.heares.2009.11.003

Tadros, S. F., Frisina, S. T., Mapes, F., Kim, S., Frisina, D. R., and Frisina, R. D. (2005). Loss of peripheral right-ear advantage in age-related hearing loss. *Audiol. Neurootol.* 10, 44–52. doi: 10.1159/000082307

Ueberfuhr, M. A., Fehlberg, H., Goodman, S. S., and Withnell, R. H. (2016). A DPOAE assessment of outer hair cell integrity in ears with age-related hearing loss. *Hear. Res.* 332, 137–150. doi: 10.1016/j.heares.2015.11.006

Vielsmeier, V., Lehner, A., Strutz, J., Steffens, T., Kreuzer, P. M., Schecklmann, M., et al. (2015). The relevance of the high frequency audiometry in tinnitus patients with normal hearing in conventional pure-tone audiometry. *BioMed Res. Int.* 2015:302515. doi: 10.1155/2015/302515

Walton, J. P., Frisina, R. D., and O'Neill, W. E. (1998). Age-related alteration in processing of temporal sound features in the auditory midbrain of the CBA mouse. *J. Neurosci.* 18, 2764–2776. doi: 10.1523/jneurosci.18-07-02764.1998

Wiley, T. L., Cruickshanks, K. J., Nondahl, D. M., Tweed, T. S., Klein, R., Klein, R., et al. (1998). Aging and high-frequency hearing sensitivity. *J. Speech Lang. Hear. Res.* 41, 1061–1072. doi: 10.1044/jslhr.4105.1061

Williamson, T. T., Zhu, X., Walton, J. P., and Frisina, R. D. (2015). Auditory brainstem gap responses start to decline in mice in middle age: a novel physiological biomarker for age-related hearing loss. *Cell Tissue Res.* 361, 359–369. doi: 10.1007/s00441-014-2003-9

Willott, J. F. (1996). Anatomic and physiologic aging: a behavioral neuroscience perspective. *J. Am. Acad. Audiol.* 7, 141–151.

Wingfield, A. (1996). Cognitive factors in auditory performance: context, speed of processing, and constraints of memory. *J. Am. Acad. Audiol.* 7, 175–182.

Wingfield, A., McCoy, S. L., Peelle, J. E., Tun, P. A., and Cox, L. C. (2006). Effects of adult aging and hearing loss on comprehension of rapid speech varying in syntactic complexity. *J. Am. Acad. Audiol.* 17, 487–497. doi: 10.3766/jaaa.17.7.4

Zeng, F.-G., Kong, Y.-Y., Michalewski, H. J., and Starr, A. (2005). Perceptual consequences of disrupted auditory nerve activity. *J. Neurophysiol.* 93, 3050–3063. doi: 10.1152/jn.00985.2004

7

The Impact of Self-Reported Hearing Difficulties on Memory Collaboration in Older Adults

Amanda J. Barnier[1,2]*, Celia B. Harris[1,2], Thomas Morris[1,3], Paul Strutt[1,2] and Greg Savage[1,4]

[1] Australian Research Council Centre of Excellence in Cognition and Its Disorders, Macquarie University, Sydney, NSW, Australia, [2] Department of Cognitive Science, Macquarie University, Sydney, NSW, Australia, [3] Dementia Centre, HammondCare, Greenwich, NSW, Australia, [4] Department of Psychology, Macquarie University, Sydney, NSW, Australia

*Correspondence:
Amanda J. Barnier
amanda.barnier@mq.edu.au

Cognitive scientists and philosophers recently have highlighted the value of thinking about people at risk of or living with dementia as intertwined parts of broader cognitive systems that involve their spouse, family, friends, or carers. By this view, we rely on people and things around us to "scaffold" mental processes such as memory. In the current study, we identified 39 long-married, older adult couples who are part of the Australian Imaging Biomarkers and Lifestyle (AIBL) Study of Ageing; all were cognitively healthy but half were subjective memory complainers. During two visits to their homes 1 week apart, we assessed husbands' and wives' cognitive performance across a range of everyday memory tasks working alone (Week 1) versus together (Week 2), including a Friends Task where they provided first and last names of their friends and acquaintances. As reported elsewhere, elderly couples recalled many more friends' names working together compared to alone. Couples who remembered successfully together used well-developed, rich, sensitive, and dynamic communication strategies to boost each other's recall. However, if one or both spouses self-reported mild-to-moderate or severe hearing difficulties (56% of husbands, 31% of wives), couples received less benefit from collaboration. Our findings imply that hearing loss may disrupt collaborative support structures that couples (and other intimate communicative partners) hone over decades together. We discuss the possibility that, cut off from the social world that scaffolds them, hearing loss may place older adults at greater risk of cognitive decline and dementia.

Keywords: memory, aging, collaborative recall, conversation, transactive memory, distributed cognition, hearing loss, presbycusis

INTRODUCTION

Across a lifetime in intimate relationships involving joint memory and action, people form expert "remembering systems" that may have (much) later cognitive payoffs (Harris et al., 2011, 2014a; Barnier et al., 2018a). Intimate partners, family members, and friends form complex, distributed "transactive memory systems" (Wegner et al., 1985; Wegner, 1987) that allow them to accomplish more together than when they work alone (Barnier et al., 2008, 2018b; Harris et al., 2014b). However, this "collaborative benefit" is not observed in all groups. In fact, most studies of memory collaboration involving either younger or older pairs of strangers demonstrate "collaborative inhibition," where individuals recalling separately outperform groups on tests of memory recall (see Basden et al., 1997; Weldon and Bellinger, 1997; Harris et al., 2008; Meade and Roediger, 2009; Rajaram, 2011; Marion and Thorley, 2016).

However, studies of collaborative memory in stranger dyads do not capture well the high levels of shared knowledge developed over the course of a lifetime of shared experiences, and rarely consider the degree to which collaborative benefits may be more (or less) related to the type of information (personal or non-personal) to be remembered (Barnier et al., 2013; Dixon, 2013). Recent work conducted by our group has sought to extend the standard collaborative recall paradigm to older, long-married couples who share a lifetime of remembering together (e.g., Harris et al., 2011, 2017; Barnier et al., 2018a); the kinds of groups that might be expected to develop transactive memory systems (Wegner, 1987; Barnier et al., 2018b). We also have investigated the degree to which tasks that involve recalling personal shared knowledge, rather than non-personal recall tasks, might lead to different patterns of collaborative success and failure. Results indicate that older, long-married couples benefit from collaboration on memory recall tasks, particularly those that require recall of personal shared knowledge (e.g., names of friends and acquaintances) (Barnier et al., 2018a). However, not all couples benefit from collaboration in the same way, despite sharing much of their adult lives together. Even among long-married couples, we find substantial individual differences in the extent to which they collaborate effectively. To gain a better understanding of why this is the case, we and other researchers have transcribed, coded, and analyzed collaborating couples' (and other dyads') conversations to identify characteristics of their communication that lead to the greatest benefits during collaborative recall (e.g., Johansson et al., 2005; Vredeveldt et al., 2016; Harris et al., 2018). In other words, it is not merely the length of a relationship that predicts collaborative success, but the ability to effectively communicate with one another (see also Harris et al., 2014b).

Given that our work so far has shown that collaboration can benefit recall performance and that communication is central to this success, it is important to consider factors that may disrupt communication. The ability to hear connects us to the world and the people around us and is fundamental to everyday cognitive and emotional health and well-being (Beechey et al., 2018). Age-related hearing loss is highly prevalent in older adults; the World Health Organization estimates that 1 in 3 people over 65 years of age are affected by disabling hearing loss (Chia et al., 2007; World Health Organization, 2019). Hearing loss also is a significant risk factor for dementia (Lin et al., 2011; Livingston et al., 2017; Jayakody et al., 2018), suggesting a possible association between hearing and memory function. Given this association, and the body of work demonstrating benefits of collaboration for memory recall in older adults, it is important to investigate whether hearing loss disrupts access to the benefits of shared remembering. If family and friends scaffold our cognition *via* joint collaborative remembering, and we in turn help to scaffold them (Harris et al., 2014b; Barnier et al., 2018a,b), we may

lose the potential cognitive and memory benefits associated with collaboration if we are less able to hear and communicate with the people around us.

In the current study, long-married older adults completed a self-report questionnaire about the extent to which they experience social and emotional difficulties related to hearing loss, and completed a series of memory tasks individually and with their spouse. We expected that if at least one member of a couple reported everyday hearing difficulties, it would disrupt their ability to remember together and reduce collaborative memory benefits. Further, we expected an association between severity of hearing loss within couples and collaborative benefits, whereby couples reporting the greatest level of hearing difficulty would benefit least from collaboration with their spouse.

METHOD

Participants

Participants were 78 men and women (39 men, 39 women) aged 68–90 years old ($M = 74.74$, $SD = 5.10$). These individuals formed 39 male–female couples, who had been married for 13–65 years ($M = 49.46$, $SD = 8.78$). Participants were a subset of those from the Australian Imaging Biomarkers and Lifestyle Study of Ageing (AIBL; Ellis et al., 2009) and had been classified as cognitively healthy based on their most recent AIBL assessment, as well as their performance on the Mini-Mental State Examination (MMSE; Folstein et al., 1975) on the day of our testing (see also Barnier et al., 2018a; Harris et al., 2018). However, half of our sample were classified as subjective memory complainers because, despite being cognitively healthy according to objective measures, they answered yes to the question "Do you have difficulties with your memory?" at their last AIBL assessment.

The AIBL Study was established in 2006 with 1,112 individuals recruited during the baseline phase. They underwent a screening interview, cognitive and mood assessments, and blood-based biomarker analyses, and completed health and lifestyle questionnaires. Approximately a quarter of the sample underwent brain imaging, including magnetic resonance imaging (MRI) and Pittsburgh compound B–positron emission tomography (PiB-PET). A clinical review panel considered all medical, psychiatric, neuropsychological, and health data and classified 768 as healthy controls, 133 as having mild cognitive impairment (MCI; Petersen et al., 1999; Winblad et al., 2004), and 211 as having Alzheimer's disease (McKhann et al., 1984). Follow-up assessments of participants have occurred approximately every 18 months, with Wave 4 testing occurring prior to our data collection, and 54 months following initial baseline testing. Further details of the study and baseline characteristics are reported in Ellis et al. (2009). For the current study, we identified 94 individuals who were being tracked as healthy controls within the AIBL sample, and who happened to be married to another AIBL participant (i.e., the whole AIBL sample contained 47 married couples). We first contacted couples *via* a letter inviting them to participate and confirmed their interest by telephone. Seventy-eight individuals (39 couples) were interested and available to participate, and these were our participants for the current study.

Measures and Procedure

The Macquarie University Human Research Ethics Committee provided ethical approval for this research and the AIBL Management Committee approved access to their participants and the study design. Prior to the experimental sessions, all participants received and completed the Hearing Handicap Inventory for the Elderly – Screening Version (HHIE-S; Ventry and Weinstein, 1983). The HHIE-S is a 10-item questionnaire measuring perceived social and emotional impacts of hearing loss using a self-report format. Responses are provided on a three-point scale "Yes" (4 points), "Sometimes" (2 points), "No" (0 points). Scores range from 0 to 40; scores of 0–8 typically indicate no (self-reported) hearing difficulties; scores of 10–24 typically indicate mild-to-moderate hearing difficulties; and scores of 26–40 typically indicate severe hearing difficulties.

On the day of testing in Week 1, participants also completed the MMSE (Folstein et al., 1975) and the Geriatric Depression Scale – Short Form (GDS-SF; Yesavage and Sheikh, 1986). The MMSE is a brief screen of general cognitive ability including items that assess orientation, registration, attention, recall, language, and visuospatial ability. The MMSE is scored out of 30; scores of 24 or above typically indicate healthy cognition. The GDS-SF is a brief measure of depressive symptoms including "yes" or "no" questions regarding how the participant felt over the last week. The GDS-SF is scored out of 15; scores of 6 or above typically indicate depressive symptoms requiring further investigation. Our participants had a mean MMSE score of 28.87 ($SD = 1.48$) and a mean GDS-SF score of 1.08 ($SD = 1.38$).

Individual and collaborative sessions were conducted in participants' homes, 1 week apart. Week 1 involved an individual recall session, while Week 2 involved a collaborative recall session. During each of the two sessions, participants completed a range of memory tasks that varied by type and degree of personal significance of the information recalled. Overall performance across these tasks is reported elsewhere (Barnier et al., 2018a). We focus in this paper on a "Mutual Friends" recall task, where participants were required to recall the names of as many mutual friends and acquaintances as possible in 2 min. In Week 1, two experimenters administered the recall tasks individually but simultaneously in separate rooms of the couples' home. In Week 2, the experimenters returned to the couples' home and tested participants together on the same recall tasks in a collaborative recall session. Participants were not reimbursed for their involvement in our study; however, morning or afternoon tea was provided by the experimenters. We focus in particular on the impact of hearing loss on couples' individual and collaborative performance.

RESULTS

Influences of Collaboration on Recall

In the collaborative recall paradigm, the impact of recalling together is indexed by comparing collaborative output with the pooled, non-redundant output of individuals recalling alone. As reported in Barnier et al. (2018a), a t-test revealed that couples recalled significantly more names of mutual friends together in Week 2 ($M_{recall} = 47.64$, $SD = 17.99$) compared to their pooled individual or "nominal" recall in Week 1 ($M_{recall} = 30.85$, $SD = 12.34$); a paired-samples t-test comparing these scores was significant, $t(38) = 10.02$, $p < 0.001$. Therefore, on average, couples showed collaborative facilitation on the Mutual Friends task, recalling 16.79 more names ($SD = 10.46$) when they remembered together compared to separately. However, underneath this group level performance, there was considerable variability in the degree of collaborative benefit achieved by each couple. We indexed individual differences in the outcomes of collaboration by assigning each couple a "collaborative benefit" score, which was the difference between the number of names couples recalled during collaboration and the combined number of names recalled by husbands and wives during their individual recall. While no couples showed inhibited recall during collaboration compared to their nominal performance, collaborative benefit scores ranged from 0 to 38 extra names. Whereas 25% of couples gained six or fewer extra names when they collaborated, 25% gained 24 or more extra names. In other words, whereas some couples collaborated very successfully, others gained little or no benefit in terms of performance when collaborating with their spouse. Do hearing difficulties help to explain why?

Impact of Hearing Difficulties on Individual Memory

On the HHIE-S, individual scores ranged from 0 to 32 (out of 40). **Table 1** presents the number of participants who reported no hearing difficulties (0–8), mild-to-moderate hearing difficulties (10–24), and severe hearing difficulties (26–40) as well as mean HHIE-S scores and other demographic information. Analysis revealed some differences in the characteristics of participants across these three hearing classifications (see **Table 1**). A chi-square analysis of frequencies indicated a trend toward gender differences, such that more men than women tended to appear in the two hearing loss categories, $\chi^2(2,78) = 5.37$, $p = 0.068$. The increased hearing difficulties reported by men may reflect a greater willingness by men to report or the fact that, within couples, husbands ($M_{age} = 76.15$, $SD = 5.44$) were slightly, but significantly, older than wives ($M_{age} = 73.33$, $SD = 4.37$), $t(38) = 5.08$, $p < 0.001$. Indeed, we found significant age differences across participants in the different hearing classifications. A one-way analysis of variance (ANOVA) of hearing group on age was significant, $F(2, 77) = 8.65$, $p < 0.001$. Follow-up comparisons (with a Bonferroni adjustment on reported p-values) suggested that each of the three hearing classifications differed from the others in age either marginally or significantly, with a pattern that hearing difficulties increased with age, all $ps < 0.073$ (see **Table 1**).

Participants across hearing classifications did not differ in cognitive measures. A one-way ANOVA of hearing group on MMSE scores was not significant, $F(2, 77) = 1.02$, $p = 0.367$, and neither was a chi-square analysis of the frequencies of subjective

TABLE 1 | Frequency of self-reported hearing difficulties, with mean HHIE-S scores, demographics, and individual recall scores.

	No Hearing Difficulties	Mild–Moderate Hearing Difficulties	Severe Hearing Difficulties
Number of participants	44	27	7
Hearing difficulties (HHIE-S)	3.41 (2.78)	14.07 (3.70)	28.57 (2.23)
Sex (% female)	61.4	37.0	28.6
Age	73.14 (4.37)	75.89 (5.12)	80.43 (4.58)
MMSE	29.00 (1.33)	28.85 (1.73)	28.14 (1.35)
Subjective memory complainers (%)	45.5	59.3	57.1
Depression (GDS)	0.84 (1.28)	1.19 (1.21)	2.14 (2.19)
Years of education	14.37 (4.23)	14.85 (4.24)	13.5 (2.88)
Individual recall	19.30 (10.08)	19.26 (7.34)	14.29 (10.19)
Range	3–46	4–33	0–25

Unless otherwise stated, values are means with standard deviations in parentheses.

memory complainers in each group, $\chi^2(2,78) = 1.38$, $p = 0.501$. There was a marginal main effect suggesting increased depression symptomatology with increased severity of hearing difficulties, $F(2, 77) = 2.94$, $p = 0.059$, but across classifications, participants' average GDS scores were well below the clinical cutoff of 6 (see **Table 1**).

On the Week 1 individual memory test, HHIE-S scores were not correlated with the number of names participants recalled, $r = -0.086$, $p = 0.452$. Instead, across our three hearing groups, a one-way ANOVA showed that participants recalled a similar number of names, $F(2, 77) = 0.88$, $p = 0.418$ (see **Table 1**). Self-reported hearing difficulties did not influence Week 1 individual memory performance on the Mutual Friends task when participants recalled alone in the presence of an experimenter.

Impact of Hearing Difficulties on Collaborative Memory

In Week 2, we explicitly instructed couples to "work together" to recall as many names as possible. Since we analyzed collaborative recall at the couple level, we classified couples into three groups to mirror our individual hearing classifications: (1) no hearing difficulties reported ($n = 12$ couples; 30.7%), (2) at least one spouse with mild hearing difficulties ($n = 20$ couples; 51.3%); and (3) at least one spouse with severe hearing difficulties ($n = 7$ couples; 17.9%). We conducted a one-way ANOVA to compare collaborative benefit scores across these three groups. This analysis yielded a significant main effect of group, $F(2, 38) = 3.57$, $p = 0.039$, and a significant linear function, $F(2, 38) = 7.14$, $p = 0.011$. Follow up comparisons (with a Bonferroni adjustment on reported p-values) indicated that couples in which at least one member reported severe hearing difficulties collaborated far less successfully ($M_{benefit} = 8.86$, $SD = 9.21$) than couples in which neither member reported hearing difficulties ($M_{benefit} = 21.33$, $SD = 11.57$), $p = 0.034$. The benefit scores for couples in which at least one member reported mild-to-moderate

difficulties ($M_{benefit} = 16.85$, $SD = 8.86$) fell in the middle and was not significantly different from the other two groups, $ps > 0.21$. The linear function suggests that collaborative benefit decreased as hearing difficulties within the couples increased.

To further examine this linear relationship between hearing difficulties and collaborative benefit within each couple, we added husbands' and wives' individual HHIE-S scores to create a measure of couple-level hearing difficulties. Higher additive scores indicate more reported hearing problems by the couples (possible range: 0–80). Couples' additive scores ranged from 4 to 56 ($M_{couple} = 18.72$, $SD = 11.69$). This range suggests that it was relatively uncommon for both partners to report very high levels of hearing difficulties. Indeed, there were no cases in which both spouses reported severe hearing difficulties, only 3 (7.7%) cases in which one spouse reported significant difficulties and the other reported mild-to-moderate difficulties, and only 4 (10.3%) cases in which both spouses reported mild-to-moderate hearing difficulties. Instead, in 20 out of 39 cases (51.3%), one of the partners reported (mild-to-moderate or severe) hearing difficulties and the other reported no difficulties. In other words, many couples showed asymmetrical profiles with one spouse struggling to hear more than the other. Consistent with the linear relationship described above, couples' combined hearing difficulty scores correlated negatively with their collaborative benefit scores, $r = -0.34$, $p = 0.033$ (two-tailed). Overall, our results suggest that greater hearing difficulties within couples' "systems" reduced the success of their memory collaboration.

DISCUSSION

In this study, we aimed to identify whether self-reported hearing difficulties reduced the benefits of collaborative recall in older, long-married couples. Because the benefits of collaboration are driven by effective communication (Harris et al., 2011, 2018; see Vredeveldt et al., 2016, for similar findings in a forensic context), we expected that hearing difficulties might reduce couples' ability to communicate and collaborate successfully. Self-reported hearing difficulties were not related to individual recall performance, and this may reflect the fact that recalling names of friends and acquaintances alone in Week 1 did not depend on discussion with anyone else. However, during collaboration in Week 2, couples benefited less from the opportunity to recall with their spouse when at least one member of the couple reported hearing difficulties. Moreover, the impact of these difficulties appeared additive, with couples' combined scores associated with less successful collaboration. Therefore, our results, while exploratory, suggest that hearing difficulties reduce the benefits of remembering with a close collaborative partner.

These results highlight the critical importance of communication in driving the outcomes of collaborative recall in intimate couples. This central role for communication was predicted by transactive memory theory (Wegner, 1987; see also Barnier et al., 2018b) and confirmed in at least two prior studies of collaborative recall of older couples (Harris et al., 2011, 2018). If strategic, sensitive, and engaged communication – such as cuing, repetition, and rapid turn-taking – supports more effective collaboration, then hearing difficulties will invariably disrupt these processes of transactive memory or "distributed cognition" (Barnier et al., 2008; Harris et al., 2014b).

To illustrate the potential impact of hearing difficulties on collaborative recall, we briefly offer the case of Paul and Irene (not their real names), one of the long-married couples who participated in this study. At the time of testing, Paul was 87 years old, Irene was 77 years old, and they had been married for 57 years. Paul's HHIE-S score was 30, representing severe self-reported hearing difficulties, whereas Irene's score was 6, representing no hearing difficulties (although their verbal interactions transcribed below suggest otherwise for Irene). On the Mutual Friends task in Week 1, Paul recalled 9 names of mutual friends and acquaintances and Irene recalled 8 when they recalled individually with the experimenters. This gave them a total (pooled, nominal) score of 17 names at Week 1. When they worked together on this task 1 week later, they again recalled 17 names, experiencing no benefit from collaboration relative to remembering alone. This stands in contrast to the average collaborative benefit for all couples of nearly 17 names and the average collaborative benefit for couples without hearing difficulties of over 21 names (reported above).

When we looked closely at Paul and Irene's conversation during the Mutual Friends task (and other tasks; see Barnier et al., 2018a), their failure of collaboration appeared to be due, at least in part, to difficulties in hearing. Based on these transcripts, individuals' hearing difficulties appeared to lead to difficulties in tracking information offered by their spouse and difficulties in successfully cueing their spouse with useful memory prompts.

Husband: I can't think of . . . Who lent you those books?
Wife: *Pardon?*
Husband: Lent you the books and magazines. We've got to get them back to her.
Wife: *I can't hear you.*
Husband: She lent you the books and magazines.
Wife: *Oh. Yeah.*
Husband: We've got to get them back to them. But I can't think of their name.
Wife: *No, I can't either.*
Husband: I'm looking at a lot of people but I just can't remember the names.

Finally, here is a segment of transcript from Paul and Irene's conversation during a second task in which we asked couples to name European countries (reported in Barnier et al., 2018a):

Husband: Scotland. Ireland. England. France. Germany. Luxembourg. Norway. Holland. Um. Sweden.
Wife: *I'm having terrible trouble hearing you.*
Husband: Sweden. Holland. I have said Luxembourg.
Wife: *Ah Switzerland. Germany. Austria.*
Husband: Austria.
Wife: *Latvia.*
Husband: Latvia.
Wife: *Ukraine. Czechoslovakia.*
Husband: Spain. Italy.
Wife: *France. Belgium. I don't know whether we said that.*

Husband: Genoa. Russia.
Wife: *Lithuania.*
Husband: Greenland.
Wife: *Hmm?*
Husband: Greenland I said.
Wife: *Speak up!*
Husband: Greenland! Turkey. No Turkey. That's not part of Europe. Belgium.
Wife: *Norway. Sweden. Finland.*
Husband: Scotland.
Wife: *I don't think we said Wales. Jutland.*
Husband: Hmm? Did you say Denmark?

Compare their collaboration to the following segment of transcript from a different couple's conversation during the Mutual Friends task. In this case, neither spouse reported hearing difficulties, and their collaboration was characterized by cross-cuing with shared knowledge, effective coordination of recall, and turn-taking:

Wife: *. . . and Glenda but I don't know what her last name is. . .*
Husband: Glenda Warren.
Wife: *Yeah. Julie Hooper.*
Husband: And Peter Hamilton.
Wife: *Yeah. And Bridget and. . .*
Husband: Bridget and James Whitmore. Yes.
Wife: *Okay where do we go now? Barry and Martha Gillis. Mirabelle and Graham Taylor. Jenny and Gary Tipper. . .*
Husband: You're going through your Christmas list, ha ha.
Wife: *Yes. Annabeth and Bill Boswell.*
Husband: Yeah. Katrina and Gomez Murray.

These examples underscore the importance of hearing and communication in successful memory collaboration.

There are several limitations to the current research, which means that these findings represent an exploratory first step in revealing a link between hearing loss and failures of memory scaffolding. Our sample was relatively small, especially when divided into hearing categories. We measured hearing difficulties *via* self-report of functional everyday impacts of hearing difficulties. Future research should include objective measures of hearing loss (e.g., audiometry, hearing performance in conversation). As is evident in the transcript above, self-report may not capture all cases or degrees of hearing loss. Whereas our measure of couple level hearing difficulties was relatively crude in simply adding spouses' hearing scores, the impact of individual hearing loss within social systems such as long-married couples may be exponential rather than additive, emergent in combination with other factors, or buffered by still other factors (for further discussion of this problem of navigating from individual to couple levels of analysis, see Barnier et al., 2016, 2018b). We need to unpack the consequences of hearing difficulties for individuals as well as their most intimate partners (i.e., the third-party disability). Finally, we cannot establish causality in the current data, and future research should examine whether treating hearing loss *via* hearing aids or implants may lead to a recovery of collaborative benefits as well as whether other demographic or health variables play an important role in links between hearing and collaborative performance.

Despite these limitations, these findings have implications for more than just an individual who experiences everyday hearing difficulties. As members of distributed cognitive systems, we rely on one another to support and extend each other's cognition (Barnier et al., 2008, 2014). For older adults in particular, the benefits of collaboration with a close family member or friend may protect (or compensate for) memory in the face of age- or disease-related decline (e.g., Kemper et al., 1995; Ross et al., 2004; Rauers et al., 2010; Hydén, 2011). However, when they are socially and cognitively cut off from the world that scaffolds them, hearing loss may place older adults at greater risk of cognitive decline. This possibility may help to explain significant, but still unexplained, links between hearing loss and increased dementia risk (e.g., Livingston et al., 2017) as well as the more recent and provocative links between marriage and reduced dementia risk (e.g., Sundström et al., 2016; Sommerlad et al., 2017). Interventions designed to support hearing, communication, and collaboration may prevent or delay cognitive decline and may even reduce dementia incidence in later life.

AUTHOR CONTRIBUTIONS

AB, CH, TM, and GS developed and designed the study. GS facilitated access to the AIBL participants. TM and AB led the conduct of the study and data collection assisted by CH and two research assistants. AB and PS led the statistical analysis assisted by CH and TM. AB and PS drafted the manuscript with contributions from CH and TM. All authors contributed to manuscript revision led by AB and CH, and read and approved the submitted version.

ACKNOWLEDGMENTS

The authors acknowledge and thank the men and women from the Australian Imaging, Biomarkers and Lifestyle Study of Ageing (AIBL; https://aibl.csiro.au) who participated in our study and whose long-term generosity and commitment to science are helping to understand trajectories of cognitive decline and predictors of dementia. The authors also acknowledge and thank Professor David Ames and Dr. Joanne Robertson from AIBL who supported this research with access to the AIBL sample and data, and Jennifer Broekhuijse, Anton Harris, Sophia Harris, Nina McIlwain, and Dr. Katya Numbers for research assistance during this project, especially during data collection (JB and KN), and data transcription and coding (JB, AH, SH, and NM).

REFERENCES

Barnier, A. J., Harris, C. B., and Congleton, A. R. (2013). Mind the gap: generations of questions in the early science of collaborative recall. *J. Appl. Res. Mem. Cogn.* 2, 124–127. doi: 10.1016/j.jarmac.2013.05.002

Barnier, A. J., Harris, C. B., Morris, T., and Savage, G. (2018a). Collaborative facilitation in older couples: successful joint remembering across memory tasks. *Front. Psychol.* 9:2385. doi: 10.3389/fpsyg.2018.02385

Barnier, A. J., Klein, L., and Harris, C. B. (2018b). Transactive memory in small, intimate groups: more than the sum of their parts. *Small Group Res.* 49, 62–97. doi: 10.1177/1046496417712439

Barnier, A. J., Harris, C. B., and Sutton, J. (2016). The hows and whys of "we" (and "I") in groups [Commentary on Baumeister, Ainsworth, & Vohs, 2016]. *Behav. Brain Sci.* 39:e138. doi: 10.1017/S0140525X15001260

Barnier, A. J., Priddis, A. C., Broekhuijse, J. M., Harris, C. B., Cox, R. E., Addis, D. R., et al. (2014). Reaping what they sow: benefits of remembering together in intimate couples. *J. Appl. Res. Mem. Cogn.* 3, 261–265. doi: 10.1016/j.jarmac.2014.06.003

Barnier, A. J., Sutton, J., Harris, C. B., and Wilson, R. A. (2008). A conceptual and empirical framework for the social distribution of cognition: the case of memory [Special Issue]. *Cogn. Syst. Res. Perspect. Soc Cogn.* 9, 33–51. doi: 10.1016/j.cogsys.2007.07.002

Basden, B. H., Basden, D. R., Bryner, S., and Thomas, R. L. (1997). A comparison of group and individual remembering: does collaboration disrupt. *J. Exp. Psychol. Learn. Mem. Cogn.* 23, 1176–1191. doi: 10.1037//0278-7393.23.5.1176

Beechey, T., Buchholz, J. M., and Keidser, G. (2018). Measuring communication difficulty through effortful speech production during conversation. *Speech Commun.* 100, 18–29. doi: 10.1016/j.specom.2018.04.007

Chia, E. M., Wang, J. J., Rochtchina, E., Cumming, R. R., Newall, P., and Mitchell, P. (2007). Hearing impairment and health-related quality of life: the blue mountains hearing study. *Ear Hear.* 28, 187–195. doi: 10.1097/aud.0b013e31803126b6

Dixon, R. A. (2013). Collaborative memory research in aging: supplemental perspectives on application. *J. Appl. Res. Mem. Cogn.* 2, 128–130. doi: 10.1016/j.jarmac.2013.05.001

Ellis, K. A., Bush, A. I., Darby, D., De Fazio, D., Foster, J., Hudson, P., et al. (2009). The australian imaging, biomarkers and lifestyle (AIBL) study of aging: methodology and baseline characteristics of 1112 individuals recruited for a longitudinal study of Alzheimer's disease. *Int. Psychogeriatr.* 21, 672–687. doi: 10.1017/s1041610209009405

Folstein, M. F., Folstein, S. E., and McHugh, P. R. (1975). Mini-mental state". A practical method for grading the cognitive state of patients for the clinician. *J. Psychiatr. Res.* 12, 189–198.

Harris, C. B., Barnier, A. J., Sutton, J., and Keil, P. G. (2014a). Couples as socially distributed cognitive systems: remembering in everyday social and material contexts. *Mem. Stud.* 7, 285–297. doi: 10.1177/1750698014530619

Harris, C. B., Rasmussen, A. S., and Berntsen, D. (2014b). The functions of autobiographical memory: an integrative approach. *Memory* 22, 559–581. doi: 10.1080/09658211.2013.806555

Harris, C. B., Barnier, A. J., Sutton, J., Keil, P. G., and Dixon, R. A. (2017). "Going episodic": collaborative inhibition and facilitation when long-married couples remember together. *Memory* 25, 1148–1159. doi: 10.1080/09658211.2016.1274405

Harris, C. B., Barnier, A. J., Sutton, J., and Savage, G. (2018). Features of successful and unsuccessful collaborative memory conversations in long-married couples. *Top. Cogn. Sci.* doi: 10.1080/09658211.2016.1274405 [Epub ahead of print].

Harris, C. B., Keil, P. G., Sutton, J., Barnier, A. J., and McIlwain, D. J. F. (2011). We remember, we forget: collaborative remembering in older couples. *Disc. Process.* 48, 267–303. doi: 10.1080/0163853X.2010.541854

Harris, C. B., Paterson, H. M., and Kemp, R. I. (2008). Collaborative recall and collective memory: what happens when we remember together? *Memory* 16, 213–230. doi: 10.1080/09658210701811862

Hydén, L. C. (2011). Narrative collaboration and scaffolding in dementia. *J. Aging Stud.* 25, 339–347. doi: 10.1016/j.jaging.2011.04.002

Jayakody, D. M. P., Friedland, P. L., Eikelboom, R. H., Martins, R. N., and Sohrabi, H. R. (2018). A novel study on association between untreated hearing loss and cognitive functions of older adults: baseline non-verbal cognitive assessment results. *Clin. Otolaryngol.* 43, 182–191. doi: 10.1111/coa.12937

Johansson, N. O., Andersson, J., and Rönnberg, J. (2005). Compensating strategies in collaborative remembering in very old couples. *Scand. J. Psychol.* 46, 349–359. doi: 10.1111/j.1467-9450.2005.00465.x

Kemper, S., Lyons, K., and Anagnopoulos, C. (1995). Joint storytelling by patients with Alzheimer's-Disease and their spouses. *Disc. Process.* 20, 205–217. doi: 10.1080/01638539509544938

Lin, F. R., Metter, E. J., O'Brien, R. J., Resnick, S. M., Zonderman, A. B., and Ferrucci, L. (2011). Hearing loss and incident dementia. *Arch. Neurol.* 68, 214–220. doi: 10.1001/archneurol.2010.362

Livingston, G., Sommerlad, A., Orgeta, V., Costafreda, S. G., Huntley, J., Ames, D., et al. (2017). Dementia prevention, intervention, and care. *Lancet* 390, 2673–2734. doi: 10.1016/s0140-6736(17)31363-6

Marion, S. B., and Thorley, C. (2016). A meta-analytic review of collaborative inhibition and post collaborative memory: testing the predictions of the retrieval strategy disruption hypothesis. *Psychol. Bull.* 142, 1141–1164. doi: 10.1037/bul0000071

McKhann, G., Drachman, D., Folstein, M., Katzman, R., Price, D., and Stadlan, E. M. (1984). Clinical diagnosis of Alzheimer's disease: report of the NINCDS-ADRDA Work Group under the auspices of Department of Health and Human Services Task Force on Alzheimer's Disease. *Neurology* 34, 939–944. doi: 10.1212/wnl.34.7.939

Meade, M. L., and Roediger, H. L. (2009). Age differences in collaborative memory: the role of retrieval manipulations. *Mem. Cogn.* 37, 962–975. doi: 10.3758/MC. 37.7.962

Petersen, R. C., Smith, G. E., Waring, S. C., Ivnik, R. J., Tangalos, E. G., and Kokmen, E. (1999). Mild cognitive impairment: clinical characterization and outcome. *Arch. Neurol.* 56, 303–308. doi: 10.1001/archneur.56.3.303

Rajaram, S. (2011). Collaboration both hurts and helps memory: a cognitive perspective. *Curr. Direct. Psychol. Sci.* 20, 76–81. doi: 10.1177/096372141 1403251

Rauers, A., Riediger, M., Schmiedek, F., and Lindenberger, U. (2010). With a little help from my spouse: does spousal collaboration compensate for the effects of cognitive aging? *Gerontology* 57, 161–166. doi: 10.1159/000317335

Ross, M., Spencer, S. J., Linardatos, L., Lam, K. C. H., and Perunovic, M. (2004). Going shopping and identifying landmarks: does collaboration improve older people's memory? *Appil. Cogn. Psychol.* 18, 683–696. doi: 10.1002/acp. 1023

Sommerlad, A., Rueggar, J., Singh-Manoux, A., Lewis, G., and Livingston, G. (2017). Marriage and risk of dementia: systematic review and meta-analysis of observational studies. *J. Neurol. Neurosurg. Psychiatry.* 89:227. doi: 10.1136/jnnp-2017-316274

Sundström, A., Westerlund, O., and Kotyrlo, E. (2016). Marital status and risk of dementia: a nationwide population-based prospective study from Sweden. *BMJ Open* 6:e008565. doi: 10.1136/bmjopen-2015-008565

Ventry, I. M., and Weinstein, B. E. (1983). Identification of elderly people with hearing problems. *ASHA* 25, 37–42.

Vredeveldt, A., Hildebrandt, A., and Van Koppen, P. J. (2016). Acknowledge, repeat, rephrase, elaborate: witnesses can help each other remember more. *Memory* 24, 669–682. doi: 10.1080/09658211.2015.1042884

Wegner, D. M. (1987). "Transactive memory: a contemporary analysis of the group mind," in *Theories of Group Behavior*, eds B. Mullen and G. R. Goethals (New York, NY: Springer), 185–208. doi: 10.1007/978-1-4612-4634-3_9

Wegner, D. M., Giuliano, T., and Hertel, P. T. (1985). "Cognitive interdependence in close relationships," in *Compatible and Incompatible Relationships*, ed. W. Ickes (New York, NY: Springer), 253–276. doi: 10.1007/978-1-4612-5044-9_12

Weldon, M. S., and Bellinger, K. D. (1997). Collective memory: collaborative and individual processes in remembering. *J. Exp. Psychol. Learn. Mem. Cogn.* 23, 1160–1175. doi: 10.1037/0278-7393.23.5.1160

Winblad, B., Palmer, K., Kivipelto, M., Jelic, V., Fratiglioni, L., Wahlund, L.-O., et al. (2004). Mild cognitive impairment—beyond controversies, towards a consensus: report of the international working group on mild cognitive impairment. *J. Intern. Med.* 256, 240–246. doi: 10.1111/j.1365-2796.2004. 01380.x

World Health Organization (2019). *Deafness and Hearing Loss*. Geneva: World Health Organization.

Yesavage, J. A., and Sheikh, J. I. (1986). Geriatric depression scale (GDS): recent evidence and development of a shorter version. *Clin. Gerontol.* 5, 165–173. doi: 10.1300/J018v05n01_09

8

Application of New Materials in Auditory Disease Treatment

Ming Li, Yurong Mu, Hua Cai, Han Wu and Yanyan Ding*

Department of Otorhinolaryngology, Union Hospital, Tongji Medical College, Huazhong University of Science and Technology, Wuhan, China

Correspondence:
Yanyan Ding
dingyanyande@163.com

Auditory diseases are disabling public health problems that afflict a significant number of people worldwide, and they remain largely incurable until now. Driven by continuous innovation in the fields of chemistry, physics, and materials science, novel materials that can be applied to hearing diseases are constantly emerging. In contrast to conventional materials, new materials are easily accessible, inexpensive, non-invasive, with better acoustic therapy effects and weaker immune rejection after implantation. When new materials are used to treat auditory diseases, the wound healing, infection prevention, disease recurrence, hair cell regeneration, functional recovery, and other aspects have been significantly improved. Despite these advances, clinical success has been limited, largely due to issues regarding a lack of effectiveness and safety. With ever-developing scientific research, more novel materials will be facilitated into clinical use in the future.

Keywords: new materials, auditory diseases, conductive hearing loss, sensorineural hearing loss, therapy

INTRODUCTION

According to the latest World Health Organization estimates, 466 million people around the world (over 5% of the world population) experience disabling hearing loss. By 2050, this number is projected to rise to approximately 900 million, and nearly 2.5 billion people are at risk of contracting auditory diseases (World Health Organization [WHO], 2021). The early detection, vaccination, accurate management, and timely treatment of auditory diseases can help improve clinical outcome. Nevertheless, therapeutic modalities and prevention strategies for the occurrence and development of auditory diseases are still limited currently. Hearing impairment caused by auditory diseases is categorized into three clinical types: conductive (CHL), sensorineural (SNHL), and mixed (MHL) hearing loss. CHL is known to result primarily from structural damage, blockage, and sclerosis of the outer and middle ear, eventually leading to aberrant signaling to the inner ear. Disruption of the inner ear, auditory nerve, central auditory nuclei, or cortex are classified as SNHL, with an elaborate pathology that includes loss of sensory hair cells, spiral ganglion neurons (SGNs), and stria vascularis cells in the inner ear, ultimately leading to the failure of auditory perception (Ma et al., 2019). The established therapy for patients suffering from conductive deafness focuses on middle-ear infection, otosclerosis, etc. Research on curative therapies for sensorineural hearing loss mainly focuses on the repair and regeneration of hair cells, stria vascularis, and nerve synapses.

The practical application of new materials is continuously undergoing considerable advancements, and substantial success has been achieved in some aspects. Whereas the new materials are being applied to treat auditory diseases, the abundant advances made in the fields of diabetes, cardiovascular disease, and neuromuscular disease using new materials are progressing. Recently, the Food and Drug Administration (FDA) approved the first RNA interference-based gene silencing technology drug—Patisiran—which regulates gene expression by the delivery of RNA to target cells, improving the prognosis of patients with rare cardiac and neurologic disease (Adams et al., 2018). For another example, with a fundamental role in the future repair or replacement of tissues defects (Zakrzewski et al., 2019), stem cells differentiate into insulin-producing cells after being implanted into the body, bringing considerable improvements to the prognosis of type 1 diabetes (Shahjalal et al., 2018). Regarding to stem cell therapy, graphene, with remarkable biocompatible and bioadhesive properties, can be fabricated as scaffolds for the proliferation and direct differentiation of stem cells (Kenry Lee et al., 2018). Some scholars even propose stem cell engraftment as a highly feasible and fundamental curing method for sensorineural deafness (Nakagawa and Ito, 2005; Cheng et al., 2019). Many prostheses formed out of new materials were reported to induce fewer immune responses and had a better overall prognosis than conventional materials after implantation (Diken Turksayar et al., 2019; Nappi et al., 2021). This review will focus on the research progress of the novel materials employed for the treatment of CHL and SNHL (see **Figure 1**).

TREATMENT ORIENTATION OF HEARING LOSS

Hearing loss is attributable to genetic factors, specific viral infections, chronic ear infections, birth complications, exposure to excessive noise, aging, and ototoxic drugs. CHL may occur as middle-ear effusion, tympanic membrane perforation, physical external trauma, infection, canal stenosis, cholesteatoma, otitis media, otosclerosis, ossicular erosions, and so on (Ontario Health, 2020). At present, treatment for CHL primarily involves surgery and drugs. Primary research directions for novel therapies are focused on new pharmaceuticals, materials, artificial auditory implantation, and other aspects. The artificial auditory implantation comprises middle-ear implant (MEI) and implantable bone-conduction devices (Chen et al., 2014). The current widespread adoption of artificial auditory implantation includes bone-anchored hearing aids (BAHAs), subcutaneous bone bridges (BBs), vibrant sound bridges (VSBs), and semi-implantable middle-ear transducers. However, due to the pathway for bone conduction being more complex than air conduction, the following areas must be considered: percutaneous attenuation of high-frequency sound after the implantation of bone-conduction hearing aid devices; the susceptibility to infection of surgical sites after BAHA implantation; vibrator displacement after MEI implantation; ossicular necrosis; the wide fluctuation of postoperative gain, and so on. Therefore, further research aimed at bone-conduction audiology and more development of audiological assist devices are still required (Ghoncheh et al., 2016).

Diseases that could contribute to SNHL are age-related hearing loss (ARHL), inherited hearing impairments, Meniere's disease (endolymphatic hydrops), autoimmune inner-ear disease, ear infection, drug-induced deafness, ear trauma, and idiopathic SNHL (Merchant and Nadol, 2001; Kanzaki et al., 2020). In addressing sudden sensorineural hearing loss (SSNHL), current SSNHL management guidelines recommend glucocorticoids, psychotherapy, and intravenous agents that can improve microcirculation and neurotrophy, besides which numerous attempts for novel therapies have been reported. For instance,

Vanwijck et al. (2019) summarized the efficacy of intratympanic injections of corticosteroids with a Silverstein tube to treat refractory SSNHL. They found that the topical application of corticosteroids with such a tube to the inner ear through the round window membrane can improve the hearing and clarity of patients who have failed in previous conventional therapies. However, therapies for SNHL remain clinically limited thus far, and the therapeutic effects remain less than satisfactory. Owing to the natural anatomical and physiological barriers of the cochlea, the supply and absorption of drugs reaching the targeting cochlea cells have been severely hindered (Zou et al., 2016; Yuan and Qi, 2018). An example is that the cochlea, surrounded by bones and located in a relatively closed environment, is difficult for drugs to access from the blood due to the presence of the blood labyrinth barrier (BLB). For local drug delivery to the cochlea, drug penetration through the oval window (OW) and round window membrane (RWM) becomes difficult due to their permselectivity. In addition, some of the drugs have a short half-life, and inter-individual differences in metabolism are marked, therefore limiting the benefits of drugs administered using traditional approaches.

In recent years, a range of new signaling pathways and genes playing essential roles in hair cell development and differentiation have been discovered that target therapies against SNHL (Diensthuber and Stover, 2018). For example, overexpressing Atoh1 can potentially reprogram supporting cells to become hair cells, subsequently promoting mammalian hair cell regeneration (Richardson and Atkinson, 2015). In cell cycle regulation, the absence of p27Kip1 drives the enhanced proliferation of supporting cells in adult mice, and inactivation of the retinoblastoma 1 (RB1) gene leads to the acquisition of newly generated hair cells originated from highly differentiated hair cells (Sage et al., 2005). For other signaling pathways, the activator of the Wnt signal pathway—β-catenin, the overexpression of which triggers Lgr5-positive cell growth and mitosis—elevates hair cell regeneration (Shi et al., 2013). When β-catenin and Atoh1 are co-expressed, the differentiation of Lg5-positive hair cells in neonatal mice is significantly advanced (Kuo et al., 2015). Furthermore, inhibition of the Notch pathway *via* γ-secretase inhibitors enables mice to regenerate hair cells in response to noise-induced damage, simultaneously gaining an improvement in their hearing level (Mizutari et al., 2013). Furthermore, there is crosstalk between Notch and Wnt signaling (Li et al., 2015; Ding et al., 2020). Hence, various predictions can be hypothesized based on these theories; that is, gene targets that can be selectively modulated using small molecules or related drugs might drive the regeneration of hair cells.

APPLICATION OF NOVEL MATERIALS IN HEARING LOSS

Treatment of New Materials in Conductive Hearing Loss

In auricle-related disorders, the microtia is a congenital craniofacial malformation, ranking only second to cleft lip

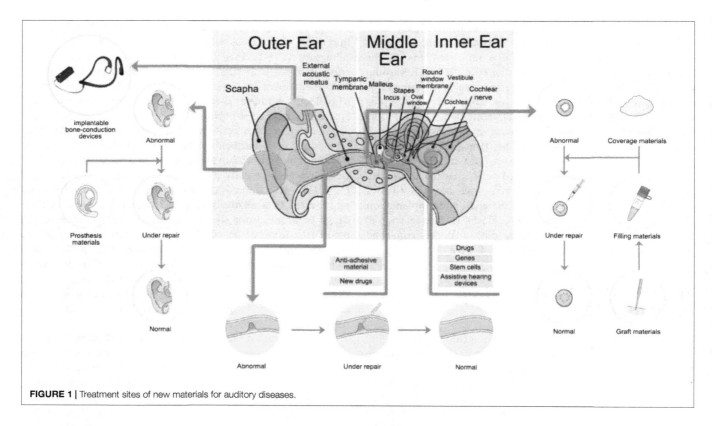

FIGURE 1 | Treatment sites of new materials for auditory diseases.

(Jiao and Zhang, 2001). Traditional healing strategies employ autologous cartilage as conventional grafts (Bichara et al., 2012). Shang et al. (2016) used 3D printing technology and medical silicone to fabricate an auricular scaffold, and they found the scaffolds were implanted *in vivo* smoothly, with excellent bio-compatibility, affordable cost, and a simple preparation process. Presently, besides adipose-derived stem cell (ADSC) application for cartilage regeneration, cartilage stem/progenitor cells (CSPCs) have also been used for the successful ear reconstruction and modeling the pathogenesis of auricular deformities (Zhou G. et al., 2018; Zucchelli et al., 2020).

In tympanic-associated disorders, tympanic membrane perforation (TMP) is a commonly seen disease in otorhinolaryngology. Although the preferred autograft materials, such as temporal muscle, cartilage, and fat, have a variety of applications, they have also been reported to be highly susceptible to infection and have pronounced dependence on nutrients from the surrounding tissue (Teh et al., 2013). Therefore, an increasing emphasis is being placed on new materials that can decrease the rate of inflammation, foster tympanic membrane regeneration, and enhance the proliferation and migration of the epithelium. The current methods for tympanic membrane repair combine autologous tissue and novel materials, the latter including platelet-rich plasma (PRP), platelet-rich fibrin (PRF), hyaluronic acid (HA), epidermal growth factor (EGF), and basic fibroblast growth factor (bFGF). Among them, PRP and PRF have gained particular interest because they are enriched in growth factors, which are effective in inducing tissue regeneration and with a lower prevalence of infections (Gur et al., 2016;

Stavrakas et al., 2016; Huang et al., 2021). Moreover, a study by Lin et al. (2013) found that recombinant human epidermal growth factor (rhEGF) in conjunction with a gelatin-based sponge scaffold can remarkably enhance the wound healing rate of chronic TMP, reduce improvement time, further improve hearing level, and has no toxic side effects on inner-ear function. Similar multiple studies have been performed for combining new materials into clinical practice, and correspondingly, an increased likelihood of TMP healing has been reported (Gisselsson-Solen et al., 2020). For example, heparin-binding epidermal growth factor (EGF)-like growth factor (Santa Maria et al., 2015), EGF-released nanofibrous patches (Seonwoo et al., 2019b), bacterial cellulose (Mandour et al., 2019), chitosan patch scaffolds incorporated with insulin-like growth factor-binding protein 2 (Seonwoo et al., 2019a), and a fibroblast growth factor (FGF)-infiltrated gelatin sponge (Omae et al., 2017; Kanemaru et al., 2018) have been documented to accelerate tympanic membrane (TM) perforation healing. As a type of novel material, Maharajan et al. (2020) have also reported that mesenchymal stem cells (MSCs) are promising candidates for therapy to treat TMP. Either separate engraftment of multipotent MSCs or a combination of these cells with biological materials and growth factors (GFs) can achieve faster TMP healing *via* increasing the activation of epidermal stem cell markers and stimulating the proliferation and migration of keratinocytes. MSCs, scaffolds, and GFs have a synergistic role in TM regeneration. The recent advancement of 3D- and 4D-printing technology has driven the development of a precise MSC-attached scaffold designed for the physical structure of patients. The direction of physical and chemical engineering may be incorporated in this advancement, further boosting the degree and rate of the target tissue regeneration (Maharajan et al., 2020). The introduction of a cobalt-chromium (Co-Cr) coronary stent into the eustachian tube potentiates middle-ear ventilation, as validated in sheep (Pohl et al., 2018). A new class of tympanostomy stent made of nickel and titanium with a TiO2 coating has previously been shown to reduce *Pseudomonas aeruginosa* biofilm formation, resulting in a lower incidence of postoperative complications, such as deafness and catheter blockage after tympanotomy tube insertion (Joe and Seo, 2018).

Tympanoplasty exerts significant actions on the treatment of auditory diseases such as chronic otitis mastoidea, tympanosclerosis, cholesteatomatous chronic otitis media, and middle-ear sound transmission defect caused by trauma. Adhesive otitis patients often require surgical interventions when they present with concomitant middle-ear atelectasis, structural adhesion in the tympanic chamber, sound transmission disorder, recurrent infection, and persistent otorrhea (Larem et al., 2016). To avoid postoperative adhesion and to clean effusion, the filler materials are required for adhesion prevention after removal of tympanic sclerotic foci and middle-ear blockage caused by pathological factors; these materials can be divided into two categories: absorbable and non-absorbable. The most recent anti-adhesive materials include chitosan hydrogel within absorbable materials (Unsaler et al., 2016) and natural polymeric biomaterials–Naso Pore (Huang et al., 2011). These two ingredients are otherwise used for nasal surgery and are of low ototoxicity, inflammatory response, and have strong anti-adhesion effects (Chen and Li, 2020). In the medical management of middle-ear cholesteatoma, traditional surgery combined with novel materials has been found to have superior efficacy. For mastoid postoperative tamponade, synthetic materials have clear advantages of easy accessibility, short procedure time, being less prone to contamination and so on, compared with traditional autologous materials, which are less accessible and unstable. Common filling synthetic materials in mastoid disorders include bioactive glass, hydroxyapatite, titanium, and silicon, with bioactive glass being most frequently used (Lee H. B. et al., 2013; Sorour et al., 2018). Tympanoplasty necessitates the use of transplanted materials, but classically employed autogenous materials are with high risk of shift, complete absorption, and residual cholesteatoma. Bartel et al. (2018) determined that total (TORP) and partial (PORP) ossicular replacement prostheses can be biosynthesized and are stiff, safe, and stable. Compared with traditional materials, the hearing improvement after ossicular chain reconstruction is almost equivalent to using biosynthesizing materials, and the curative effect of myringoplasty is even superior to that of traditional autologous grafting materials (Bartel et al., 2018; Li et al., 2021).

The ear is one of the predilection sites for keloids, frequently following trauma, surgery, burns, and ear piercing. Due to the high rate of recurrence, the search for excellent postoperative coverage materials and preventing recurrence has become a particular research hotspot in the treatment of keloids (Du and Zhu, 2015). Park et al. proposed that employing hydrocolloid dressing as a wound coverage and pressurizing with a magnet during the early postoperative period, compared with traditional dressings used to cover wounds, could protect the wound tissue, facilitate the healing process, and reduce the water content inside the wound tissue (Park and Chang, 2013). Besides, more coverage materials to promote wound healing and reduce inflammation will become available in the coming years. For patients with CHL but normal hearing function of the inner ear, other assistive hearing devices are increasingly promising in addition to the aforementioned BAHA, BB, vibrant sound-bridge (VSB), and middle-ear transducers, such as ADHEAR–a new non-invasive bone-conduction hearing-assistive device, which uses a cohesive adaptor affixed to the skin surface behind the ear and applies no pressure to the skin (Brill et al., 2019).

Treatment of New Materials in Sensorineural Hearing Loss

The loss of outer hair cells and spiral ganglion cell degeneration are major causes of sensorineural hearing loss (Wong and Ryan, 2015). The loss of hair cells, spiral ganglion cells, and auditory nerve fibers in the adult ear is irreversible, leading to permanent SNHL. The surgical implantation of a cochlear implant (CI) is envisaged as one of means to restore hearing, but the function of artificial cochlea is highly reliant on residue numbers of spiral ganglion cells. A recent study has found that superparamagnetic iron oxide (SPIO) nanoparticles can direct spiral ganglion neurites to orient to a CI electrode under the application of magnetic field modulation and maintain the survival of SGNs, producing a positive CI treatment effect (Hu et al., 2021). Various other *in vitro* experiments have newly demonstrated that the cGMP-dependent atrial natriuretic peptide (ANP) and the permissive environment created by novel silicon micro-pillar substrates (MPS) could facilitate the survival and growth of SGNs (Mattotti et al., 2015; Sun et al., 2020). Through *in vivo* experiments, mesenchymal stem cells (Maharajan et al., 2021), valproic acid (VPA; 2-propylpentanoic acid) with growth factors (Wakizono et al., 2021), as well as neural stem cells (He et al., 2021) have been found to be beneficial for SGN growth.

Additionally, to achieve more SGNs and hair cell regeneration, researchers have been studying drug delivery systems (DDSs), gene therapy, and cell therapy from different perspectives (Ma et al., 2019) (see **Figure 2**).

The clinical advancement of DDS has been hindered by a short biological half-life, poor pharmacokinetics, and low permeability through the biological barriers of nerve growth factor (NGF). Hence, developing highly efficient and inexpensive materials is of substantial importance (Bartus, 2012; Khalin et al., 2015). Currently, the nanotechnology-based ongoing development of novel NGF delivery systems covers nanogels, hydrogels, micelles, microspheres, electrospun nanofibers, nanoparticles, and supraparticles. NGF could be immobilized in nanomaterials *via* physical trapping, adsorption, or electrostatic interactions, then the sustained release can be obtained using diffusion of NGF and/or degradation of carriers, with the aim of local, sustained drug release (Ma et al., 2019). One such nanoscaled drug delivery system could be used in targeted drug delivery. By constructing degradable and non-toxic nanoparticle loading

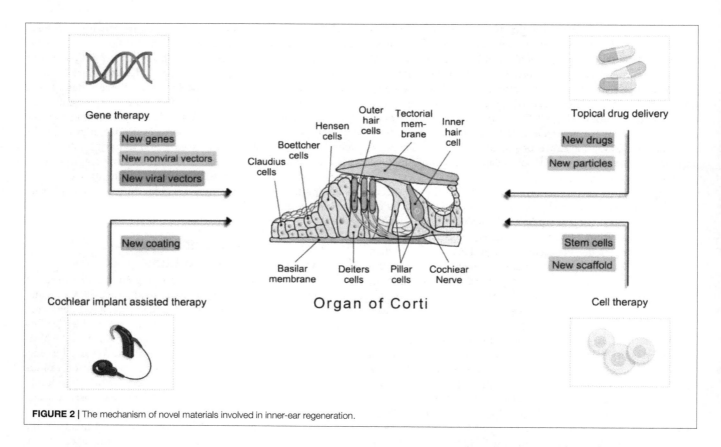

FIGURE 2 | The mechanism of novel materials involved in inner-ear regeneration.

drugs, ligands for the specific recognition and delivery into targeted organs or tissues, nanoscaled drug delivery systems show the stability and property of sustained release (Ding et al., 2019; An and Zha, 2020). Moreover, supraparticles have increased volume in comparison to nano-onions, which have yet to be fully translated into clinical practice. The supraparticles have a larger capacity for the delivery of drugs and provide sustained drug release, concurrently spreading to particular targeted areas (Ma et al., 2018). However, several challenges persist for the clinical application of nanoparticle drug delivery systems, such as drug delivery risk assessments through the RWM or OW routes and the implementation of controlled release and targeted nano-drug delivery. For example, intratympanic medication injection or nanoparticle delivery may access the inner ear more through the RWM approach (Du et al., 2013; Liu et al., 2013), but OW shows higher permeability than RWM (King et al., 2011, 2013; Zou et al., 2012). Chen et al. also found similar results in that fluorescence traceable chitosan nanoparticles (CS-NPs) were more quickly transported into the inner ear through OW, with less damage exhibited (Ding et al., 2019), but further validation regarding nanomaterials and loaded drugs for optimum routes of delivery is still necessary. In gene therapy, the introgressed gene in the inner ear typically involves the basic helix-loop-helix (bHLH) family transcription factor (Shou et al., 2003) as well as neurotrophic (Sun et al., 2011), anti-apoptotic (Chan et al., 2007; Pfannenstiel et al., 2009), antioxidant (Kawamoto et al., 2004), connexin (Birkenhager et al., 2006; Sun et al., 2009), cochlear protein-related, interleukin, and other (Zhuo et al., 2008) genes.

To cross the BBB and blood labyrinth barrier successfully and transfer functional genes into the mammalian inner ear, both viral and non-viral vectors are the most common tools for transgene delivery. Viral vectors consist of adenovirus (AV), adeno-associated virus (AAV), herpes simplex virus type I, vaccinia virus, and so on. Non-viral vectors can be categorized into liposomes, cationic polymers, peptide-based nanoparticles, and other synthetic vectors (Sun and Wu, 2013). Other vectors, such as viral and non-viral composite carriers, as well as bacterial vectors, are being studied (Akin et al., 2007). AAV2/Anc80L65, a recently discovered synthetic viral vector, targets the inner and outer hair cells of the cochlea with high efficiency and elicits only a weak immune response when compared to other viral vectors with low transfection ability (Zinn et al., 2015). Tan et al. designed a variant of AAV—AAV-inner ear (AAV-ie). The variant not only achieved 90% successful transfection to supporting cells but also expanded the number of mice hair cells *via* carrying the Atoh1 gene, which did not affect the numbers of hair cells or hearing level (Tan et al., 2019). MicroRNA regulates gene expression *in vivo* by means of inhibiting protein translation and promoting mRNA degradation, the primary function of which is to play a suppressor role post-transcriptionally (Wu et al., 2020). Luo et al. constructed MicroRNA-146a (miR-146a) lentiviral recombinant vectors and found that miR-146a could significantly mitigate inflammatory injury and auditory dysfunctions of the inner ear after being injected into the inner ear through the scala tympani (Luo et al., 2016). A single microRNA can regulate hundreds of different transcription processes, by which the regeneration of damaged hair cells in the inner ear and treating hearing loss are major focuses of much recent research (Zhou W. et al., 2018). Autoimmune inner ear disease (AIED) is an independent disorder, the main clinical manifestation of which is bilateral, rapidly progressive sensorineural hearing loss. Distinct from conventional systemic glucocorticoid treatment, Cai et al. injected adenoviral-mediated interleukin-10 (IL-10) through the RWM. The authors found that adenoviral carrying IL-10 can be imported into the inner ear of guinea pigs and express the gene products, consequently attenuating inflammatory injury and impairment in the auditory function of the inner ear to some extent (Cai and Tan, 2015). Therapies for sensorineural hearing loss by replacement of damaged or lost cells and secreting neurotrophic factors, cytokines, immunoregulatory protein, etc., with the transplanted cells hold promise in a wide variety of fields (Mehrabani et al., 2016; Kanzaki, 2018). Mesenchymal (MSCs), embryonic (ESCs), and induced pluripotent (iPSCs) stem cells are the most frequently used sources for regenerative medicine in the field of otology. Nevertheless, in contrast, the potential tumorigenicity and immune rejection response caused by ESCs and iPSCs, MSCs have a higher safety profile, anti-apoptotic properties, and characteristics of easy amplification; hence, MSCs have become a particular focus of regenerative medicine research (Kaboodkhani et al., 2021). The application of MSCs promotes BDNF secretion and increases the expression of connexin26 and connexin30, contributing to the alleviation of inflammation, oxidative stress, and apoptosis, the recovery of cell-cell junctions, an increased number of SGNs differentiated into neural progenitor cells and specific lineages of neurons, and significantly decreased hearing threshold and improved audial function (Matsuoka et al., 2007; Jang et al., 2015; Young et al., 2018; Mittal et al., 2020). In regenerative medicine, scaffolds are essential for cell growth and could provide a three-dimensional structure for cell differentiation and migration to restore the normal function of damaged organs (Khodakaram-Tafti et al., 2017). The preparation of scaffolds can be accomplished with various source materials, including decellularizing tissue (Hashemi et al., 2018), 3D printing technologies (Wang and Yang, 2021), tailored hydrogels (Slaughter et al., 2009), and electrospinning (Malik et al., 2021). Recent studies have used biological scaffolds comprising 3D graphene and artificial photonic crystals for stem cell culture. Scaffolds mimicking the microenvironment of cell growth *in vivo* can positively regulate stem cell growth, proliferation, and differentiation (Yang et al., 2013; Ankam et al., 2015; Fang et al., 2019). Other novel materials yielding similarly supportive effects for stem cells include 3D polydopamine-functionalized carbon microfibrous scaffolds (Yang et al., 2020), $Ti_3C_2T_x$Mxene membranes (Guo et al., 2020), microfluidic chip platforms (Park et al., 2014), and anisotropy inverse opals (Pettinato et al., 2015). Suggested mechanisms of the aforementioned materials include the promotion of cell growth, expansion, development and cell-cell adhesion, alignment, and connection.

In terms of hearing ancillary equipment, the application of CI for bilateral severe-to-profound SNHL has also reached maturity. However, implantation surgery can potentially cause invasive damage. Recent studies have increasingly found that degradable cell coatings for CI electrodes can increase neuronal survival by persistently releasing BDNF from cell-coated surfaces (Richardson et al., 2009). In addition, the local delivery of dexamethasone into the inner ear or coating *Cis* with dexamethasone during cochlear implantation may alleviate inflammation in the surgical sites (Farhadi et al., 2013; Lee J. et al., 2013).

OTHER NOVEL MATERIALS FOR TREATING AUDITORY-RELATED CONDITIONS

The control of tinnitus by external noise stimuli has become a therapy of particular interest. Tinnitus afflicts approximately 15% of the general population worldwide, and there is currently no cure for this disorder. Attempts have been made to ameliorate tinnitus with individually applied spectrally optimized near-threshold noise (Schilling et al., 2021), with most patients stating that subjective tinnitus loudness was suppressed during the noise stimulation.

The discovery of novel pharmaceuticals is one of the important directions for future research. Today, drug candidates with potential therapeutic applications for hearing loss include antioxidants, regulators of mitochondrial function, ion channel modulators, hair-cell protectants, and anti-inflammatory drugs (Ji et al., 2021). Other potentially effective drugs that have been experimentally validated are N-acetylcysteine (NAC) (Marie et al., 2018), melatonin (Serra et al., 2020), resveratrol (Xiong et al., 2015), mineralocorticoid aldosterone (ALD) (Campos-Banales et al., 2015; Halonen et al., 2016), teprenone (GGA) (Mikuriya et al., 2008), aspirin (Verschuur et al., 2014), and salicylic acid (Li et al., 2020) et al. One example is age-related hearing loss (ARHL); SAMP8 mice models demonstrated notably decreased auditory brainstem response (ABR) thresholds, increased distortion product otoacoustic emission (DPOAE) amplitudes, and memory improvement after the administration of NAC, suggesting that NAC has protective effects on hair cells and neurons of the central nervous system (CNS) (Li et al., 2020). Some systemic diseases are accompanied by damage to the inner ear, such as the microvascular and nerve damage caused by long-term diabetes, further leading to neurovascular injury in the cochlear. Gao et al. (2018) found resveratrol to be effective in preventing cell apoptosis and reducing diabetes damage to the inner ear by hypoglycemic activities, anti-dyslipidemic effects, and inhibiting anti-oxidative stress, ICAM-1, and VEGF expression. GGA was found to up-regulate heat-shock proteins (HSPs), and many experimental studies have demonstrated the protective effect of HSPs against cochlear damage induced by noise exposure, ototoxic drugs, and heat stress. In addition, a decline of ABR thresholds was observed in presbycusis mice (Mikuriya et al., 2008). ARHL models of DBA/2J mice were given injections of 200 mg/kg salicylic acid, and the expression of prestin, hair-cell survival, and function of the cochlea were significantly better than in saline-treated controls (Li et al., 2020). However, although antioxidants, such as resveratrol, ferulic acid (Fetoni et al., 2010), and glutathione

(Ohinata et al., 2000) are currently under active research, Sha Suhua et al. expressed caution that long-term or excessive intake of exogenous antioxidants or vitamin supplements is not only hazardous to hearing but also increases the risk of developing cancer (Sha and Schacht, 2017). Additionally, Kashio et al. (2009) and Polanski et al. identified that various antioxidants such as Ginkgo biloba extract (GBE), alpha-lipoic acid (AL), and vitamins A, E, and C do not result in hearing improvement (Polanski and Cruz, 2013). For other novel agents, bioactive peptides from Rapana venosa were found to exert an antioxidant effect, as demonstrated *via* the diminishing hair-cell uptake of gentamicin, activating Nrf2-Kcap1-ARE, up-regulation of Nrf2, and the expression of related antioxidant genes without damaging mechanoelectrical transduction channels (Yan, 2021). It has been suggested that rapamycin can slow the onset of ARHL through the inhibition of mTORC1 hyperactivation (Fu et al., 2018). Multiple previous studies have also shown that rapamycin reduces cisplatin- and gentamicin-induced nephrotoxicity (Fang and Xiao, 2014; Ebnoether et al., 2017) and alleviates noise-induced hearing loss (NIHL) by reducing oxidative stress (Yuan et al., 2015). However, rapamycin has many side effects as an immunosuppressant. New drugs can simulate the antioxidant activity of rapamycin with fewer side effects, and such classes of drugs are currently undergoing clinical experimentation. Traditional herbal medicines have been used in China for thousands of years. However, to date, the efficacy of these medicines has yet to be confirmed, and their action mechanisms remain unclear. Modern pharmacological studies have also spurred intense research programs targeting the auditory diseases. For instance, Xuan et al. (2018) demonstrated that composite Jianer formulations, mainly consisting of Puerariae Lobatae Radix (Gegen in Chinese), Scutellariae Radix (Huangqin in Chinese), and Salvia miltiorrhiza (Danshen in Chinese), reduced the level of malondialdehyde (MDA), the main product of lipid peroxidation, to exhibit an antioxidant effect in adult mice. Besides, the composite Jianer formulations ameliorated mtDNA damage and the release of Cyt-c, thereby attenuating caspase-mediated apoptosis through the mitochondrial pathway and playing a protective role against age-related decline in hair cells and spiral ganglion neurons. Furthermore, traditional Chinese herbal medicine (TCHM) seems to be associated with few adverse effects (Xuan et al., 2018). Another active ingredient extracted from traditional Chinese medicine Flos puerariae (Gehua in Chinese)—total flavonoids of Pueraria lobata—has been found to suppress the inflammatory response. The total flavonoids of Pueraria lobata reduce isoprenaline-induced damage to the inner ear of the rat *via* inhibiting the expression of TNF-α, IL-4, and Bax and up-regulating ACTH proteins, at the same time regulating auditory system homeostasis and improving the microvasculature circulation

of the inner ear and the ischemia conditions of tissue cells in rats (Zhao and Liang, 2018). Thus, TCHM has substantial potential for treating auditory diseases. The development of new classes of novel antibiotics is valuable for the treatment of hearing loss. For example, for severe chronic suppurative otitis media, new antibiotics are required for effective anti-infectious therapeutics owing to the constant emergence of drug-resistant bacteria. A kind of new cephalosporin— "ceftolozane-tazobactam"—has particularly good therapeutic benefits for moderate to severe suppurative otitis media caused by multidrug- and extensively drug-resistant (MDR and XDR) *P. aeruginosa* (Saraca et al., 2019).

This study has highlighted some bottlenecks in the application of therapeutic materials for auditory diseases, such as the tumorigenicity of repair-promoting substances, immune reaction to implanted materials, high cost, and a difficult fabrication process. More research combining materials science, basic medicine, and clinical medicine is required to address these bottlenecks, with the aim of obtaining more cost-effective and safer new materials for treating hearing loss.

CONCLUSION

Presently, various deficiencies still exist regarding insufficient treatment options and their modest efficacy for auditory diseases, leading to CHL and SNHL. Nevertheless, the development and application of novel materials are gradually improving the condition. The novel materials are able to hasten perforated tympanic membrane healing, tympanoplasty of the middle ear, and repair of the microtia, as well as promote the regeneration of inner hair cells, spiral ganglion cells, and the synaptic ribbons, decrease inflammation level, and modify hearing level adjunctively. Although the efficacy and safety of novel materials in clinical application remain to be verified, with more progression of research and substantial technological innovation, these novel materials will be continuously improved, and more refined materials could be employed to treat hearing loss clinically.

AUTHOR CONTRIBUTIONS

ML conceived and wrote the manuscript. YD modified the manuscript. All authors contributed to the article and approved the submitted version.

ACKNOWLEDGMENTS

The authors thank Yang Zhang for his assistance in the preparation of all figures.

REFERENCES

Adams, D., Gonzalez-Duarte, A., O'Riordan, W. D., Yang, C. C., Ueda, M., Kristen, A. V., et al. (2018). Patisiran, an RNAi therapeutic, for hereditary transthyretin amyloidosis. *N. Engl. J. Med.* 379, 11–21. doi: 10.1056/NEJMoa1716153

Akin, D., Sturgis, J., Ragheb, K., Sherman, D., Burkholder, K., Robinson,

J. P., et al. (2007). Bacteria-mediated delivery of nanoparticles and cargo into cells. *Nat. Nanotechnol.* 2, 441–449. doi: 10.1038/nnano.2007.149

An, X., and Zha, D. (2020). Advances in research on nanoparticle delivery systems for inner ear targeted drug delivery and therapy. *Chin. J. Otol.* 18, 409–413.

Ankam, S., Lim, C. K., and Yim, E. K. (2015). Actomyosin contractility plays a role in MAP2 expression during nanotopography-directed neuronal differentiation of human embryonic stem cells. *Biomaterials* 47, 20–28. doi: 10.1016/j.biomaterials.2015.01.003

Bartel, R., Cruellas, F., Hamdan, M., Gonzalez-Compta, X., Cisa, E., Domenech, I., et al. (2018). Hearing results after type III tympanoplasty: incus transposition versus PORP. A systematic review. *Acta Otolaryngol.* 138, 617–620. doi: 10.1080/00016489.2018.1425901

Bartus, R. T. (2012). Translating the therapeutic potential of neurotrophic factors to clinical 'proof of concept': a personal saga achieving a career-long quest. *Neurobiol. Dis.* 48, 153–178. doi: 10.1016/j.nbd.2012.04.004

Bichara, D. A., O'Sullivan, N. A., Pomerantseva, I., Zhao, X., Sundback, C. A., Vacanti, J. P., et al. (2012). The tissue-engineered auricle: past, present, and future. *Tissue Eng. Part B Rev.* 18, 51–61. doi: 10.1089/ten.TEB.2011.0326

Birkenhager, R., Zimmer, A. J., Maier, W., and Schipper, J. (2006). [Pseudodominants of two recessive connexin mutations in non-syndromic sensorineural hearing loss?]. *Laryngorhinootologie* 85, 191–196. doi: 10.1055/s-2005-870302

Brill, I. T., Brill, S., and Stark, T. (2019). [New options for rehabilitation of conductive hearing loss: tests on normal-hearing subjects with simulated hearing loss]. *HNO* 67, 698–705. doi: 10.1007/s00106-019-0685-8

Cai, W., and Tan, W. (2015). Adenovirus-mediated IL-10 gene for the treatment of autoimmune inner ear disease——an experimental study. *J. Audiol. Speech Pathol.* 23, 602–606.

Campos-Banales, E. M., Lopez-Campos, D., de Serdio-Arias, J. L., Esteban-Rodriguez, J., Garcia-Sainz, M., Munoz-Cortes, A., et al. (2015). [A comparative study on efficacy of glucocorticoids, mineralocorticoids and vasoactive drugs on reversing hearing loss in patients suffering idiopathic sensorineural cochlear hypoacusis. A preliminary clinical trial]. *Acta Otorrinolaringol. Esp.* 66, 65–73. doi: 10.1016/j.otorri.2014.05.008

Chan, D. K., Lieberman, D. M., Musatov, S., Goldfein, J. A., Selesnick, S. H., and Kaplitt, M. G. (2007). Protection against cisplatin-induced ototoxicity by adeno-associated virus-mediated delivery of the X-linked inhibitor of apoptosis protein is not dependent on caspase inhibition. *Otol. Neurotol.* 28, 417–425. doi: 10.1097/01.mao.0000247826.28893.7a

Chen, K., Dai, P., Yang, L., and Zhang, T. (2014). Progress in middle ear implants. *Progr.Biomed. Eng.* 35, 23–27.

Chen, M., and Li, S. (2020). Advances in diagnosis and treatment of adhesive otitis media. *Chin. J. Ophthalmol. Otorhinolaryngol.* 20, 493–497.

Cheng, C., Wang, Y., Guo, L., Lu, X., Zhu, W., Muhammad, W., et al. (2019). Age-related transcriptome changes in Sox2+ supporting cells in the mouse cochlea. *Stem Cell Res. Ther.* 10:365. doi: 10.1186/s13287-019-1437-0

Diensthuber, M., and Stover, T. (2018). Strategies for a regenerative therapy of hearing loss. *HNO* 66(Suppl. 1), 39–46. doi: 10.1007/s00106-017-0467-0

Diken Turksayar, A. A., Saglam, S. A., and Bulut, A. C. (2019). Retention systems used in maxillofacial prostheses: a review. *Niger. J. Clin. Pract.* 22, 1629–1634. doi: 10.4103/njcp.njcp_92_19

Ding, S., Xie, S., Chen, W., Wen, L., Wang, J., Yang, F., et al. (2019). Is oval window transport a royal gate for nanoparticle delivery to vestibule in the inner ear? *Eur. J. Pharm. Sci.* 126, 11–22. doi: 10.1016/j.ejps.2018.02.031

Ding, Y., Meng, W., Kong, W., He, Z., and Chai, R. (2020). The role of FoxG1 in the inner ear. *Front. Cell. Dev. Biol.* 8:614954. doi: 10.3389/fcell.2020.614954

Du, G., and Zhu, J. (2015). Ear keloid and clinical research progress. *J. Clin. Otorhinolaryngol. Head Neck Surg. (China)* 29, 770–772.

Du, X., Chen, K., Kuriyavar, S., Kopke, R. D., Grady, B. P., Bourne, D. H., et al. (2013). Magnetic targeted delivery of dexamethasone acetate across the round window membrane in guinea pigs. *Otol. Neurotol.* 34, 41–47. doi: 10.1097/MAO.0b013e318277a40e

Ebnoether, E., Ramseier, A., Cortada, M., Bodmer, D., and Levano-Huaman, S. (2017). Sesn2 gene ablation enhances susceptibility to gentamicin-induced hair cell death via modulation of AMPK/mTOR signaling. *Cell Death Discov.* 3:17024. doi: 10.1038/cddiscovery.2017.24

Fang, B., and Xiao, H. (2014). Rapamycin alleviates cisplatin-induced ototoxicity in vivo. *Biochem. Biophys. Res. Commun.* 448, 443–447. doi: 10.1016/j.bbrc.2014.04.123

Fang, Q., Zhang, Y., Chen, X., Li, H., Cheng, L., Zhu, W., et al. (2019). Three-dimensional graphene enhances neural stem cell proliferation through metabolic regulation. *Front. Bioeng. Biotechnol.* 7:436. doi: 10.3389/fbioe.2019.00436

Farhadi, M., Jalessi, M., Salehian, P., Ghavi, F. F., Emamjomeh, H., Mirzadeh, H., et al. (2013). Dexamethasone eluting cochlear implant: histological study in animal model. *Cochlear Implants Int.* 14, 45–50. doi: 10.1179/1754762811Y.0000000024

Fetoni, A. R., Mancuso, C., Eramo, S. L., Ralli, M., Piacentini, R., Barone, E., et al. (2010). In vivo protective effect of ferulic acid against noise-induced hearing loss in the guinea-pig. *Neuroscience* 169, 1575–1588. doi: 10.1016/j.neuroscience.2010.06.022

Fu, X., Sun, X., Zhang, L., Jin, Y., Chai, R., Yang, L., et al. (2018). Tuberous sclerosis complex-mediated mTORC1 overactivation promotes age-related hearing loss. *J. Clin. Invest.* 128, 4938–4945. doi: 10.1172/JCI98058

Gao, H., Qu, Y., Zhang, X., Mu, J., Zhang, P., Wang, X., et al. (2018). The protective effects and its mechanisms of resveratrol on inner ear damage in diabetes rats. *J. Audiol. Speech Pathol.* 29, 409–413.

Ghoncheh, M., Lilli, G., Lenarz, T., and Maier, H. (2016). Outer ear canal sound pressure and bone vibration measurement in SSD and CHL patients using a transcutaneous bone conduction instrument. *Hear. Res.* 340, 161–168. doi: 10.1016/j.heares.2015.12.019

Gisselsson-Solen, M., Tahtinen, P. A., Ryan, A. F., Mulay, A., Kariya, S., Schilder, A. G. M., et al. (2020). Panel 1: biotechnology, biomedical engineering and new models of otitis media. *Int. J. Pediatr. Otorhinolaryngol.* 130(Suppl. 1):109833. doi: 10.1016/j.ijporl.2019.109833

Guo, R., Xiao, M., Zhao, W., Zhou, S., Hu, Y., Liao, M., et al. (2020). 2D Ti3C2TxMXene couples electrical stimulation to promote proliferation and neural differentiation of neural stem cells. *Acta Biomater.* S1742-7061, 30749-30752. doi: 10.1016/j.actbio.2020.12.035

Gur, O. E., Ensari, N., Ozturk, M. T., Boztepe, O. F., Gun, T., Selcuk, O. T., et al. (2016). Use of a platelet-rich fibrin membrane to repair traumatic tympanic membrane perforations: a comparative study. *Acta Otolaryngol.* 136, 1017–1023. doi: 10.1080/00016489.2016.1183042

Halonen, J., Hinton, A. S., Frisina, R. D., Ding, B., Zhu, X., and Walton, J. P. (2016). Long-term treatment with aldosterone slows the progression of age-related hearing loss. *Hear. Res.* 336, 63–71. doi: 10.1016/j.heares.2016.05.001

Hashemi, S. S., Jowkar, S., Mahmoodi, M., Rafati, A. R., Mehrabani, D., Zarei, M., et al. (2018). Biochemical methods in production of three-dimensional scaffolds from human skin: a window in aesthetic surgery. *World J. Plast. Surg.* 7, 204–211.

He, Z., Ding, Y., Mu, Y., Xu, X., Kong, W., Chai, R., et al. (2021). Stem cell-based therapies in hearing loss. *Front. Cell. Dev. Biol.* 9:730042. doi: 10.3389/fcell.2021.730042

Hu, Y., Li, D., Wei, H., Zhou, S., Chen, W., Yan, X., et al. (2021). Neurite extension and orientation of spiral ganglion neurons can be directed by superparamagnetic iron oxide nanoparticles in a magnetic field. *Int. J. Nanomed.* 16, 4515–4526. doi: 10.2147/IJN.S313673

Huang, G., Chen, X., and Jiang, H. (2011). Effects of NasoPore packing in the middle ear cavity of the guinea pig. *Otolaryngol. Head Neck Surg.* 145, 131–136. doi: 10.1177/0194599811400834

Huang, J., Yuan, Z., Hu, S., Lv, C., Hu, Y., and Shen, Y. (2021). The effectiveness and research progress of platelet-rich concentrate products in tympanic membrane perforation. *Chin. J. Cell Biol.* 43, 1700–1704.

Jang, S., Cho, H. H., Kim, S. H., Lee, K. H., Jun, J. Y., Park, J. S., et al. (2015). Neural-induced human mesenchymal stem cells promote cochlear cell regeneration in deaf Guinea pigs. *Clin. Exp. Otorhinolaryngol.* 8, 83–91. doi: 10.3342/ceo.2015.8.2.83

Ji, L., Shen, Q., and Zhao, L. (2021). Progress in treatment of presbycusis. *J. Otol.* 19, 662–665.

Jiao, T., and Zhang, F. (2001). The present situation of auricular prostheses. *Chin. J. Dent. Mater. Devices* 10, 213–215.

Joe, H., and Seo, Y. J. (2018). A newly designed tympanostomy stent with TiO2 coating to reduce *Pseudomonas aeruginosa* biofilm formation. *J. Biomater. Appl.* 33, 599–605. doi: 10.1177/0885328218802103

Kaboodkhani, R., Mehrabani, D., and Karimi-Busheri, F. (2021). Achievements and challenges in transplantation of mesenchymal stem cells in otorhinolaryngology. *J. Clin. Med.* 10:2940. doi: 10.3390/jcm10132940

Kanemaru, S. I., Kanai, R., Yoshida, M., Kitada, Y., Omae, K., and Hirano, S. (2018). Application of regenerative treatment for tympanic membrane perforation with cholesteatoma, tumor, or severe calcification. *Otol. Neurotol.* 39, 438–444. doi: 10.1097/MAO.0000000000001701

Kanzaki, S. (2018). Gene delivery into the inner ear and its clinical implications for hearing and balance. *Molecules* 23:2507. doi: 10.3390/molecules23102507

Kanzaki, S., Toyoda, M., Umezawa, A., and Ogawa, K. (2020). Application of mesenchymal stem cell therapy and inner ear regeneration for hearing loss: a review. *Int. J. Mol. Sci.* 21:5764. doi: 10.3390/ijms21165764

Kashio, A., Amano, A., Kondo, Y., Sakamoto, T., Iwamura, H., Suzuki, M., et al. (2009). Effect of vitamin C depletion on age-related hearing loss in SMP30/GNL knockout mice. *Biochem. Biophys. Res. Commun.* 390, 394–398. doi: 10.1016/j.bbrc.2009.09.003

Kawamoto, K., Sha, S. H., Minoda, R., Izumikawa, M., Kuriyama, H., Schacht, J., et al. (2004). Antioxidant gene therapy can protect hearing and hair cells from ototoxicity. *Mol. Ther.* 9, 173–181. doi: 10.1016/j.ymthe.2003.11.020

Kenry, Lee, W. C., Loh, K. P., and Lim, C. T. (2018). When stem cells meet graphene: opportunities and challenges in regenerative medicine. *Biomaterials* 155, 236–250. doi: 10.1016/j.biomaterials.2017.10.004

Khalin, I., Alyautdin, R., Kocherga, G., and Bakar, M. A. (2015). Targeted delivery of brain-derived neurotrophic factor for the treatment of blindness and deafness. *Int. J. Nanomedicine.* 10, 3245–3267. doi: 10.2147/IJN.S77480

Khodakaram-Tafti, A., Mehrabani, D., and Shaterzadeh-Yazdi, H. (2017). An overview on autologous fibrin glue in bone tissue engineering of maxillofacial surgery. *Dent. Res. J. (Isfahan)* 14, 79–86.

King, E. B., Salt, A. N., Eastwood, H. T., and O'Leary, S. J. (2011). Direct entry of gadolinium into the vestibule following intratympanic applications in Guinea pigs and the influence of cochlear implantation. *J. Assoc. Res. Otolaryngol.* 12, 741–751. doi: 10.1007/s10162-011-0280-5

King, E. B., Salt, A. N., Kel, G. E., Eastwood, H. T., and O'Leary, S. J. (2013). Gentamicin administration on the stapes footplate causes greater hearing loss and vestibulotoxicity than round window administration in guinea pigs. *Hear. Res.* 304, 159–166. doi: 10.1016/j.heares.2013.07.013

Kuo, B. R., Baldwin, E. M., Layman, W. S., Taketo, M. M., and Zuo, J. (2015). In vivo cochlear hair cell generation and survival by coactivation of beta-catenin and atoh1. *J. Neurosci.* 35, 10786–10798. doi: 10.1523/JNEUROSCI.0967-15.2015

Larem, A., Haidar, H., Alsaadi, A., Abdulkarim, H., Abdulraheem, M., Sheta, S., et al. (2016). Tympanoplasty in adhesive otitis media: a descriptive study. *Laryngoscope* 126, 2804–2810. doi: 10.1002/lary.25987

Lee, H. B., Lim, H. J., Cho, M., Yang, S. M., Park, K., Park, H. Y., et al. (2013). Clinical significance of beta-tricalcium phosphate and polyphosphate for mastoid cavity obliteration during middle ear surgery: human and animal study. *Clin. Exp. Otorhinolaryngol.* 6, 127–134. doi: 10.3342/ceo.2013.6.3.127

Lee, J., Ismail, H., Lee, J. H., Kel, G., O'Leary, J., Hampson, A., et al. (2013). Effect of both local and systemically administered dexamethasone on long-term hearing and tissue response in a Guinea pig model of cochlear implantation. *Audiol. Neurootol.* 18, 392–405. doi: 10.1159/000353582

Li, C., Wang, B., Zhang, H., Yang, S., Yang, T., Han, X., et al. (2021). Advances in the surgical treatment of cholesteatoma of the middle ear. *J. Clin. Otorhinolaryngol. Head Neck Surg. (China)* 35, 952–956.

Li, S., Wu, K., and Ji, Y. (2020). Protective effect of long-term injection of salicylic acid on presbycusis. *Chin. J. Otol.* 18, 755–762.

Li, W., Wu, J., Yang, J., Sun, S., Chai, R., Chen, Z. Y., et al. (2015). Notch inhibition induces mitotically generated hair cells in mammalian cochleae *via* activating the Wnt pathway. *Proc. Natl. Acad. Sci. U.S.A.* 112, 166–171. doi: 10.1073/pnas.1415901112

Lin, Y., Yin, F., Chen, J., Bai, Z., Liu, S., and Zhang, J. (2013). The clinical effect of recombinant human epidermal growth factor in treatment of chronic tympanic membrane perforation. *J. Kunming Med. Univ.* 34, 102–104, 109.

Liu, H., Chen, S., Zhou, Y., Che, X., Bao, Z., Li, S., et al. (2013). The effect of surface charge of glycerol monooleate-based nanoparticles on the round window membrane permeability and cochlear distribution. *J. Drug Target.* 21, 846–854. doi: 10.3109/1061186X.2013.829075

Luo, C., Li, T., Tan, C., and Huang, H. (2016). Local injection of the microRNA-146a recombinant lentiviral vector into the inner ear for immune-mediated inner ear disease in guinea pigs. *J. Med. Postgra* 29, 801–807.

Ma, Y., Bjornmalm, M., Wise, A. K., Cortez-Jugo, C., Revalor, E., Ju, Y., et al. (2018). Gel-mediated electrospray assembly of silica supraparticles for sustained drug delivery. *ACS Appl. Mater. Interfaces* 10, 31019–31031. doi: 10.1021/acsami.8b10415

Ma, Y., Wise, A. K., Shepherd, R. K., and Richardson, R. T. (2019). New molecular therapies for the treatment of hearing loss. *Pharmacol. Ther.* 200, 190–209.

doi: 10.1016/j.pharmthera.2019.05.003

Maharajan, N., Cho, G. W., and Jang, C. H. (2020). Application of mesenchymal stem cell for tympanic membrane regeneration by tissue engineering approach. *Int. J. Pediatr. Otorhinolaryngol.* 133:109969. doi: 10.1016/j.ijporl.2020.109969

Maharajan, N., Cho, G. W., and Jang, C. H. (2021). Therapeutic application of mesenchymal stem cells for cochlear regeneration. *In Vivo* 35, 13–22. doi: 10.21873/invivo.12227

Malik, S., Sundarrajan, S., Hussain, T., Nazir, A., and Ramakrishna, S. (2021). Role of block copolymers in tissue engineering applications. *Cells Tissues Organs* 1–14. doi: 10.1159/000511866

Mandour, Y. M. H., Mohammed, S., and Menem, M. O. A. (2019). Bacterial cellulose graft versus fat graft in closure of tympanic membrane perforation. *Am. J. Otolaryngol.* 40, 168–172. doi: 10.1016/j.amjoto.2018.12.008

Marie, A., Meunier, J., Brun, E., Malmstrom, S., Baudoux, V., Flaszka, E., et al. (2018). N-acetylcysteine treatment reduces age-related hearing loss and memory impairment in the senescence-accelerated prone 8 (SAMP8) mouse model. *Aging Dis.* 9, 664–673. doi: 10.14336/AD.2017.0930

Matsuoka, A. J., Kondo, T., Miyamoto, R. T., and Hashino, E. (2007). Enhanced survival of bone-marrow-derived pluripotent stem cells in an animal model of auditory neuropathy. *Laryngoscope* 117, 1629–1635. doi: 10.1097/MLG.0b013e31806bf282

Mattotti, M., Micholt, L., Braeken, D., and Kovacic, D. (2015). Characterization of spiral ganglion neurons cultured on silicon micro-pillar substrates for new auditory neuro-electronic interfaces. *J. Neural Eng.* 12:026001. doi: 10.1088/1741-2560/12/2/026001

Mehrabani, D., Mojtahed Jaberi, F., Zakerinia, M., Hadianfard, M. J., Jalli, R., Tanideh, N., et al. (2016). The healing effect of bone marrow-derived stem cells in knee osteoarthritis: a case report. *World J. Plast. Surg.* 5, 168–174.

Nadol, J. B. Jr., and Merchant, S. N. (2001). Histopathology and molecular genetics of hearing loss in the human. *Int. J. Pediatr. Otorhinolaryngol.* 61, 1–15. doi: 10.1016/s0165-5876(01)00546-8

Mikuriya, T., Sugahara, K., Sugimoto, K., Fujimoto, M., Takemoto, T., Hashimoto, M., et al. (2008). Attenuation of progressive hearing loss in a model of age-related hearing loss by a heat shock protein inducer, geranylgeranylacetone. *Brain Res.* 1212, 9–17. doi: 10.1016/j.brainres.2008.03.031

Mittal, R., Ocak, E., Zhu, A., Perdomo, M. M., Pena, S. A., Mittal, J., et al. (2020). Effect of bone marrow-derived mesenchymal stem cells on cochlear function in an experimental rat model. *Anat. Rec. (Hoboken)* 303, 487–493. doi: 10.1002/ar.24065

Mizutari, K., Fujioka, M., Hosoya, M., Bramhall, N., Okano, H. J., Okano, H., et al. (2013). Notch inhibition induces cochlear hair cell regeneration and recovery of hearing after acoustic trauma. *Neuron* 77, 58–69. doi: 10.1016/j.neuron.2012.10.032

Nakagawa, T., and Ito, J. (2005). Cell therapy for inner ear diseases. *Curr. Pharm. Des.* 11, 1203–1207. doi: 10.2174/1381612053507530

Nappi, F., Iervolino, A., and Singh, S. S. A. (2021). The new challenge for heart endocarditis: from conventional prosthesis to new devices and platforms for the treatment of structural heart disease. *Biomed. Res. Int.* 2021:7302165. doi: 10.1155/2021/7302165

Ohinata, Y., Yamasoba, T., Schacht, J., and Miller, J. M. (2000). Glutathione limits noise-induced hearing loss. *Hear. Res.* 146, 28–34. doi: 10.1016/s0378-5955(00)00096-4

Omae, K., Kanemaru, S. I., Nakatani, E., Kaneda, H., Nishimura, T., Tona, R., et al. (2017). Regenerative treatment for tympanic membrane perforation using gelatin sponge with basic fibroblast growth factor. *Auris Nasus Larynx* 44, 664–671. doi: 10.1016/j.anl.2016.12.005

Ontario Health. (2020). Implantable devices for single-sided deafness and conductive or mixed hearing loss: a health technology assessment. *Ont. Health Technol. Assess. Ser.* 20, 1–165.

Park, J., Kim, S., Park, S. I., Choe, Y., Li, J., and Han, A. (2014). A microchip for quantitative analysis of CNS axon growth under localized biomolecular treatments. *J. Neurosci. Methods* 221, 166–174. doi: 10.1016/j.jneumeth.2013.09.018

Park, T. H., and Chang, C. H. (2013). Early postoperative magnet application combined with hydrocolloid dressing for the treatment of earlobe keloids. *Aesthetic Plast. Surg.* 37, 439–444. doi: 10.1007/s00266-013-0076-6

Pettinato, G., Wen, X., and Zhang, N. (2015). Engineering strategies for the formation of embryoid bodies from human pluripotent stem cells. *Stem Cells Dev.* 24, 1595–1609. doi: 10.1089/scd.2014.0427

Pfannenstiel, S. C., Praetorius, M., Plinkert, P. K., Brough, D. E., and Staecker, H. (2009). Bcl-2 gene therapy prevents aminoglycoside-induced degeneration of auditory and vestibular hair cells. *Audiol. Neurootol.* 14, 254–266. doi: 10.1159/000192953

Pohl, F., Schuon, R. A., Miller, F., Kampmann, A., Bultmann, E., Hartmann, C., et al. (2018). Stenting the eustachian tube to treat chronic otitis media - a feasibility study in sheep. *Head Face Med.* 14:8. doi: 10.1186/s13005-018-0165-5

Polanski, J. F., and Cruz, O. L. (2013). Evaluation of antioxidant treatment in presbyacusis: prospective, placebo-controlled, double-blind, randomised trial. *J. Laryngol. Otol.* 127, 134–141. doi: 10.1017/S0022215112003118

Richardson, R. T., and Atkinson, P. J. (2015). Atoh1 gene therapy in the cochlea for hair cell regeneration. *Expert Opin. Biol. Ther.* 15, 417–430. doi: 10.1517/14712598.2015.1009889

Richardson, R. T., Wise, A. K., Thompson, B. C., Flynn, B. O., Atkinson, P. J., Fretwell, N. J., et al. (2009). Polypyrrole-coated electrodes for the delivery of charge and neurotrophins to cochlear neurons. *Biomaterials* 30, 2614–2624. doi: 10.1016/j.biomaterials.2009.01.015

Sage, C., Huang, M., Karimi, K., Gutierrez, G., Vollrath, M. A., Zhang, D. S., et al. (2005). Proliferation of functional hair cells in vivo in the absence of the retinoblastoma protein. *Science* 307, 1114–1118. doi: 10.1126/science.1106642

Santa Maria, P. L., Kim, S., Varsak, Y. K., and Yang, Y. P. (2015). Heparin binding-epidermal growth factor-like growth factor for the regeneration of chronic tympanic membrane perforations in mice. *Tissue Eng. Part A* 21, 1483–1494. doi: 10.1089/ten.TEA.2014.0474

Saraca, L. M., Di Giuli, C., Sicari, F., Priante, G., Lavagna, F., and Francisci, D. (2019). Use of ceftolozane-tazobactam in patient with severe medium chronic purulent otitis by XDR *Pseudomonas aeruginosa. Case Rep. Infect. Dis.* 2019:2683701. doi: 10.1155/2019/2683701

Schilling, A., Krauss, P., Hannemann, R., Schulze, H., and Tziridis, K. (2021). [Reducing tinnitus intensity: pilot study to attenuate tonal tinnitus using individually spectrally optimized near-threshold noise]. *HNO* 69, 891–898. doi: 10.1007/s00106-020-00963-5

Seonwoo, H., Shin, B., Jang, K. J., Lee, M., Choo, O. S., Park, S. B., et al. (2019b). Epidermal growth factor-releasing radially aligned electrospun nanofibrous patches for the regeneration of chronic tympanic membrane perforations. *Adv. Healthc. Mater.* 8:e1801160. doi: 10.1002/adhm.201801160

Seonwoo, H., Kim, S. W., Shin, B., Jang, K. J., Lee, M., Choo, O. S., et al. (2019a). Latent stem cell-stimulating therapy for regeneration of chronic tympanic membrane perforations using IGFBP2-releasing chitosan patch scaffolds. *J. Biomater. Appl.* 34, 198–207. doi: 10.1177/0885328219845082

Serra, L. S. M., Araujo, J. G., Vieira, A. L. S., Silva, E. M. D., Andrade, R. R., Kuckelhaus, S. A. S., et al. (2020). Role of melatonin in prevention of age-related hearing loss. *PLoS One* 15:e0228943. doi: 10.1371/journal.pone.0228943

Sha, S. H., and Schacht, J. (2017). Emerging therapeutic interventions against noise-induced hearing loss. *Expert Opin. Investig. Drugs* 26, 85–96. doi: 10.1080/13543784.2017.1269171

Shahjalal, H. M., Abdal Dayem, A., Lim, K. M., Jeon, T. I., and Cho, S. G. (2018). Generation of pancreatic beta cells for treatment of diabetes: advances and challenges. *Stem Cell Res. Ther.* 9:355. doi: 10.1186/s13287-018-1099-3

Shang, J., Jiang, T., Tang, L., and Wang, Z. (2016). Key technology of transplantable human auricular scaffold based on 3D printing. *J. Natl. Univ. Defense Technol.* 38, 175–180.

Shi, F., Hu, L., and Edge, A. S. (2013). Generation of hair cells in neonatal mice by beta-catenin overexpression in Lgr5-positive cochlear progenitors. *Proc. Natl. Acad. Sci. U.S.A.* 110, 13851–13856. doi: 10.1073/pnas.1219952110

Shou, J., Zheng, J. L., and Gao, W. Q. (2003). Robust generation of new hair cells in the mature mammalian inner ear by adenoviral expression of Hath1. *Mol. Cell. Neurosci.* 23, 169–179. doi: 10.1016/s1044-7431(03)00066-6

Slaughter, B. V., Khurshid, S. S., Fisher, O. Z., Khademhosseini, A., and Peppas, N. A. (2009). Hydrogels in regenerative medicine. *Adv. Mater.* 21, 3307–3329. doi: 10.1002/adma.200802106

Sorour, S. S., Mohamed, N. N., Abdel Fattah, M. M., Elbary, M. E. A., and El-Anwar, M. W. (2018). Bioglass reconstruction of posterior meatal wall after canal wall down mastoidectomy. *Am. J. Otolaryngol.* 39, 282–285. doi: 10.1016/j.amjoto.2018.03.007

Stavrakas, M., Karkos, P. D., Markou, K., and Grigoriadis, N. (2016). Platelet-rich plasma in otolaryngology. *J. Laryngol. Otol.* 130, 1098–1102. doi: 10.1017/S0022215116009403

Sun, F., Zhou, K., Tian, K. Y., Wang, J., Qiu, J. H., and Zha, D. J. (2020). Atrial natriuretic peptide improves neurite outgrowth from spiral ganglion neurons in vitro through a cGMP-dependent manner. *Neural Plast.* 2020:8831735. doi: 10.1155/2020/8831735

Sun, H., and Wu, X. (2013). Current status and prospects of non-viral vector in inner ear gene therapy. *J. Clin. Otorhinolaryngol. Head Neck Surg. (China)* 27, 1339–1342.

Sun, H., Huang, A., and Cao, S. (2011). Current status and prospects of gene therapy for the inner ear. *Hum. Gene Ther.* 22, 1311–1322. doi: 10.1089/hum.2010.246

Sun, Y., Tang, W., Chang, Q., Wang, Y., Kong, W., and Lin, X. (2009). Connexin30 null and conditional connexin26 null mice display distinct pattern and time course of cellular degeneration in the cochlea. *J. Comp. Neurol.* 516, 569–579. doi: 10.1002/cne.22117

Tan, F., Chu, C., Qi, J., Li, W., You, D., Li, K., et al. (2019). AAV-ie enables safe and efficient gene transfer to inner ear cells. *Nat. Commun.* 10:3733. doi: 10.1038/s41467-019-11687-8

Teh, B. M., Marano, R. J., Shen, Y., Friedland, P. L., Dilley, R. J., and Atlas, M. D. (2013). Tissue engineering of the tympanic membrane. *Tissue Eng. Part B Rev.* 19, 116–132. doi: 10.1089/ten.TEB.2012.0389

Unsaler, S., Basaran, B., Ozturk Sari, S., Kara, E., Deger, K., Wormald, P. J., et al. (2016). Safety and efficacy of chitosan-dextran hydrogel in the middle ear in an animal model. *Audiol. Neurootol.* 21, 254–260. doi: 10.1159/000447623

Vanwijck, F., Rogister, F., Pierre Barriat, S., Camby, S., and Lefebvre, P. (2019). Intratympanic steroid therapy for refractory sudden sensory hearing loss: a 12-year experience with the Silverstein catheter. *Acta Otolaryngol.* 139, 111–116. doi: 10.1080/00016489.2018.1532107

Verschuur, C., Agyemang-Prempeh, A., and Newman, T. A. (2014). Inflammation is associated with a worsening of presbycusis: evidence from the MRC national study of hearing. *Int. J. Audiol.* 53, 469–475. doi: 10.3109/14992027.2014.891057

Wakizono, T., Nakashima, H., Yasui, T., Noda, T., Aoyagi, K., Okada, K., et al. (2021). Growth factors with valproic acid restore injury-impaired hearing by promoting neuronal regeneration. *JCI Insight* 6:e139171. doi: 10.1172/jci.insight.139171

Wang, Z., and Yang, Y. (2021). Application of 3D printing in implantable medical devices. *Biomed. Res. Int.* 2021:6653967. doi: 10.1155/2021/6653967

Wong, A. C., and Ryan, A. F. (2015). Mechanisms of sensorineural cell damage, death and survival in the cochlea. *Front. Aging Neurosci.* 7:58. doi: 10.3389/fnagi.2015.00058

World Health Organization [WHO] (2021). *WHO: 1 in 4 People Projected to Have Hearing Problems by 2050.* Available online at: https://www.who.int/news/item/02-03-2021-who-1-in-4-people-projected-to-have-hearing-problems-by-2050 (accessed March 2, 2021).

Wu, X., Zou, S., Wu, F., He, Z., and Kong, W. (2020). Role of microRNA in inner ear stem cells and related research progress. *Am. J. Stem Cells* 9, 16–24.

Xiong, H., Pang, J., Yang, H., Dai, M., Liu, Y., Ou, Y., et al. (2015). Activation of miR-34a/SIRT1/p53 signaling contributes to cochlear hair cell apoptosis: implications for age-related hearing loss. *Neurobiol. Aging* 36, 1692–1701. doi: 10.1016/j.neurobiolaging.2014.12.034

Xuan, Y., Ding, D., Xuan, W., Huang, L., Tang, J., Wei, Y., et al. (2018). A traditional Chinese medicine compound (Jian Er) for presbycusis in a mouse model: Reduction of apoptosis and protection of cochlear sensorineural cells and hearing. *Int. J. Herb. Med.* 6, 127–135.

Yan, G. (2021). Studies on the Protective Effects on Sensory Hair Cells of Bioactive Peptides from Rapana venosa, Vol. 10. 69. Jinan: Qilu University of Technology.

Yang, K., Jung, K., Ko, E., Kim, J., Park, K. I., Kim, J., et al. (2013). Nanotopographical manipulation of focal adhesion formation for enhanced differentiation of human neural stem cells. *ACS Appl. Mater. Interfaces* 5, 10529–10540. doi: 10.1021/am402156f

Yang, Y., Zhang, Y., Chai, R., and Gu, Z. (2020). A polydopamine-functionalized carbon microfibrous scaffold accelerates the development of neural stem cells. *Front. Bioeng. Biotechnol.* 8:616. doi: 10.3389/fbioe.2020.00616

Young, E., Westerberg, B., Yanai, A., and Gregory-Evans, K. (2018). The olfactory mucosa: a potential source of stem cells for hearing regeneration. *Regen. Med.* 13, 581–593. doi: 10.2217/rme-2018-0009

Yuan, F., and Qi, W. (2018). Development of drug delivery to inner ear. *Chin. J. Otol.* 16, 575–580.

Yuan, H., Wang, X., Hill, K., Chen, J., Lemasters, J., Yang, S. M., et al. (2015). Autophagy attenuates noise-induced hearing loss by reducing oxidative stress. *Antioxid. Redox Signal.* 22, 1308–1324. doi: 10.1089/ars.2014.6004

Zakrzewski, W., Dobrzynski, M., Szymonowicz, M., and Rybak, Z. (2019). Stem cells: past, present, and future. *Stem Cell Res. Ther.* 10:68. doi: 10.1186/s13287-019-1165-5

Zhao, J., and Liang, Y. (2018). Experimental study on the effect of total flavonoids of *Pueraria lobata* on inflammatory cytokines in rats with inner ear injury induced by iso-proterenol. *Chin. J. Clin. Pharmacol. Ther.* 23, 1003–1007.

Zhou, G., Jiang, H., Yin, Z., Liu, Y., Zhang, Q., Zhang, C., et al. (2018). In vitro regeneration of patient-specific ear-shaped cartilage and its first clinical application for auricular reconstruction. *EBioMedicine* 28, 287–302. doi: 10.1016/j.ebiom.2018.01.011

Zhou, W., Du, J., Jiang, D., Wang, X., Chen, K., Tang, H., et al. (2018). microRNA183 is involved in the differentiation and regeneration of Notch signalingprohibited hair cells from mouse cochlea. *Mol. Med. Rep.* 18, 1253–1262. doi: 10.3892/mmr.2018.9127

Zhuo, X. L., Wang, Y., Zhuo, W. L., Zhang, Y. S., Wei, Y. J., and Zhang, X. Y. (2008). Adenoviral-mediated up-regulation of Otos, a novel specific cochlear gene, decreases cisplatin-induced apoptosis of cultured spiral ligament fibrocytes *via* MAPK/mitochondrial pathway. *Toxicology* 248, 33–38. doi: 10.1016/j.tox.2008.03.004

Zinn, E., Pacouret, S., Khaychuk, V., Turunen, H. T., Carvalho, L. S., Andres-Mateos, E., et al. (2015). In silico reconstruction of the viral evolutionary lineage yields a potent gene therapy vector. *Cell Rep.* 12, 1056–1068. doi: 10.1016/j.celrep.2015.07.019

Zou, J., Poe, D., Ramadan, U. A., and Pyykko, I. (2012). Oval window transport of Gd-dOTA from rat middle ear to vestibulum and scala vestibuli visualized by in vivo magnetic resonance imaging. *Ann. Otol. Rhinol. Laryngol.* 121, 119–128. doi: 10.1177/000348941212100209

Zou, J., Pyykko, I., and Hyttinen, J. (2016). Inner ear barriers to nanomedicine-augmented drug delivery and imaging. *J. Otol.* 11, 165–177. doi: 10.1016/j.joto.2016.11.002

Zucchelli, E., Birchall, M., Bulstrode, N. W., and Ferretti, P. (2020). Modeling normal and pathological ear cartilage in vitro using somatic stem cells in three-dimensional culture. *Front. Cell. Dev. Biol.* 8:666. doi: 10.3389/fcell.2020.00666

9

LGR5-Positive Supporting Cells Survive Ototoxic Trauma in the Adult Mouse Cochlea

Natalia Smith-Cortinez[1,2†], Rana Yadak[1,2†], Ferry G. J. Hendriksen[1], Eefje Sanders[1], Dyan Ramekers[1,2], Robert J. Stokroos[1,2], Huib Versnel[1,2] and Louise V. Straatman[1,2*]

[1] Department of Otorhinolaryngology and Head & Neck Surgery, University Medical Center Utrecht, Utrecht, Netherlands,
[2] UMC Utrecht Brain Center, University Medical Center Utrecht, Utrecht University, Utrecht, Netherlands

*Correspondence:
Louise V. Straatman
L.V.Straatman@umcutrecht.nl

†These authors share first authorship

Sensorineural hearing loss is mainly caused by irreversible damage to sensory hair cells (HCs). A subgroup of supporting cells (SCs) in the cochlea express leucine-rich repeat-containing G-protein coupled receptor 5 (LGR5), a marker for tissue-resident stem cells. LGR5+ SCs could be used as an endogenous source of stem cells for regeneration of HCs to treat hearing loss. Here, we report long-term presence of LGR5+ SCs in the mature adult cochlea and survival of LGR5+ SCs after severe ototoxic trauma characterized by partial loss of inner HCs and complete loss of outer HCs. Surviving LGR5+ SCs (confirmed by GFP expression) were located in the third row of Deiters' cells. We observed a change in the intracellular localization of GFP, from the nucleus in normal-hearing to cytoplasm and membrane in deafened mice. These data suggests that the adult mammalian cochlea possesses properties essential for regeneration even after severe ototoxic trauma.

Keywords: inner ear regeneration, deafness, LGR5+ supporting cells, ototoxicity, adult mammalian cochlea

INTRODUCTION

Hearing loss affects almost 500 million people worldwide, including 34 million children (World Health Organization, 2021), and it has been estimated that 900 million people could have disabling hearing loss by 2050 (Wilson et al., 2017; Chadha et al., 2018). Diverse etiologies, including aging, trauma, noise exposure, ototoxic drugs or genetic diseases, cause irreversible damage to sensory hair cells (HCs) in the cochlea (Edge and Chen, 2008; Mittal et al., 2017). While hearing aids and cochlear implants often result in recovery of hearing in hearing-impaired patients, a key problem is limited quality of the auditory percept (Caldwell et al., 2017; Lesica, 2018; Peters et al., 2018). Regeneration of cochlear HCs from endogenous cochlear stem cells could be a novel approach to improve hearing without the need of an electronic device.

In non-mammalian vertebrates, HC loss triggers spontaneous regeneration through re-entry of supporting cells (SCs) into cell cycle and transdifferentiation into new HCs (Dooling et al., 1997). In mammals, it has been described that a subset of SCs from the mouse and human cochlea have stem cell characteristics, and possess the potential to differentiate into new HCs *in vitro* and *in vivo* (Warchol et al., 1993; Li et al., 2003; White et al., 2006; McLean et al., 2017; Shu et al., 2019). The differentiation of SCs into HCs is mainly controlled by the Notch and Wnt signaling pathways which promote cell proliferation and differentiation (Chai et al., 2011, 2012; Mizutari et al., 2013; Li et al., 2015; Żak et al., 2015). The leucine-rich repeat-containing G-protein coupled receptor 5 (LGR5) is a membrane receptor in the Wnt pathway, which has been described as a stem-cell marker in different organs including the cochlea. It is expressed in a subgroup of SCs which give rise to HCs during murine embryonic development (Groves, 2010; Shi et al., 2012, 2013; Bramhall et al., 2014; Żak et al., 2016). Potentially these LGR5 positive (LGR5+) SCs can be utilized as endogenous stem cells for HC regeneration to treat hearing loss including deafness (severe hearing loss).

The differentiation into sensory HCs has been achieved by different experimental approaches using 3D-grown inner ear organoids derived from human pluripotent stem cells (Koehler et al., 2013), mouse embryonic stem cells (Koehler and Hashino, 2014) and human fetal cochlear progenitors (Roccio et al., 2018). Moreover, the differentiation of LGR5+ SCs into sensory HCs has also been observed by culturing 3D-grown cochlear organoids from the neonatal mouse cochlea after manipulation of the Wnt and/or Notch signaling pathways (Chai et al., 2012; Shi et al., 2012; McLean et al., 2017; Roccio and Edge, 2019). Preliminary results of one study demonstrated that myosin VIIA positive hair cell-like cells can even be regenerated from human adult inner ear epithelium *in vitro* (McLean et al., 2017).

Interestingly, neonatal LGR5+ SCs have been shown to survive and retain regeneration potential after an ototoxic trauma with neomycin *in vitro* (Zhang et al., 2017). Moreover, after selective ablation of HCs, LGR5+ SCs act as region-specific HC progenitors and are capable of both mitotic and non-mitotic HC regeneration in the neonatal mouse cochlea (Wang et al., 2015). Although it is known that LGR5+ SCs are still present in the organ of Corti in the adult mouse (Chai et al., 2011; Shi et al., 2012) their long-term presence in the mature mouse (after p60) has not been elucidated. Moreover, and critical toward therapeutic applications, it is unknown whether the LGR5+ SCs survive an ototoxic trauma in the adult cochlea. Therefore, we examined LGR5 expression in the organ of Corti 1 week after ototoxic medication in adult Lgr5^{GFP} mice.

Here, we report for the first time the survival of LGR5+ SCs in the deafened adult cochlea, using a mouse model of ototoxicity previously established in our lab (Jansen et al., 2013) in adult Lgr5^{GFP} transgenic mice. LGR5+ SCs might therefore be target cells for therapeutic treatment to regenerate HCs even in adulthood.

RESULTS

Auditory Brainstem Responses and Cochlear Anatomical Organization Are Similar in Normal-Hearing Lgr5^{GFP} and Wild Type Adult Mice (p30 and p100)

To determine the hearing performance of the Lgr5^{GFP} transgenic adult mice relative to WT mice, we recorded click-evoked auditory brainstem responses (ABRs) in both groups. The p30 WT and Lgr5^{GFP} mice had similar ABR waveforms and their ABR thresholds were similar (difference smaller than 5 dB, data not shown). Immunofluorescence microscopy of whole-mount dissections of the cochlea of WT (p30) and Lgr5^{GFP} mice (p30 and p100) showed the typical image of one row of inner hair cells (IHCs) and three rows of outer hair cells (OHCs) in the apex, middle and base of the cochlea, expressed as MYO7A+ cells (in

red, **Figure 1**). Moreover, we could clearly observe LGR5+ SCs in the apex, middle and base of the cochlea of all Lgr5^{GFP} adult mice, even until p100 (in green, **Figure 1**). The LGR5+ SCs were located in the third row of Deiters' cells (DC3s) as well as, to a lesser extent, in the inner pillar cells (IPCs) in the cochlea of p30 and p100 Lgr5^{GFP} mice (**Figure 1**).

Ototoxic Trauma Causes Severe Hearing Loss, Extensive Loss of Outer Hair Cells but Survival of LGR5+ SCs

Animals had normal thresholds before deafening (approximately 45 dB peak equivalent sound pressure level, peSPL), as observed in click-evoked ABRs (**Figure 2A**). One week after ototoxic trauma, mice showed little or no click-evoked ABR (**Figure 2A**), so the ABR thresholds were near the upper limitation of the recordings (>90 dB peSPL), confirming successful deafening after 7 days. Two animals with significant residual hearing (threshold shifts < 25 dB) were excluded from the analyses. Immunofluorescence microscopy of cochlear whole-mount dissections showed that the ototoxic medication destroyed all OHCs in the apex, middle and base (**Figures 2B,C**) and the expression of MYO7A (in red, **Figure 2B**) indicated an average survival of 60–80% of IHCs (**Figures 2B,C**). Interestingly, LGR5 (GFP) was still expressed in DC3s in the apex, middle and base of cochleas from deafened mice (in green, **Figures 2B,C**). However, IPCs seemed to have lost the LGR5 (GFP) expression (**Figure 2B**). Notably, some of the deafened cochleas showed two rows of LGR5+ SCs and these were located significantly closer to IHCs than in cochleas from normal-hearing mice [$p < 0.001$, $F(1, 9) = 27$; **Figure 2D**]. Furthermore, we observed no changes in the number of LGR5+ SCs located in DC3s after deafening [$p = 0.17$, $F(1, 9) = 2.2$; **Figure 2C**, right panel].

Analysis of MYO7A and LGR5 (GFP) expression in cryosections showed that in control cochleas (up to p100) LGR5 (GFP) was present in DC3s and IPCs, and after deafening LGR5 (GFP) was present only in DC3s (**Figure 3**). Furthermore, MYO7A expression was observed mainly in IHCs in cochleas from deafened mice and in IHC and OHC in cochleas from normal-hearing mice (**Figure 3**).

GFP Changes Its Subcellular Localization After Deafening

In the immunofluorescence data, we observed that GFP expression was mainly localized in the nuclei and cytoplasm of SCs in cochleas from normal-hearing mice and in the cytoplasm and plasma membrane (PM) of SCs in cochleas from deafened mice. To quantify the subcellular localization of GFP, we calculated Pearson's correlation coefficient (PCC) in z-stacks taken for GFP (green) and DAPI (blue) in apex, middle and base of normal and deafened cochleas. We observed that GFP is present in the nuclei and to a lesser extent in the cytoplasm of SCs in control cochleas (**Figure 4A**, top panels) and mainly in the cytoplasm and PM of SCs in the deafened cochlea (**Figure 4A**, bottom panels). After plotting the green intensities vs. blue intensities of images in **Figure 4A** we can observe that in the normal conditions there is a gradient of

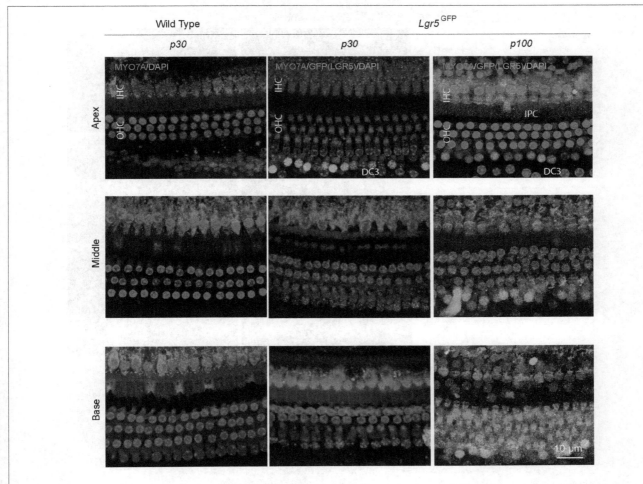

FIGURE 1 | Anatomy of the organ of Corti in normal-hearing wild type (WT) and Lgr5^{GFP} adult mice. Representative images of immunofluorescence microscopy of apex, middle and base in whole mount dissections of the cochlea of WT and Lgr5^{GFP} adult (p30 and p100) mice stained with myosin VII A (MYO7A) in red, GFP (LGR5) in green and DAPI in blue. GFP (LGR5) was detected particularly in the 3rd row of Deiters' cells (DC3s) and, to a lesser extent, in the inner pillar cells (IPCs). No changes in GFP (LGR5) expression were found between p30 and p100 mice. Bar = 10 μm. n_{WT} = 3; $n_{Lgr5GFP(p30)}$ = 7; $n_{Lgr5GFP(p100)}$ = 3 (representative images of 1 cochlea per group).

pixels that co-localize in both channels (square 1, **Figure 4B**) whereas in deafened conditions there are pixels that either express DAPI or GFP but not both (square 2, **Figure 4B**). According to PCC, which is independent from fluorophore intensity, the co-localization was significantly lower in deafened mice (characterized by a low PCC in the apex, middle and base) than in normal-hearing mice (characterized by a high PCC in the apex, middle and base) [$F(1, 9)$ = 39, $p < 0.001$; **Figure 4C**]. These results suggest that the subcellular localization of GFP is mainly nuclear in SCs of the normal-hearing mice and non-nuclear after deafening.

DISCUSSION

In this study the presence of LGR5+ SCs in cochleas of adult normal-hearing and deafened mice was evaluated *in vivo*. In normal-hearing adult Lgr5^{GFP} transgenic mice, with a hearing

threshold similar to wild type (WT) littermates, LGR5+ SCs were found in the DC3s and, to a lesser extent, in the IPCs. One week after deafening, using a single dose of ototoxic co-medication of kanamycin and furosemide, there was survival of LGR5+ SCs in adult Lgr5^{GFP} transgenic mice, even though there was extensive loss of OHCs and substantial loss of IHCs. Interestingly, a change in subcellular localization of GFP in SCs was observed, which was expressed in the nuclei of SCs in normal cochleas and in the cytoplasm of SCs in deafened cochleas.

Potential Endogenous Cochlear Stem Cells During Adulthood

Since the generation of the Lgr5^{GFP} transgenic mice (Barker et al., 2007) the LGR5 expression has been described in many tissues with known or previously unknown regeneration potential. In the neonatal mouse cochlea some SCs that express LGR5 have progenitor potential and can regenerate into new HCs *in vitro* and *in vivo* (Chai et al., 2012; Li et al., 2015;

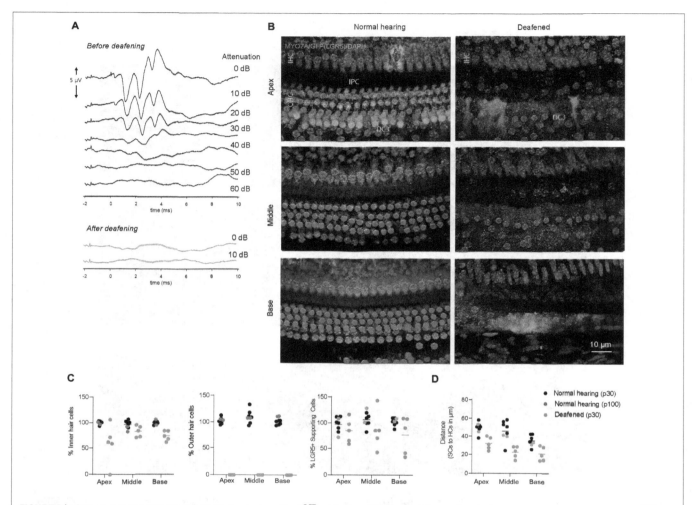

FIGURE 2 | LGR5+ supporting cells are detected in the deafened Lgr5^{GFP} adult mice. **(A)** Representative auditory brain stem responses (ABRs) of one Lgr5^{GFP} mouse before (in black) and 1 week after (in red) deafening. **(B)** Representative images of immunofluorescence microscopy of apex, middle and base in whole-mount dissections of the cochlea of Lgr5^{GFP} normal-hearing and deafened mice stained with myosin VIIA (MYO7A) in red, GFP (LGR5) in green and DAPI in blue. MYO7A stainings showed that the outer hair cells (OHCs) were completely abolished after deafening, with partial preservation of inner hair cells (IHCs). Compared to the normal cochlea, the GFP (LGR5) expression after deafening was still present in the third row of Deiters' cells (DC3s) and showed a cytoplasmic sublocalization and a more diffuse staining. **(C)** Cell counts, in percentage, for apex, middle and base of the cochlea of normal-hearing (p30 in black and p100 in gray) and deafened (p30) Lgr5^{GFP} mice. **(D)** Distance in μm from GFP + SCs to MYO7A+ IHCs. Bar = 10 μm. n$_{normal\ hearing(p30)}$ = 6; n$_{normal\ hearing(p100)}$ = 2 n$_{deafened(p30)}$ = 5, mean.

Ni et al., 2016; Chen et al., 2017). However, cochlear LGR5 expression has not been thoroughly described for adult mice, which is important since the majority of hearing-disabled people are adults (Cunningham and Tucci, 2017), so studying the role of LGR5+ SCs in adulthood is clinically very relevant. It has been shown that LGR5 expression gradually decreases until the second postnatal week and that it remains detectable only in the DC3s in the adult (p30) cochlea (Chai et al., 2011). Chai et al. (2011) also described that LGR5 expression is only detected in IPCs until p12. In contrast, another study showed that LGR5 is expressed in the adult (p30 and p60) mouse cochlea in the DC3s as well as in the IPCs (Shi et al., 2012). Our data further confirm these latter findings since we observed LGR5 expression even at p100 in DC3s and IPCs. As Shi et al., we performed immunofluorescence stainings using anti-GFP antibodies to increase the detection of LGR5, whereas Chai et al. (2011) did

not use anti-GFP antibodies in their immunofluorescence, which potentially resulted in absence of a detectable LGR5 signal in the IPCs in mice older than p12. Moreover, in the present study no deterioration was found of LGR5 expression between p30 and p100. To our knowledge, this is the first study showing LGR5 expression in both DC3s and IPCs until p100 in Lgr5^{GFP} transgenic mice. This indicates that LGR5 expression in the cochlear SCs does not deteriorate during adulthood and suggests long-term availability of target cells for regenerative therapy for the adult cochlea.

LGR5+ Cell Survival and Regenerative Capacities After Severe Ototoxic Trauma

Interestingly, in neonatal mouse cochlear tissue, it has been shown that after application of neomycin *in vitro* to induce HC

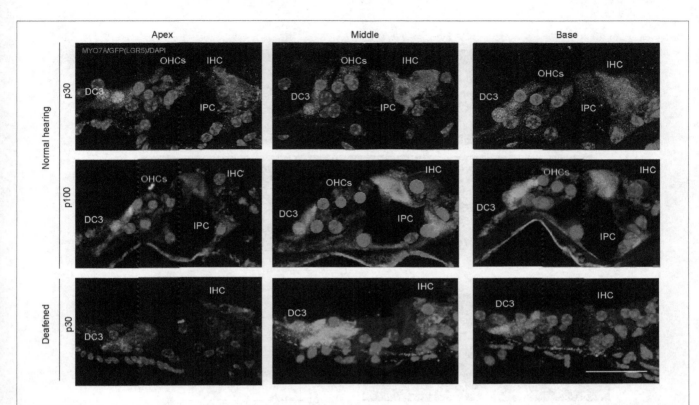

FIGURE 3 | After deafening inner pillar cells (IPCs) lose LGR5 expression. Representative images of immunofluorescence microscopy of cryosections of the cochlea of normal-hearing (p30 and p100) and deafened Lgr5^{GFP} mice stained with myosin VII A (MYO7A) in red, GFP (LGR5) in green and DAPI in blue. IPCs of normal-hearing animals showed LGR5 expression, which disappeared after deafening. Bar = 10 μm. $n_{normal\ hearing(p30)}$ = 6; $n_{normal\ hearing(p100)}$ = 1 $n_{deafened(p30)}$ = 5 (representative images of 1 cochlea per group).

loss, LGR5+ progenitors showed increased ability to proliferate and regenerate HCs 4 days after the ototoxic trauma (Zhang et al., 2017). For the adult mouse cochlea, this is the first study showing survival of LGR5+ SCs after deafening, which were located in the DC3s after deafening. This strongly suggests that the deafened mammalian cochlea retains regenerative potential, and hence therapeutic opportunities targeting the LGR5+ SCs could arise. A pioneering clinical trial has already shown that modulating the Wnt and Notch signaling pathway with a recently commercialized drug (FX322) in patients with sensorineural hearing loss improves speech recognition (both in quiet and in noise) 90 days after treatment (McLean et al., 2021). This report, including only patients with noise-induced or idiopathic sudden SNHL, supports the hypothesis that Wnt-responsive SCs with regeneration potential are present in human, even after deafness. The fact that we also found surviving LGR5+ progenitors after ototoxic trauma opens an opportunity for this treatment of ototoxically induced hearing loss as well.

The survival of SCs 1 week after an ototoxic event, even when resulting in extensive HC loss, is in accordance with previous studies and indicates that these are potentially less susceptible to ototoxic trauma. This is probably a result of less uptake of aminoglycoside (like kanamycin) in SCs, compared to HCs (Aran et al., 1995; Richardson et al., 1997;

1999; Young and Raphael, 2007; Taylor et al., 2012). Also in long-term experiments with mice deafened with 1 dose of kanamycin and bumetanide, survival of SCs 6 months after ototoxic trauma was shown, even when there was complete loss of IHCs and OHCs; however, it was not determined if the surviving SCs had progenitor potential (Taylor et al., 2012). Some other studies supported the hypothesis that there are SCs with regenerative capacities after ototoxic trauma: In adult guinea pigs treated with neomycin, the loss of HCs was accompanied by increasing number of dividing SCs 4 days after treatment, suggesting SCs were proliferating (Young and Raphael, 2007). Furthermore, in deafened adult guinea pigs, ototoxic trauma was accompanied by loss of IHCs and OHCs and survival of SCs. In these animals Atoh1 gene therapy improved regeneration and differentiation of new HCs 4 days (Izumikawa et al., 2005), 30 and 60 days (Kawamoto et al., 2003) after gene therapy.

In our study, we assessed expression of LGR5 1 week after deafening which represents an intermediate step between an acute and a chronic model. Further experiments need to be performed to assess the long-term effects of deafening on LGR5 expression and hence translate these findings into the patient's situation, which are usually chronically injured and establish the best therapeutic window for the treatment. However, based on previous studies showing long term (up to 1 year)

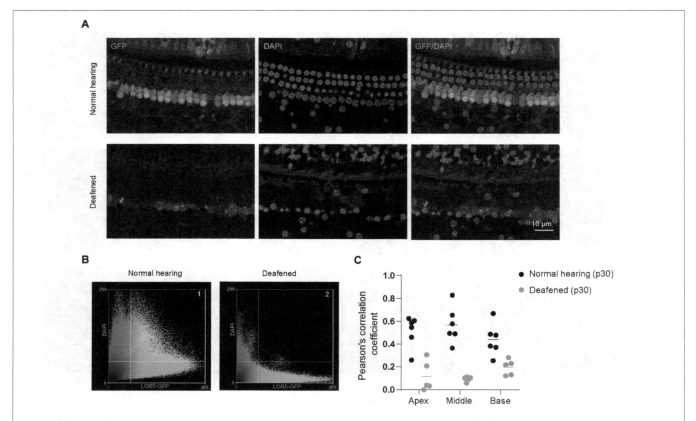

FIGURE 4 | GFP expression is located in different subcellular compartments in the cochlea of normal-hearing and deafened mice. **(A)** Representative images of immunofluorescence microscopy of whole-mount dissections of the cochlea of normal-hearing and deafened Lgr5^{GFP} mice stained with GFP in green, DAPI in blue and merged images. **(B)** Scatter plot of green intensity vs. blue intensity of images in panel (A). Square 1 represents the pixels that are expressed in both channels in normal hearing and square 2 represents the pixels that are expressed in both channels in deafened. **(C)** Pearson's correlation coefficient (PCC) calculated for the apex, middle and base of the cochlea of normal-hearing and deafened Lgr5^{GFP} mice. Bar = 10 μm. $n_{normal\ hearing(p30)}$ = 6; $n_{deafened(p30)}$ = 5.

survival of SOX2 + SCs in the mouse cochlea, even after injection of high concentrations of kanamycin and furosemide (Oesterle et al., 2008), long term survival of LGR5+ SCs is expected.

Change in Subcellular Localization of GFP After Deafening: From Nucleus to Cytoplasm

In the present study a change in the intracellular localization of GFP was found in the SCs after deafening. It must be taken into account that Lgr5^{GFP} mice allow for visualization of LGR5+ cells due to a genetic modification that produces EGFP controlled by the promoter of LGR5 (Barker et al., 2007), however, GFP is not fused to LGR5. In the normal cochlea, the GFP expression was mainly localized in the nucleus of SCs. Interestingly, a nuclear localization of GFP is also visible in data of other studies using the Lgr5^{GFP} animal model: in the normal cochlea of Lgr5^{GFP} mice (p0-p19) GFP staining was localized in the nuclei of DC3s (Chai et al., 2011; Shi et al., 2012), and it colocalized with Prox1 (Chai et al., 2011), a transcription factor that is expressed in the nuclei of DCs and pillar cells (PCs) (Bermingham-McDonogh et al., 2006) and with SOX2

(Shi et al., 2012), a transcription factor that controls inner ear development and is expressed in the nuclei of some SCs (Steevens et al., 2019). The observations above further confirm the hypothesis that in both the neonatal and mature organ of Corti in normal-hearing mice, GFP localizes in the nuclei of SCs. After deafening there was a shift of GFP expression to the cytoplasm. The accumulation of GFP or EGFP in the cell nucleus has been previously reported in other models (Seibel et al., 2007) and it is known to occur due to the low molecular weight of the protein which, with only 27 kDa, is able to passively diffuse to the nuclei (Macara, 2001). Nuclear translocation of proteins is a mechanism that occurs in physiological conditions to control gene expression. Many proteins that move to the nuclei have a conserved nuclear localization sequence to signal the translocation through nuclear pore complexes or receptor-mediated import pathways. However, no nuclear localization sequences have been found for GFP or EGFP (Seibel et al., 2007). The change in intracellular localization from nuclei to cytoplasm after deafening could suggest that the nuclear membrane is becoming more permeable, thus promoting leakage of EGFP to the cytoplasm. It could also be due to changes in the concentration of EGFP molecules, which could suggest more EGFP production after deafening.

CONCLUSION

In conclusion, this study showed the presence of LGR5+ SCs in the cochlea of adult mice up to p100, which indicates potential endogenous cochlear stem cells with proliferative and regenerative capacities in adulthood. *In vivo* survival of these progenitor cells, after a severe ototoxic event, indicates the availability of target cells for future therapeutic approaches for ototoxic-induced deafness by manipulation of the Wnt- and Notch-signaling pathways. Furthermore, a change in the subcellular localization of GFP after deafening was reported. This report gives further insight into the regeneration potential of the adult deafened cochlea and sets the basis of future therapy to improve hair cell regeneration in hearing-impaired patients.

MATERIALS AND METHODS

Animals

We used 4 C57BL/6 WT mice and 18 heterozygous LGR5-EGFP-CreERT2 (Jackson Laboratory, Stock 008875) mice (Lgr5^{GFP}). Nineteen mice were used at postnatal day 30 (p30) and three Lgr5^{GFP} mice at p100. Mice were housed in open cages with food and water *ad libitum* and standard laboratory conditions. All surgical and experimental procedures were approved by the Dutch Central Authority for Scientific Procedures on Animals (CCD:1150020186105).

Deafening Procedure

Mice were deafened as described previously (Jansen et al., 2013). Non-treated mice were used as normal-hearing controls and consisted of 8 Lgr5^{GFP} and 4 WT p30 mice. The deafened group consisted of 7 Lgr5^{GFP} p30 mice. Normal hearing was confirmed by recordings of ABRs, as described below. Then, 700 mg/kg kanamycin sulfate was injected subcutaneously (stock solution 100 mg/ml in saline). Within 5 min after kanamycin administration, 100 mg/kg furosemide was infused into the tail vein (stock solution 100 mg/ml). Mice were weighed before the deafening procedure and daily after the deafening, since substantial loss of weight can indicate kanamycin-induced kidney failure.

Auditory Brainstem Responses

ABRs were recorded under general anesthesia using three subcutaneously positioned needle electrodes. The active electrode was placed behind the right pinna, the reference electrode was placed anteriorly on the skull, and the ground electrode was placed in the hind limb. Stimulus generation and data acquisition were controlled by custom-written software involving a personal computer and a Multi-I/O processor (RZ6; Tucker-Davis Technologies, Alachua, FL, United States). Acoustic stimuli consisted of trains of 20-µs clicks with an interstimulus interval of 33 ms. Sounds were presented in an open-field configuration with an electrostatic speaker (TDT ES1) positioned at 3 cm from the pinna. Sound levels were varied from approximately 90 dB peSPL down to below threshold in 10 dB steps. Calibration was performed with Bruel and Kjaer equipment (2203 sound level meter; 1-inch condenser microphone 4132).

Genotyping

Lgr5^{GFP} transgenic mice were genotyped by isolating DNA from ear tissue. Genomic DNA isolation was performed with DirectPCR lysis reagent (Viagen, Biotech, Los Angeles, CA, United States) according to the manufacturer's instructions. The primers for PCR amplification were: GFP, forward: CACTGCATTCTAGTTGTGG; and reverse: CGGTGCCCGCAGCGAG. Amplicons were separated by electrophoresis in a 3% agarose gel.

Cryosectioning and Whole Mount Sample Preparation

Mouse cochleas were harvested after termination by decapitation. Tissues were prepared as described previously (Żak et al., 2016). Briefly, tissues were fixed in 2% paraformaldehyde (Sigma–Aldrich) in phosphate-buffered saline (PBS, pH 7.4) and stored in 2% PFA in PBS at 4°C. Cochleas were decalcified in 270 mM (=10%) EDTA-2Na (Sigma–Aldrich: ED2SS) in dH$_2$O at room temperature under constant agitation for 7 days. Cryoprotection of tissues was performed using solutions of increasing concentrations of sucrose (Merck: 1.07653.1000), up to 30%, in PBS (pH 7.4). After subsequent infiltration in a mixture (1:1) of 30% sucrose/OCT compound (Sakura Finetek Europe B.V., Alphen aan den Rijn, The Netherlands) and pure OCT compound, tissues were embedded in OCT and stored at −80°C. Cryosections of 12 µm were cut using a Leica CM3050 cryostat and mounted on microscope slides. For whole-mount samples, tissues were fixed and decalcified as described above. After decalcification, the otic capsule was opened, the lateral wall, Reissner's membrane, tectorial membrane and modiolus were removed and the basilar membrane containing the organ of Corti was dissected into individual half-turns.

Immunofluorescence Microscopy

Immunofluorescence staining was performed on cryosections and whole-mount dissections. The tissues and slides were washed with blocking solution (2% donkey serum and 0.1% triton X-100 in PBS). Specimens were incubated with primary antibodies, anti-myosin VIIA (MYO7A, 1/300, rabbit, Proteus Biosciences, 25-6790) and anti-GFP (1/200, goat, Abcam, ab5450) overnight at 4°C. Later, slides and tissues were washed with blocking solution and incubated with secondary antibodies donkey-anti Rabbit-Alexa 594 (1/500, Invitrogen, A-21207), donkey-anti Goat-Alexa 488 (1/200, Abcam, AB150129), and DAPI solution (1/500, Abcam, AB228549) for 90 min at room temperature. Lastly, specimens were washed in PBS and mounted in Vectashield Antifade Mounting Medium (Vector laboratories, H-1000). Slides were imaged using a Zeiss LSM700 Scanning Confocal Microscope. Apical, middle, and basal regions were calculated by measuring the total length of each cochlear duct in the whole-mount dissections and calculating 25% (apex), 50% (middle), and 75% (basal) distance from the apical end. Three-dimensional image reconstruction of Z-stacks and PCC analyses of DAPI and GFP signals were performed using ImageJ software.

Cell Counting

Cells were counted by three independent raters using whole-mount dissection immunofluorescence staining images. The total number of IHCs and OHCs were counted by analyzing MYO7A+ cells. SCs were counted by assessing LGR5+ cells located in the DC3s. Cells were counted in each of three cochlear segments (apical, middle and basal). Density (cells per 100 μm) was then calculated for each segment and numbers were normalized vs. normal-hearing littermates and shown in percentages.

Statistical Analysis

Significance of differences in cochlear tissues between the deafened and normal-hearing mice was tested by repeated measures ANOVA with ototoxic treatment as between-group factor and cochlear location (basal, middle, apical) as within-animal factor. These analyses were performed in SPSS

statistics version 27 for windows (IBM Corp., Armonk, NY, United States). Results were considered statistically different when the p-value <0.05.

AUTHOR CONTRIBUTIONS

NS-C, RY, and LS: conceptualization. RY, FH, and HV: methodology. NS-C, RY, FH, ES, DR, and LS: investigation. NS-C and HV: formal analysis. HV, RS, and LS: resources, project administration, and funding. NS-C, HV, and LS: writing—original draft. HV and LS: writing—revision and editing and project supervision. All authors contributed to the article and approved the submitted version.

ACKNOWLEDGMENTS

We thank Corlinda ten Brink from the Cell Microscopy Core, Department of Cell Biology, Center for Molecular Medicine, UMC Utrecht for support in the confocal microscopy. We thank Jacco van Rheenen from the Netherlands Cancer Institute for providing p100 transgenic mice.

REFERENCES

Aran, J. M., Chappert, C., Dulon, D., Erre, J. P., and Aurousseau, C. (1995). Uptake of amikacin by hair cells of the guinea pig cochlea and vestibule and ototoxicity: comparison with gentamicin. *Hear. Res.* 82, 179–183. doi: 10.1016/0378-5955(94)00175-P

Barker, N., Van Es, J. H., Kuipers, J., Kujala, P., Van Den Born, M., Cozijnsen, et al. (2007). Identification of stem cells in small intestine and colon by marker gene Lgr5. *Nature* 449, 1003–1007. doi: 10.1038/nature06196

Bermingham-McDonogh, O., Oesterle, E. C., Stone, J. S., Hume, C. R., Huynh, H. M., and Hayashi, T. (2006). Expression of Prox1 during mouse cochlear development. *J. Comp. Neurol.* 496, 172–186. doi: 10.1002/cne.20944

Bramhall, N. F., Shi, F., Arnold, K., Hochedlinger, K., and Edge, A. S. B. (2014). Lgr5-positive supporting cells generate new hair cells in the postnatal cochlea. *Stem Cell Rep.* 2, 311–322. doi: 10.1016/j.stemcr.2014.01.008

Caldwell, M. T., Jiam, N. T., and Limb, C. J. (2017). Assessment and improvement of sound quality in cochlear implant users. *Laryngoscope Investigative Otolaryngol. Laryngoscope Investig Otolaryngol.* 2, 119–124. doi: 10.1002/lio2.71

Chadha, S., Cieza, A., and Krug, E. (2018). Global hearing health: future directions. *Bull. World Health Organ.* 96:146. doi: 10.2471/BLT.18.209767

Chai, R., Kuo, B., Wang, T., Liaw, E. J., Xia, A., Jan, T. A., et al. (2012). Wnt signaling induces proliferation of sensory precursors in the postnatal mouse cochlea. *Proc. Natl. Acad. Sci. U S A.* 109, 8167–8172. doi: 10.1073/pnas.1202774109

Chai, R., Xia, A., Wang, T., Jan, T. A., Hayashi, T., Bermingham-McDonogh, O., et al. (2011). Dynamic expression of Lgr5, a Wnt target gene, in the developing and mature mouse cochlea. *J. Assoc. Res. Otolaryngol.* 12, 455–469. doi: 10.1007/s10162-011-0267-2

Chen, Y., Lu, X., Guo, L., Ni, W., Zhang, Y., Zhao, L., et al. (2017). Hedgehog signaling promotes the proliferation and subsequent hair cell formation of progenitor cells in the neonatal mouse cochlea. *Front. Mol. Neurosci.* 10:426. doi: 10.3389/fnmol.2017.00426

Cunningham, L. L., and Tucci, D. L. (2017). Hearing loss in adults. *N. Engl. J. Med.* 377, 2465–2473. doi: 10.1056/NEJMra1616601

Dooling, R. J., Ryals, B. M., and Manabe, K. (1997). Recovery of hearing and vocal behavior after hair-cell regeneration. *Proc. Natl. Acad. Sci. U S A.* 94, 14206–14210. doi: 10.1073/pnas.94.25.14206

Edge, A. S., and Chen, Z. Y. (2008). Hair cell regeneration. *Curr. Opin. Neurobiol.* 18, 377–382. doi: 10.1016/j.conb.2008.10.001

Groves, A. K. (2010). The challenge of hair cell regeneration. *Exp. Biol. Med. (Maywood)* 235, 434–446. doi: 10.1258/ebm.2009.009281

Izumikawa, M., Minoda, R., Kawamoto, K., Abrashkin, K. A., Swiderski, D. L., Dolan, D. F., et al. (2005). Auditory hair cell replacement and hearing improvement by Atoh1 gene therapy in deaf mammals. *Nat. Med.* 11, 271–276. doi: 10.1038/nm1193

Jansen, T. T. G., Bremer, H. G., Topsakal, V., Hendriksen, F. G. J., Klis, S. F. L., and Grolman, W. (2013). Deafness induction in mice. *Otol. Neurotol.* 34, 1496–1502. doi: 10.1097/MAO.0b013e318291c610

Kawamoto, K., Ishimoto, S. I., Minoda, R., Brough, D. E., and Raphael, Y. (2003). Math1 gene transfer generates new cochlear hair cells in mature guinea pigs in vivo. *J. Neurosci.* 23, 4395–4400. doi: 10.1523/jneurosci.23-11-04395.2003

Koehler, K. R., and Hashino, E. (2014). 3D mouse embryonic stem cell culture for generating inner ear organoids. *Nat. Protoc.* 9, 1229–1244. doi: 10.1038/nprot.2014.100

Koehler, K. R., Mikosz, A. M., Molosh, A. I., Patel, D., and Hashino, E. (2013). Generation of inner ear sensory epithelia from pluripotent stem cells in 3D culture. *Nature* 500, 217–221. doi: 10.1038/nature12298

Lesica, N. A. (2018). Why do hearing aids fail to restore normal auditory perception? *Trends Neurosci.* 41, 174–185. doi: 10.1016/j.tins.2018.01.008

Li, H., Liu, H., and Heller, S. (2003). Pluripotent stem cells from the adult mouse inner ear. *Nat. Med.* 9, 1293–1299. doi: 10.1038/nm925

Li, W., Wu, J., Yang, J., Sun, S., Chai, R., Chen, Z. Y., et al. (2015). Notch inhibition induces mitotically generated hair cells in mammalian cochleae via activating the Wnt pathway. *Proc. Natl. Acad. Sci. U S A.* 112, 166–171. doi: 10.1073/pnas.1415901112

Macara, I.G. (2001). Transport into and out of the nucleus. *Microbiol. Mol. Biol. Rev.* 65, 570–594. doi: 10.1128/mmbr.65.4.570-594

McLean, W. J., Hinton, A. S., Herby, J. T. J., Salt, A. N., Hartsock, J. J., Wilson, S., et al. (2021). Improved speech intelligibility in subjects with stable sensorineural hearing loss following intratympanic dosing of FX-322 in a phase 1b study. *Otol. Neurotol.* 42, e849–e857.

McLean, W. J., Yin, X., Lu, L., Lenz, D. R., McLean, D., Langer, R., et al. (2017). Clonal expansion of Lgr5-Positive cells from mammalian cochlea and high-purity generation of sensory hair cells. *Cell Rep.* 18, 1917–1929. doi: 10.1016/j.celrep.2017.01.066

Mittal, R., Nguyen, D., Patel, A. P., Debs, L. H., Mittal, J., Yan, D., et al. (2017). Recent advancements in the regeneration of auditory hair cells and hearing restoration. *Front. Mol. Neurosci.* 10:236. doi: 10.3389/fnmol.2017.00236

Mizutari, K., Fujioka, M., Hosoya, M., Bramhall, N., Okano, H. J., Okano, H., et al. (2013). Notch inhibition induces cochlear hair cell regeneration and recovery of hearing after acoustic trauma. *Neuron* 77, 58–69. doi: 10.1016/j.neuron.2012. 10.032

Ni, W., Zeng, S., Li, W., Chen, Y., Zhang, S., Tang, M., et al. (2016). Wnt activation followed by Notch inhibition promotes mitotic hair cell regeneration in the postnatal mouse cochlea. *Oncotarget* 7, 66754–66768.

Oesterle, E. C., Campbell, S., Taylor, R. R., Forge, A., and Hume, C. R. (2008). Sox2 and Jagged1 expression in normal and drug-damaged adult mouse inner ear. *JARO - J. Assoc. Res. Otolaryngol.* 9, 65–89. doi: 10.1007/s10162-007-0106-7

Peters, J. P. M., Wendrich, A. W., Van Eijl, R. H. M., Rhebergen, K. S., Versnel, H., and Grolman, W. (2018). The sound of a cochlear implant investigated in patients with single-sided deafness and a cochlear implant. *Otol. Neurotol.* 39, 707–714. doi: 10.1097/MAO.0000000000001821

Richardson, G. P., Forge, A., Kros, C. J., Fleming, J., Brown, S. D. M., and Steel, K. P. (1997). Myosin VIIA is required for aminoglycoside accumulation in cochlear hair cells. *J. Neurosci.* 17, 9506–9519. doi: 10.1523/jneurosci.17-24-09506.1997

Richardson, G. P., Forge, A., Kros, C. J., Marcotti, W., Becker, D., Williams, D. S., et al. (1999). A missense mutation in myosin VIIA prevents aminoglycoside accumulation in early postnatal cochlear hair cells. *Ann. N. Y. Acad. Sci.* 884, 110–11024.

Roccio, M., and Edge, A. S. B. (2019). Inner ear organoids: new tools to understand neurosensory cell development, degeneration and regeneration. *Development* 146:dev177188. doi: 10.1242/dev.177188

Roccio, M., Perny, M., Ealy, M., Widmer, H. R., Heller, S., and Senn, P. (2018). Molecular characterization and prospective isolation of human fetal cochlear hair cell progenitors. *Nat. Commun.* 9:4027. doi: 10.1038/s41467-018-06334-7

Seibel, N. M., Eljouni, J., Nalaskowski, M. M., and Hampe, W. (2007). Nuclear localization of enhanced green fluorescent protein homomultimers. *Anal. Biochem.* 368, 95–99.

Shi, F., Hu, L., and Edge, A. S. B. (2013). Generation of hair cells in neonatal mice by β-catenin overexpression in Lgr5-positive cochlear progenitors. *Proc. Natl. Acad. Sci. U S A.* 110, 13851–13856. doi: 10.1073/pnas.1219952110

Shi, F., Kempfle, J. S., and Edge, A. S. B. (2012). Wnt-responsive Lgr5-expressing stem cells are hair cell progenitors in the cochlea. *J. Neurosci.* 32, 9639–9684. doi: 10.1523/JNEUROSCI.1064-12.2012

Shu, Y., Li, W., Huang, M., Quan, Y. Z., Scheffer, D., Tian, C., et al. (2019). Renewed proliferation in adult mouse cochlea and regeneration of hair cells. *Nat. Commun.* 10:5530. doi: 10.1038/s41467-019-13157-7

Steevens, A. R., Glatzer, J. C., Kellogg, C. C., Low, W. C., Santi, P. A., and Kiernan, A. E. (2019). SOX2 is required for inner ear growth and cochlear nonsensory formation before sensory development. *Development* 146:dev170522. doi: 10. 1242/dev.170522

Taylor, R. R., Jagger, D. J., and Forge, A. (2012). Defining the cellular environment in the organ of corti following extensive hair cell loss: a basis for future sensory cell replacement in the cochlea. *PLoS One* 7:e30577. doi: 10.1371/journal.pone. 0030577

Wang, T., Chai, R., Kim, G. S., Pham, N., Jansson, L., Nguyen, et al. (2015). Lgr5+ cells regenerate hair cells via proliferation and direct transdifferentiation in damaged neonatal mouse utricle. *Nat. Commun.* 6:6613. doi: 10.1038/ncomms7613

Warchol, M. E., Lambert, P. R., Goldstein, B. J., Forge, A., and Corwin, J. T. (1993). Regenerative proliferation in inner ear sensory epithelia from adult guinea pigs and humans. *Science* 259, 1619–1622. doi: 10.1126/science.845 6285

White, P. M., Doetzlhofer, A., Lee, Y. S., Groves, A. K., and Segil, N. (2006). Mammalian cochlear supporting cells can divide and trans-differentiate into hair cells. *Nature* 441, 984–987. doi: 10.1038/nature04849

World Health Organization (2021). *Deafness and Hearing Loss*. Available online at: https://www.who.int/news-room/fact-sheets/detail/deafness-and-hearing-loss (accessed April 1, 2021).

Wilson, B. S., Tucci, D. L., Merson, M. H., and O'Donoghue, G. M. (2017). Global hearing health care: new findings and perspectives. *Lancet* 390, 2503–2515. doi: 10.1016/S0140-6736(17)31073-5

Young, H. K., and Raphael, Y. (2007). Cell division and maintenance of epithelial integrity in the deafened auditory epithelium. *Cell Cycle* 6, 612–619. doi: 10. 4161/cc.6.5.3929

Żak, M., Klis, S. F. L., and Grolman, W. (2015). The Wnt and Notch signalling pathways in the developing cochlea: formation of hair cells and induction of regenerative potential. *Int. J. Dev. Neurosci.* 47(Pt B), 247–258. doi: 10.1016/j. ijdevneu.2015.09.008

Żak, M., Van Oort, T., Hendriksen, F. G., Garcia, M. I., Vassart, G., and Grolman, W. (2016). LGR4 and LGR5 regulate hair cell differentiation in the sensory epithelium of the developing mouse cochlea. *Front. Cell. Neurosci.* 10:186. doi: 10.3389/fncel.2016.00186

Zhang, S., Zhang, Y., Yu, P., Hu, Y., Zhou, H., Guo, L., et al. (2017). Characterization of Lgr5+ progenitor cell transcriptomes after neomycin injury in the neonatal mouse cochlea. *Front. Mol. Neurosci.* 10:213. doi: 10.3389/fnmol.2017.00213

10

Superparamagnetic Iron Oxide Nanoparticles and Static Magnetic Field Regulate Neural Stem Cell Proliferation

Dan Li[1,2,3†], Yangnan Hu[2,3†], Hao Wei[4†], Wei Chen[2,3], Yun Liu[2,3], Xiaoqian Yan[2,3], Lingna Guo[2,3,5], Menghui Liao[2,3], Bo Chen[6], Renjie Chai[2,3*] and Mingliang Tang[2,7*]

[1] School of Biology, Food and Environment, Hefei University, Hefei, China, [2] Co-innovation Center of Neuroregeneration, Nantong University, Nantong, China, [3] School of Life Sciences and Technology, Southeast University, Nanjing, China, [4] Department of Otorhinolaryngology Head and Neck Surgery, Drum Tower Clinical Medical College, Nanjing Medical University, Nanjing, China, [5] Department of Otolaryngology Head and Neck Surgery, The Second Affiliated Hospital of Anhui Medical University, Hefei, China, [6] Materials Science and Devices Institute, Suzhou University of Science and Technology, Suzhou, China, [7] Department of Cardiovascular Surgery of the First Affiliated Hospital and Institute for Cardiovascular Science, Medical College, Soochow University, Suzhou, China

*Correspondence:
Renjie Chai
renjiec@seu.edu.cn
Mingliang Tang
mltang@suda.edu.cn

† These authors have contributed equally to this work

Neural stem cells (NSCs) transplantation is a promising approach for the treatment of various neurodegenerative diseases. Superparamagnetic iron oxide nanoparticles (SPIOs) are reported to modulate stem cell behaviors and are used for medical imaging. However, the detailed effects of SPIOs under the presence of static magnetic field (SMF) on NSCs are not well elucidated. In this study, it was found that SPIOs could enter the cells within 24 h, while they were mainly distributed in the lysosomes. SPIO exhibited good adhesion and excellent biocompatibility at concentrations below 500 µg/ml. In addition, SPIOs were able to promote NSC proliferation in the absence of SMF. In contrast, the high intensity of SMF (145 ± 10 mT) inhibited the expansion ability of NSCs. Our results demonstrate that SPIOs with SMF could promote NSC proliferation, which could have profound significance for tissue engineering and regenerative medicine for SPIO applications.

Keywords: SPIO, SMF, neural stem cells, proliferation, regulation

INTRODUCTION

Neural stem cells (NSCs) act as one of the adult stem cells that are typically considered capable of giving rise to neurons and glia cell lineages (Gage, 2000). Currently, they have been widely used for spinal cord repairing and for the treatment of various neurodegenerative diseases in animal models (Gage, 2000; Madhavan and Collier, 2010; Mathieu et al., 2010; Carletti et al., 2011; Yoneyama et al., 2011; He et al., 2012; Reekmans et al., 2012). Nowadays, numerous reports have suggested that biomaterials could provide a tremendous opportunity to influence stem cell behaviors. For instance, the physicochemical properties of biomaterials, including substrate mechanical stiffness (Engler et al., 2006; Lee et al., 2013), nanometer-scale topography (Dalby et al., 2007; Yim et al., 2010; McMurray et al., 2011), and simple chemical functionality (Benoit et al., 2008; Saha et al., 2011), could regulate the stem cell fate. In particular, a previous study has shown that superparamagnetic iron oxide nanoparticles (SPIOs) promoted the proliferation of human mesenchymal stem cells (MSCs) through diminishing intracellular H_2O_2 and accelerating cell cycle progression (Huang et al., 2009). Furthermore, recent research has indicated that SPIOs promoted osteogenic differentiation of human bone-derived mesenchymal stem cells (hBMSCs) (Wang et al., 2016). Similarly, it has also been reported that SPIOs could promote osteogenic differentiation of adipose-derived mesenchymal stem cells (ASCs) (Xiao et al., 2015). These findings suggest that SPIOs may have the potential to modulate stem cell behaviors.

Stem cell fate is determined by the complex interactions between stem cells and their surroundings, including biochemical factors, extracellular matrix components, intercellular interactions, and physical factors (Allazetta and Lutolf, 2015). A magnetic field is an effective physical factor that has been reported to modulate cell proliferation as earlier as 1999 (Fanelli et al., 1999). Meanwhile, it was reported to mediate the osteogenic differentiation of human ASCs (Kang et al., 2013) and induce MSC differentiation into osteoblasts and cartilage (Ross et al., 2015). In addition, the magnetic fields and magnetic nanomaterials were used together to induce the growth direction of neurons (Riggio et al., 2014) and facilitate drug delivery (Qiu et al., 2017). However, there is no report to explore the biological effects of SPIO under the presence of a magnetic field on NSC behaviors.

MATERIALS AND METHODS

Synthesis of Superparamagnetic Iron Oxide Nanoparticles

The SPIOs were coated by polyglucose-sorbitol-carboxymethylether (PSC) as modified in this experiment. The method to synthesize SPIOs was applied to the classic chemical coprecipitation combined with an excellent alternating-current magnetic field (ACMF)-induced internal-heat mode (Chen et al., 2016). Briefly, 40 mg PSC was dissolved in 2 ml of deionized water, then the mixture of the 6 mg $FeCl_3$ with 3 mg $FeCl_2$ dissolved in 15 ml of deionized water was added. After cooling the mixture to 5°C, 1 g 28% (w/v) ammonium hydroxide was added with stirring for over 2 min. The mixture was then heated at 80°C for 1 h, then the deionized water was purified with five cycles of ultrafiltration using a 100 kDa membrane.

Characterization of Superparamagnetic Iron Oxide Nanoparticles

The core of synthesized SPIOs was detected by transmission electron microscopy (TEM; JEOL/JEM-200CX, Japan). The size distribution was analyzed by dynamic light scattering (DLS) with a particle size analyzer (Malvern Zetasizer Nano ZS90, United Kingdom). The hysteresis loop of SPIOs was measured using a vibrating sample magnetometer (LS 7307-9309, Lakeshore Cryotronic, United States). The final concentrations of iron in the aqueous solution were measured by inductively coupled plasma mass spectrometry (ICP-MS) on an Optima 5300DV instrument.

Neural Stem Cell Culture

Neural stem cell isolation and culture were described in the previously published protocol [32]. Briefly, NSCs were cultured in mixed DMEM-F12 medium (Gibco, Grand Island, NY)

containing 2% B-27 (Gibco), 100 U/ml penicillin, and 100 μg/ml streptomycin (Sigma-Aldrich, St. Louis, MO, United States) in the condition of 5% CO_2 at 37°C. NSCs were passaged every 3–5 days during culturing. For the determination of NSC proliferation, cells were seeded with a concentration of 5×10^4 cells/ml in DMEM-F12 medium with 2% B-27, 20 ng/ml EGF (R&D Systems, Minneapolis, MN, United States), and 20 ng/ml FGF-2 (R&D Systems, Minneapolis, MN, United States). For NSC differentiation assays, cells were seeded in an NSC differentiation kit (Stem Cell, Hangzhou, China). The care and use of animals in these experiments followed the guidelines and protocol approved by the Care and Use of Animals Committee of Southeast University. All efforts were made to minimize the number of animals used and their suffering.

Cellular Uptake of Superparamagnetic Iron Oxide Nanoparticles by Inductively Coupled Plasma Mass Spectrometry

Cells were seeded in 25 cm² flasks at the concentration of 1×10^5 to 1×10^6 per flask and incubated with SPIOs at the indicated concentrations. After 1, 2, 3, or 4 days of treatment, cells were harvested and counted. Then, the cell suspension was dissociated by hydrochloric acid with a final concentration of 60%. The concentration of iron in cell lysates was measured by ICP-MS according to PerkinElmer's operating procedures.

Cell Viability Assay

Neural stem cells were seeded in 96-well cell culture plates at the concentration of 1×10^5 cells per well ($n = 6$) and cultured overnight. The cells were then incubated with differentiation concentrations of SPIOs at indicated concentrations. After culturing for 12 or 24 h, cell viability was measured by CCK-8 assay (Beyotime, Shanghai, China) according to the manufacturer's instructions. The NSCs cultured with the ordinary medium were considered as the control.

Immunostaining

Neural stem cells were fixed with 4% paraformaldehyde for 1 h at room temperature, following treatment with blocking medium for 1 h. Next, the cells were incubated with primary antibody diluted solution overnight at 4°C. Then, each sample was washed with phosphate buffer solution [0.1% Triton X-100 in phosphate buffer solution (PBST) twice per 5 min]. The samples were further incubated with a secondary antibody for 1 h at room temperature. Finally, samples were washed with PBST, and an antifade fluorescence mounting medium (DAKO) was added. The antibodies used were Nestin (Beyotime, China). Cell proliferation was detected by Click-it EdU imaging kit (Invitrogen). All the images were captured by a Zeiss LSM 700 confocal microscope, and ImageJ (NIH) was used for image analysis.

Scanning Electron Microscope and Transmission Electron Microscopy Examination

Neural stem cells were seeded in 24-well cell culture plates at the concentration of 1×10^4 cells per well and incubated

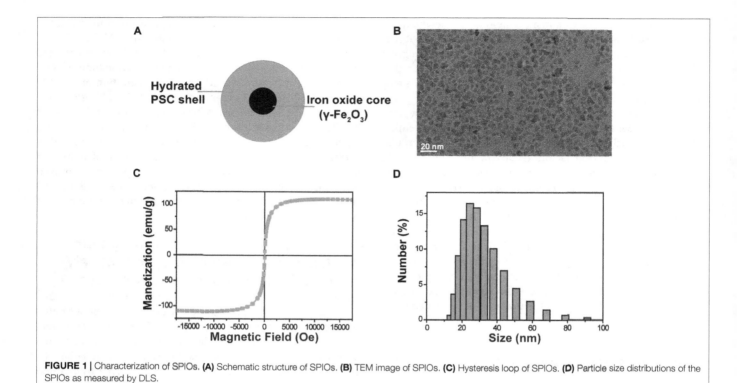

FIGURE 1 | Characterization of SPIOs. **(A)** Schematic structure of SPIOs. **(B)** TEM image of SPIOs. **(C)** Hysteresis loop of SPIOs. **(D)** Particle size distributions of the SPIOs as measured by DLS.

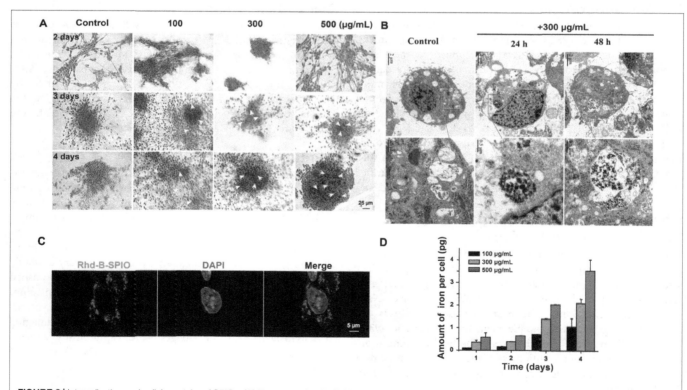

FIGURE 2 | Internalization and cellular uptake of SPIOs. **(A)** Representative Perl's blue staining images of SPIOs-treated NSCs. Scale bar = 25 μm. **(B)** TEM images of NSCs under SPIOs treatment (300 μg/ml for 24 and 48 h). A higher-magnification image of the indicated portion is shown in the inferior panel. **(C)** Laser confocal images of NSCs with Rhd-B-SPIOs treatment for 24 or 48 h. Red, Rhd-B, blue, nucleus. Scale bar = 5 μm. **(D)** The amount of intracellular iron uptake in NSCs after SPIOs treatment for different concentrations at the indicated time.

with a differentiation concentration of SPIOs at indicated concentrations. After incubation for 3 days, cells were washed two times with $1 \times$ PBS (pH 7.4); 2.5% glutaraldehyde solution (Alfa Aesar, Tewksbury, MA, United States) was added to each sample. Cells were co-incubated for 1 h at 37°C. Then, cells were dehydrated overnight, and the cell morphology was detected by scanning electron microscope (SEM) (Ultra Plus, Zeiss, Oberkochen, Germany).

Neural stem cells were seeded in 25 cm^2 flasks at the concentration of 1×10^6 and incubated with SPIOs at the concentration of 100 μg/ml. After 12- or 24-h treatment, the cells were harvested and washed two times with PBS; 2.5% glutaraldehyde solution was added to each sample, and cells were co-incubated overnight at 4°C to fix the cells. Then, the samples were transferred to 1% osmium tetroxide, dehydrated in ethanol, and embedded in Epon (Sigma–Aldrich). Finally, uranyl acetate and lead citrate were used for staining of ultrathin slices (60–80 nm). The images were captured by TEM (JEOL/JEM-200CX, Tokyo, Japan).

Statistical Analysis

All data are shown as mean and SD. Statistical analyses were conducted using GraphPad Prism 6 software. For all experiments, n represents the number of replicates, and at least three individual experiments were conducted. One- or two-way ANOVA analysis followed by a Tukey's *post hoc* test was used to determine the statistical significance between multiple groups, and Student's *t*-test was used for comparisons between two groups. A value of $p < 0.05$ was considered to be statistically significant.

RESULTS

Synthesis and Characterization of Superparamagnetic Iron Oxide Nanoparticles

The SPIOs were composed of a γ-Fe$_2$O$_3$ core and PSC shell (**Figure 1A**). The size of the γ-Fe$_2$O$_3$ core is about 6–8 nm (**Figure 1B**). The hysteresis loop of SPIOs is about 105 emu/g (**Figure 1C**), which indicates that it has a good superparamagnetic property. The average diameter of whole SPIOs measured by DLS is about 30 nm (**Figure 1D**). These results suggest that the SPIOs synthesized by this method have a uniform particle size, stable structure, good dispersion (PDI of 0.154), and stronger magnetic properties than the conventional coprecipitation method.

Internalization and Cellular Uptake of Superparamagnetic Iron Oxide Nanoparticles

Superparamagnetic iron oxide could enter the cells after co-incubation for 1 day (**Figure 2A**). The amount of SPIO could

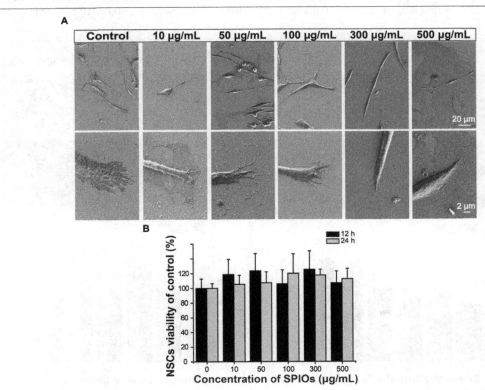

FIGURE 3 | Biocompatibility of SPIOs. **(A)** SEM images of NSCs after culturing with SPIO for 3 days at indicated concentrations. **(B)** Cell viability was detected by the CCK-8 assay. The cells were treated with SPIOs for 12–24 h at indicated concentrations. Data were normalized to the control group (no SPIOs exposure). Data are presented as mean ± SD. Student's *t*-test.

increase with time and concentrations of SPIO (**Figure 2D**). It was noticed that there was no significant difference between the 3- and 4-day groups, indicating that the uptake by a single cell was stale within 3 days. Furthermore, TEM and fluorescence imaging were employed to examine the internalization of SPIOs in NSCs. TEM results revealed that SPIOs were located in the lysosomes after 24 and 48 h of exposure (**Figure 2B**). It was further verified that SPIOs were located outside the cell nucleus after 24 h of exposure (**Figure 2C**).

The morphology of NSCs was observed by SEM after 3-day co-incubation with various concentrations of SPIOs. Cells in all groups presented normal phenotypes (**Figure 3A**). Importantly, SPIOs exposure did not affect NSC viability at concentrations up to 500 μg/ml for 24 h (**Figure 3B**), indicating the good biocompatibility of SPIOs.

Effects of Superparamagnetic Iron Oxide Nanoparticle and Static Magnetic Field on Neural Stem Cell Proliferation

Neural stem cell proliferation was first evaluated by neurosphere formation assay. NSCs from higher concentrations of SPIOs (300 and 500 μg/ml) had a significantly higher rate of neurosphere formation compared to the control group, while lower concentrations of SPIOs (10, 50, and 100 μg/ml) or 50 ± 10 mT SMF treatment had no obvious effect on the number of neurosphere formation (**Figures 4A,B**). In contrast, SPIOs at different concentrations (100, 300, and 500 μg/ml)

simultaneously exposed to SMF (50 ± 10 mT) resulted in a slower rate of neurosphere formation (**Figures 4A,B**). Although more neurospheres were generated from NSCs treated with higher concentration SPIOs, there was no significant effect on the diameters of the neurospheres compared to the control group (**Figures 4A,C**). Notably, when the NSCs were simultaneously exposed to SMF, the neurospheres exhibited a larger diameter at concentrations of 100–500 μg/ml.

Since the low concentration of SPIOs (10 and 50 μg/ml) had no effect on NSC proliferation regardless of SMF presence, these two concentrations were not included in the subsequent experiments. Next, EdU$^+$/DAPI cells were counted to further examine NSC proliferation. NSCs treated with 100, 300, and 500 μg/ml SPIOs generated significantly more EdU$^+$/DAPI cells than those from the control group (control group: 38.60 ± 6.11%; 100 μg/ml: 46.61 ± 6.16; 300 μg/ml: 46.13 ± 6.62; 500 μg/ml: 53.57 ± 7.49%; $p < 0.001$) (**Figures 5A,C**). Furthermore, SMF (145 ± 10 mT) presence inhibited the ratio of EdU$^+$/DAPI cells when compared to the control (0 μg/ml: 71.62 ± 3.93%; SMF: 66.58 ± 4.98%; $p < 0.001$). Next, when NSCs were cultured in the presence of SPIOs (100, 300, and 500 μg/ml) plus SMF (145 ± 10 mT) for 3 days, significantly lower ratio of EdU$^+$/DAPI cells was observed (100 μg/ml: 54.92 ± 6.03%; 300 μg/ml: 43.79 ± 6.93%; 500 μg/ml: 38.37 ± 7.39%) (**Figures 5B,D**).

Interestingly, when the SMF intensity was reduced to 50 ± 10 mT, the exposure of SPIOs at concentrations of 100–300 μg/ml failed to reduce the ratio of EdU$^+$/DAPI cells (**Figures 6A,C**). However, 100 ± 10 mT SMF could significantly

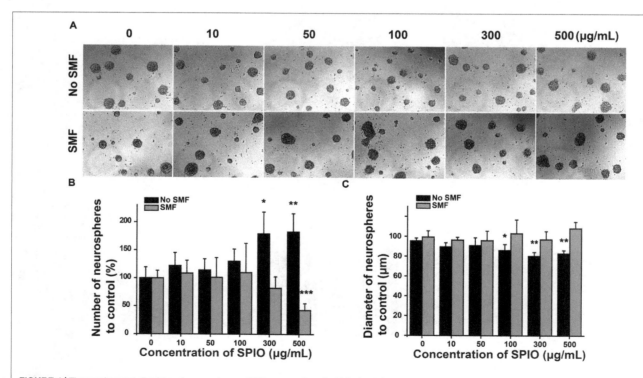

FIGURE 4 | The number and diameter of neurospheres. NSCs were cultured with indicated concentrations of SPIO (10, 50, 100, 300, and 500 μg/ml) with or without SMF for 3 days. **(A)** Representative optical images of neurospheres. **(B)** Quantification of the neurospheres number. **(C)** Quantification of the neurospheres diameter in the experimental groups. Data are presented as mean ± SD, *$p < 0.05$, **$p < 0.01$, and ***$p < 0.001$.

suppress NSC proliferation when SPIO concentration was more than 500 μg/ml, as evidenced by the decreased ratio of EdU$^+$/DAPI cells (**Figures 6B,D**).

DISCUSSION

Stem cells have a wide application prospect in the biomedical fields. NSCs have been verified for their potential in the treatment of various diseases, especially neural diseases [3–9]. The stem cell niche is the interaction between stem cells and their microenvironment which is regarded as key players in stem cell fate decisions. The niche includes several physical factors, biochemical factors, and extracellular matrix components (Allazetta and Lutolf, 2015). Many biomaterials have been proposed to modulate the stem cell niche to further regulate stem cell fate. For example, SPIOs have been reported to be able to modulate stem cell behaviors, including proliferation and differentiation (Huang et al., 2009; Xiao et al., 2015; Wang et al., 2016). Meanwhile, the magnetic field is also confirmed as one of the physical factors that affect stem cell

fate decisions. In this research, we introduced SPIOs and magnetic fields together to explore whether they could affect NSC proliferation.

Some types of SPIOs have been reported to exert excellent biocompatibility, while the potential toxicity under certain conditions (e.g., surface modification) is still under debate. Numerous studies focus on SPIO cytotoxicity on different types of cells. SPIO labeling was found not to alter MSC viability and apoptosis (Schafer et al., 2009; Zhang et al., 2014; Singh et al., 2019; Xu et al., 2020). It was further revealed that SPIOs coated with unfractionated heparin did not affect MSC survival (Lee et al., 2012). Furthermore, histological examination showed that silica-coated SPIOs induced no obvious tissue impairments or abnormal inflammation and pathology in major organs (Ledda et al., 2020). Our results were consistent with the above reports that SPIOs at concentrations less than 500 μg/ml did not affect NSC adhesion or induce cell death. SPIO toxicity is believed to be highly correlated with the cores and coatings. Usually, the SPIO core should have a magnetic responsive component. Some high-magnetic materials such as nickel are easy to be oxidized, thus leading to certain toxicity

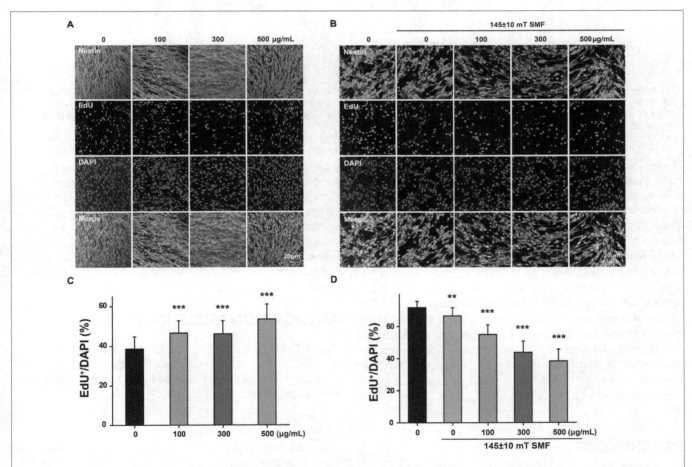

FIGURE 5 | Neural stem cells proliferation was measured by EdU labeling. NSCs were cultured with indicated concentrations of SPIO (100, 300, and 500 μg/ml) with or without 145 ± 10 SMF for 3 days. EdU was added to the culture from day 2 to day 3. Representative images for EdU staining in **(A)** control group and **(B)** 145 ± 10 mT SMF group with or without SPIO treatment at indicated concentrations (100, 300, and 500 μg/ml). The ratio of EdU + /DAPI was shown in **(C,D)**, respectively. Data are presented as mean ± SD, **p < 0.01, ***p < 0.001.

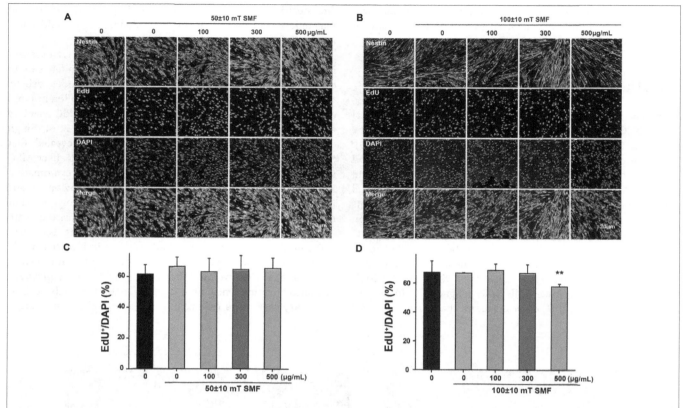

FIGURE 6 | Neural stem cells proliferation was measured by EdU labeling. NSCs were cultured with indicated concentrations of SPIO (100, 300, and 500 µg/ml) with or without SMF for 3 days. EdU was added to the culture from day 2 to day 3. Representative images for EdU staining in **(A)** 50 ± 10 mT group and **(B)** 100 ± 10 mT SMF group with or without SPIO treatment at indicated concentrations (100, 300, and 500 µg/ml). The ratio of EdU + /DAPI was shown in **(C,D)**, respectively. Data are presented as mean ± SD, **$p < 0.01$.

(Tartaj and Serna, 2003; Mahmoudi et al., 2011). The main iron oxides, hematite (α-Fe_2O_3), maghemite (γ-Fe_2O_3), and magnetite (Fe_3O_4) are superparamagnetic and also have good biocompatibility. In this study, SPIOs were prepared by an alternating-current magnetic field (ACMF)-induced internal-heat mode that was described previously (Chen et al., 2016). The SPIOs synthesized in this study were composed of a γ-Fe_2O_3 core and PSC shell. This type of SPIOs has good biosafety, as evidenced by our results. In addition, size could be a critical factor to determine SPIO cytotoxicity. It is believed that SPIOs with a diameter ranging from 10 to 100 nm are considered to be optimal for the purpose of systemic administration (Wahajuddin and Arora, 2012). SPIO toxicity was also reported with a particle size within this range. In this study, the SPIO size was within 20–40 nm, and no obvious cytotoxicity was observed at this range.

In summary, we found that SPIOs are a potential regulator for NSC expansion. SPIOs at appropriate concentrations can elevate the proliferation ability of NSCs. In the meantime, our results also indicate that SMF may suppress NSC proliferation at high intensity. In the future, we will make the best effort to uncover the biological effects of SPIOs on NSC behaviors, including migration and differentiation. Also, the detailed mechanisms underlying the observed effects will be explored as well.

AUTHOR CONTRIBUTIONS

DL, YH, HW, WC, YL, XY, LG, ML, and BC conducted the experiments and analyzed the data. RC and MT supervised the study and acquired the funding. All authors wrote the manuscript.

REFERENCES

Allazetta, S., and Lutolf, M. P. (2015). Stem cell niche engineering through droplet microfluidics. *Curr. Opin. Biotechnol.* 35, 86–93. doi: 10.1016/j.copbio.2015. 05.003

Benoit, D. S. W., Schwartz, M. P., Durney, A. R., and Anseth, K. S. (2008).

Small functional groups for controlled differentiation of hydrogel-encapsulated human mesenchymal stem cells. *Nat. Mater.* 7, 816–823. doi: 10.1038/nmat2269

Carletti, B., Piemonte, F., and Rossi, F. (2011). Neuroprotection: the Emerging Concept of Restorative Neural Stem Cell Biology for the Treatment of Neurodegenerative Diseases. *Curr. Neuropharmacol.* 9, 313–317. doi: 10.2174/157015911795596603

Chen, B., Li, Y., Zhang, X. Q., Liu, F., Liu, Y. L., Ji, M., et al. (2016). An efficient synthesis of ferumoxytol induced by alternating-current magnetic field. *Mater. Lett.* 170, 93–96.

Dalby, M. J., Gadegaard, N., Tare, R., Andar, A., Riehle, M. O., Herzyk, P., et al. (2007). The control of human mesenchymal cell differentiation using nanoscale symmetry and disorder. *Nat. Mater.* 6, 997–1003. doi: 10.1038/nmat2013

Engler, A. J., Sen, S., Sweeney, H. L., and Discher, D. E. (2006). Matrix elasticity directs stem cell lineage specification. *Cell* 126, 677–689. doi: 10.1016/j.cell.2006.06.044

Fanelli, C., Coppola, S., Barone, R., Colussi, C., Gualandi, G., Volpe, P., et al. (1999). Magnetic fields increase cell survival by inhibiting apoptosis *via* modulation of Ca2+ influx. *FASEB J.* 13, 95–102. doi: 10.1096/fasebj.13.1.95

Gage, F. H. (2000). Mammalian neural stem cells. *Science* 287, 1433–1438. doi: 10.1126/science.287.5457.1433

He, X., Knepper, M., Ding, C., Li, J., Castro, S., Siddiqui, M., et al. (2012). Promotion of spinal cord regeneration by neural stem cell-secreted trimerized cell adhesion molecule L1. *PLoS One* 7:e46223. doi: 10.1371/journal.pone.0046223

Huang, D. M., Hsiao, J. K., Chen, Y. C., Chien, L. Y., Yao, M., Chen, Y. K., et al. (2009). The promotion of human mesenchymal stem cell proliferation by superparamagnetic iron oxide nanoparticles. *Biomaterials* 30, 3645–3651. doi: 10.1016/j.biomaterials.2009.03.032

Kang, K. S., Hong, J. M., Kang, J. A., Rhie, J. W., Jeong, Y. H., and Cho, D. W. (2013). Regulation of osteogenic differentiation of human adipose-derived stem cells by controlling electromagnetic field conditions. *Exp. Mol. Med.* 45:e6. doi: 10.1038/emm.2013.11

Ledda, M., Fioretti, D., Lolli, M. G., Papi, M., Di Gioia, C., Carletti, R., et al. (2020). Biocompatibility assessment of sub-5 nm silica-coated superparamagnetic iron oxide nanoparticles in human stem cells and in mice for potential application in nanomedicine. *Nanoscale* 12, 1759–1778. doi: 10.1039/c9nr09683c

Lee, J., Abdeen, A. A., Zhang, D., and Kilian, K. A. (2013). Directing stem cell fate on hydrogel substrates by controlling cell geometry, matrix mechanics and adhesion ligand composition. *Biomaterials* 34, 8140–8148. doi: 10.1016/j.biomaterials.2013.07.074

Lee, J. H., Jung, M. J., Hwang, Y. H., Lee, Y. J., Lee, S., Lee, D. Y., et al. (2012). Heparin-coated superparamagnetic iron oxide for *in vivo* MR imaging of human MSCs. *Biomaterials* 33, 4861–4871. doi: 10.1016/j.biomaterials.2012.03.035

Madhavan, L., and Collier, T. J. (2010). A synergistic approach for neural repair: cell transplantation and induction of endogenous precursor cell activity. *Neuropharmacology* 58, 835–844. doi: 10.1016/j.neuropharm.2009.10.005

Mahmoudi, M., Sant, S., Wang, B., Laurent, S., and Sen, T. (2011). Superparamagnetic iron oxide nanoparticles (SPIONs): development, surface modification and applications in chemotherapy. *Adv. Drug Deliv. Rev.* 63, 24–46. doi: 10.1016/j.addr.2010.05.006

Mathieu, P., Battista, D., Depino, A., Roca, V., Graciarena, M., and Pitossi, F. (2010). The more you have, the less you get: the functional role of inflammation on neuronal differentiation of endogenous and transplanted neural stem cells in the adult brain. *J. Neurochem.* 112, 1368–1385. doi: 10.1111/j.1471-4159.2009.06548.x

McMurray, R. J., Gadegaard, N., Tsimbouri, P. M., Burgess, K. V., Mcnamara, L. E., Tare, R., et al. (2011). Nanoscale surfaces for the long-term maintenance of mesenchymal stem cell phenotype and multipotency. *Nat. Mater.* 10, 637–644. doi: 10.1038/nmat3058

Qiu, Y., Tong, S., Zhang, L., Sakurai, Y., Myers, D. R., Hong, L., et al. (2017). Magnetic forces enable controlled drug delivery by disrupting endothelial cell-cell junctions. *Nat. Commun.* 8:15594. doi: 10.1038/ncomms15594

Reekmans, K., Praet, J., Daans, J., Reumers, V., Pauwels, P., Van Der Linden, A., et al. (2012). Current challenges for the advancement of neural stem cell biology and transplantation research. *Stem Cell Rev. Rep.* 8, 262–278.

Riggio, C., Calatayud, M. P., Giannaccini, M., Sanz, B., Torres, T. E., Fernandez-Pacheco, R., et al. (2014). The orientation of the neuronal growth process can be directed *via* magnetic nanoparticles under an applied magnetic field. *Nanomed. Nanotechnol. Biol. Med.* 10, 1549–1558. doi: 10.1016/j.nano.2013.12.008

Ross, C. L., Siriwardane, M., Almeida-Porada, G., Porada, C. D., Brink, P., Christ, G. J., et al. (2015). The effect of low-frequency electromagnetic field on human bone marrow stem/progenitor cell differentiation. *Stem Cell Res.* 15, 96–108. doi: 10.1016/j.scr.2015.04.009

Saha, K., Mei, Y., Reisterer, C. M., Pyzocha, N. K., Yang, J., Muffat, J., et al. (2011). Surface-engineered substrates for improved human pluripotent stem cell culture under fully defined conditions. *Proc. Natl. Acad. Sci. U. S. A.* 108, 18714–18719. doi: 10.1073/pnas.1114854108

Schafer, R., Kehlbach, R., Muller, M., Bantleon, R., Kluba, T., Ayturan, M., et al. (2009). Labeling of human mesenchymal stromal cells with superparamagnetic iron oxide leads to a decrease in migration capacity and colony formation ability. *Cytotherapy* 11, 68–78. doi: 10.1080/14653240802666043

Singh, A. V., Dad Ansari, M. H., Dayan, C. B., Giltinan, J., Wang, S., Yu, Y., et al. (2019). Multifunctional magnetic hairbot for untethered osteogenesis, ultrasound contrast imaging and drug delivery. *Biomaterials* 219:119394. doi: 10.1016/j.biomaterials.2019.119394

Tartaj, P., and Serna, C. J. (2003). Synthesis of monodisperse superparamagnetic Fe/silica nanospherical composites. *J. Am. Chem. Soc.* 125, 15754–15755.

Wahajuddin, and Arora, S. (2012). Superparamagnetic iron oxide nanoparticles: magnetic nanoplatforms as drug carriers. *Int. J. Nanomedicine* 7, 3445–3471. doi: 10.2147/IJN.S30320

Wang, Q. W., Chen, B., Cao, M., Sun, J. F., Wu, H., Zhao, P., et al. (2016). Response of MAPK pathway to iron oxide nanoparticles *in vitro* treatment promotes osteogenic differentiation of hBMSCs. *Biomaterials* 86, 11–20. doi: 10.1016/j.biomaterials.2016.02.004

Xiao, H. T., Wang, L., and Yu, B. (2015). Superparamagnetic iron oxide promotes osteogenic differentiation of rat adipose-derived stem cells. *Int. J. Clin. Exp. Med.* 8, 698–705.

Xu, L., Yuan, S., Chen, W., Ma, Y., Luo, Y., Guo, W., et al. (2020). Transplantation and Tracking of the Human Umbilical Cord Mesenchymal Stem Cell Labeled with Superparamagnetic Iron Oxide in Deaf Pigs. *Anat. Rec.* 303, 494–505. doi: 10.1002/ar.24346

Yim, E. K. F., Darling, E. M., Kulangara, K., Guilak, F., and Leong, K. W. (2010). Nanotopography-induced changes in focal adhesions, cytoskeletal organization, and mechanical properties of human mesenchymal stem cells. *Biomaterials* 31, 1299–1306. doi: 10.1016/j.biomaterials.2009.10.037

Yoneyama, M., Shiba, T., Hasebe, S., and Ogita, K. (2011). Adult Neurogenesis Is Regulated by Endogenous Factors Produced During Neurodegeneration. *J. Pharmacol. Sci.* 115, 425–432. doi: 10.1254/jphs.11r02cp

Zhang, R., Li, J., Li, J., and Xie, J. (2014). Efficient *In vitro* labeling rabbit bone marrow-derived mesenchymal stem cells with SPIO and differentiating into neural-like cells. *Mol. Cells* 37, 650–655. doi: 10.14348/molcells.2014.0010

11

The Risk of Hearing Impairment from Ambient Air Pollution and the Moderating Effect of a Healthy Diet: Findings from the United Kingdom Biobank

Lanlai Yuan[1][†], Dankang Li[2,3][†], Yaohua Tian[2,3] and Yu Sun[1]*

[1] Department of Otorhinolaryngology, Union Hospital, Tongji Medical College, Huazhong University of Science and Technology, Wuhan, China, [2] Department of Maternal and Child Health, School of Public Health, Tongji Medical College, Huazhong University of Science and Technology, Wuhan, China, [3] Ministry of Education Key Laboratory of Environment and Health, State Key Laboratory of Environmental Health (Incubating), School of Public Health, Tongji Medical College, Huazhong University of Science and Technology, Wuhan, China

*Correspondence:
Yu Sun
sunyu@hust.edu.cn
[†] These authors share first authorship

The link between hearing impairment and air pollution has not been established, and the moderating effect of a healthy diet has never been investigated before. The purpose of this study was to investigate the association between air pollution and hearing impairment in British adults aged 37–73 years, and whether the association was modified by a healthy diet. We performed a cross-sectional population-based study with 158,811 participants who provided data from United Kingdom Biobank. A multivariate logistic regression model was used to investigate the link between air pollution and hearing impairment. Subgroup and effect modification analyses were carried out according to healthy diet scores, gender, and age. In the fully adjusted model, we found that exposure to PM_{10}, NO_X, and NO_2 was associated with hearing impairment [PM_{10}: odds ratio (OR) = 1.15, 95% confidence interval (95% CI) 1.02–1.30, $P = 0.023$; NO_X: OR = 1.02, 95% CI 1.00–1.03, $P = 0.040$; NO_2: OR = 1.03, 95% CI 1.01–1.06, $P = 0.044$], while $PM_{2.5}$ and $PM_{2.5}$ absorbance did not show similar associations. We discovered an interactive effect of age and air pollution on hearing impairment, but a healthy diet did not. The findings suggested that exposure to PM_{10}, NO_X and NO_2 was linked to hearing impairment in British adults, whereas $PM_{2.5}$ and $PM_{2.5}$ absorbance did not show similar associations. These may help researchers focus more on the impact of air pollution on hearing impairment and provide a basis for developing effective prevention strategies.

Keywords: hearing impairment, air pollution, digit triplet test (DTT), United Kingdom Biobank (UKB), healthy diet

INTRODUCTION

Hearing impairment is one of the most common age-related chronic health problems (Vos et al., 2016). The rate of clinically significant hearing impairment is doubling approximately every decade (Lin et al., 2011; Goman and Lin, 2016). Hearing impairment has been reported to be the second most prevalent disorder and the dominant cause of years lived with disability among global non-infectious diseases (Vos et al., 2016). In contrast with normal hearing adults of the same age, those with hearing impairment have a greater incidence of hospitalization (Genther et al., 2013), death (Contrera et al., 2015), falls (Lin and Ferrucci, 2012), cardiovascular disorders (McKee et al., 2018), depression (Li et al., 2014), and dementia (Lin et al., 2013). Consequently, hearing impairment causes a huge burden on the emotional and physical wellbeing of individuals (Dawes et al., 2014b). It is predicted that one-fifth of the population of the United Kingdom will suffer from hearing impairment by 2035 (Taylor et al., 2020). Accordingly, the key is to prevent hearing impairment. Hearing impairment is caused by a combination of hereditary and environmental factors (Cunningham and Tucci, 2017). The identification of modifiable risk factors is critical to provide the basis for preventive strategies.

Global trends in urbanization and industrialization have led to a growing problem of air pollution (Landrigan, 2017), which has become the main public health issue across the world (Brunekreef and Holgate, 2002). Of note, growing evidence demonstrates that air pollution exposure is not only connected with respiratory disorders, such as lung cancer (Xing et al., 2019), but also with cardiovascular diseases (Lelieveld et al., 2019; Hayes et al., 2020), inflammatory diseases (Chang et al., 2016), diabetes (Strak et al., 2017), and neurodegenerative diseases (Chen et al., 2017). Besides, the main environmental risk factor for human death is air pollution (Gordon et al., 2014). Lately, there have been reports that air pollution may impact hearing health, but available data is limited. A recent study (Tsai et al., 2020) found that participants exposed to fine particulate matter ($PM_{2.5}$: particulate matter ≤ 2.5 μm in diameter) and nitrogen dioxide (NO_2) had a substantially increased risk of sudden sensorineural hearing loss (SSNHL). Another study (Chang et al., 2020) showed that increased concentrations of NO_2 were linked to a higher risk of sensorineural hearing loss, while in a nested case-control study (Choi et al., 2019), SSNHL was associated with NO_2 exposure, but particulate matter with a diameter of 10 μm or less (PM_{10}) was not associated with SSNHL. Similarly, another study (Lee et al., 2019) also found no association between PM_{10} and number of SSNHL patient. Although these studies explored the association of air pollution with sensorineural hearing loss, the results remained controversial.

A healthy diet might preserve hearing (Spankovich and Le Prell, 2013; Curhan et al., 2018, 2020), as described by their role in preventing chronic illnesses (Yevenes-Briones et al., 2021). A healthy diet includes multiple components that support antioxidant function and protect against free radical damage (Curhan et al., 2020), thereby regulating oxidative stress and delaying mitochondrial dysfunction (Yevenes-Briones et al., 2021). In addition, a healthy diet might be beneficial to hearing impairment by protecting microvascular and macrovascular damage to cochlear blood flow (Appel et al., 2006; Fung et al., 2008), providing the essential nutrients for an adequate cochlear blood supply (Yevenes-Briones et al., 2021), and reducing inflammation (Neale et al., 2016). According to previous research, dietary patterns could modify the relationship between air pollution and health-related outcomes, such as cardiovascular disease mortality risk (Lim et al., 2019) and cognitive function (Zhu et al., 2022). However, the moderating effect of a healthy diet on the link between hearing impairment and air pollution has not been investigated before. Therefore, in this cross-sectional study, we aimed to explore the link between air pollution and hearing impairment and to analyze whether a healthy diet has moderating effects on this link.

MATERIALS AND METHODS

Study Subjects

The United Kingdom Biobank is an international and accessible data resource[1] containing data on more than half a million people aged from 37 to 73 years (99.5% were between 40 and 69 years) in England, Scotland, and Wales (Collins, 2012). Adults living within a 25-mile radius of one of 22 Biobank Assessment Centers in the United Kingdom were invited by email to join the United Kingdom Biobank between 2006 and 2010, achieving a response rate of approximately 5.5% (Sudlow et al., 2015). Participants completed a computer touch screen questionnaire (which included questions on topics such as population, health, lifestyle, environment as well as medical history, etc.) and underwent physical measurements, including a hearing test. Written informed consent was signed by all the participants. The research was carried out with the general approval of the National Health Service and the National Research Ethics Service. The subjects of the current study were all those participants for whom data on both air pollution measures and hearing test results were available.

Hearing Test

The speech-in-noise hearing test (i.e., digit triplet test, DTT) of the United Kingdom Biobank provided participants with 15 groups of English monosyllabic numbers to evaluate the listening thresholds (i.e., signal-to-noise ratio) at different sound levels.[2] Each ear was examined separately, in the order that the participants were allocated at random. Participants first wore circumaural headphones and selected the most comfortable volume. Then, they started the speech-in-noise hearing test to identify and type the three numbers they had heard by touching the screen interface. The noise level of the subsequent triple would increase if the triplet was correctly recognized; otherwise, it would reduce. The speech reception threshold (SRT) was defined as the signal-to-noise ratio of correctly understanding half of the presented speech. The SRT ranged from −12 to +8 dB, with a lower score representing better performance. Based on the cutoff point established by Dawes et al. (2014b), the better performance ear was chosen for this study, and participants were divided into normal (SRT < −5.5 dB) and hearing impairment (SRT $\geq$ −5.5 dB) groups.

The DTT shows a very good correlation with the pure tone hearing test ($r = 0.77$) (Jansen et al., 2010), so it can be considered as a measure of hearing impairment (Dawes et al., 2014b). There are some advantages to the DTT, for example, there is no need for a sound booth and the test can be delivered *via* the internet (Moore et al., 2014). The most common hearing complaint is difficulty in hearing over background noise (Pienkowski, 2017), so the speech-in-noise hearing test used to evaluate hearing

---

[1] www.UKbiobank.ac.UK

[2] https://biobank.ctsu.ox.ac.UK/crystal/label.cgi?id=100049

function represents an ecologically effective as well as objective hearing indicator (Couth et al., 2019).

Measures of Air Pollution

The air pollution data recorded in the United Kingdom Biobank were from the Small Area Health Statistics Unit,[3] a part of the BioShaRE-EU Environmental Determinants of Health Project.[4] The Land Use Regression model was applied to assess air pollution in 2010 by modeling at each residential address of the participants, which was developed as part of the European Study of Cohorts for Air Pollution Effects.[5] The Land Use Regression model used to calculate the spatial distribution of air pollutants was based on geographic predictors such as traffic, land use, and topography in the geographical information system. In this study, the air pollutants assessed were $PM_{2.5}$, PM_{10}, $PM_{2.5}$ absorbance, NO_X, and NO_2, of which all were annual average concentrations in $\mu g/m^3$. More details about the air pollution data used in the United Kingdom Biobank are available elsewhere.[6]

Assessment of Other Variables

Age, gender, ethnicity, educational background, employment, smoking status, and alcohol intake were utilized as baseline data. The ethnic background of participants was divided into six categories: White, Black, Asian, Chinese, Mixed, and other. The educational background was divided into six categories: higher national diploma (HND), national vocational qualification (NVQ), higher national certificate (HNC), or equivalent; A levels or AS levels (including the higher school certificate), or equivalent; O levels (including the school certificate), general certificate of secondary educations (GCSEs), or equivalent; certificate of secondary educations (CSEs), or equivalent; college or university degree; and other professional qualification. Employment status was divided into seven categories: retired; unable to work because of sickness or disability; looking after home and/or family; unemployed; in paid employment or self-employed; student (full-time or part-time); or doing unpaid or voluntary work. Smoking status (Dawes et al., 2014a) was divided into three categories: never-smokers, current and former smokers. Alcohol consumption frequency was divided into five categories: daily or almost daily; three or four times a week; once or twice a week; occasional drinking; and never. Body mass index (BMI) was categorized as obese (BMI ≥ 30), overweight (25 ≤ BMI < 30), normal weight (18.5 ≤ BMI < 25), and underweight (BMI < 18.5). Evaluation of physical activity was conducted through the questions in the International Physical Activity Questionnaire, which graded activity into three degrees: low, moderate, and high.[7] A questionnaire[8] containing the usual dietary intake was completed by United Kingdom Biobank participants during the baseline assessment. The intake of fruits (fresh fruit intake and dried fruit intake), vegetables (cooked vegetable intake and salad/raw vegetable intake), fish (oily fish

intake and non-oily fish intake), processed meat and unprocessed red meat (beef intake, lamb/mutton intake, and pork intake) from the United Kingdom Biobank food intake questionnaire was used to calculate the health diet scores (Wang et al., 2021): fruit intake ≥ three pieces per day, vegetable intake ≥ four tablespoons per day, fish intake ≥ twice per week, processed meat intake ≤ twice per week, unprocessed red meat intake ≤ twice per week. Each favorable dietary factor gave a point, so the healthy diet scores were 0–5. The serum concentrations of glycosylated hemoglobin and total cholesterol were regarded as continuous variables. Vascular problems included angina, heart attack, stroke, and high blood pressure.

Data Analysis

All analyses were performed using R version 4.0.2. The data are summarized descriptively. Continuous variables are represented as mean (standard deviation) and comparison between the two groups was performed by independent sample t test. The classification variables are represented as percentages (%) and the rate was compared by χ^2 test. The link between air pollution and hearing impairment was investigated using a multivariate logistic regression model with and without adjusting for other variables. Model 1 was unadjusted, Model 2 was adjusted for age and gender, and Model 3 was further adjusted for race, educational level, employment, smoking status and alcohol consumption frequency, BMI, physical activity, glycosylated hemoglobin, total cholesterol, and vascular diseases (heart attack, stroke, angina, and hypertension). Moreover, we evaluated the association between subgroups stratified by healthy diet scores (low: 0–2, and high: 3–5), gender (female and male) and age (≤50, 51–60, and >60). The Wald test was used to test interactions among subgroups. $P < 0.05$ (two-sided test) was considered statistically significant.

RESULTS

In total, 158,811 subjects were enrolled in this study, including 18,881 (11.9%) with hearing impairment and 139,930 (88.1%) with normal hearing, 54.5% were female ($n = 86,516$), 91.7% were white ($n = 145,633$), with the mean (standard deviation) age of 56.68 (8.15) years. The distribution of baseline characteristics and air pollution in the two groups is shown in **Table 1**. Except for physical activity, other variables were significantly distributed in the two groups ($P < 0.05$). In comparison to the group of people with normal hearing, the subjects in the hearing impairment group were older on average, non-whites. In addition, they were more likely to be obese and to have cardiovascular problems. Furthermore, the hearing impairment group was exposed to higher mean annual concentrations of air pollutants than the normal hearing group (**Table 1**).

Table 2 shows the risks of several air pollutants and hearing impairment. Model 1 (without adjustment for any confounders) showed significant associations between air pollutants and hearing impairment ($P < 0.001$) [$PM_{2.5}$: odds ratio (OR) = 2.03, 95% confidence interval (95% CI) 1.73–2.40; PM_{10}: OR = 1.64, 95% CI 1.51–1.78; $PM_{2.5}$ absorbance: OR = 1.48, 95% CI 1.40–1.56; NO_X: OR = 1.06, 95% CI 1.05–1.07; NO_2: OR = 1.17,

[3] http://www.sahsu.org/
[4] http://www.bioshare.eu/
[5] http://www.escapeproject.eu/
[6] https://biobank.ndph.ox.ac.uk/showcase/ukb/docs/EnviroExposEst.pdf
[7] https://biobank.ndph.ox.ac.uk/showcase/ukb/docs/ipaq_analysis.pdf
[8] https://biobank.ndph.ox.ac.uk/showcase/label.cgi?id=100052

TABLE 1 | Characteristics of participants (N = 158,811).

	Normal hearing	Hearing impairment	P
N	139,930	18,881	
Age (years), mean (SD)	56.21 (8.13)	60.13 (7.40)	<0.001
Gender (%)			0.004
Female	76,414 (54.6)	10,102 (53.5)	
Male	63,516 (45.4)	8,779 (46.5)	
Race (%)			<0.001
White ethnicity	129,996 (93.2)	15,637 (83.3)	
Mixed ethnicity	1,053 (0.8)	137 (0.7)	
Asian ethnicity	3,541 (2.5)	1,328 (7.1)	
Black ethnicity	3,019 (2.2)	1,026 (5.5)	
Chinese ethnicity	462 (0.3)	123 (0.7)	
Other ethnicity	1,336 (1.0)	523 (2.8)	
Education (%)			<0.001
Other professional qualification	7,113 (5.9)	1,191 (8.6)	
College or university degree	48,983 (40.7)	5,098 (36.8)	
O level/GCSEs or equivalent	30,497 (25.4)	3,580 (25.9)	
CSEs or equivalent	8,280 (6.9)	845 (6.1)	
A/AS levels or equivalent	16,528 (13.7)	1,670 (12.1)	
NVQ or HND or HNC or equivalent	8,876 (7.4)	1,465 (10.6)	
Employment (%)			<0.001
Inpaid employment or self-employed	81,816 (59.0)	7,467 (40.1)	
Retired	44,969 (32.4)	9,136 (49.1)	
Looking after home and/or family	4,195 (3.0)	474 (2.5)	
Unable to work because of sickness or disability	3,575 (2.6)	883 (4.7)	
Unemployed	2,996 (2.2)	478 (2.6)	
Doing unpaid or voluntary work	678 (0.5)	115 (0.6)	
Full-time or part-time student	384 (0.3)	66 (0.4)	
BMI (%), kg/m^2			<0.001
Underweight	721 (0.5)	121 (0.6)	
Normal weight	46,225 (33.2)	5,590 (30.0)	
Overweight	58,610 (42.1)	7,817 (41.9)	
Obesity	33,548 (24.1)	5,127 (27.5)	
Smoke (%)			<0.001
Never	77,310 (55.4)	10,140 (54.0)	
Previous	48,353 (34.7)	6,572 (35.0)	
Current	13,839 (9.9)	2,054 (10.9)	
Drink frequency (%)			<0.001
Daily or almost daily	29,132 (20.8)	3,327 (17.7)	
Three or four times a week	32,246 (23.1)	3,443 (18.3)	
Once or twice a week	35,588 (25.5)	4,367 (23.2)	
Occasional drinkers	32,275 (23.1)	5,095 (27.0)	
Never	10,551 (7.5)	2,609 (13.8)	
Physical activity (%)			0.061
Low	20,316 (17.6)	2,658 (18.1)	
Moderate	46,945 (40.7)	5,839 (39.7)	
High	48,013 (41.7)	6,198 (42.2)	
HbA1c, mean (SD), mmol/mol	36.02 (6.50)	37.55 (8.10)	<0.001
TC, mean (SD), mmol/L	5.71 (1.14)	5.60 (1.20)	<0.001
Vascular problems (%)			<0.001
None	10,0638 (73.8)	11,826 (64.9)	
Hypertension	29,376 (21.5)	4,868 (26.7)	
Heart attack, angina, or stroke	3,184 (2.3)	703 (3.9)	
High blood pressure and heart attack, angina, or stroke	3,235 (2.4)	813 (4.5)	

(Continued)

TABLE 1 | Continued

	Normal	Hearing impairment	P
Air pollution			
$PM_{2.5}$, mean (SD), $\mu g/m^3$	9.88 (0.91)	9.94 (0.95)	<0.001
PM_{10}, mean (SD), $\mu g/m^3$	16.28 (1.82)	16.45 (1.85)	<0.001
$PM_{2.5}$ absorbance, mean (SD), per-meter	1.21 (0.27)	1.24 (0.29)	<0.001
NO_X, mean (SD), $\mu g/m^3$	43.52 (14.44)	44.92 (15.83)	<0.001
NO_2, mean (SD), $\mu g/m^3$	26.88 (7.21)	27.72 (7.70)	<0.001

Abbreviations: N, number; SD, standard deviation; GCSEs, general certificate of secondary educations; CSEs, certificate of secondary educations; NVQ, national vocational qualification; HND, higher national diploma; HNC, higher national certificate; BMI, body mass index; HbA1c, glycosylated hemoglobin; TC, total cholesterol; PM, particulate matter; NO_2, nitrogen dioxides; NO_X, nitrogen oxides.

TABLE 2 | Association of air pollution and hearing impairment.

	Model 1		Model 2		Model 3	
	OR (95% CI)	P	OR (95% CI)	P	OR (95% CI)	P
$PM_{2.5}$	2.03 (1.73–2.40)	<0.001	3.02 (2.56–3.57)	<0.001	1.01 (0.79–1.29)	0.970
PM_{10}	1.64 (1.51–1.78)	<0.001	1.82 (1.67–1.97)	<0.001	1.15 (1.02–1.30)	0.023
$PM_{2.5}$ absorbance	1.48 (1.40–1.56)	<0.001	1.67 (1.59–1.77)	<0.001	1.08 (0.99–1.18)	0.063
NO_X	1.06 (1.05–1.07)	<0.001	1.09 (1.08–1.10)	<0.001	1.02 (1.001–1.03)	0.040
NO_2	1.17 (1.14–1.19)	<0.001	1.24 (1.21–1.26)	<0.001	1.03 (1.01–1.06)	0.044

Abbreviations: OR, odds ratio; CI, confidence interval; PM, particulate matter; NO_2, nitrogen dioxides; NO_X, nitrogen oxides.
Model 1: unadjusted.
Model 2: adjusted for age and gender.
Model 3: adjusted for age, gender, race, education, employment, smoking, drink frequency, body mass index, physical activity, glycosylated hemoglobin, total cholesterol, and vascular disease (heart attack, stroke, angina, and hypertension).

95% CI 1.41–1.19]. After adjusting for age and gender, Model 2 showed that air pollutants were still significantly associated with hearing impairment ($P < 0.001$), and all OR values were larger than Model 1 ($PM_{2.5}$: OR = 3.02, 95% CI 2.56–3.57; PM_{10}: OR = 1.82, 95% CI 1.67–1.97; $PM_{2.5}$ absorbance: OR = 1.67, 95% CI 1.59–1.77; NO_X: OR = 1.09, 95% CI 1.08–1.10; NO_2: OR = 1.24, 95% CI 1.21–1.26). Except for $PM_{2.5}$ and $PM_{2.5}$ absorbance, which showed no significant associations with hearing impairment ($P = 0.970$ and $P = 0.063$, respectively), we observed that the associations between the other pollutants and hearing impairment remained in Model 3 after further adjusting for other confounders on the basis of Model 2 (PM_{10}: OR = 1.15, 95% CI 1.02–1.30, $P = 0.023$; NOx: OR = 1.02, 95% CI 1.00–1.03, $P = 0.040$; NO_2: OR = 1.03, 95% CI 1.01–1.06, $P = 0.044$), even though the estimates were lower than those in Models 1 and 2.

Table 3 shows the associations between several air pollutants and hearing impairment, stratified by healthy diet scores. In this study, no significant associations and moderating effects were observed. After stratification by age (**Table 4**), we found that PM_{10}, $PM_{2.5}$ absorbance, NO_X, and NO_2 were associated with hearing impairment in participants up to and including 50 years of age (PM_{10}: OR = 1.62, 95% CI 1.20–2.18, $P = 0.002$; $PM_{2.5}$ absorbance: OR = 1.32, 95% CI 1.08–1.61, $P = 0.006$; NO_X: OR = 1.04, 95% CI 1.01–1.08, $P = 0.014$; NO_2: OR = 1.09, 95% CI 1.01–1.17, $P = 0.031$). In participants aged 51 to 60 years and above 60, there was no connection between air pollution and hearing impairment. Additionally, there was a statistically significant interaction between age and air pollution with hearing impairment ($P < 0.05$). Further, after stratifying by gender

(**Table 5**), we found that NO_X and NO_2 were correlated with hearing impairment in men.

DISCUSSION

In this cross-sectional study, we investigated the association between hearing impairment and air pollution (comprising $PM_{2.5}$, PM_{10}, $PM_{2.5}$ absorbance, NO_X, and NO_2) using United Kingdom Biobank data. We found that exposure to PM_{10}, NO_X, and NO_2 was linked to hearing impairment after adjusting for confounding factors, while $PM_{2.5}$ and $PM_{2.5}$ absorbance showed no similar correlations. Furthermore, there was no modification of these associations by a healthy diet. Regarding age, interaction effects were observed.

The relationship between air pollution and hearing impairment has not been fully established yet. Several studies indicated that exposure to NO_2 could be related to hearing problems. Chang et al. (2020) found that people exposed to moderate (hazard ratio, HR = 1.40, 95% CI 1.27–1.54) and high levels of NO_2 (HR = 1.63, 95% CI 1.48–1.81) were at higher risk of developing sensorineural hearing loss than those exposed to the low level. The results of Tsai et al. (2020) were similar, finding a significantly increased risk of SSNHL in those exposed to high concentrations of NO_2 (adjusted HR = 1.02, 95% CI 1.01–1.04). Likewise, Choi et al. (2019) discovered that SSNHL was associated with short-term exposure to NO_2 (14 days) (adjusted OR = 3.12, 95% CI 2.16–4.49). Consistent with previous studies, NO_2 was associated with hearing impairment

TABLE 3 | Associations of air pollution and hearing impairment in subgroups stratified by healthy diet scores.

	Low (N = 58324)		High (N = 94414)		P-interaction
	OR (95% CI)	P	OR (95% CI)	P	
$PM_{2.5}$	1.05 (0.69, 1.61)	0.823	0.84 (0.62, 1.14)	0.271	0.403
PM_{10}	1.20 (0.97, 1.49)	0.086	1.14 (0.98, 1.32)	0.094	0.688
$PM_{2.5}$ absorbance	1.10 (0.95, 1.27)	0.191	1.10 (0.99, 1.22)	0.060	0.902
NO_X	1.02 (0.99, 1.05)	0.147	1.01 (0.99, 1.03)	0.498	0.300
NO_2	1.04 (0.99, 1.10)	0.161	1.02 (0.98, 1.06)	0.315	0.377

Abbreviations: OR, odds ratio; CI, confidence interval; PM, particulate matter; NO_2, nitrogen dioxides; NO_X, nitrogen oxides.
All models were adjusted for age, gender, race, education, employment, smoking, drink frequency, body mass index, physical activity, glycosylated hemoglobin, total cholesterol, and vascular disease (heart attack, stroke, angina, and hypertension).
This subgroup included 152,738 participants because of the missing data of dietary information for 6,073 participants.

TABLE 4 | Associations of air pollution and hearing impairment in subgroups stratified by age.

	≤50 (N = 40,978)		51–60 (N = 53,844)		>60 (N = 63,989)		P-interaction
	OR (95% CI)	P	OR (95% CI)	P	OR (95% CI)	P	
$PM_{2.5}$	1.74 (0.96–3.14)	0.067	1.02 (0.66–1.59)	0.918	0.80 (0.57–1.13)	0.198	0.013
PM_{10}	1.62 (1.20–2.18)	0.002	1.15 (0.92–1.43)	0.215	1.04 (0.88–1.23)	0.647	0.005
$PM_{2.5}$ absorbance	1.32 (1.08, 1.61)	0.006	1.04 (0.89–1.21)	0.626	1.05 (0.93–1.18)	0.417	0.029
NO_X	1.04 (1.01–1.08)	0.014	1.02 (0.99–1.05)	0.247	1.00 (0.98–1.02)	0.921	0.005
NO_2	1.09 (1.01–1.17)	0.031	1.03 (0.97–1.09)	0.292	1.01 (0.97–1.06)	0.641	0.017

Abbreviations: OR, odds ratio; CI, confidence interval; PM, particulate matter; NO_2, nitrogen dioxides; NO_X, nitrogen oxides.
All models were adjusted for gender, race, education, employment, smoking, drink frequency, body mass index, physical activity, glycosylated hemoglobin, total cholesterol, and vascular disease (heart attack, stroke, angina, and hypertension).

TABLE 5 | Associations of air pollution and hearing impairment in subgroups stratified by gender.

	Female (N = 86516)		Male (N = 72295)		P-interaction
	OR (95% CI)	P	OR (95% CI)	P	
$PM_{2.5}$	0.86 (0.61–1.22)	0.406	1.19 (0.83–1.69)	0.346	0.191
PM_{10}	1.16 (0.98–1.38)	0.085	1.15 (0.97–1.37)	0.118	0.914
$PM_{2.5}$ absorbance	1.10 (0.98–1.23)	0.112	1.07 (0.95–1.21)	0.261	0.920
NO_X	1.01 (0.98–1.02)	0.879	1.03 (1.01–1.05)	0.011	0.061
NO_2	1.02 (0.97–1.06)	0.489	1.05 (1.00–1.09)	0.049	0.216

Abbreviations: OR, odds ratio; CI, confidence interval; PM, particulate matter; NO_2, nitrogen dioxides; NO_X, nitrogen oxides.
All models were adjusted for age, race, education, employment, smoking, drink frequency, body mass index, physical activity, glycosylated hemoglobin, total cholesterol, and vascular disease (heart attack, stroke, angina, and hypertension).

in our study. Moreover, NO_X, a term that contains several nitrogen compounds but is mainly composed of nitrogen oxide and NO_2, showed an association with hearing impairment.

In contrast to our expectations, we found a significant association between PM_{10} and hearing impairment but not $PM_{2.5}$. Conversely, previous studies (Choi et al., 2019; Lee et al., 2019) showed no correlation between PM_{10} and hearing impairment. A study reported (Tsai et al., 2020) a significantly higher risk of developing SSNHL with moderate (adjusted HR = 1.58, 95% CI 1.21–2.06) or high (adjusted HR = 1.32, 95% CI 1.00–1.74) level exposure to $PM_{2.5}$ compared to those exposed to the low level. And another study discovered a slight negative association between the maximum $PM_{2.5}$ concentration and the admission rate of SSNHL (Lee et al., 2019). In 2017, a study (Strak et al., 2017) in a large national health survey

reported that oxidative potential of $PM_{2.5}$ rather than $PM_{2.5}$, was associated with diabetes prevalence, indicating that the impact of particulate matter on diabetes might vary with the compositions. According to a study (Yin and Harrison, 2008) conducted at three sites (urban roadside, central urban background, and rural) in Birmingham, United Kingdom, organics, nitrate, and sulfate accounted for a substantial amount of the overall mass for both PM_{10} and $PM_{2.5}$. This research also showed that proportions of these three major parts and other secondary compositions like iron-rich dust and sodium chloride varied in both. Although discrepancies in associations with diseases after $PM_{2.5}$ and PM_{10} exposure could be explained by different compositions of particulate matter, the evidence may still be limited. More research is required to clarify this issue in the future.

Oxidative stress and mitochondrial dysfunction play a crucial role in hearing impairment (Yamasoba et al., 2013). Air pollution might be involved in oxidative stress by producing or directly acting as reactive oxygen species (Kelly, 2003), which can then induce mitochondrial damage (Rodríguez-Martínez et al., 2013). Dysfunctional mitochondria increase reactive oxygen species generation and accumulation, reducing the mitochondrial membrane potential, activating the apoptosis pathway, and causing the death of inner ear hair cells (Park et al., 2016). What's more, air pollution might indirectly be associated with hearing impairment by causing cardiovascular diseases through pro-inflammatory pathways and the production of reactive oxygen species (Simkhovich et al., 2008; Brook et al., 2010). It has been demonstrated that cardiovascular diseases are risk factors for hearing impairment (Oron et al., 2014; Tan et al., 2018). Nonetheless, the link between air pollution and hearing impairment was still evident after adjusting for related vascular problems in Model 3, suggesting that other mechanisms may also be involved in the link between air pollution and hearing impairment.

There was evidence that a healthy diet could protect against hearing impairment by reducing vascular damage, decreasing inflammation, and inhibiting oxidative damage (Curhan et al., 2020; Yevenes-Briones et al., 2021). Based on similar mechanistic pathways, modifying the health effects of air pollution by diet may be possible. But in our study, no effect modification of diet was observed. Studies previously showed an interaction between dietary patterns and air pollution exposure on health-related outcomes. In a birth cohort in Northeast China, animal foods pattern was found to significantly modify the association between exposure to NO_2 and carbon monoxide and gestational diabetes mellitus, with higher intake related to a higher rate of gestational diabetes mellitus following exposure to air pollution (Hehua et al., 2021). A Mediterranean diet reduced cardiovascular disease mortality risk related to long-term exposure to air pollutants in a large prospective US cohort (Lim et al., 2019). A prospective cohort study of Chinese older adults reported that a plant-based dietary pattern mitigated the adverse effects of air pollution on cognitive function (Zhu et al., 2022).

It seems to be accepted that hearing impairment becomes more common with increasing age (Díaz et al., 2016). Nevertheless, the association between air pollution and hearing impairment was only found in participants younger under or equal to 50 years of age in this study. An interaction effect between age and air pollution on hearing impairment was also observed. Age is an unmodifiable risk factor for hearing impairment, which could lead to cochlear aging (Yamasoba et al., 2013). However, modifiable risk factors play a significant part in the development of hearing impairment at a relatively young age (i.e., <85 years old), while their effects decrease in the oldest people (i.e., ≥85 years old) (Zhan et al., 2010). Therefore, we speculated that air pollution, a modifiable risk factor, might have a greater impact on people younger than or equal to 50 years old compared to those over 50 years old, even if our study subjects were all under 85 years old.

Our research used data from the United Kingdom Biobank, a national cohort with good quality control. Additionally, the hearing test was based on the DTT data in the United Kingdom Biobank, which represented an ecologically effective and objective hearing indicator. We also adjusted for many confounders (including demographic information, lifestyle, and related diseases affecting hearing) to reduce their potential impact. However, our research also had some limitations. Above all, the cross-sectional design of this study was inadequate to account for the cause and effect between air pollution and hearing impairment, and further longitudinal studies are needed. Second, the sample of participants in United Kingdom Biobank was suggested to be unrepresentative of the general population because of the bias toward recruiting participants who were generally healthier and had a higher socioeconomic status (Fry et al., 2017). Hence, the subsample from United Kingdom Biobank and estimated hearing impairment rate in this study might not be representative of the general population. Third, like other epidemiological studies of air pollution, there might be potential misclassifications of air pollution exposure in this study because air pollution exposure was evaluated at the place of residence. Fourth, in the United Kingdom, where emissions regulations are strict and average pollution level is relatively low, it is not clear to what extent this study can be generalizable to other settings. Finally, in spite of adjusting for many confounders in our study, the potential effects of residual confounds of unmeasured variables could not be excluded, such as the use of ototoxic drugs, which was not considered due to lack of data.

CONCLUSION

In conclusion, we found that exposure to PM_{10}, NO_X, and NO_2 was associated with hearing impairment in British adults, while $PM_{2.5}$ and $PM_{2.5}$ absorbance did not show similar correlations. Our findings may help researchers pay more attention to the impact of air pollution on hearing impairment and provide a basis for developing effective prevention strategies.

AUTHOR CONTRIBUTIONS

YS, YT, and LY conceived the overall project and developed the methods as well as procedures throughout the study. DL and LY managed the data collection and data entry and carried out data verification and statistical analyses. LY drafted the first version of the manuscript. All authors oversaw statistical analysis, involved in the interpretation of the results, reviewed, and approved the final manuscript.

ACKNOWLEDGMENTS

We are grateful to all the participants of United Kingdom Biobank. We also sincerely thank those who participated in data collection and management of United Kingdom Biobank. This study has been carried out with the use of the United Kingdom Biobank resource (application number 69741).

REFERENCES

Appel, L. J., Brands, M. W., Daniels, S. R., Karanja, N., Elmer, P. J., Sacks, F. M., et al. (2006). Dietary approaches to prevent and treat hypertension: a scientific statement from the American Heart Association. *Hypertension* 47, 296–308. doi: 10.1161/01.HYP.0000202568.01167.B6

Brook, R. D., Rajagopalan, S., Pope, C. A. III, Brook, J. R., Bhatnagar, A., Diez-Roux, A. V., et al. (2010). Particulate matter air pollution and cardiovascular disease: an update to the scientific statement from the American Heart Association. *Circulation* 121, 2331–2378. doi: 10.1161/CIR.0b013e3181dbece1

Brunekreef, B., and Holgate, S. T. (2002). Air pollution and health. *Lancet* 360, 1233–1242. doi: 10.1016/s0140-6736(02)11274-8

Chang, K. H., Hsu, C. C., Muo, C. H., Hsu, C. Y., Liu, H. C., Kao, C. H., et al. (2016). Air pollution exposure increases the risk of rheumatoid arthritis: a longitudinal and nationwide study. *Environ. Int.* 94, 495–499. doi: 10.1016/j.envint.2016.06.008

Chang, K. H., Tsai, S. C., Lee, C. Y., Chou, R. H., Fan, H. C., Lin, F. C., et al. (2020). Increased Risk of Sensorineural Hearing Loss as a Result of Exposure to Air Pollution. *Int. J. Environ. Res. Public Health* 17:1969. doi: 10.3390/ijerph17061969

Chen, C. Y., Hung, H. J., Chang, K. H., Hsu, C. Y., Muo, C. H., Tsai, C. H., et al. (2017). Long-term exposure to air pollution and the incidence of Parkinson's disease: a nested case-control study. *PLoS One* 12:e0182834. doi: 10.1371/journal.pone.0182834

Choi, H. G., Min, C., and Kim, S. Y. (2019). Air pollution increases the risk of SSNHL: a nested case-control study using meteorological data and national sample cohort data. *Sci. Rep.* 9:8270. doi: 10.1038/s41598-019-44618-0

Collins, R. (2012). What makes UK Biobank special? *Lancet* 379, 1173–1174. doi: 10.1016/s0140-6736(12)60404-8

Contrera, K. J., Betz, J., Genther, D. J., and Lin, F. R. (2015). Association of hearing impairment and mortality in the National Health and Nutrition Examination Survey. *JAMA Otolaryngol. Head Neck Surg.* 141, 944–946. doi: 10.1001/jamaoto.2015.1762

Couth, S., Mazlan, N., Moore, D. R., Munro, K. J., and Dawes, P. (2019). Hearing Difficulties and Tinnitus in Construction, Agricultural, Music, and Finance Industries: contributions of Demographic, Health, and Lifestyle Factors. *Trends Hear.* 23:2331216519885571. doi: 10.1177/2331216519885571

Cunningham, L. L., and Tucci, D. L. (2017). Hearing Loss in Adults. *N. Engl. J. Med.* 377, 2465–2473. doi: 10.1056/NEJMra1616601

Curhan, S. G., Halpin, C., Wang, M., Eavey, R. D., and Curhan, G. C. (2020). Prospective Study of Dietary Patterns and Hearing Threshold Elevation. *Am. J. Epidemiol.* 189, 204–214. doi: 10.1093/aje/kwz223

Curhan, S. G., Wang, M., Eavey, R. D., Stampfer, M. J., and Curhan, G. C. (2018). Adherence to Healthful Dietary Patterns Is Associated with Lower Risk of Hearing Loss in Women. *J. Nutr.* 148, 944–951. doi: 10.1093/jn/nxy058

Dawes, P., Fortnum, H., Moore, D. R., Emsley, R., Norman, P., Cruickshanks, K., et al. (2014b). Hearing in middle age: a population snapshot of 40- to 69-year olds in the United Kingdom. *Ear and Hearing* 35, e44–e51. doi: 10.1097/AUD.0000000000000010

Dawes, P., Cruickshanks, K. J., Moore, D. R., Edmondson-Jones, M., McCormack, A., Fortnum, H., et al. (2014a). Cigarette smoking, passive smoking, alcohol consumption, and hearing loss. *J. Assoc .Res. Otolaryngol.* 15, 663–674. doi: 10.1007/s10162-014-0461-0

Díaz, C., Goycoolea, M., and Cardemil, F. (2016). Hipoacusia: trascendencia, Incidencia Y Prevalencia. *Revista. Médica. Clínica. Las Condes* 27, 731–739. doi: 10.1016/j.rmclc.2016.11.003

Fry, A., Littlejohns, T. J., Sudlow, C., Doherty, N., Adamska, L., Sprosen, T., et al. (2017). Comparison of Sociodemographic and Health-Related Characteristics of UK Biobank Participants With Those of the General Population. *Am. J. Epidemiol.* 186, 1026–1034. doi: 10.1093/aje/kwx246

Fung, T. T., Chiuve, S. E., McCullough, M. L., Rexrode, K. M., Logroscino, G., and Hu, F. B. (2008). Adherence to a DASH-style diet and risk of coronary heart disease and stroke in women. *Arch. Intern. Med.* 168, 713–720. doi: 10.1001/archinte.168.7.713

Genther, D. J., Frick, K. D., Chen, D., Betz, J., and Lin, F. R. (2013). Association of hearing loss with hospitalization and burden of disease in older adults. *J. Am. Med. Assoc.* 309, 2322–2324. doi: 10.1001/jama.2013.5912

Goman, A. M., and Lin, F. R. (2016). Prevalence of Hearing Loss by Severity in the United States. *Am. J. Public health* 106, 1820–1822. doi: 10.2105/ajph.2016.303299

Gordon, S. B., Bruce, N. G., Grigg, J., Hibberd, P. L., Kurmi, O. P., Lam, K. B., et al. (2014). Respiratory risks from household air pollution in low and middle income countries. *Lancet Respir. Med.* 2, 823–860. doi: 10.1016/s2213-2600(14)70168-7

Hayes, R. B., Lim, C., Zhang, Y., Cromar, K., Shao, Y., Reynolds, H. R., et al. (2020). PM2.5 air pollution and cause-specific cardiovascular disease mortality. *Int. J. Epidemiol.* 49, 25–35. doi: 10.1093/ije/dyz114

Hehua, Z., Yang, X., Qing, C., Shanyan, G., and Yuhong, Z. (2021). Dietary patterns and associations between air pollution and gestational diabetes mellitus. *Environ. Int.* 147:106347. doi: 10.1016/j.envint.2020.106347

Jansen, S., Luts, H., Wagener, K. C., Frachet, B., and Wouters, J. (2010). The French digit triplet test: a hearing screening tool for speech intelligibility in noise. *Int. J. Audiol.* 49, 378–387. doi: 10.3109/14992020903431272

Kelly, F. J. (2003). Oxidative stress: its role in air pollution and adverse health effects. *Occupat. Environ. Med.* 60, 612–616. doi: 10.1136/oem.60.8.612

Landrigan, P. J. (2017). Air pollution and health. *Lancet Public health* 2, e4–e5. doi: 10.1016/s2468-2667(16)30023-8

Lee, H. M., Kim, M. S., Kim, D. J., Uhm, T. W., Yi, S. B., Han, J. H., et al. (2019). Effects of meteorological factor and air pollution on sudden sensorineural hearing loss using the health claims data in Busan, Republic of Korea. *Am. J. Otolaryngol.* 40, 393–399. doi: 10.1016/j.amjoto.2019.02.010

Lelieveld, J., Klingmüller, K., Pozzer, A., Pöschl, U., Fnais, M., Daiber, A., et al. (2019). Cardiovascular disease burden from ambient air pollution in Europe reassessed using novel hazard ratio functions. *Eur. Heart J.* 40, 1590–1596. doi: 10.1093/eurheartj/ehz135

Li, C. M., Zhang, X., Hoffman, H. J., Cotch, M. F., Themann, C. L., and Wilson, M. R. (2014). Hearing impairment associated with depression in US adults, National Health and Nutrition Examination Survey 2005–2010. *Otolaryngol. Head Neck Surg.* 140, 293–302. doi: 10.1001/jamaoto.2014.42

Lim, C. C., Hayes, R. B., Ahn, J., Shao, Y., Silverman, D. T., Jones, R. R., et al. (2019). Mediterranean Diet and the Association Between Air Pollution and Cardiovascular Disease Mortality Risk. *Circulation* 139, 1766–1775. doi: 10.1161/CIRCULATIONAHA.118.035742

Lin, F. R., and Ferrucci, L. (2012). Hearing loss and falls among older adults in the United States. *Arch. Intern. Med.* 172, 369–371. doi: 10.1001/archinternmed.2011.728

Lin, F. R., Thorpe, R., Gordon-Salant, S., and Ferrucci, L. (2011). Hearing loss prevalence and risk factors among older adults in the United States. *J. Gerontol. Series Biol. Sci. Med. Sci.* 66, 582–590. doi: 10.1093/gerona/glr002

Lin, F. R., Yaffe, K., Xia, J., Xue, Q. L., Harris, T. B., Purchase-Helzner, E., et al. (2013). Hearing loss and cognitive decline in older adults. *JAMA Intern. Med.* 173, 293–299. doi: 10.1001/jamainternmed.2013.1868

McKee, M. M., Stransky, M. L., and Reichard, A. (2018). Hearing loss and associated medical conditions among individuals 65 years and older. *Disab. Health J.* 11, 122–125. doi: 10.1016/j.dhjo.2017.05.007

Moore, D. R., Edmondson-Jones, M., Dawes, P., Fortnum, H., McCormack, A., Pierzycki, R. H., et al. (2014). Relation between speech-in-noise threshold, hearing loss and cognition from 40-69 years of age. *PLoS One* 9:e107720. doi: 10.1371/journal.pone.0107720

Neale, E. P., Batterham, M. J., and Tapsell, L. C. (2016). Consumption of a healthy dietary pattern results in significant reductions in C-reactive protein levels in adults: a meta-analysis. *Nutr. Res.* 36, 391–401. doi: 10.1016/j.nutres.2016.02.009

Oron, Y., Elgart, K., Marom, T., and Roth, Y. (2014). Cardiovascular risk factors as causes for hearing impairment. *Audiol. Neuro-otol.* 19, 256–260. doi: 10.1159/000363215

Park, Y. H., Shin, S. H., Byun, S. W., and Kim, J. Y. (2016). Age- and Gender-Related Mean Hearing Threshold in a Highly-Screened Population: the Korean National Health and Nutrition Examination Survey 2010–2012. *PLoS One* 11:e0150783. doi: 10.1371/journal.pone.0150783

Pienkowski, M. (2017). On the Etiology of Listening Difficulties in Noise Despite Clinically Normal Audiograms. *Ear Hear.* 38, 135–148. doi: 10.1097/aud.0000000000000388

Rodríguez-Martínez, E., Martínez, F., Espinosa-García, M. T., Maldonado, P., and Rivas-Arancibia, S. (2013). Mitochondrial dysfunction in the hippocampus of rats caused by chronic oxidative stress. *Neuroscience* 252, 384–395. doi: 10.1016/j.neuroscience.2013.08.018

Simkhovich, B. Z., Kleinman, M. T., and Kloner, R. A. (2008). Air pollution and cardiovascular injury epidemiology, toxicology, and mechanisms. *J. Am. Coll. Cardiol.* 52, 719–726. doi: 10.1016/j.jacc.2008.05.029

Spankovich, C., and Le Prell, C. G. (2013). Healthy diets, healthy hearing: National Health and Nutrition Examination Survey, 1999–2002. *Int. J. Audiol.* 52, 369–376. doi: 10.3109/14992027.2013.780133

Strak, M., Janssen, N., Beelen, R., Schmitz, O., Vaartjes, I., Karssenberg, D., et al. (2017). Long-term exposure to particulate matter, NO(2) and the oxidative potential of particulates and diabetes prevalence in a large national health survey. *Environ. Int.* 108, 228–236. doi: 10.1016/j.envint.2017.08.017

Sudlow, C., Gallacher, J., Allen, N., Beral, V., Burton, P., Danesh, J., et al. (2015). UK biobank: an open access resource for identifying the causes of a wide range of complex diseases of middle and old age. *PLoS medicine* 12:e1001779. doi: 10.1371/journal.pmed.1001779

Tan, H. E., Lan, N. S. R., Knuiman, M. W., Divitini, M. L., Swanepoel, D. W., Hunter, M., et al. (2018). Associations between cardiovascular disease and its risk factors with hearing loss-A cross-sectional analysis. *Clin. Otolaryngol.* 43, 172–181. doi: 10.1111/coa.12936

Taylor, H., Shryane, N., Kapadia, D., Dawes, P., and Norman, P. (2020). Understanding ethnic inequalities in hearing health in the UK: a cross-sectional study of the link between language proficiency and performance on the Digit Triplet Test. *BMJ Open* 10:e042571. doi: 10.1136/bmjopen-2020-042571

Tsai, S. C.-S., Hsu, Y.-C., Lai, J.-N., Chou, R.-H., Fan, H.-C., Lin, F. C.-F., et al. (2020). Long-Term Exposure to Air Pollution and The Risk of Developing Sudden Sensorineural Hearing Loss. *J. Transl. Med.* doi: 10.21203/rs.3.rs-72326/v1

Vos, T., Allen, C., Arora, M., Barber, R. M., Bhutta, Z. A., Brown, A., et al. (2016). Global, regional, and national incidence, prevalence, and years lived with disability for 310 diseases and injuries, 1990–2015: a systematic analysis for the Global Burden of Disease Study 2015. *Lancet* 388, 1545–1602. doi: 10.1016/s0140-6736(16)31678-6

Wang, M., Zhou, T., Song, Y., Li, X., Ma, H., Hu, Y., et al. (2021). Joint exposure to various ambient air pollutants and incident heart failure: a prospective analysis in UK Biobank. *Eur. Heart J.* 42, 1582–1591. doi: 10.1093/eurheartj/ehaa1031

Xing, D. F., Xu, C. D., Liao, X. Y., Xing, T. Y., Cheng, S. P., Hu, M. G., et al. (2019). Spatial association between outdoor air pollution and lung cancer incidence in China. *BMC public health* 19:1377. doi: 10.1186/s12889-019-7740-y

Yamasoba, T., Lin, F. R., Someya, S., Kashio, A., Sakamoto, T., and Kondo, K. (2013). Current concepts in age-related hearing loss: epidemiology and mechanistic pathways. *Hear. Res.* 303, 30–38. doi: 10.1016/j.heares.2013.01.021

Yevenes-Briones, H., Caballero, F. F., Struijk, E. A., Machado-Fragua, M. D., Ortola, R., Rodriguez-Artalejo, F., et al. (2021). Diet Quality and the Risk of Impaired Speech Reception Threshold in Noise: the UK Biobank cohort. *Ear Hear.* doi: 10.1097/AUD.0000000000001108

Yin, J., and Harrison, R. M. (2008). Pragmatic mass closure study for PM1.0, PM2.5 and PM10 at roadside, urban background and rural sites. *Atmospher. Environ.* 42, 980–988. doi: 10.1016/j.atmosenv.2007.10.005

Zhan, W., Cruickshanks, K. J., Klein, B. E., Klein, R., Huang, G. H., Pankow, J. S., et al. (2010). Generational differences in the prevalence of hearing impairment in older adults. *Am. J. Epidemiol.* 171, 260–266. doi: 10.1093/aje/kwp370

Zhu, A., Chen, H., Shen, J., Wang, X., Li, Z., Zhao, A., et al. (2022). Interaction between plant-based dietary pattern and air pollution on cognitive function: a prospective cohort analysis of Chinese older adults. *Lancet Reg. Health West. Pac.* 20:100372. doi: 10.1016/j.lanwpc.2021.100372

12

Gray Matter Atrophy is Associated with Cognitive Impairment in Patients with Presbycusis

Fuxin Ren[1], Wen Ma[2], Muwei Li[3], Huaiqiang Sun[4], Qian Xin[5], Wei Zong[1], Weibo Chen[6], Guangbin Wang[1], Fei Gao[1]* and Bin Zhao[1]*

[1] Shandong Medical Imaging Research Institute, Shandong University, Jinan, China, [2] Department of Otolaryngology, Jinan Central Hospital, Shandong University, Jinan, China, [3] Vanderbilt University Institute of Imaging Science, Vanderbilt University, Nashville, TN, United States, [4] Huaxi MR Research Center, Department of Radiology, West China Hospital of Sichuan University, Chengdu, China, [5] Central Laboratory, The Second Hospital of Shandong University, Jinan, China, [6] Philips Healthcare, Shanghai, China

*Correspondence:
Fei Gao
feigao6262@163.com
Bin Zhao
qpqpoo6262@163.com

Presbycusis (PC) is characterized by bilateral sensorineural hearing loss at high frequencies and speech-perception difficulties in noisy environments and has a strikingly detrimental impact on cognitive function. As the neural consequences of PC may involve the whole brain, we hypothesized that patients with PC would show structural alterations not only in the auditory cortex but also in the cortexes involved in cognitive function. The purpose of this study was to use surface-based morphometry (SBM) analysis to elucidate whole-brain structural differences between patients with PC and age-matched normal hearing controls. Three-dimensional T1-weighted MR images of 26 patients with mild PC and 26 age-, sex- and education-matched healthy controls (HCs) were acquired. All participants underwent a battery of neuropsychological tests. Our results revealed gray matter atrophy in several auditory cortical areas, nodes of the default mode network (DMN), including the bilateral precuneus and inferior parietal lobule, the right posterior cingulate cortex (PCC), and the right insula of patients with PC compared to that in the HCs. Our findings also revealed that hearing loss was associated with reduced gray matter volume in the right primary auditory cortex of patients with PC. Moreover, structural alterations in the nodes of the DMN were associated with cognitive impairments in PC patients. Additionally, this study provides evidence that a thicker right insula is associated with better speech perception in patients with PC. Based on these findings, we argue that the onset of PC seems to trigger its own cascade of conditions, including a need for increased cognitive resources during speech comprehension, which might lead to auditory and cognition-related cortical reorganization.

Keywords: presbycusis, cognitive impairment, hearing loss, GM atrophy, surface-based morphometry

INTRODUCTION

Age-related hearing loss, also known as presbycusis (PC), is characterized by bilateral sensorineural hearing loss at high frequencies, slowed central processing of acoustic information and speech-perception difficulties in noisy environments (Gates and Mills, 2005). PC is the most common sensory deficit in the aging population and is associated with a diminished quality of life. Recently, many large population-based longitudinal studies have suggested that age-related hearing loss is independently associated with cognitive decline and that patients with PC are more likely to develop dementia (Lin et al., 2011a,b; Gurgel et al., 2014). For instance, one cross-sectional study found that patients with PC showed worse performance than normal hearing controls on the Digit Symbol Substitution Test, which evaluates psychomotor speed and executive function (Lin, 2011). Moreover, compared with normal hearing controls, PC patients with mild, moderate and severe hearing loss are, respectively, two, three and five times as likely to develop dementia (Lin et al., 2011a). In line with these findings, researchers have realized that PC may have a strikingly detrimental impact on cognitive function (Mudar and Husain, 2016; Hewitt, 2017; Jayakody et al., 2018). Given that hearing loss is relatively easier to remediate than other risk factors for dementia and Alzheimer's disease (Mudar and Husain, 2016), it is highly important to illuminate the neural mechanisms that underlie PC-related cognitive decline.

Magnetic resonance imaging (MRI) has become a novel and widely used technique to investigate the pathogenesis of various neuropsychiatric disorders. In one structural MRI study, patients with PC exhibited decreases in gray matter (GM) volume and thickness in the bilateral auditory cortexes compared with normal hearing young adults (Profant et al., 2014). Other studies have reported decreases in GM volume in the right primary auditory cortex that correlated with poorer hearing ability in older adults (Peelle et al., 2011). In one functional magnetic resonance imaging (fMRI) study, compared with normal hearing young adults, patients with PC showed higher blood-oxygen-level-dependent activation responses to acoustical stimuli in the temporal lobes (Ouda et al., 2015). However, these studies lacked age-matched normal hearing controls; thus, the further validation of these findings is required. In our previous studies using proton magnetic resonance spectroscopy, compared with age-matched normal hearing controls, decreased concentrations of gamma-aminobutyric acid (GABA), the main inhibitory neurotransmitter in the central auditory system, have been found in the bilateral auditory cortexes in patients with PC (Gao et al., 2015). However, the aforementioned studies and our studies have mainly focused on structural, functional and metabolic changes in the auditory cortex.

The strong connection between PC and cognitive decline has been explained by several hypotheses (Humes et al., 2013; Wayne and Johnsrude, 2015). Several researchers have suggested that even relatively mild levels of hearing loss can lead to increased listening effort, including the need for increased cognitive resources to understand acoustically degraded speech, and that reduced hearing ability has cascading consequences for the neural processes supporting both speech perception and cognition (Wingfield and Peelle, 2012; Peelle and Wingfield, 2016). As the neural consequences of PC may involve the whole brain, we should also consider neural alterations in nonauditory cortical regions. Therefore, the purpose of this study was to use surface-based morphometric (SBM) analysis to elucidate structural differences in the whole brain between patients with PC and age-matched

normal hearing controls. Furthermore, the relationships between structural changes and cognitive decline in patients with PC were analyzed. We hypothesized that patients with PC would present structural alterations not only in the auditory cortex but also in the cortical regions involved in cognitive functions.

MATERIALS AND METHODS

Participants

The study was approved by the Shandong University institutional review board and each participant provided informed consent. Twenty-six patients with mild PC (PC group, 14 males/12 females, mean age, 64.38 ± 3.24 years) visiting the Department of Otolaryngology at our local hospital were recruited for this study (**Table 1**). Hearing loss was assessed by the speech-frequency pure tone average (PTA) of thresholds at 0.5, 1, 2, and 4 kHz (air conduction) in the better hearing ear as per the definition of hearing loss adjudicated by the World World Health Organization [WHO], 1991. The PTA value of 25 decibels hearing level (dB HL) was accepted as the normal hearing threshold limit (Lin et al., 2011b). Inclusion criteria were the following: (1) hearing loss: PTA> 25 dB HL in the better hearing ear; (2) age≥ 60 years. Exclusion criteria were the following: (1) ear diseases that affected hearing thresholds and sensorineural hearing losses other than PC; (2) previous history of otologic surgery, ototoxic drug therapy, noise exposure, or hearing aid use; (3) asymmetric hearing loss with a difference in air conduction thresholds exceeding 20 dB at least two frequencies between 0.5, 1, 2, and 4 kHz; (4) conductive hearing loss (a mean air-bone difference at 0.5, 1, 2, and 4 kHz) > 10 dB in one or both

TABLE 1 | Participants' demographic and clinical data.

Characteristics	PC (n = 26)	HCs (n = 26)	p-value
Gender (male/female)	14/12	13/13	0.781
Age (years)	64.38 ± 3.24	64.96 ± 3.00	0.508
Education (years)	11.31 ± 2.17	11.15 ± 2.68	0.821
Disease duration (years)	5.23 ± 2.08	–	–
PTA	32.65 ± 5.34	14.69 ± 3.86	<0.001*
SRT	32.63 ± 4.31	15.90 ± 4.49	<0.001*
MMSE	27.35 ± 0.98	27.73 ± 0.83	0.132
MoCA	25.77 ± 1.11	26.19 ± 0.69	0.105
Anxiety	3.92 ± 1.57	3.46 ± 2.04	0.366
Depression	3.73 ± 1.76	3.38 ± 1.83	0.490
AVLT	57.08 ± 4.51	59.88 ± 8.53	0.144
Stroop	135.88 ± 11.18	125.69 ± 11.10	0.002*
SDMT	42.31 ± 9.30	51.31 ± 13.07	0.006*
TMT-A	42.08 ± 5.84	38.15 ± 8.88	0.066
TMT-B	106.58 ± 13.34	96.08 ± 19.05	0.026*

*The data are presented as means ± standard deviations. *Indicates p < 0.05. PC, presbycusis; HCs, healthy controls; PTA, pure tone average; SRT, speech reception threshold; MMSE, Mini Mental State Examination; MoCA, Montreal Cognitive Assessment; AVLT, Auditory Verbal Learning Test; SDMT, Symbol Digit Modalities Test; TMT, Trail-Making Test; levels of anxiety and depression were assessed according to the Hospital Anxiety and Depression Scale (HADS).*

ears; and (5) tinnitus, head trauma, lesions of the facial nerve, disorders of the cervical spine, or neurological or psychiatric diseases.

Twenty-six age-, sex- and education-level matched healthy controls (HCs; control group, 13 males/13 females, mean age, 64.96 ± 3.0 years; PTA ≤ 25 dB HL in the better hearing ear) were recruited for this study (Table 1). All controls were in good health and had no history of neurological or psychiatric diseases. All participants were right-handed, as determined by the Li's handedness inventory (Gong et al., 2005; Hatta, 2007).

Assessment of Auditory Function

An otoscopic examination was performed for all participants to remove cerumen and confirm the presence of an intact tympanic membrane. The auditory function of all participants was evaluated using tympanometry and pure tone audiometry. Tympanometry was performed with a GSI Tympstar to confirm optimal middle ear conditions. Pure tone audiometry was performed with a GSI AudioStar Pro audiometer coupled with TDH-50P Telephonics headphones. Bone conduction thresholds were measured at 0.25, 0.5, 1, 2, and 4 kHz, and air conduction thresholds were measured at 0.125, 0.25, 0.5, 1, 2, 4, and 8 kHz. Hearing thresholds were detected with a resolution of 5 dB steps. The PTA values for all participants' ears were calculated.

Speech reception threshold (SRT) was measured in quiet conditions. SRT testing was conducted using the automated HOPE software for the presentation and scoring of spondee words. The SRT testing in this software is conducted according to the American Speech-language Hearing Association recommended SRT testing guidelines. The process is as follows: first, an initial sound intensity is determined based on the PTA hearing threshold where five spondee words are correctly identified. If these words are not identified correctly, the software will prompt "Increase initial sound intensity". Then, the software will automatically control the playback intensity steps: 5 dB decreases for every five words played. When the patient fails to recognize the five words at certain intensity, the test is terminated. The software counts the number of words that the patient successfully recognized during the entire step-down process and subtracts this from the initial intensity, plus a 2.5 dB correction factor, which is the patient's SRT.

Assessment of Cognitive Function

The participants' cognitive status were tested using the Mini Mental State Examination (MMSE) and Montreal Cognitive Assessment (MoCA) for general cognitive function (Galea and Woodward, 2005; Nasreddine et al., 2005), the Auditory Verbal Learning Test (AVLT, Chinese version) for verbal learning and memory (Zhao et al., 2012), the Stroop color word interference test for attention (Savitz and Jansen, 2003), the Symbol Digit Modalities Test (SDMT) for psychomotor speed (Van Schependom et al., 2014), and the Trail-Making Test for executive control (Sanchez-Cubillo et al., 2009). Levels of anxiety and depression were assessed according to the Hospital Anxiety and Depression Scale (HADS) (Zigmond and Snaith, 1983). Each

participant took approximately 60 min to complete all tests, which were completed in a fixed order.

MRI Acquisition

All participants were scanned on a 3T scanner (Philips Achieva TX, Best, Netherlands) using an eight-channel phased-array head coil as a receiver. T1-weighted three-dimensional TFE images were used as a localizer and acquired with the following parameters: TR = 8.1 ms; TE = 3.7 ms; slice thickness = 1 mm; field of view = 24 cm × 24 cm; and flip angle = 8°. Images were reconstructed with 1 mm × 1 mm × 1 mm isotropic voxels.

Surface-Based Morphometric Analysis

All the T1-weighted images were processed with surface stream and volume stream that were integrated in FreeSurfer software (version 5.3[1]). The surface stream constructs the boundary models of white matter, gray matter as well as the pial surface, from which, the anatomical measurements, such as cortical thickness and curvature, could be obtained at each point on the cortex. Then the cortex was segmented into 74 regions of interest (ROIs) using the volume stream, which consists three major steps. First, T1 image is spatially aligned to a standard coordinate, namely, Montreal Neurological Institute (MNI) space, using affine registration which is insensitive to local anatomical difference and used to maximize the accuracy of final segmentation. This is followed by a refined high-dimensional nonlinear registration, which warps the T1 image to an MNI-space atlas whose cortical area has been manually segmented to 74 ROIs. The non-linear registration allows for the point-to-point correspondence between T1 image and the atlas, and therefore enable the automatic segmentation of the T1 image. Consequently, the normalized volume [dividing by intracranial volume (ICV)], average thickness and average curvature within each ROI could be obtained for accurate characterization of local anatomical morphometry of cortical areas. The Shapiro-Wilk normality test was used to test for normality of distribution. For each ROI, group differences in these measurements between the PC and HCs groups were assessed by two-sample t-test (Gutiérrez-Galve et al., 2010; Vainik et al., 2018). The age, sex and education level were modeled as covariates. The analysis was corrected for multiple comparisons using the FDR criterion and the statistical significance was set at $p < 0.05$.

Statistical Analysis

We used the two-tailed t-test to assess group differences in demographic and clinical characteristics. Gender-specific group differences were analyzed using the chi-square test. P-values of less than 0.05 were accepted as significant. Partial correlation analyses were performed to explore the potential relationships between structural changes and cognitive impairments or audiological outcomes in the PC group (controlled for age, sex, education level). All statistical analyses

---

[1] https://surfer.nmr.mgh.harvard.edu

were conducted using PASW software (version 17.0, Chicago, IL, United States).

RESULTS

Demographic and Clinical Characteristics

The demographic and clinical characteristics are listed in **Table 1**. The two groups did not exhibit significant differences in age, gender or education level. Compared to the HCs, patients with PC performed worse on the Stroop, SDMT and TMT-B tests ($p < 0.05$) (**Table 1**). All participants had a type A curve (normal middle ear function) on tympanometry. There was no significant difference in PTA or SRT between the left and right ears in the PC and HCs groups, thus the thresholds of both ears were averaged in each group. Average hearing thresholds of the PC and HCs groups were shown in **Figure 1**. The PTA and SRT were significantly higher in patients with PC than in HCs (PTA, $p < 0.001$; SRT, $p < 0.001$) (**Table 1**).

Group Differences in Cortical Morphology

All cortical variables were normal distribution ($p > 0.05$) except the cortex thickness of the right insular of PC group. The quantile–quantile plot (Wilk and Gnanadesikan, 1968) was used to check for major deviations from the normal distribution, then one patient's data was excluded from the cortex thickness of the right insular. The significant parcel-wise differences between the PC and HCs groups in cortical volume are illustrated in **Figure 2**. Compared with the HCs group, the PC group showed decreased volume in the left superior temporal sulcus; the right posterior cingulate cortex (PCC) and transverse temporal sulcus; and the bilateral precuneus, temporal plane of the superior temporal gyrus and subparietal sulcus.

The significant parcel-wise differences between the PC and HCs groups in cortical thickness are illustrated in **Figure 3**.

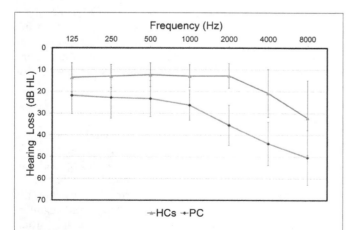

FIGURE 1 | Hearing thresholds of the presbycusis (PC) and healthy controls (HCs) groups (means ± standard deviation) in air conduction. Hearing thresholds from both ears are averaged.

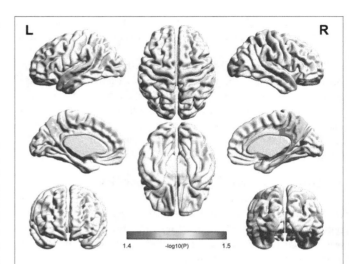

FIGURE 2 | Compared with healthy controls, patients with presbycusis showed decreased volume in the left superior temporal sulcus; the right posterior cingulate cortex and transverse temporal sulcus; and the bilateral precuneus, temporal plane of the superior temporal gyrus and subparietal sulcus ($p < 0.05$, false discovery rate corrected).

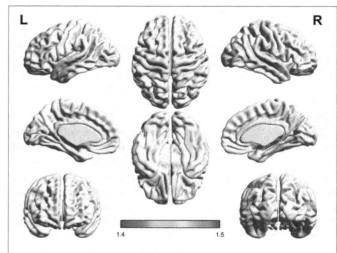

FIGURE 3 | Compared with healthy controls, patients with presbycusis showed reduced thickness in the left Heschl's gyrus; the right insular gyrus and planum polare of the superior temporal gyrus; and bilateral superior temporal sulcus ($p < 0.05$, false discovery rate corrected).

Compared with the HCs group, the PC group showed reduced thickness in the left Heschl's gyrus (HG); the right insular gyrus and planum polare of the superior temporal gyrus; and bilateral superior temporal sulcus. There were no significant parcel-wise differences between the PC and HCs groups in cortical curvature.

Correlations Between Clinical Characteristics and Cortical Morphology

In the PC group (**Figure 4**), partial correlation analyses revealed that Stroop scores were negatively correlated with the cortical thickness of the right insula ($r = -0.570$, $p = 0.006$);

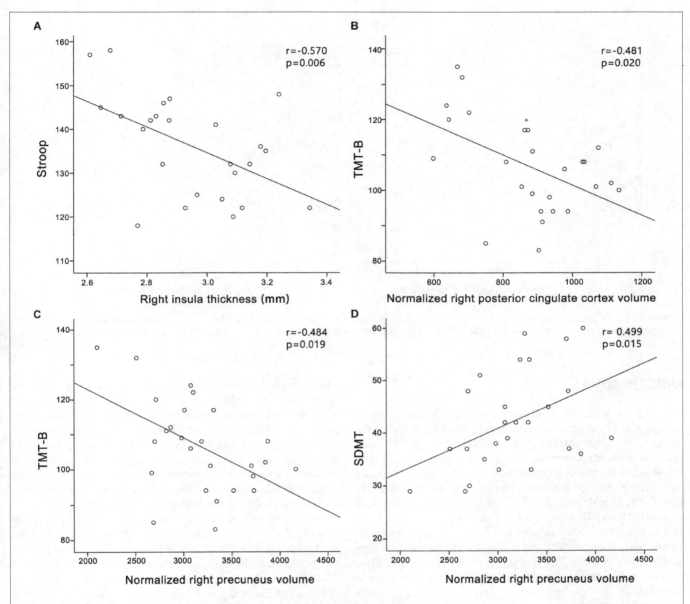

FIGURE 4 | Correlations between structural changes and cognitive impairments in the presbycusis group. **(A)** Stroop scores were negatively correlated with the cortical thickness of the right insula ($r = -0.570$, $p = 0.006$); **(B)** TMT-B scores were negatively correlated with the cortical volume of the right posterior cingulate cortex ($r = -0.481$, $p = 0.020$); **(C)** TMT-B scores were negatively correlated with the cortical volume of the right precuneus ($r = -0.484$, $p = 0.019$); **(D)** SDMT scores were positively associated with the cortical volume of the right precuneus ($r = 0.499$, $p = 0.015$). Normalized cortical volume = (cortical volume/intracranial volume) $*10^6$.

TMT-B scores were negatively correlated with the cortical volume of the right PCC ($r = -0.481$, $p = 0.020$); TMT-B scores were negatively correlated with the cortical volume of the right precuneus ($r = -0.484$, $p = 0.019$); SDMT scores were positively associated with the cortical volume of the right precuneus ($r = 0.499$, $p = 0.015$). In the HCs group (**Supplementary Figure S1**), no correlations were observed between cognitive scores and cortical morphology. In all participants (**Supplementary Figure S3**), Stroop scores were negatively correlated with the cortical thickness of the right insula ($r = -0.394$, $p = 0.006$).

In the PC group (**Figure 5**), partial correlation analyses revealed that PTA was negatively correlated with the cortical thickness of the left HG ($r = -0.439$, $p = 0.036$), and a trend toward correlation was seen between SRT and the cortical thickness of the right insula ($r = -0.387$, $p = 0.075$). In the HCs group (**Supplementary Figure S2**), PTA was negatively correlated with the cortical thickness of the left HG ($r = -0.460$, $p = 0.027$). In all participants (**Supplementary Figure S4**), PTA was negatively correlated with the cortical thickness of the left HG ($r = -0.556$, $p < 0.001$); SRT was negatively correlated with the cortical thickness of the right insula ($r = -0.552$, $p < 0.001$).

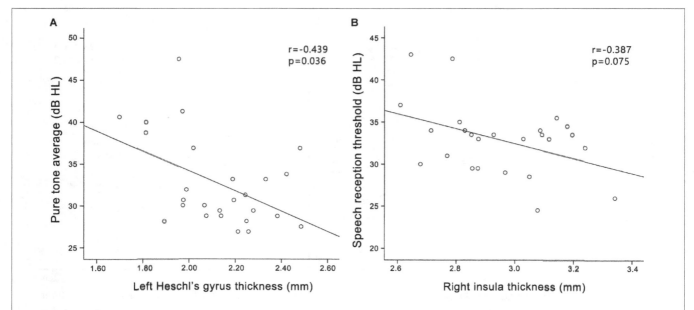

FIGURE 5 | Correlations between structural changes and audiological outcomes in the presbycusis group. **(A)** PTA was negatively correlated with the cortical thickness of the left HG ($r = -0.439$, $p = 0.036$); **(B)** A trend toward correlation was seen between SRT and the cortical thickness of the right insula ($r = -0.387$, $p = 0.075$).

DISCUSSION

Our study demonstrated GM atrophy in several auditory cortical areas; nodes of the default mode network (DMN), including the bilateral precuneus, inferior parietal lobule and right PCC; and the right insula of patients with PC compared to those of age- and sex-matched normal hearing controls. Our findings also revealed that hearing loss was associated with reduced cortical thickness in the left HG of patients with PC. Moreover, structural alterations in nodes of the DMN were associated with cognitive impairments in PC patients. Additionally, a trend toward correlation was demonstrated between SRT and the cortical thickness of the right insula in patients with PC. To the best of our knowledge, this is the first study to systematically elucidate structural differences in the whole brain of patients with PC and their correlations with cognitive impairments.

The plastic reorganization of sensory cortexes often occurs when sensory input is degraded. In our study, decreased cortical volume and/or thickness in patients with PC were observed in several auditory cortical areas, such as the left HG, the right planum polare of the superior temporal gyrus and bilateral temporal plane of the superior temporal gyrus. These findings could demonstrate corresponding brain dysfunctions that are related to long-term hearing loss. To our knowledge, only one study has reported structural changes in the GM of patients with PC. In that study, the GM volume and thickness of bilateral HG and the planum temporale were decreased in patients with mild PC in comparison with young control subjects (Profant et al., 2014). Therefore, alterations in auditory cortical areas may be mainly caused by aging rather than hearing loss. Intriguingly, our findings revealed that hearing loss was associated with reduced cortical thickness in the left HG of patients with PC,

which suggests a link between hearing ability and the structural integrity of the auditory cortex. These results are consistent with previous studies indicating cortical reorganization when peripheral auditory acuity is moderately decreased in older adults (Peelle et al., 2011). HG is a crucial brain structure as it contains the primary auditory cortex, which plays an important role in auditory information processing (Langers et al., 2007; Wong et al., 2008). For patients with PC, long-term hearing loss may impair the ability of the primary auditory cortex to respond to auditory signals. Significant correlations were also observed between the cortical morphology and hearing thresholds both in the HCs group and all participants. In our study, hearing loss was assessed by the speech-frequency PTA of thresholds at 0.5, 1, 2, and 4 kHz in the better hearing ear. However, healthy controls had high frequency hearing losses, especially in 8 kHz, which were not been fully evaluated by speech-frequency PTA. Moreover, the relationships between the cortical morphology and hearing thresholds in all participants were more robust than those in PC or HCs group. One possible reason for the result could be an increase in the sample size.

Previous studies on PC have indicated that hearing loss contributes to cognitive decline (Lin, 2011; Lin et al., 2011a,b; Gurgel et al., 2014). In our study, patients with PC showed poorer performances than the HCs in most of the cognitive tests, such as the Stroop, SDMT and TMT-B tests, which indicates that patients exhibited attention, information processing speed and executive function dysfunctions. These results may possibly explain the finding of morphological alterations that involved not only the auditory cortex but also cognitive areas. The DMN is a large-scale brain network of interacting brain regions that shows increased activity at rest and plays a critical role in modulating consciousness (Raichle et al., 2001; Mantini et al., 2007). In this study, several nodes in the DMN of PC patients showed decreased cortical volume and/or thickness. These areas included the right PCC, which has been found to be associated with attention and cognitive control (Leech et al., 2011; Leech and Sharp, 2014); the bilateral precuneus, which is responsible for episodic memory and visuospatial processing (Cavanna and Trimble, 2006); and the bilateral inferior parietal lobules, which are involved in maintaining attentive control and interpretation of sensory information (Singh-Curry and Husain, 2009). The complexity of an acoustic signal such as speech requires the involvement of nonauditory cortexes for correct processing (Ouda et al., 2015). PC-related hearing loss increases listening effort, including a need for increased cognitive resources to understand acoustically degraded speech, especially in noisy places (Peelle and Wingfield, 2016). Therefore, our results presumably indicate a plastic reorganization of neural systems in patients with PC in which some nodes of the DMN become overused to compensate for the lost ability to inhibit irrelevant stimuli such as background noise. The chronic overuse of nodes of the DMN in patients with PC may eventually lead to structural modifications in these nodes, as seen in our study. Moreover, our analysis showed that impaired cognitive function scores were related to decreased cortical volume in the right precuneus and PCC. Structural alterations in the nodes of the DMN in patients with PC were associated with cognitive decline, suggesting that brain morphometry might be a potential imaging marker for PC-associated cognitive impairments.

We also found significant cortical thickness decreases in the right insula in patients with PC. Moreover, a trend toward correlation was demonstrated between SRT and the cortical thickness of the right insula in PC patients, indicating a thicker right insula is associated with better speech perception. These findings suggest that in addition to peripheral structures and the auditory cortex, cognitive areas also contribute to the ability to perceive speech in patients with PC. Virtually all high-level auditory information processes rely on the control and conditioning of cognitive processes (Cardin, 2016). The insula, a key node in cognitive control network (CCN), participates in several key auditory processes, such as auditory attention allocation and focusing on novel auditory stimuli, temporal processing, phonological processing and visual-auditory information integration (Bamiou et al., 2003; Cole and Schneider, 2007). Thus, our findings may suggest that a remodeling in cognitive control areas is necessary for auditory processing in PC patients. Previous fMRI studies of patients with USNHL have shown increased regional homogeneity (ReHo) in the right anterior insula, and functional connectivity analyses showed an enhanced relationship between the right insula and several key nodes of the DMN (Wang et al., 2014). Additionally, stroop scores were negatively correlated with the cortical thickness of the right insula in this study. Taken together with the current data showing the altered integrity of GM in key nodes of the CCN and DMN, these results indicate a functional reorganization both within and between cognitive networks in

patients with PC; these findings encourage further investigations using resting-state fMRI.

There are some limitations to our study design. First, as it was a cross-sectional study, although relationships between structural changes and cognitive decline were found in patients with PC, it is still not clear whether improving hearing ability through the use of hearing aids might help preserve cognitive function. Second, there is a lack of evaluation of how the freesurfer measurements would change when using a different atlas for registration. Morphological change of elderly population, for example, larger ventricle and atrophied cortical areas, might reduce the registration accuracy when using a universal atlas. Therefore, an elderly population-specific atlas is highly expected to yield unbiased measurement and further increase the statistic power. Third, our sample size is small, and the results require confirmation in larger samples. Fourth, a more comprehensive neuropsychological battery including measures of visual memory, semantic memory, as well as additional executive processes (e.g., verbal fluency, working memory and concept formation/problem solving) is another limitation of the study.

CONCLUSION

Our findings indicate that GM atrophy of key nodes in the DMN may be imaging markers for PC-related cognitive decline. Moreover, this study provides evidence that a thicker right insula is associated with better speech perception in patients with PC. Based on these findings, we argue that the onset of PC appears to trigger its own cascade of conditions, including the need for increased cognitive resources for speech comprehension, which might lead to auditory and cognition-related cortical reorganization.

AUTHOR CONTRIBUTIONS

FG and BZ designed the experiments. FR, WM, and QX carried out the experiments. WZ and WC analyzed experimental results. ML and HS analyzed MRI data and developed analysis tools. GW assisted with. FR and FG wrote the manuscript.

FUNDING

This work was supported by the National Natural Science Foundation of China for Young Scholars (No. 81601479); Shandong Provincial Key Research and Development Plan of China (No. 2016GSF201090); Shandong Provincial Natural Science Foundation of China (No. BS2015YY003); Shandong Provincial Medical and Healthy Technology Development Program of China (Nos. 2015WS0176 and 2017WS610); and China Postdoctoral Science Foundation funded project (No. 2017M621089).

REFERENCES

Bamiou, D. E., Musiek, F. E., and Luxon, L. M. (2003). The insula (Island of Reil) and its role in auditory processing. Literature review. *Brain Res. Brain Res. Rev.* 42, 143–154. doi: 10.1016/S0165-0173(03)00172-3

Cardin, V. (2016). Effects of aging and adult-onset hearing loss on cortical auditory regions. *Front. Neurosci.* 10:199. doi: 10.3389/fnins.2016.00199

Cavanna, A. E., and Trimble, M. R. (2006). The precuneus: a review of its functional anatomy and behavioural correlates. *Brain* 129(Pt 3), 564–583. doi: 10.1093/brain/awl004

Cole, M. W., and Schneider, W. (2007). The cognitive control network: integrated cortical regions with dissociable functions. *Neuroimage* 37, 343–360. doi: 10.1016/j.neuroimage.2007.03.071

Galea, M., and Woodward, M. (2005). Mini-Mental State Examination (MMSE). *Aust. J. Physiother.* 51:198. doi: 10.1016/S0004-9514(05)70034-9

Gao, F., Wang, G., Ma, W., Ren, F., Li, M., Dong, Y., et al. (2015). Decreased auditory GABA + concentrations in presbycusis demonstrated by edited magnetic resonance spectroscopy. *Neuroimage* 106, 311–316. doi: 10.1016/j.neuroimage.2014.11.023

Gates, G. A., and Mills, J. H. (2005). Presbycusis. *Lancet* 366, 1111–1120. doi: 10.1016/s0140-6736(05)67423-5

Gong, G., Jiang, T., Zhu, C., Zang, Y., He, Y., Xie, S., et al. (2005). Side and handedness effects on the cingulum from diffusion tensor imaging. *Neuroreport* 16, 1701–1705. doi: 10.1097/01.wnr.0000183327.98370.6a

Gurgel, R. K., Ward, P. D., Schwartz, S., Norton, M. C., Foster, N. L., and Tschanz, J. T. (2014). Relationship of hearing loss and dementia: a prospective, population-based study. *Otol. Neurotol.* 35, 775–781. doi: 10.1097/mao.0000000000000313

Gutiérrez-Galve, L., Wheeler-Kingshott, C. A., Altmann, D. R., Price, G., Chu, E. M., Leeson, V. C., et al. (2010). Changes in the frontotemporal cortex and cognitive correlates in first-episode psychosis. *Biol. Psychiatry* 68, 51–60. doi: 10.1016/j.biopsych.2010.03.019

Hatta, T. (2007). Handedness and the brain: a review of brain-imaging techniques. *Magn. Reson. Med. Sci.* 6, 99–112. doi: 10.2463/mrms.6.99

Hewitt, D. (2017). Age-related hearing loss and cognitive decline: you haven't heard the half of it. *Front. Aging Neurosci.* 9:112. doi: 10.3389/fnagi.2017.00112

Humes, L. E., Busey, T. A., Craig, J., and Kewley-Port, D. (2013). Are age-related changes in cognitive function driven by age-related changes in sensory processing? *Atten. Percept. Psychophys.* 75, 508–524. doi: 10.3758/s13414-012-0406-9

Jayakody, D. M. P., Friedland, P. L., Martins, R. N., and Sohrabi, H. R. (2018). Impact of aging on the auditory system and related cognitive functions: a narrative review. *Front. Neurosci.* 12:125. doi: 10.3389/fnins.2018.00125

Langers, D. R., Backes, W. H., and van Dijk, P. (2007). Representation of lateralization and tonotopy in primary versus secondary human auditory cortex. *Neuroimage* 34, 264–273. doi: 10.1016/j.neuroimage.2006.09.002

Leech, R., Kamourieh, S., Beckmann, C. F., and Sharp, D. J. (2011). Fractionating the default mode network: distinct contributions of the ventral and dorsal posterior cingulate cortex to cognitive control. *J. Neurosci.* 31, 3217–3224. doi: 10.1523/jneurosci.5626-10.2011

Leech, R., and Sharp, D. J. (2014). The role of the posterior cingulate cortex in cognition and disease. *Brain* 137(Pt 1), 12–32. doi: 10.1093/brain/awt162

Lin, F. R. (2011). Hearing loss and cognition among older adults in the United States. *J. Gerontol. A Biol. Sci. Med. Sci.* 66, 1131–1136. doi: 10.1093/gerona/glr115

Lin, F. R., Metter, E. J., O'Brien, R. J., Resnick, S. M., Zonderman, A. B., and Ferrucci, L. (2011a). Hearing loss and incident dementia. *Arch. Neurol.* 68, 214–220. doi: 10.1001/archneurol.2010.362

Lin, F. R., Thorpe, R., Gordon-Salant, S., and Ferrucci, L. (2011b). Hearing loss prevalence and risk factors among older adults in the United States. *J. Gerontol. A Biol. Sci. Med. Sci.* 66, 582–590. doi: 10.1093/gerona/glr002

Mantini, D., Perrucci, M. G., Del Gratta, C., Romani, G. L., and Corbetta, M. (2007). Electrophysiological signatures of resting state networks in the human brain. *Proc. Natl. Acad. Sci. U.S.A.* 104, 13170–13175. doi: 10.1073/pnas.0700668104

Mudar, R. A., and Husain, F. T. (2016). Neural alterations in acquired age-related hearing loss. *Front. Psychol.* 7:828. doi: 10.3389/fpsyg.2016.00828

Nasreddine, Z. S., Phillips, N. A., Bedirian, V., Charbonneau, S., Whitehead, V., Collin, I., et al. (2005). The Montreal Cognitive Assessment, MoCA: a brief screening tool for mild cognitive impairment. *J. Am. Geriatr. Soc.* 53, 695–699. doi: 10.1111/j.1532-5415.2005.53221.x

Ouda, L., Profant, O., and Syka, J. (2015). Age-related changes in the central auditory system. *Cell Tissue Res.* 361, 337–358. doi: 10.1007/s00441-014-2107-2

Peelle, J. E., Troiani, V., Grossman, M., and Wingfield, A. (2011). Hearing loss in older adults affects neural systems supporting speech comprehension. *J. Neurosci.* 31, 12638–12643. doi: 10.1523/jneurosci.2559-11.2011

Peelle, J. E., and Wingfield, A. (2016). The neural consequences of age-related hearing loss. *Trends Neurosci.* 39, 486–497. doi: 10.1016/j.tins.2016.05.001

Profant, O., Skoch, A., Balogova, Z., Tintera, J., Hlinka, J., and Syka, J. (2014). Diffusion tensor imaging and MR morphometry of the central auditory pathway and auditory cortex in aging. *Neuroscience* 260, 87–97. doi: 10.1016/j.neuroscience.2013.12.010

Raichle, M. E., MacLeod, A. M., Snyder, A. Z., Powers, W. J., Gusnard, D. A., and Shulman, G. L. (2001). A default mode of brain function. *Proc. Natl. Acad. Sci. U.S.A.* 98, 676–682. doi: 10.1073/pnas.98.2.676

Sanchez-Cubillo, I., Perianez, J. A., Adrover-Roig, D., Rodriguez-Sanchez, J. M., Rios-Lago, M., Tirapu, J., et al. (2009). Construct validity of the trail making test: role of task-switching, working memory, inhibition/interference control, and visuomotor abilities. *J. Int. Neuropsychol. Soc.* 15, 438–450. doi: 10.1017/S1355617709090626

Savitz, J. B., and Jansen, P. (2003). The stroop color-word interference test as an indicator of ADHD in poor readers. *J. Genet. Psychol.* 164, 319–333. doi: 10.1080/00221320309597986

Singh-Curry, V., and Husain, M. (2009). The functional role of the inferior parietal lobe in the dorsal and ventral stream dichotomy. *Neuropsychologia* 47, 1434–1448. doi: 10.1016/j.neuropsychologia.2008.11.033

Vainik, U., Baker, T. E., Dadar, M., Zeighami, Y., Michaud, A., Zhang, Y., et al. (2018). Neurobehavioral correlates of obesity are largely heritable. *Proc. Natl. Acad. Sci. U.S.A.* 115, 9312–9317. doi: 10.1073/pnas.1718206115

Van Schependom, J., D'Hooghe, M. B., Cleynhens, K., D'Hooge, M., Haelewyck, M. C., De Keyser, J., et al. (2014). The symbol digit modalities test as sentinel test for cognitive impairment in multiple sclerosis. *Eur. J. Neurol.* 21:1219-e72. doi: 10.1111/ene.12463

Wang, X., Fan, Y., Zhao, F., Wang, Z., Ge, J., Zhang, K., et al. (2014). Altered regional and circuit resting-state activity associated with unilateral hearing loss. *PLoS One* 9:e96126. doi: 10.1371/journal.pone.0096126

Wayne, R. V., and Johnsrude, I. S. (2015). A review of causal mechanisms underlying the link between age-related hearing loss and cognitive decline. *Ageing Res. Rev.* 23, 154–166. doi: 10.1016/j.arr.2015.06.002

Wilk, M. B., and Gnanadesikan, R. (1968). Probability plotting methods for the analysis for the analysis of data. *Biometrika* 55, 1–17. doi: 10.2307/2334448

Wingfield, A., and Peelle, J. E. (2012). How does hearing loss affect the brain? *Aging Health* 8, 107–109. doi: 10.2217/ahe.12.5

Wong, P. C., Warrier, C. M., Penhune, V. B., Roy, A. K., Sadehh, A., Parrish, T. B., et al. (2008). Volume of left Heschl's Gyrus and linguistic pitch learning. *Cereb. Cortex* 18, 828–836. doi: 10.1093/cercor/bhm115

World Health, and Organization. (1991). *Report of the Informal Working Group on Prevention of Deafness and Hearing Impairment Programme Planning.* Geneva: WHO.

Zhao, Q., Lv, Y., Zhou, Y., Hong, Z., and Guo, Q. (2012). Short-term delayed recall of auditory verbal learning test is equivalent to long-term delayed recall for identifying amnestic mild cognitive impairment. *PLoS One* 7:e51157. doi: 10.1371/journal.pone.0051157

Zigmond, A. S., and Snaith, R. P. (1983). The hospital anxiety and depression scale. *Acta Psychiatr. Scand.* 67, 361–370. doi: 10.1111/j.1600-0447.1983.tb09716.x

13

Hearing Loss in Offspring Exposed to Antiretrovirals during Pregnancy and Breastfeeding

J. Riley DeBacker [1,2]*, Breanna Langenek [3] and Eric C. Bielefeld [3]

[1]VA RR&D National Center for Rehabilitative Auditory Research, VA Portland Healthcare System, Portland, OR, United States, [2]Oregon Hearing Research Center, Oregon Health and Science University, Portland, OR, United States, [3]Department of Speech and Hearing Science, The Ohio State University, Columbus, OH, United States

*Correspondence:
J. Riley DeBacker
debacker.2@osu.edu

Over 27 million people worldwide currently receive daily antiretroviral therapy for the management of HIV/AIDS. In order to prevent the continued spread of HIV, the World Health Organization (WHO) recommends the use of highly active antiretroviral therapy by pregnant and nursing women. There is currently little research into the auditory effects of this therapy on children exposed during pregnancy and breastfeeding, and research to date on the direct effects of antiretroviral exposure on the auditory system is inconclusive. The current study examined the effects of WHO-recommended first-line antiretrovirals in a well-controlled animal model to evaluate the potential for auditory damage and dysfunction following these exposures. Female breeding mice were each exposed to one of four antiretroviral cocktails or a vehicle control once daily during pregnancy and breastfeeding. Offspring of these mice had their auditory status evaluated after weaning using auditory brainstem responses and distortion-product otoacoustic emissions (DPOAEs). Auditory brainstem response thresholds following antiretroviral exposure during gestation and breastfeeding showed elevated thresholds and increased wave latencies in offspring of exposed mice when compared to unexposed controls, but no corresponding decrease in DPOAE amplitude. These differences in threshold were small and so may explain the lack of identified hearing loss in antiretroviral-exposed children during hearing screenings at birth. Minimal degrees of hearing impairment in children have been correlated with decreased academic performance and impaired auditory processing, and so these findings, if also seen in human children, suggest significant implications for children exposed to antiretrovirals during development despite passing hearing screenings at birth.

Keywords: antiretroviral therapy, ototoxicity, HIV, translational model, sensorineural hearing loss, auditory brainstem response

Abbreviations: 3TC, lamivudine; ABR, auditory brainstem response; AIDS, acquired immunodeficiency syndrome; ANOVA, analysis of variance; AZT, zidovudine; ARV, antiretroviral; DPOAE, distortion product otoacoustic emissions; EFV, efavirenz; HAART, highly-active antiretroviral therapy; HIV, human immunodeficiency virus; NRTI, nucleoside reverse transcriptase inhibitor; NVP, nevirapine; OHC, outer hair cell; PaB, pregnancy and breastfeeding; TDF, tenofovir disoproxil fumarate; TDT, Tucker Davis Technologies; WHO, World Health Organization.

INTRODUCTION

Human immunodeficiency virus (HIV) is an acquired viral infection that suppresses the immune system and leaves those infected more prone to opportunistic and latent disease. The World Health Organization (WHO) estimates that, at the end of 2020, there were nearly 38 million people living with HIV and that more than 27 million of those individuals were taking lifelong antiretroviral (ARV) therapy for HIV management (WHO, 2020). Highly-active antiretroviral therapy (HAART), also commonly referred to as "combination antiretroviral therapy," has been used since 1996 to manage symptoms of HIV and prevent disease progression and seroconversion to acquired immunodeficiency syndrome (AIDS). HAART typically consists of two nucleoside reverse transcriptase inhibitors (NRTIs) and one or more other drugs that have been shown to be effective not only at disease management but also at lowering disease burden to a point that prevents transmission (Cohen et al., 2011). As the WHO and other public health entities have a goal of preventing HIV transmission, HAART is recommended for all people living with HIV, and special focus has been paid to preventing the spread of HIV from mother to child during pregnancy (vertical transmission). While the use of HAART during pregnancy and breastfeeding has been shown to be effective in preventing the spread of HIV, exposure to HIV and HAART during development has been found to have negative impacts on cognitive development (Blanche et al., 1999; Tardieu et al., 2005; Brogly et al., 2007; Coelho et al., 2017; McHenry et al., 2019), language development (Rice et al., 2013), and auditory function (Poblano et al., 2004; Fasunla et al., 2014; Torre et al., 2017).

Current evidence regarding the auditory effects of HAART on perinatally HIV exposed but uninfected (PHEU) children has been inconclusive. Fasunla et al. (2014) found that *in utero* HIV exposure was more likely to result in failed hearing screening and confirmed hearing loss on a diagnostic auditory brainstem response (ABR), with a significant relationship between maternal viral load during pregnancy and hearing loss, but no relationship between CD4+ cell count and hearing loss. This study suggests that there may be some relationship between pre- and peri-natal HIV exposure and congenital hearing loss, but it did not control for whether or not mothers in the study were taking ARV therapy during pregnancy. Another study found significant delays in the Wave I latency and I-III interpeak latency on the ABR for PHEU infants exposed to the HAART drug zidovudine (AZT) alone or in combination with lamivudine (3TC; Poblano et al., 2004). In contrast, Torre and colleagues found that no specific HAART drug was related to an increased likelihood of hearing screening failure in PHEU children and that exposure to the drug tenofovir disoproxil fumarate (TDF) during the first trimester was associated with a lower odds ratio for a failed hearing screening. The authors also noted that a number of HAART drugs demonstrated an incredibly wide range of variability in auditory outcomes for newborns, even after controlling for factors that often contribute to failed hearing screenings (Torre et al., 2017). Despite the lack of differences in hearing screening results at birth, the Torre group also found that PHEU young adults were more likely to have impaired words-in-noise performance with otherwise normal cognition than young adults with HIV, suggesting an effect of exposure to these drugs during pregnancy and breastfeeding (PaB) not seen from post-natal exposures (Torre et al., 2020).

A prospective controlled human study of the relative contributions of HIV and HAART to hearing loss would be unethical, due to the high efficacy of HAART in preventing vertical HIV transmission, and so this question should first be explored in a well-controlled non-human model. Our group undertook an initial exploration of this modeling by exposing C57BL6/J female mice to AZT and 3TC during PaB (DeBacker et al., 2022). When offspring of these mice underwent ABR threshold testing at three weeks old, they had higher thresholds than control offspring at five of six tested frequencies. This indicates that exposure to AZT+3TC during PaB can lead to auditory dysfunction during development in a mouse model. AZT+3TC alone is not a currently recommended first-line management regimen for HIV, however, and so there is interest in understanding if these effects are seen across different currently-recommended ARV combinations. The current study seeks to expand upon our previous work by evaluating the auditory system of animals exposed to several different currently-recommended ARV combinations.

The current study used a well-characterized model of ototoxicity, the CBA/CaJ mouse, to investigate the auditory effects of HAART exposure during PaB. This model was used due to its stable hearing thresholds over the projected length of the study, in contrast to models with earlier onset of presbycusis like the C57BL6/J used previously. The authors hypothesized that exposure to HAART would lead to increased ABR and distortion product otoacoustic emissions (DPOAE) thresholds at wean in exposed offspring when compared to unexposed controls, with the greatest threshold elevation resulting from exposure to AZT and efavirenz (EFV). This hypothesis was based upon the previously-discussed findings on PHEU children and a study of the effects of ARV compounds on auditory cell (HEI-OC1) lines by Thein et al. (2014). This study found that exposure to moderate- and high-dose EFV resulted in almost 100% cell death and that even low-dose exposures cause significant cell death. While TDF was more toxic than AZT in the Thein et al. (2014) study, Torre et al. (2017) found a decrease in reported hearing screening failures following TDF exposure, and so it was predicted that AZT would have greater auditory effects than TDF. When combined with previous work by Thein et al. (2014) and our lab (DeBacker et al., 2022) on combination ARVs, it was anticipated that this study of WHO-recommended first-line HAART cocktails would result in greater auditory impairment than was observed in our previous study. By using currently-recommended HAART cocktails, this model provides a clinically translatable model of HAART exposure and contributes significant pre-clinical evidence toward the understanding of the auditory effects of HAART exposure during PaB.

METHODS

Subjects

One hundred CBA/CaJ mice were used in this study. Of these mice, 20 were breeding mice obtained from Jackson Labs (Las Vegas, NV) and housed in a vivarium at The Ohio State University. The breeding mice were divided into breeding pairs and then assigned to one of five experimental groups. The other 80 mice were offspring of those pairs. Each experimental group consisted of four breeding mice and 10–16 offspring. In order to exclude confounding variables, the male breeder mice were not exposed to HAART or any other manipulation during the study. Breeding pairs were allowed to generate no more than five litters before removal from the study. The mice were kept in a quiet colony, in which the 24-h dB Leq level never exceeded 45 dB SPL. Animals were acclimatized to the colony for at least 7 days before beginning experiments. All procedures involving the animals were approved by The Ohio State University's Institutional Animal Care and Use Committee.

Antiretroviral Exposures

For all experimental arms and conditions, the following groups were used: one group's (Group 1) breeder females received volume-matched distilled water vehicle; the other four groups' (Groups 2–5) breeder females received 3TC combined with the following drugs: Group (2) TDF and EFV; Group (3) AZT and EFV; Group (4) TDF and nevirapine (NVP); Group (5) AZT and NVP. These drug cocktails correspond to permutations of HAART currently recommended by WHO for first-line therapy for pregnant and nursing women, though emtricitabine is also recommended as an alternative to 3TC, which was used in this study. The combinations were chosen because significant differences were seen in cellular toxicity between EFV and NVP and TDF and AZT, respectively, but no such differences were observed between emtricitabine and 3TC (Thein et al., 2014).

All drugs used in this study were obtained as capsules or tablets through The Ohio State University Wexner Medical Center Pharmacy. AZT and TDF tablets were crushed using a mortar and pestle, and distilled water was added to dissolve them and create stock solutions with a concentration of 10 mg/ml. 3TC tablets were crushed using a mortar and pestle, and distilled water was added to create a stock solution with a concentration of 50 mg/ml. Suspensions were made using the combinations of 3TC with AZT or TDF, depending on the experimental group. For groups receiving NVP, tablets were crushed and added to the suspension. For groups receiving EFV, capsules were emptied directly into the suspension. After adding EFV or NVP, 4 ml of water were added to each suspension, and they were thoroughly mixed to minimize particulate in each jar. All jars were agitated prior to administration to minimize particulate in the suspensions. Suspensions were refrigerated between administrations. Each day, suspensions were monitored for an irregularity in appearance prior to administration. After 28 days, any remaining suspension was discarded, and new suspensions were mixed.

Because the female breeder mice grew in size and weight over the course of the study, the doses of the HAART compounds increased as well. However, best practice standards set the maximum fluid volume that could be delivered to the mice through oral gavage at 0.20 ml. Therefore, in order to deliver the required doses without exceeding the maximum fluid volume, the concentrations in mg/ml of the compounds needed to increase, and so after 3 months, concentrations of the HAART suspensions were recalculated to reflect the higher weight of the animals at that time. After this recalculation, concentrations of AZT and TDF were 13 mg/ml, concentrations of EFV and NVP were 83 mg/ml, and concentration of 3TC was 68.2 mg/ml. Preparations were otherwise unchanged from the above procedure.

Each female breeding mouse was given a once-daily dose *via* oral gavage of one of the four cocktails of antiretroviral agents listed earlier in this section or a matched volume of vehicle solution for control subjects in Group 1. Daily doses were administered beginning after baseline testing and continued until the final group of offspring used for the study was weaned. As such, female mice were exposed during the mating period, pregnancy, and nursing of all offspring. Weights to determine dosing were collected on the first day of each week and were used for the duration of that week unless a mouse gave birth. After giving birth, the previous week's weight was used for the remaining doses during that week. All gavage doses were delivered in a sterile environment under a biosafety hood in the University Laboratory Animal Resource housing vivarium.

Auditory Brainstem Responses

For this study, all animals were anesthetized using an inhaled mixture of gaseous isoflurane (2.5% for induction, 1.2% for maintenance) and oxygen (2 L/min for induction, 1 L/min for maintenance) during both ABR and DPOAE collection. ABR and DPOAE testing was performed in a sound-attenuating booth (Controlled Acoustical Environments, Bronx, NY).

For eliciting the ABRs, tone bursts were presented beginning at 90 dB SPL and in decreasing 5 dB steps to 20 dB SPL or until no repeatable waveform was observed. Test frequencies were 4, 8, 12, 16, 24, and 32 kHz. The stimuli were generated using Tucker Davis Technologies (TDT, Gainesville, FL) SigGen software. Each tone burst was 1 ms in duration and had a 0.5 ms rise/fall time with no plateau. Stimuli were presented at a rate of 19/s. Signals were routed to a speaker (TDT Model MF1) positioned at 90 degrees azimuth (directly next to the right ear), 3 cm from the vertex of each mouse's head. The levels were calibrated with a SoundTrack LxT1 sound level meter (Larson Davis, Depew, NY) with a $\frac{1}{4}$ in condenser microphone (model 7016 and model 4016, ACO Pacific, Inc.), placed at the level of the animal's head. For recording electrical responses from the mice, three 6-mm platinum electrodes (Rochester Electro-Medical, Lutz, FL) were inserted subdermally behind the right pinna (inverting), behind the left pinna (non-inverting), and in the right rear leg (ground) of each anesthetized mouse. The evoked responses of the mice were amplified with a gain of 50,000× using a TDT RA4LI headstage connected to a TDT RA4PA preamplifier. ABRs were averaged across 300 responses at each level. Responses were processed through a 300–3,000 Hz band-pass filter as recommended by the software manufacturer

(TDT). Post-acquisition analyses were performed using TDT BioSig RZ software. ABR P1 latencies were obtained by placing cursors at the positive P1 peak, and P3 latencies were obtained using the same process for the third positive peak.

Distortion-Product Otoacoustic Emissions

While still under the isoflurane anesthesia after the ABR recording, DPOAEs were measured. Prior to recording DPOAEs, all animals were visually inspected for signs of middle ear infection or cerumen buildup within the external auditory canal. DPOAE measurements were collected at the same f_2 frequencies as for ABR (4, 8, 12, 16, 24, and 32 kHz) with a ratio of f_2/f_1 constant at 1.25 and a ratio of L1/L2 constant at 1.2. At each frequency, stimuli began at 80 dB SPL for L1 and decreased in 10-dB steps to 20 dB SPL or until no cubic DPOAE ($2f_1$-f_2) response was observed. A cubic DPOAE was considered to be present if there was a visible spike at $2f_1$-f_2 that exceeded the noise floor at nearby frequencies, as can be seen in the example in **Figure 1**. The lowest intensity at which a visible cubic DPOAE could be detected was recorded at each tested frequency and was defined as the DPOAE threshold for that frequency. The stimuli were generated using TDT SigGen software. Signals were routed to two speakers (TDT Model MF1) in a closed field configuration that were coupled to the microphone tip of the Etymotic Research ER10B+ low noise microphone system (Elk Grove Village, IL) using 1/16" inner diameter, 1/8" outer diameter plastic tubing (McMaster-Carr, Cleveland, OH). The microphone tip was coupled to the ear of each mouse using a pipet tip that was trimmed to fit the ear. For each level, DPOAE recordings were averaged across 128 responses at each level as recommended by the software manufacturer (TDT). Gain for responses was set at 0.00001 so that plot outputs matched dBv for simple conversion to dB SPL and F1, F2, and DP ($2f_1$-f_2) were labeled for all collected responses.

For breeding pairs, ABRs and DPOAEs were recorded prior to assigning each mouse to an experimental group, and then 1, 3, and 6 months after pairing the mice and beginning HAART exposure. For offspring, ABRs and DPOAEs were recorded at 28 days post-birth. Day 28 was selected as the test date because the mice were weaned from their birth cages at 21 days, and then the additional week was given for them to acclimatize to their new cages before undergoing anesthetized auditory testing. All auditory testing was performed during the day (between 9 a.m. and 6 p.m. Eastern time).

Statistical Analyses

For the breeder females', a three-way analysis of variance (ANOVA) comparing group × frequency × test time (0, 3, or 6 months since enrollment) was used. Frequency and test time were treated as within-subjects factors, with the group as the between-subjects factor. ABR and DPOAE thresholds were analyzed for differences by exposure group at wean using a two-factor ANOVA (group*frequency). When significant effects were observed, all *post hoc* analyses for the group used Tukey A pairwise comparisons. Significance was assigned at $p < 0.05$ for all analyses. All statistical analyses were performed using IBM SPSS version 25 (IBM, Armonk, NY) and all associated

figures were created using SigmaPlot (Systat Software Inc., San Jose, CA).

RESULTS

Breeding Pairs

At the beginning of the study, the auditory status of all 20 breeding animals was evaluated *via* ABR. No animals were found to have abnormally high baseline ABR thresholds at enrollment, as can be seen in **Figure 2**. For the pre-exposure ABR thresholds, a two-factor ANOVA (frequency*ARV exposure group) was performed to determine differences in baseline hearing between groups' breeder females. There was neither a two-way interaction of frequency and group ($F_{1,20} = 1.106$, $p = 0.401$) nor a main effect of group ($F_{1,4} = 0.608$, $p = 0.675$). This lack of differences between breeding mice across groups indicates that any differences seen in offspring are likely the result of ARV exposures and not the result of obvious inherent differences. While the female breeding mice were being exposed to daily antiretrovirals by gavage, their ABR thresholds were monitored throughout the duration of the study. ABRs were collected at 1, 3, and 6 months (see **Figure 2** for means) after beginning the exposures in order to monitor any auditory changes resulting from HAART. A three-way repeated measures ANOVA (time*frequency*group) was performed to evaluate threshold changes across groups and frequencies over time in the HAART-exposed female breeding animals. There was no three-way interaction of group, frequency, and time ($F_{1,40} = 0.846$, $p = 0.693$) nor any two-way interaction of frequency and group ($F_{1,20} = 0.662$, $p = 0.808$). The only significant interaction was a two-way interaction of time and frequency ($F_{1,10} = 2.734$, $p = 0.016$). Evaluation of this effect showed a significant change in the mean threshold at 16 kHz between the 3-month and 6-month time points across groups. No other significant differences were observed, as can be seen in **Figure 2**. Overall, the results indicate that the daily ARV gavages did not create significant hearing threshold changes and that the mice exhibited generally stable thresholds, consistent with expectations for the CBA/CaJ mouse.

Offspring

The target group size for each exposure group (Groups 1–5) was eight mice. Due to differences in litter sizes, this number served as a target, but the achieved group sizes for each exposure group varied slightly. ABRs and DPOAEs were measured 7 days after wean (28 days of age) for all offspring in the study. This timepoint is referred to as "wean" throughout the rest of this manuscript, and it reflects the auditory status as it was first measured after weaning these animals. Mean ABR and DPOAE thresholds at wean are depicted below in **Figure 3**, and group comparisons are described below.

For the ABR thresholds at this wean time point, a two-factor ANOVA (frequency*group) was performed. There was no two-way interaction ($F_{(1,17.685)} = 1.222$, $p = 0.241$). To account for a lack of sphericity, a Huynh-Feldt correction was run on the reported two-way interaction. A significant main effect was seen for the group ($F_{(1,4)} = 4.749$, $p = 0.002$). When evaluating the

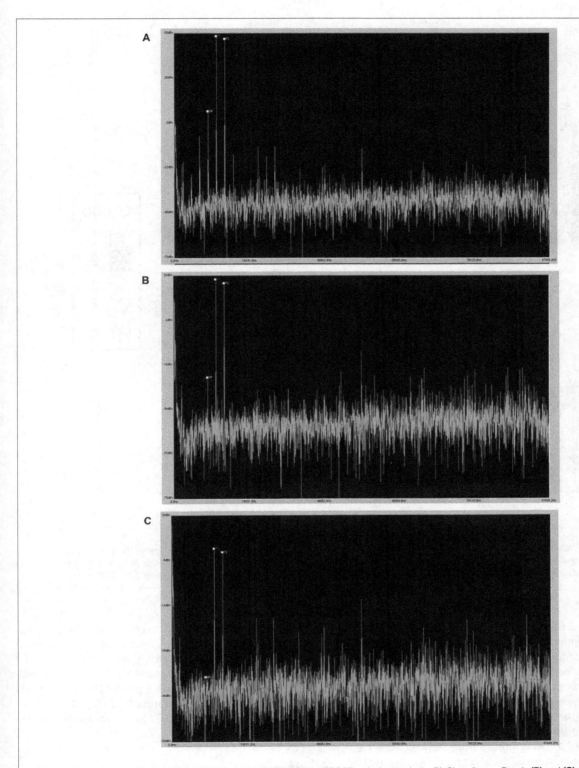

FIGURE 1 | DPOAE example. Panel **(A)** provides an example of a robust DPOAE as it displays in the BioSig software. Panels **(B)** and **(C)** provide examples of the visual indication of a DPOAE at the threshold and the absence of a DPOAE at lower levels.

wean average threshold across frequencies by group with Tukey A *post hoc* comparison, the control group (Group 1) had lower thresholds than Group 2 (5.63 dB mean difference, $p = 0.043$), Group 3 (9.39 dB, $p = 0.001$), and Group 5 (5.83 dB, $p = 0.049$). DPOAE thresholds for this time point were analyzed using a two-factor ANOVA (frequency*group). There was no two-way

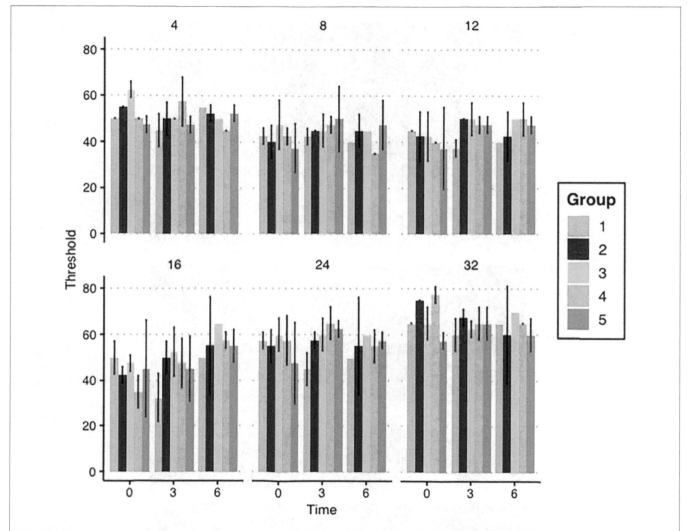

FIGURE 2 | Breeder ABR results. Mean ABR thresholds for each group of female breeding mice are depicted by the bars in each panel. Thresholds are grouped with the first set in each panel depicting mean thresholds before enrollment in the study and the next sets indicating the ABR thresholds at 3 and 6 months, respectively. Each panel represents a tested frequency. No significant differences exist between groups. Error bars represent ±1 standard deviation (SD).

interaction of group and frequency ($F_{(1,13.810)} = 1.1622, p = 0.073$) and there was no significant effect of group ($F_{(1,4)} = 2.363$, $p = 0.059$). To account for a lack of sphericity, a Huynh-Feldt correction was run on the reported two-way interaction with no change in the significance.

To physiologically evaluate the consequences of HAART exposure during PaB on the afferent synaptic pathway and auditory brainstem, P1 and P3 latencies, and P1-P3 interpeak latencies were evaluated for all responses from 70 to 90 dB SPL at 16 kHz for all animals at wean. 16 kHz was chosen for this measure because it had robust responses and low thresholds in all experimental groups, and so was considered likely to indicate if there were any suprathreshold effects across groups. A one-way ANOVA (group) found a significant effect of group for P1 latency at 75 dB SPL ($p = 0.036$) and for P3 latency and P1-P3 interpeak latency at 75 ($p = <0.001, 0.021$), 80

($p = 0.001, <0.001$), and 85 dB SPL ($p = 0.001, .011$). When evaluating these differences using Tukey A *post hoc* analysis, Group 4 had a greater P1 latency than Group 3 at 75 dB SPL, a greater P3 latency than Groups 2, 3, and 5 at 75–85 dB SPL and than Group 1 at 75–80 dB SPL, and a greater P1-P3 interpeak latency than Group 1 at 75 dB SPL, Groups 1, 2, 3, and 5 at 80 dB SPL, and than Groups 3 and 5 at 85 dB SPL. These results can be seen in greater detail in **Figure 4**.

DISCUSSION

Exposure to AZT and EFV During PaB Leads to Elevated ABR Thresholds at Wean
This study represents the first evaluation of the risk associated with exposure to specific controlled antiretrovirals during PaB.

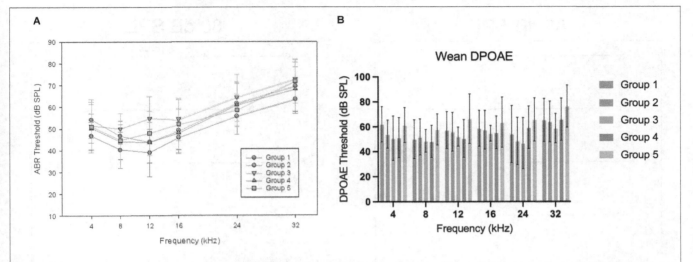

FIGURE 3 | Wean ABR and OAE. Panel **(A)** shows the mean ABR thresholds for each group of offspring mice at wean. No frequency-specific differences were reported at this time point. Mean thresholds for Group 1 were lower than in Groups 2, 3, and 5 ($p < 0.05$). Panel **(B)** shows the mean DPOAE thresholds for each group of offspring mice at wean. No significant differences were seen at this time point. Error bars represent ±1 SD.

The authors hypothesized that antiretroviral exposure during PaB would cause elevated ABR thresholds, with the greatest elevation arising from exposure to AZT and EFV. The results indicate that this hypothesis was correct, as both groups receiving either AZT or EFV had higher thresholds than controls. The group receiving both EFV and AZT saw an additional roughly 4-dB threshold mean increase over the groups receiving only one of those drugs. It is important to acknowledge that while Group 3 (AZT+EFV+3TC) saw higher thresholds than any other group in the study, those thresholds did not reach the level of statistical significance when compared to other ARV-exposed groups. While Group 4 (TDF+NVP+3TC) did not see elevated thresholds when compared to the control group, this group saw increased P3 and interpeak latencies when compared to all other groups. This indicates that different antiretroviral combinations may have different auditory impacts related to exposure during pregnancy and breastfeeding, and the differences across auditory measures may help to distinguish the site of lesion for these exposures.

The hypotheses of this study were largely driven by findings of toxicity to auditory cell lines *in vitro* (Thein et al., 2014). In that study, the authors investigated the mechanisms driving observed ototoxicity and were able to state that auditory cell losses seemed to be caspase 3/7-independent, indicating that those pro-apoptotic pathways did not appear to be the drivers of cell death. They hypothesized that, since EFV did not bind to mitochondrial DNA polymerase-y, EFV-induced damage was likely the result of endoplasmic reticulum stress. Subsequent exploration of the mechanisms of EFV-driven cytotoxicity has found that EFV causes significant cellular instability through the permeabilization of the mitochondrial outer membrane and induces changes in the mitochondrial membrane potential (Ganta et al., 2017). Changes in the mitochondrial membrane potential lead to cytochrome c release and mitochondrial-mediated apoptosis, both known causes of outer hair cell loss

(Wang et al., 2004). ARV exposures have also shown toxicity to the placenta (Collier et al., 2003) and other organs throughout the body (Benbrik et al., 1997), which may lead to auditory impacts as a result of this damage. While the current study did not directly evaluate the cellular mechanisms driving threshold elevation, these results when combined with the current literature, suggest that one or more mechanisms may be synergistically combining to damage the auditory system of those exposed to these drugs during PaB.

The lack of significant differences in DPOAE thresholds for this study indicates that the ABR threshold elevations were not the result of damage to the OHCs and were instead the result of damage to the inner hair cells, auditory nerve, and/or auditory brainstem. This is in line with previous work on the auditory impacts of ARVs that found abnormalities in the morphology of the ABR thought to be indicative of central auditory system pathology (Matas et al., 2010) and our previous experiment in the C57Bl6/J mouse (DeBacker et al., 2022). While this contradicts the findings of Thein et al. (2014), it is possible that differences in route of administration, cochlear supporting structures, or *in utero* delivery vs. direct administration to *ex vivo* samples may have caused these differences. This is further supported by the differences in P3 latency and P1-P3 interpeak latency seen in Group 4 when compared to other exposure groups. Especially since Group 4 had no significant differences in ABR threshold at wean, these significant differences in ABR morphology indicate that antiretroviral exposure during PaB may be causing auditory dysfunction that is not detected using conventional hearing screening methods.

Likely the most significant implication of this work is that ARV exposure during PaB causes auditory dysfunction that would not be detected in the most common newborn hearing screenings with ABRs or DPOAEs. This may help to clarify the currently mixed findings in the literature for PHEU children. The Torre group found impaired auditory processing in young

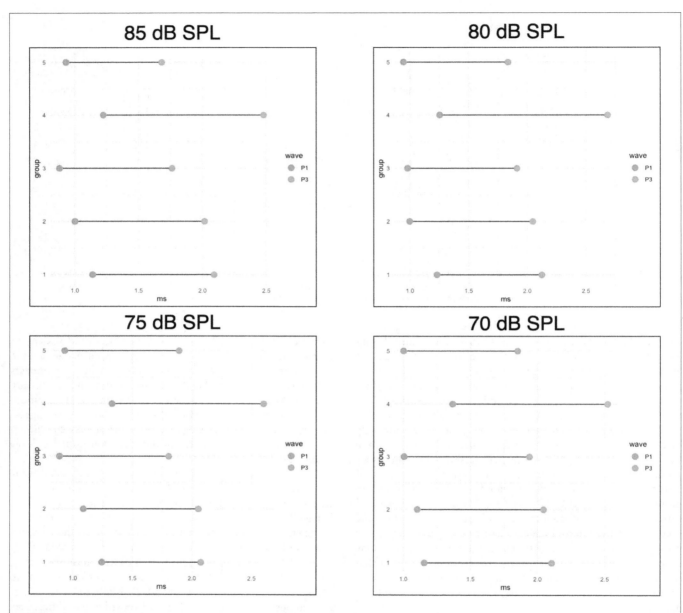

FIGURE 4 | Wean ABR latencies. This figure shows the mean P1 and P3 latencies for offspring measured at wean for four intensities (90 dB SPL is not pictured, but no significant differences were seen at this level). P1-P3 interpeak latencies are represented by the bars connecting the points for each group. Group 4 had a greater P1 latency than Group 3 at 75 dB SPL, a greater P3 latency than groups 2, 3, and 5 at 75–85 dB SPL and than Group 1 at 75–80 dB SPL, and a greater P1-P3 interpeak latency than Group 1 at 75 dB SPL, Groups 1, 2, 3, and 5 at 80 dB SPL, and than Groups 3 and 5 at 85 dB SPL. All significant differences are $p < 0.05$.

adults who had been exposed to HIV and HAART *in utero* (Torre et al., 2020), but did not find an increased rate of failed hearing screenings in children exposed to HIV and HAART *in utero* (Torre et al., 2017). These findings could indicate that children exposed to HAART *in utero* are not at increased risk for clinically-significant hearing loss, but are at risk for other auditory processing difficulties. It is important to note, however, that hearing screening at birth is not as sensitive as other auditory measures, like diagnostic threshold ABRs, and so is likely to miss subtle differences resulting from *in utero* HAART exposure. The

small threshold elevations seen in the mice in this study would be unlikely to cause a failed hearing screening, especially given the lack of impact on DPOAEs, which are frequently used in newborn hearing screenings. As such, it is possible that if such minimal hearing losses are also occurring in PHEU children, they are being missed on early hearing evaluations. PHEU children are therefore unable to benefit from the early intervention they would have received had these hearing differences been caught at birth. There is evidence linking short-term minimal hearing losses from otitis media to long-term auditory processing difficulties (Moore et al., 2020), and so it is possible that persistent minimal hearing losses like those seen in this study could result in the auditory processing difficulties described by Torre et al. (2020).

No Threshold Shifts Were Seen in Adult Mice

No auditory differences were seen in adult mice as a result of ARV exposure during the study. This is in agreement with previous studies of ARV exposure in mice (Bektas et al., 2008), and it is consistent with a model that indicates ARV exposure is causing subtle, even sub-clinical, changes in hearing during development. The CBA/CaJ mouse has "golden ears," a term used to indicate that they develop little age-related hearing loss. Certainly, within the time window of the breeding for the experiments, the female breeder mice would not have been expected to develop age-related hearing loss, and indeed they did not. Our previous work in this area used the C57Bl6/J mouse (DeBacker et al., 2022), which develops age-related hearing loss within weeks of its wean age (Willott et al., 1991). The variability in thresholds of those mice makes it difficult to interpret small mean differences of less than 10 dB. However, the same differences were detected in the CBA/CaJ mouse, which significantly reinforces the earlier finding. There was no reason to expect the HAART-exposed CBA/CaJ mice to be different from the control group unless the HAART exposure during PaB was indeed affecting the auditory system.

Limitations

It is of course important to recognize that the current study was a pre-clinical model of hearing using the CBA/CaJ mouse. While this is a well-studied model of audition and ototoxicity and every effort was made to design this study to be translational in nature, there are limitations inherent to non-human animal studies when applying the results to human populations. As such, further study in humans is required to confirm these findings are applicable across species. Additionally, it should be recognized that this was a model of HAART exposure only and not of the combined effects of HIV and HAART on the developing offspring. As such, differences may exist when introducing the variable of HIV infection alongside these exposures, and future studies should evaluate these exposures concurrently to determine if the addition of HIV impacts the auditory effects seen in this study. Lastly, it should be recognized that the mean threshold elevations

seen in this study are small (5–9 dB SPL). Despite the small degree of hearing impairment, the literature on language and cognitive development in children discussed above indicates that even these minimal hearing losses can have significant impacts on outcomes in children. This impact on outcomes is particularly concerning given the fact that minimal hearing losses like those observed in this study are less likely to be detected, even in settings with robust early hearing screening protocols.

CONCLUSIONS

The current study found that exposure to HAART, especially cocktails including AZT and EFV, during PaB was associated with increased ABR thresholds and differences in ABR wave latencies at wean when compared to unexposed offspring. These same threshold elevations were not seen on DPOAEs. Due to the minimal degree of threshold elevation (5–9 dB SPL) and lack of impact on DPOAEs, these hearing losses would be unlikely to be detected with common newborn hearing screenings. This may explain some of the discrepancies in the current literature relating to auditory function at birth in PHEU children (Poblano et al., 2004; Fasunla et al., 2014; Torre et al., 2017). Further study in models of concurrent HIV and HAART exposure and in human subjects is warranted to confirm the clinical relevance of these results.

AUTHOR CONTRIBUTIONS

JD and EB contributed to the conception and design of this study. JD and BL performed experiments and collected data. JD performed statistical analyses and wrote the first draft of the manuscript. BL and EB wrote sections of the manuscript. All authors contributed to the article and approved the submitted version.

ACKNOWLEDGMENTS

We would like to thank Drs. Christina Roup, Eric Healy, and Ruili Xie for editorial feedback, Dr. Aaron Roman for assistance in generating figures, and Dr. Cara Hollander for sparking this particular line of research.

REFERENCES

Bektas, D., Martin, G. K., Stagner, B. B., and Lonsbury-Martin, B. L. (2008). Noise-induced hearing loss in mice treated with antiretroviral drugs. Hear. Res. 239, 69–78. doi: 10.1016/j.heares.2008.01.016

Benbrik, E., Chariot, P., Bonavaud, S., Ammi-Saïd, M., Frisdal, E., Rey, C., et al. (1997). Cellular and mitochondrial toxicity of zidovudine (AZT), didanosine (ddI) and zalcitabine (ddC) on cultured human muscle cells. J. Neurol. Sci. 149, 19–25. doi: 10.1016/s0022-510x(97)05376-8

Blanche, S., Tardieu, M., Rustin, P., Slama, A., Barret, B., Firtion, G., et al. (1999). Persistent mitochondrial dysfunction and perinatal exposure to antiretroviral nucleoside analogues. The Lancet 354, 1084–1089. doi: 10.1016/S0140-6736(99)07219-0

Brogly, S. B., Ylitalo, N., Mofenson, L. M., Oleske, J., Van Dyke, R., Crain, M. J., et al. (2007). In utero nucleoside reverse transcriptase inhibitor exposure and signs of possible mitochondrial dysfunction in HIV-uninfected children. AIDS 21, 929–938. doi: 10.1097/QAD.0b013e3280d5a786

Coelho, A., Tricarico, P., Celsi, F., and Crovella, S. (2017). Antiretroviral treatment in HIV-1-positive mothers: neurological implications in virus-free children. Int. J. Mol. Sci. 18:423. doi: 10.3390/ijms18020423

Cohen, M. S., Chen, Y. Q., McCauley, M., Hosseinipour, M. C., Kumarasamy, N., Hakim, J. G., et al. (2011). Prevention of HIV-1 infection with early antiretroviral therapy. N. Engl. J. Med. 365, 493–505. doi: 10.1056/NEJMoa1105243

Collier, A. C., Helliwell, R. J. A., Keelan, J. A., Paxton, J. W., Mitchell, M. D., Tingle, M. D., et al. (2003). 3'-azido-3'-deoxythymidine (AZT) induces apoptosis and alters metabolic enzyme activity in human placenta. *Toxicol. Appl. Pharmacol.* 192, 164–173. doi: 10.1016/s0041-008x(03)00274-6

DeBacker, J. R., Hu, B. H., and Bielefeld, E. C. (2022). Mild hearing loss in C57BL6/J mice after exposure to antiretroviral compounds during gestation and nursing. *Int. J. Audiol.* 25, 1–7. doi: 10.1080/14992027.2022.2067081

Fasunla, A. J., Ogunbosi, B. O., Odaibo, G. N., Nwaorgu, O. G. B., Taiwo, B., Olaleye, D. O., et al. (2014). Comparison of auditory brainstem response in HIV-1 exposed and unexposed newborns and correlation with the maternal viral load and CD4+ cell counts. *AIDS* 28, 2223–2230. doi: 10.1097/QAD.0000000000000393

Ganta, K. K., Mandal, A., and Chaubey, B. (2017). Depolarization of mitochondrial membrane potential is the initial event in non-nucleoside reverse transcriptase inhibitor efavirenz induced cytotoxicity. *Cell Biol. Toxicol.* 33, 69–82doi: 10.1007/s10565-016-9362-9

Matas, C. G., Silva, S. M., de Almeida Macron, B., and Gonçalves, I. C. (2010). Electrophysiological manifestations in adults with HIV/AIDS submitted and not submitted to antiretroviral therapy. *Pró-Fono R. Atual. Cient.* 22, 107–113. doi: 10.1590/s0104-56872010000200007

McHenry, M. S., Balogun, K. A., McDonald, B. C., Vreeman, R. C., Whipple, E. C., Serghides, L., et al. (2019). *In utero* exposure to HIV and/or antiretroviral therapy: a systematic review of preclinical and clinical evidence of cognitive outcomes. *J. Int. AIDS Soc.* 22:e25275. doi: 10.1002/jia2.25275

Moore, D. R., Zobay, O., and Ferguson, M. A. (2020). Minimal and mild hearing loss in children: association with auditory perception, cognition and communication problems. *Ear Hear.* 41, 720–732. doi: 10.1097/AUD.0000000000000802

Poblano, A., Figueroa, L., Figueroa-Damián, R., and Schnaas, L. (2004). Effects of prenatal exposure to Zidovudine and Lamivudine on brainstem auditory evoked potentials in infants from HIV-infected women. *Proc. West. Pharmacol. Soc.* 47, 46–49.

Rice, M. L., Zeldow, B., Siberry, G. K., Purswani, M., Malee, K., Hoffman, H. J., et al. (2013). Evaluation of risk for late language emergence after *in utero* antiretroviral drug exposure in HIV-exposed uninfected infants. *Pediatr. Infect. Dis. J.* 32, e406–e413. doi: 10.1097/INF.0b013e31829b80ee

Tardieu, M., Brunelle, F., Raybaud, C., Ball, W., Barret, B., Pautard, B., et al. (2005). Cerebral MR imaging in uninfected children born to HIV-seropositive mothers and perinatally exposed to zidovudine. *Am. J. Neuroradiol.* 7, 695–701.

Thein, P., Kalinec, G. M., Park, C., and Kalinec, F. (2014). *In vitro* assessment of antiretroviral drugs demonstrates potential for ototoxicity. *Hear. Res.* 310, 27–35. doi: 10.1016/j.heares.2014.01.005

Torre, P., Russell, J. S., Smith, R., Hoffman, H. J., Lee, S., Williams, P. L., et al. (2020). Words-in-noise test performance in young adults perinatally HIV infected and exposed, uninfected. *Am. J. Audiol.* 29, 68–78. doi: 10.1044/2019_AJA-19-00042

Torre, P., Zeldow, B., Yao, T., Hoffman, H., Siberry, G., Purswani, M., et al. (2017). Newborn hearing screenings in human immunodeficiency virus-exposed uninfected infants. *J. AIDS Immune Res.* 10:102.

Wang, J., Ladrech, S., Pujol, R., Brabet, P., Van De Water, T. R., Puel, J.-L., et al. (2004). Caspase inhibitors, but not c-Jun NH2-terminal kinase inhibitor treatment, prevent cisplatin-induced hearing loss. *Cancer Res* 64, 9217–9224. doi: 10.1158/0008-5472.CAN-04-1581

WHO (2020). *HIV/AIDS Fact Sheet [WWW Document].* Available online at: http://www.who.int/mediacentre/factsheets/fs360/en/.

Willott, J. F., Parham, K., and Hunter, K. P. (1991). Comparison of the auditory sensitivity of neurons in the cochlear nucleus and inferior colliculus of young and aging C57BL/6J and CBA/J mice. *Hear Res.* 53, 78–94. doi: 10.1016/0378-5955(91)90215-u

14

The Expression and Roles of the Super Elongation Complex in Mouse Cochlear Lgr5+ Progenitor Cells

Yin Chen[1†], Ruiying Qiang[2†], Yuan Zhang[2†], Wei Cao[3†], Leilei Wu[2], Pei Jiang[2], Jingru Ai[2], Xiangyu Ma[2], Ying Dong[2], Xia Gao[1], He Li[4*], Ling Lu[1*], Shasha Zhang[2*] and Renjie Chai[2,5,6,7*]

[1] Jiangsu Provincial Key Medical Discipline (Laboratory), Department of Otolaryngology Head and Neck Surgery, Drum Tower Hospital Clinical College of Nanjing Medical University, Nanjing, China, [2] State Key Laboratory of Bioelectronics, Jiangsu Province High-Tech Key Laboratory for Bio-Medical Research, School of Life Sciences and Technology, Southeast University, Nanjing, China, [3] Department of Otorhinolaryngology, Head and Neck Surgery, The Second Hospital of Anhui Medical University, Hefei, China, [4] Department of Otolaryngology, The First Affiliated Hospital of Wenzhou Medical University, Wenzhou, China, [5] Co-innovation Center of Neuroregeneration, Nantong University, Nantong, China, [6] Institute for Stem Cell and Regeneration, Chinese Academy of Sciences, Beijing, China, [7] Beijing Key Laboratory of Neural Regeneration and Repair, Capital Medical University, Beijing, China

*Correspondence:
Renjie Chai
renjiec@seu.EdU.cn
Shasha Zhang
zhangss5576@163.com
Ling Lu
entluling60@126.com
He Li
lihewuyao@163.com

† These authors have contributed equally to this work

The super elongation complex (SEC) has been reported to play a key role in the proliferation and differentiation of mouse embryonic stem cells. However, the expression pattern and function of the SEC in the inner ear has not been investigated. Here, we studied the inner ear expression pattern of three key SEC components, AFF1, AFF4, and ELL3, and found that these three proteins are all expressed in both cochlear hair cells (HCs)and supporting cells (SCs). We also cultured Lgr5+ inner ear progenitors in vitro for sphere-forming assays and differentiation assays in the presence of the SEC inhibitor flavopiridol. We found that flavopiridol treatment decreased the proliferation ability of Lgr5+ progenitors, while the differentiation ability of Lgr5+ progenitors was not affected. Our results suggest that the SEC might play important roles in regulating inner ear progenitors and thus regulating HC regeneration. Therefore, it will be very meaningful to further investigate the detailed roles of the SEC signaling pathway in the inner ear in vivo in order to develop effective treatments for sensorineural hearing loss.

Keywords: super elongation complex (SEC), inner ear, expression, proliferation, differentiation

INTRODUCTION

Hearing loss occurs mainly due to noise exposure, aging, ototoxic drugs, and genetic factors (Sun et al., 2017). There were around 466 million people worldwide with disabling hearing loss in 2020, and the World Health Organization [WHO] (2019) estimates that by 2050 over 900 million people will have disabling hearing loss. Deafness has become a major global health problem, and sensorineural hearing loss is the most common type of hearing impairment (Youm and Li, 2018). However, due to the lack of effective drugs and a non-invasive method for targeted delivery of drugs to the inner ear, the treatment options for sensorineural hearing loss are limited (Mittal et al., 2019). Cochlear hair cells (HCs) in adult mammals lose the ability to regenerate, thus hearing deficits caused by HC loss are permanent (Warchol et al., 1993; Ryan, 2003; Cox et al., 2014; Xu et al., 2017; Chen et al., 2019). Therefore, induction of HC regeneration after injury by stimulating quiescent inner ear progenitor cells has been a main focus of auditory research in recent years.

The super elongation complex (SEC) is extremely important in the transcriptional elongation checkpoint control stage of transcription and is composed mainly of P-TEFb (positive transcription elongation factor), ELL (11–19 lysine-rich leukemia gene) family proteins, AFF (AF4/FMR2) family proteins, ENL (11–19 leukemia), AF9 (ALL1-fused gene from chromosome 9), and many other transcription factors (Luo et al., 2012b). P-TEFb and ELL are RNA polymerase II (Pol II)-related elongation factors (Shilatifard et al., 2003). AFF family proteins act as transcriptional activators with a positive action on RNA elongation (Melko et al., 2011). ENL and AF9 are homologous, and they can connect the SEC to RNA Pol II-related factors (He et al., 2011). P-TEFb is composed of cyclin-dependent kinase 9 (CDK9) and cyclin T (CycT), and it promotes the transition into productive elongation by phosphorylating RNA polymerase II (Peng et al., 1998). It has been reported that the SEC plays an important role in regulating mouse embryonic stem cell proliferation and differentiation (Lin et al., 2011), and mis-regulation of the SEC leads to the uncontrolled regulation of gene expression during the differentiation of embryonic stem cells, which results in a variety of diseases such as acute lymphoblastic leukemia, cerebellar ataxia, and diffuse midline glioma (Lin et al., 2011; Dahl et al., 2020). ELL3, one of the key factors of the SEC, can protect differentiated cells from apoptosis by promoting the degradation of p53, enhancing the differentiation of mouse embryonic stem cells, and regulating the proliferation and survival of embryonic stem cells (Ahn et al., 2012). However, the roles of the SEC in the inner ear remain unclear.

Flavopiridol is a semi-synthetic flavonoid that has been used in the treatment of acute myeloid leukemia (Zeidner and Karp, 2015), chronic lymphocytic leukemia (Wiernik, 2016), and other chronic diseases. Flavopiridol binds directly to CDK9, which is a component of P-TEFb, and inhibits its kinase activity (Chao et al., 2000). In turn, P-TEFb, as an important component of the SEC, can activate RNA polymerase II and transcriptional elongation (Hnisz et al., 2013). Thus, the most common method for blocking SEC function is to directly inhibit CDK9 with flavopiridol (Morales and Giordano, 2016), and we used flavopiridol to inhibit the function of the SEC as previously reported (Lin et al., 2011).

Recent studies have shown that Lgr5+ supporting cells (SCs) are inner ear progenitors and that they have the ability to regenerate new HCs in the neonatal stage (Shi et al., 2012). The activation of Wnt/β-catenin signaling and inhibition of Notch signaling can induce Lgr5+ progenitors to regenerate Myo7a+ HCs (Chai et al., 2012; Korrapati et al., 2013; Mizutari et al., 2013), and several recent studies have also shown that Lgr5+ progenitors can be regulated by many other factors and signaling pathways such as Shh, Foxg1, and Hippo (Gregorieff et al., 2015; Chen et al., 2017; Zhang et al., 2020). However, the regeneration efficiency of Lgr5+ progenitors is still very limited, which suggests that there

are other factors or signaling pathways involved in the HC regeneration process. Because the transcription extension stage is the main stage of gene expression regulation, transcriptional regulation of developmental regulatory genes is the core link between embryonic stem cell differentiation and organ formation (Smith and Shilatifard, 2010; Levine, 2011). Therefore, we speculate that the SEC may also play important roles in cochlear progenitor cells.

Here we measured the expression of the key SEC factors AFF1, AFF4, and ELL3 in the neonatal mouse cochlea, the function of SEC inhibitor flavopiridol in House Ear Institute-Organ of Corti 1 (HEI-OC1) cell line, and we assessed the proliferation and differentiation ability of Lgr5+ progenitors after treatment with the SEC inhibitor flavopiridol. Our results suggest important roles for the SEC in Lgr5+ progenitors *in vitro*, and further *in vivo* studies need to be done to elucidate the roles of the SEC in the inner ear. These studies will form the experimental basis for using cochlear progenitors to regenerate functional HCs in order to treat patients with sensorineural hearing loss.

MATERIALS AND METHODS

Experimental Animals

Lgr5-EGFP-Ires-CreERT2 (Lgr5-EGFP) mice (Barker et al., 2007) (Jackson Laboratory, Stock No. 00887) and FVB mice used as wide-type mice were raised in a comfortable environment with suitable temperature and light and fed with standard laboratory food and water *ad libitum*. We are approved by the Animal Care and Use Committee of Southeast University and were consistent with the National Institutes of Health Guide for the Care and Use of Laboratory Animals. All the operations were carried out in accordance with the procedures.

RNA Extraction and Reverse Transcription-Polymerase Chain Reaction

About 20 wild-type mouse cochleae were dissected to extract total RNA, which was reverse transcribed into cDNA with the cDNA Synthesis Kit (Thermo Fisher Scientific, K1622). Gene expression was measured by reverse transcription-polymerase chain reaction (RT-PCR) with GAPDH as the endogenous reference gene. The RT-PCR conditions were as follow for a total of 35 cycles: initial denaturation at 95°C for 15 s, denaturation at 95°C for 15 s, annealing at 60°C for 60 s, and extension at 72°C. The primers were as follows: GAPDH: (F) 5′-AGG TCG GTG TGA ACG GAT TTG-3′; (R) 5′-TGT AGA CCA TGT AGT TGA GGT CA-3′; AFF1: (F) 5′-GAA GGA AAG ACG CAA CCA AGA-3′; (R) 5′-TAG CTC ATC GCC TTT TGC AGT-3′; AFF4: (F) 5′-ATG AAC CGT GAA GAC CGG AAT-3′; (R) 5′-TGC TAG TGA CTT TGT ATG GCT CA-3′; ELL3: (F) 5′-GAC CAG CCT CCT GAT GCT AAG-3′; (R) 5′-GCC ACC ATT AGT GCC CTC TTG-3′.

Western Blotting

About 10 cochleae from postnatal day (P)3 mice were dissected in order to extract proteins. GAPDH was used as the reference protein. The primary antibodies were anti-AFF1 (Sigma-Aldrich,

#SAB2106246), anti-AFF4 (Santa Cruz, #sc135337), and anti-ELL3 (Abcam, #ab67415). Peroxidase-conjugated goat anti-rabbit (Life, A-31572) and goat anti-mouse (Invitrogen, A21202) were used as the secondary antibodies. The gray levels were measured by Image-J.

Cell Culture

HEI-OC1 cells were cultured in Dulbecco's modified Eagle's medium (DMEM) with 10% fetal bovine serum and 1% ampicillin at 37°C and 5% CO_2. The cells were divided into two groups. The experimental group was treated with flavopiridol (AbMole M1710) at the concentration of 10 μM. Control cells were treated with dimethyl sulfoxide (DMSO) in the same culture medium. After 12-h culture, cells were treated with 0.25% trypsin/ethylene diamine tetraacetic acid (EDTA) and then ultrasonicated (Bioruptor™ UCD-200) for CDK9 kinase detection.

Cyclin-Dependent Kinase 9 Kinase Assay

HEI-OC1 cells with or without flavopiridol treatment were used after ultrasonication to detect the CDK9 activity by using CDK9 Cyclin K Kinase Assay kit (Promega, V4104) and ADP-Glo Kinase Assay kit (Promega, V6930). To initiate the CDK9 reaction, CDK9 substrate PDKtides and adenosine triphosphate (ATP) were added into each group for 120 min at room temperature to produce adenosine diphosphate (ADP) according to the manufacturer's instruction (Promega, #TM313). And then ADP-Glo Reagent was added for 40 min at room temperature to deplete the remaining ATP. The Kinase Detection Reagent was added to convert the ADP produced at the first step to ATP with luminescence. Finally, the luminescence was recorded by BioTek CYTATION 5 (Integration time 1 s) to determine the CDK9 activity in each sample. The relative light units were calculated to represent the activity of CDK9.

Isolation of Lgr5+ Progenitors *via* Flow Cytometry

About 50–60 cochleae were isolated from P0 to P3 Lgr5-EGFP mice and then treated with 0.125% trypsin/EDTA (Invitrogen, 25200114) at 37°C. Trypsin inhibitor (10 mg/ml, Worthington Biochem) was added after 10 min to terminate the reaction. The trypsinized cochleae were pipetted up and down 80–100 times to obtain single cells, and the cells were then filtered through a 40 μM cell strainer (BD Biosciences, 352340). Dissociated cells were sorted on a flow cell sorter (BD FACS Aria III). The EGFP+ cells were collected as Lgr5+ progenitors for further *in vitro* cell culture experiments.

Sphere-Forming Assay and Differentiation Assay

Sorted Lgr5+ cells were cultured in DMEM/F12 medium at a density of 2 cells/μl (200 cells per well) for 5 days for sphere forming. The formula of DMEM/F12 medium was the same in previous study (Zhang et al., 2020). Spheres were identified with the Live Cell Imaging System and quantified using Image J. For differentiation, cells were cultured in the DMEM/F12 medium described above at a density of 20 cells/μl (2,000 cells per well)

for 10 days. EdU [10 μM (Invitrogen, C10420)] was added to label proliferating cells from day 4 to day 7. Flavopiridol (AbMole, M1710) was added to the experimental group from day 1 to day 10 at a concentration of 10 μM, while DMSO was added to the control group. Differentiated neurospheres were analyzed by immunofluorescent staining.

Immunofluorescent Staining

The cochleae were dissected in cold Hanks Balanced Salt Solution (HBSS) in order to prevent protein degradation and then fixed with 4% paraformaldehyde (PFA) for 1 h at room temperature. *In vitro* cultured neurospheres were also fixed with 4% PFA for 1 h at room temperature. After washing with phosphate buffered saline with tween (PBST) three times, the cochleae or neurospheres were blocked with blocking solution for 1 h at room temperature and then incubated overnight at 4°C with primary antibodies. The primary antibodies used were anti-Myosin7a (Myo7a; Proteus Bioscience, #25-6790; 1:1,000 dilution), anti-Sox2 (1:400 dilution), anti-AFF1 (1:400 dilution), anti-AFF4 (1:50 dilution), and anti-ELL3 (1:400 dilution). After washing again three times, the cochleae or neurospheres were further incubated with secondary antibodies (Invitrogen, A21131, A21124) diluted 1:400 in PBT2 for 1 h at room temperature. After washing three times, the cochleae or neurospheres were mounted on slides with anti-fade fluorescence mounting medium (DAKO, S3023). Images were captured by Zeiss LSM 710 confocal microscope and analyzed by Image J software.

Tissue Embedment

The P40 temporal bones were dissected and put in 4% PFA to be shaken for 1–2 h and sit overnight at 4°C. Later, the temporal bones were put in 0.5 M EDTA for decalcification for 2 days. After washing with PBST three times, the temporal bones were transferred into 15% sucrose solution, vacuum for 1 h, 4°C overnight. Afterward, the temporal bones were put in 20% sucrose solution, vacuum for 1 h, then transferred to 30% sucrose solution, vacuum 1 h, 4°C overnight. Then, the temporal bones were put into a 1:1 solution of 30% sucrose in optimum cutting temperature (OCT) medium (Sakura 4583), vacuum for 1 h, overnight at 4°C. The following day, temporal bones were put in a 3:7 solution of 30% sucrose in OCT medium, vacuum for 1 h, then the 3:17 solution of 30% sucrose in OCT medium, vacuum for 1 h, and lastly the 100% OCT medium (adjust position as round window and ellipse window are toward on the ground), vacuum for 1 h, 4°C overnight. For the last step, the temporal bones were put in 100% OCT into vacuum for 1 h adjust position, then in cryostat (Microm HM525) for a 20-min quick-freeze, and restored in −80°C. For slicing, adjust the cryostat half an hour in advance; secondly, adjust the blade temperature and internal temperature to −20°C. The selected sections were stained using the method described above.

Statistical Analysis

All the data in this research are presented as means ± SEM, and all experiments were repeated at least three times. All statistical analyses were performed in GraphPad Prism 5. P-values were calculated using a two-tailed, unpaired Student's t-test, and a p-value < 0.05 was considered statistically significant.

RESULTS

AFF1, AFF4, and ELL3 Are Expressed in the Cochlea

We first measured the expression of the three key SEC subunits AFF1, AFF4, and ELL3 by RT-PCR (**Figure 1A**) and Western blotting analysis (**Figures 1B,C**), and we found that AFF1, AFF4, and ELL3 were all highly expressed in the cochlea. Moreover, we measured the expression of AFF1, AFF4, and ELL3 in Lgr5+ cells (**Figure 1D**), and we found those three expressions in both cochlea and Lgr5+ cells were similar. We further studied the expression pattern from both the obverse and lateral sides of AFF1, AFF4, and ELL3 in the cochlea of P3 and P40 mice

and found that AFF1, AFF4, and ELL3 were all expressed in the cochlear HCs and SCs (**Figures 2A–D**). However, the immunostaining intensities of these three subunits in the SCs were weaker than in the HCs.

Flavopiridol Treatment Inhibited the Activity of Cyclin-Dependent Kinase 9 in House Ear Institute-Organ of Corti 1 Cells

Flavopiridol has been reported to be an inhibitor of CDK9 which is an indispensable part of SEC and the low level of its kinase activity prevents the recruitment of other elongation factors in

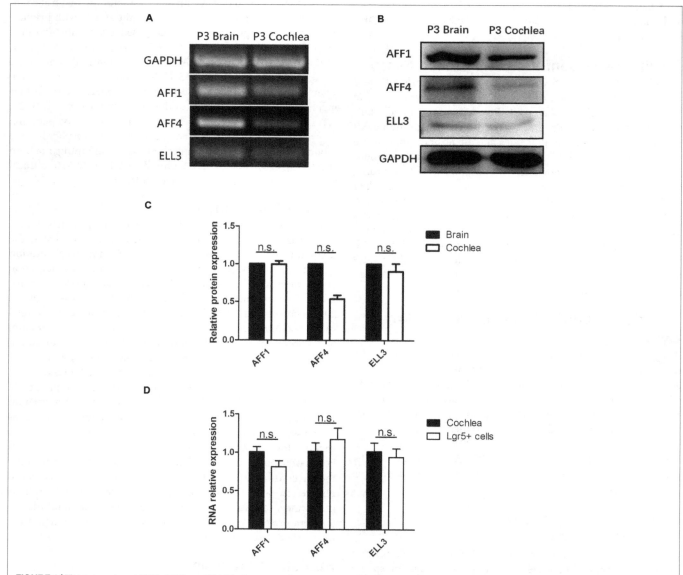

FIGURE 1 | The expression of AFF1, AFF4, and ELL3 in the neonatal mouse cochlea. **(A,B)** The mRNA and protein expression of AFF1, AFF4, and ELL3 in P3 mouse cochleae were detected by RT-PCR **(A)** and western blotting **(B)**, respectively. **(C)** The gray levels comparison of western blot. **(D)** The mRNA expression of AFF1, AFF4, and ELL3 in Lgr5+ cells. Brain samples of P3 mice were used as the positive control, and GAPDH was used as the internal reference. n.s., not significant.

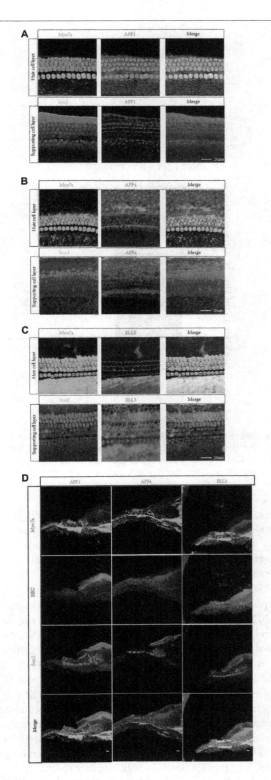

FIGURE 2 | Immunofluorescent staining of AFF1, AFF4, and ELL3 in the mouse cochlea. **(A–C)** The whole-mount basilar membrane of P3 was immunostained by antibodies against AFF1 **(A)**, AFF4 **(B)**, and ELL3 **(C)**. **(D)** Frozen sections of P40 were immunostained by antibodies against AFF1, AFF4, and ELL3. Myo7a and Sox2 were used to label hair cells (HCs) and supporting cells (SCs), respectively. Scale bar = 20 μM.

SEC (Peng et al., 1998). However, the function of flavopiridol has not been verified in inner ear. Here, we used ADP-Glo Kinase Assay to detect the activity of CDK9. After the kinase reaction, the remaining ATP was depleted and the ADP was converted to luminescent ATP (**Figure 3A**). HEI-OC1 cells were cultured for 3 days, and then treated by 10 μM flavopiridol which was diluted in the culture medium for 12 h. Images of cells were taken before and after flavopiridol treatment (**Figure 3B**). After flavopiridol treatment, the number and diameter of cells visually decrease in comparison with the control group with no change in shapes. The luminescent ATP was recorded and the relative light units was calculated to represent the activity of CDK9 (**Figure 3C**). The results showed that flavopiridol could also function as the CDK9 inhibitor to inhibit SEC activity in HEI-OC1 cells.

Flavopiridol Treatment Decreased the Sphere-Forming Ability of Lgr5+ Progenitors *in vitro*

Flavopiridol was previously used to inhibit SEC transcription activity (Lin et al., 2011). Here we also used flavopiridol to inhibit SEC activity in Lgr5+ progenitors in order to determine whether the SEC plays roles in the proliferation and differentiation ability of Lgr5+ progenitors. In order to determine the effect of the SEC on the sphere-forming ability of Lgr5+ progenitors, Lgr5+ cells were isolated from Lgr5-EGFP mice by flow cytometry and then cultured *in vitro* for 5 days to form spheres with or without 10 μM flavopiridol treatment (**Figures 4A,B**). The flavopiridol treatment decreased both the number (**Figure 4C**) and diameter of the spheres (**Figure 4D**), which suggested that inhibition of the SEC could decrease the sphere-forming ability and proliferation ability of Lgr5+ progenitors *in vitro*.

No Difference Was Observed in the Differentiation Assay After Flavopiridol Treatment

In order to further evaluate the effect of the SEC on the differentiation ability of Lgr5+ progenitors, we isolated Lgr5+ cells by flow cytometry and cultured them *in vitro* for the differentiation assay with or without 10 μM flavopiridol treatment (**Figure 5A**). The cells were immunostained with Myo7a, EdU, and DAPI (**Figure 5B**), and the Myo7a+ cells and EdU+ cells inside and outside the colonies were quantified. There were more EdU+ cells in the flavopiridol treatment group than in the control group (**Figure 5C**), while the numbers of Myo7a+ cells were almost the same in the flavopiridol treatment group and the control group (**Figure 5D**). These results suggested that inhibition of the SEC did not affect the differentiation ability of Lgr5+ cells *in vitro*.

In summary, our results showed that the key SEC factors AFF1, AFF4, and ELL3 are all highly expressed in the cochlea. And we verified that flavopiridol could inhibit SEC by inhibiting CDK9 activity in HEI-OC1 cell line. We used flavopiridol as an SEC inhibitor to investigate the effect of the SEC on the proliferation and differentiation ability of Lgr5+ progenitors and found that the number and diameter of spheres of Lgr5+ progenitors were both decreased after SEC inhibitor treatment,

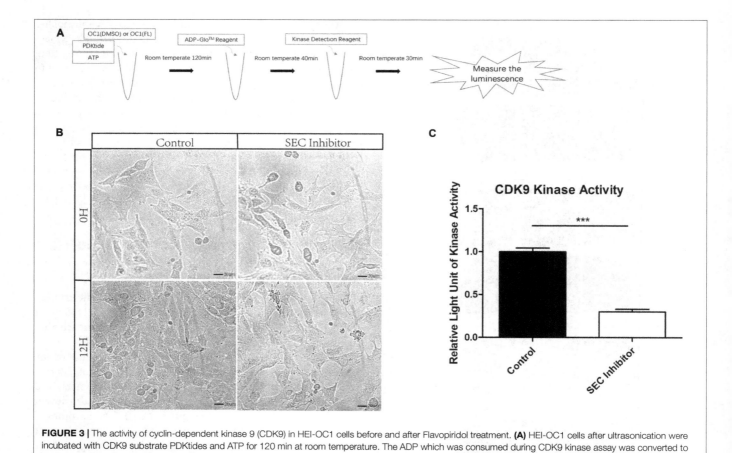

FIGURE 3 | The activity of cyclin-dependent kinase 9 (CDK9) in HEI-OC1 cells before and after Flavopiridol treatment. **(A)** HEI-OC1 cells after ultrasonication were incubated with CDK9 substrate PDKtides and ATP for 120 min at room temperature. The ADP which was consumed during CDK9 kinase assay was converted to ATP and could be quantitated by luciferase assay. **(B)** Images of HEI-OC1 cells before and after 10 µM Flavopiridol treatment. DMSO was added as control treatment in the Control group. Scale bar = 20 µM. **(C)** Fold change of CDK9 kinase activity in HEI-OC1 cells with or without Flavopiridol treatment. $n = 3$, $***p < 0.001$.

while the differentiation ability of Lgr5+ progenitors was not affected. Therefore, the SEC appears to promote the proliferation ability of Lgr5+ progenitors, but not their differentiation ability.

DISCUSSION

Irreversible damage to HCs in the mammalian cochlea is the main cause of sensorineural hearing loss. Previous studies have reported that Lgr5+ cells are cochlear progenitors with the ability to regenerate HCs (Shi et al., 2012), and it has been documented that the SEC plays an important role in the process of gene transcription and extension and that it is necessary for the differentiation of mouse embryonic stem cells (Lin et al., 2011). Therefore, we speculated that the SEC also plays an important role in the proliferation and differentiation of mouse cochlear progenitors. Besides, it has also been reported that AFF proteins and ELL proteins increase the diversity and regulatory potential of the SEC family in mammals (Luo et al., 2012a). Furthermore, AFF1 and AFF4 are the backbones of the SEC (Mück et al., 2016) and ELL3 has the ability to associate with other translocation partners of the SEC (Lin et al., 2011). Thus we chose to investigate the expression of AFF1, AFF4, and ELL3 in the inner ear. Our results showed that AFF1, AFF4, and ELL3,

were all highly expressed in the cochlea and that the SEC inhibitor flavopiridol could induce the proliferation of Lgr5+ progenitors *in vitro*, but not their differentiation. This study thus provides an experimental foundation for the clinical application of HC regeneration for treating hearing loss.

The SEC is known to be widely expressed in most tissues, and it plays important roles during development (Kapushesky et al., 2010). However, its expression in the inner ear has not been studied. We found that AFF1, AFF4, and ELL3 were highly expressed in the cochlea, and this suggests that the SEC functions in the inner ear. Furthermore, we found that AFF1, AFF4, and ELL3 were all expressed in the cochlear HCs and SCs by immunostaining, but the expression of SEC proteins in SCs was lower than that in HCs. In addition to its role in Lgr5+ progenitors studied in our research, the SEC likely plays an essential role in cochlear HCs. However, due to the lack of studies of the SEC in the inner ear and the lack of mouse models, the specific role of the SEC in HCs awaits further study.

Flavopiridol, a potent inhibitor of CDK9, is reported to inhibit transcription (Blagosklonny, 2004; Lee and Zeidner, 2019). CDKs combine with cyclins to play important roles in transcription and stem cell self-renewal (Lim and Kaldis, 2013), and P-TEFb (composed of CDK9 and CycT) is an indispensable part of the SEC that phosphorylates RNA polymerase II and thus

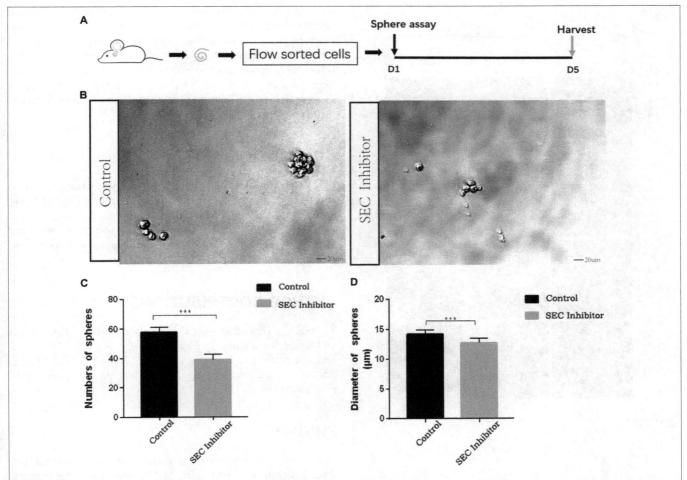

FIGURE 4 | The sphere-forming assay of Lgr5+ progenitors after inhibition of the super elongation complex (SEC). **(A)** Schematic of the sphere-forming assay. The cochleae of neonatal Lgr5-EGFP-CreER mice were trypsinized for FAC sorting, and the sorted Lgr5+ progenitors were cultured *in vitro* for 5 days to form spheres with or without 10 μM flavopiridol treatment. **(B)** The spheres (indicated by black arrows) formed by Lgr5+ progenitors with 10 μM flavopiridol added as the SEC inhibitor. DMSO was added as control treatment in the Control group. Scale bar = 20 μM. **(C,D)** Quantification of the sphere number per well **(C)** and the sphere diameter **(D)**. $n = 3$. ***$P < 0.001$.

activates transcription elongation of important genes involved in cell proliferation and survival (Zhu et al., 1997; Zeidner and Karp, 2015). Flavopiridol can inhibit the function of the SEC by inactivating CDK9 (Chao and Price, 2001), and thus we chose flavopiridol as the SEC inhibitor as previously reported (Lin et al., 2011).

In addition, our results suggest that inhibition of the SEC by flavopiridol could reduce the sphere-forming ability and proliferating cell number of Lgr5+ progenitors in the differentiation assay, which is consistent with previous reports that AFF1 promotes leukemia cell proliferation (Fioretti et al., 2019), that AFF4 enhances the sphere-forming capacity and tumor-initiation capacity in head and neck squamous cell carcinoma (Deng et al., 2018), and that ELL3 stimulates the proliferation and stem cell properties of breast cancer cells (Ahn et al., 2013).

ELL3 has also been shown to promote the differentiation of mouse embryonic stem cells by regulating the epithelial-mesenchymal transition and apoptosis (Ahn et al., 2012), and the overexpression of AFF1 impairs the differentiation of mesenchymal stem cells, while overexpression of AFF4 enhances their differentiation (Zhou et al., 2017). In our results, inhibition of the SEC did not affect the differentiation ability of Lgr5+ progenitors *in vitro*, which might be because of the different regulatory roles of these three proteins in cell differentiation.

The different roles of SEC in the proliferation and differentiation ability of Lgr5 progenitors might have been expected. SEC was first systematically studied for being associated with infant acute lymphoblastic and mixed lineage leukemia (Lin et al., 2010). Then it has since been studied in other neoplastic models (Hashizume et al., 2014; Narita et al., 2017; Liang et al., 2018). While transcriptional regulation is a complex process, it has been sure that the role of SEC is essential in transcriptional elongation. The SEC incorporates the CDK9 to promote rapid transcriptional elongation facilitates cell growth

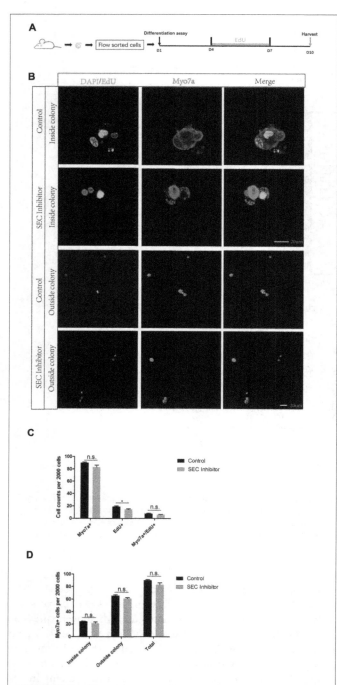

FIGURE 5 | The differentiation assay of Lgr5+ cells after inhibition of the super elongation complex (SEC). **(A)** Schematic of the differentiation assay. The cochleae of neonatal Lgr5-EGFP-CreER mice were trypsinized for FAC sorting, and the sorted Lgr5+ progenitors were cultured *in vitro* for 10 days with or without 10 μM flavopiridol. EdU was added during day 4–7 to label proliferating cells. **(B)** Immunofluorescence images of colonies and single cells formed from Lgr5+ progenitors with 10 μM flavopiridol added as the SEC inhibitor. DMSO was used as the control treatment in the Control group. Myo7a and Sox2 were used to label hair cells (HCs) and supporting cells (SCs), respectively, and EdU was used to label proliferating cells. Scale bar = 20 μM. **(C,D)** Quantification of the total numbers of Myo7a+ and EdU+ cells **(C)** and the number of Myo7a+ cells inside and outside the colonies **(D)**. *n* = 3. n.s., not significant. *P < 0.05.

(Dahl et al., 2020). However, speaking of the differentiation ability of SEC, totally different results were found concerning the different components of this complex. Our paper first studied the differentiation ability of the total complex and found that the whole SEC cannot change the differentiation in Lgr5 progenitors. There is a certain possibility that this finding may also apply to other stem cells. The detailed mechanisms behind this need further exploration.

CONCLUSION

In conclusion, we show here that the SEC is expressed in cochlear HCs and SCs in neonatal mice and that the SEC can induce the proliferation ability of Lgr5+ progenitors but not their differentiation. Our study thus provides new candidates for regulating inner ear progenitor cells as a step toward HC regeneration.

AUTHOR CONTRIBUTIONS

YC, HL, LL, SZ, and RC conceived and designed the experiments and wrote the manuscript. YC, RQ, YZ, WC, YD, LW, PJ, JA, and XM performed the experiments. YC, RQ, YZ, WC, XG, LL, SZ, and RC analyzed the data. All authors read and approved the final manuscript.

FUNDING

This work was supported by grants from the National Key R&D Program of China (No. 2017YFA0103903), the Strategic Priority Research Program of the Chinese Academy of Sciences (XDA16010303), the National Natural Science Foundation of China (Nos. 82171149, 81970882, 81970892, and 81700913), the Natural Science Foundation of Jiangsu Province (BE2019711, BE2018605, and BK20190062), the Jiangsu Provincial Medical Youth Talent of the Project of Invigorating Health Care through Science, Technology and Education (QNRC2016002), the Fundamental Research Funds for the Central Universities for the Support Program of Zhishan Youth Scholars of Southeast University (2242021R41136), and the Zhejiang Provincial Natural Science Foundation of China (LY19H130004).

REFERENCES

Ahn, H.-J., Cha, Y., Moon, S.-H., Jung, J.-E., and Park, K.-S. (2012). Ell3 enhances differentiation of mouse embryonic stem cells by regulating epithelial-mesenchymal transition and apoptosis. *PLoS One* 7:e40293. doi: 10.1371/journal.pone.0040293

Ahn, H.-J., Kim, G., and Park, K.-S. (2013). Ell3 stimulates proliferation, drug resistance, and cancer stem cell properties of breast cancer cells *via* a MEK/ERK-dependent signaling pathway. *Biochem. Biophys. Res. Commun.* 437, 557–564. doi: 10.1016/j.bbrc.2013.06.114

Barker, N., van Es, J. H., Kuipers, J., Kujala, P., van den Born, M., Cozijnsen, M., et al. (2007). Identification of stem cells in small intestine and colon by marker gene Lgr5. *Nature* 449, 1003–1007.

Blagosklonny, M. V. (2004). Flavopiridol, an inhibitor of transcription: implications, problems and solutions. *Cell Cycle* 3, 1537–1542. doi: 10.4161/cc.3.12.1278

Chai, R., Kuo, B., Wang, T., Liaw, E. J., Xia, A., Jan, T. A., et al. (2012). Wnt signaling induces proliferation of sensory precursors in the postnatal mouse cochlea. *Proc. Natl. Acad. Sci. U.S.A.* 109, 8167–8172. doi: 10.1073/pnas.1202774109

Chao, S. H., Fujinaga, K., Marion, J. E., Taube, R., Sausville, E. A., Senderowicz, A. M., et al. (2000). Flavopiridol inhibits P-TEFb and blocks HIV-1 replication. *J. Biol. Chem.* 275, 28345–28348. doi: 10.1074/jbc.C000446200

Chao, S. H., and Price, D. H. (2001). Flavopiridol inactivates P-TEFb and blocks most RNA polymerase II transcription *in vivo*. *J. Biol. Chem.* 276, 31793–31799. doi: 10.1074/jbc.M102306200

Chen, Y., Lu, X., Guo, L., Ni, W., Zhang, Y., Zhao, L., et al. (2017). Hedgehog signaling promotes the proliferation and subsequent hair cell formation of progenitor cells in the neonatal mouse cochlea. *Front. Mol. Neurosci.* 10:426. doi: 10.3389/fnmol.2017.00426

Chen, Y., Zhang, S., Chai, R., and Li, H. (2019). Hair cell regeneration. *Adv. Exper. Med. Biol.* 1130, 1–16. doi: 10.1007/978-981-13-6123-4_1

Cox, B. C., Chai, R., Lenoir, A., Liu, Z., Zhang, L., Nguyen, D.-H., et al. (2014). Spontaneous hair cell regeneration in the neonatal mouse cochlea *in vivo*. *Development* 141, 816–829. doi: 10.1242/dev.103036

Dahl, N. A., Danis, E., Balakrishnan, I., Wang, D., Pierce, A., Walker, F. M., et al. (2020). Super elongation complex as a targetable dependency in diffuse midline glioma. *Cell Rep.* 31:107485. doi: 10.1016/j.celrep.2020.03.049

Deng, P., Wang, J., Zhang, X., Wu, X., Ji, N., Li, J., et al. (2018). AFF4 promotes tumorigenesis and tumor-initiation capacity of head and neck squamous cell carcinoma cells by regulating SOX2. *Carcinogenesis* 39, 937–947. doi: 10.1093/carcin/bgy046

Fioretti, T., Cevenini, A., Zanobio, M., Raia, M., Sarnataro, D., Salvatore, F., et al. (2019). Crosstalk between 14-3-3θ and AF4 enhances MLL-AF4 activity and promotes leukemia cell proliferation. *Cell Oncol.* 42, 829–845. doi: 10.1007/s13402-019-00468-6

Gregorieff, A., Liu, Y., Inanlou, M. R., Khomchuk, Y., and Wrana, J. L. (2015). Yap-dependent reprogramming of Lgr5(+) stem cells drives intestinal regeneration and cancer. *Nature* 526, 715–718. doi: 10.1038/nature15382

Hashizume, R., Andor, N., Ihara, Y., Lerner, R., Gan, H., Chen, X., et al. (2014). Pharmacologic inhibition of histone demethylation as a therapy for pediatric brainstem glioma. *Nat. Med.* 20, 1394–1396. doi: 10.1038/nm.3716

He, N., Chan, C. K., Sobhian, B., Chou, S., Xue, Y., Liu, M., et al. (2011). Human Polymerase-Associated Factor complex (PAFc) connects the Super Elongation Complex (SEC) to RNA polymerase II on chromatin. *Proc. Natl. Acad. Sci. U.S.A.* 108, E636–E645. doi: 10.1073/pnas.1107107108

Hnisz, D., Abraham, B. J., Lee, T. I., Lau, A., Saint-André, V., Sigova, A. A., et al. (2013). Super-enhancers in the control of cell identity and disease. *Cell* 155, 934–947. doi: 10.1016/j.cell.2013.09.053

Kapushesky, M., Emam, I., Holloway, E., Kurnosov, P., Zorin, A., Malone, J., et al. (2010). Gene expression atlas at the European bioinformatics institute. *Nucleic Acids Res.* 38, D690–D698. doi: 10.1093/nar/gkp936

Korrapati, S., Roux, I., Glowatzki, E., and Doetzlhofer, A. (2013). Notch signaling limits supporting cell plasticity in the hair cell-damaged early postnatal murine cochlea. *PLoS One* 8:e73276. doi: 10.1371/journal.pone.0073276

Lee, D. J., and Zeidner, J. F. (2019). Cyclin-dependent kinase (CDK) 9 and 4/6 inhibitors in acute myeloid leukemia (AML): a promising therapeutic approach. *Expert Opin. Investig. Drugs* 28, 989–1001. doi: 10.1080/13543784.2019.1678583

Levine, M. (2011). Paused RNA polymerase II as a developmental checkpoint. *Cell* 145, 502–511. doi: 10.1016/j.cell.2011.04.021

Liang, K., Smith, E. R., Aoi, Y., Stoltz, K. L., Katagi, H., Woodfin, A. R., et al. (2018). Targeting processive transcription elongation *via* SEC disruption for MYC-induced cancer therapy. *Cell* 175, 766–779.e717. doi: 10.1016/j.cell.2018.09.027

Lim, S., and Kaldis, P. (2013). Cdks, cyclins and CKIs: roles beyond cell cycle regulation. *Development* 140, 3079–3093. doi: 10.1242/dev.091744

Lin, C., Garrett, A. S., De Kumar, B., Smith, E. R., Gogol, M., Seidel, C., et al. (2011). Dynamic transcriptional events in embryonic stem cells mediated by the super elongation complex (SEC). *Genes Dev.* 25, 1486–1498. doi: 10.1101/gad.2059211

Lin, C., Smith, E. R., Takahashi, H., Lai, K. C., Martin-Brown, S., Florens, L., et al. (2010). AFF4, a component of the ELL/P-TEFb elongation complex and a shared subunit of MLL chimeras, can link transcription elongation to leukemia. *Mol. Cell* 37, 429–437. doi: 10.1016/j.molcel.2010.01.026

Luo, Z., Lin, C., and Shilatifard, A. (2012b). The super elongation complex (SEC) family in transcriptional control. *Nat. Rev. Mol. Cell Biol.* 13, 543–547. doi: 10.1038/nrm3417

Luo, Z., Lin, C., Guest, E., Garrett, A. S., Mohaghegh, N., Swanson, S., et al. (2012a). The super elongation complex family of RNA polymerase II elongation factors: gene target specificity and transcriptional output. *Mol. Cell Biol.* 32, 2608–2617. doi: 10.1128/mcb.00182-12

Melko, M., Douguet, D., Bensaid, M., Zongaro, S., Verheggen, C., Gecz, J., et al. (2011). Functional characterization of the AFF (AF4/FMR2) family of RNA-binding proteins: insights into the molecular pathology of FRAXE intellectual disability. *Hum. Mol. Genet.* 20, 1873–1885. doi: 10.1093/hmg/ddr069

Mittal, R., Pena, S. A., Zhu, A., Eshraghi, N., Fesharaki, A., Horesh, E. J., et al. (2019). Nanoparticle-based drug delivery in the inner ear: current challenges, limitations and opportunities. *Artific. Cells Nanomed. Biotechnol.* 47, 1312–1320. doi: 10.1080/21691401.2019.1573182

Mizutari, K., Fujioka, M., Hosoya, M., Bramhall, N., Okano, H. J., Okano, H., et al. (2013). Notch inhibition induces cochlear hair cell regeneration and recovery of hearing after acoustic trauma. *Neuron* 77, 58–69. doi: 10.1016/j.neuron.2012.10.032

Morales, F., and Giordano, A. (2016). Overview of CDK9 as a target in cancer research. *Cell Cycle* 15, 519–527. doi: 10.1080/15384101.2016.1138186

Mück, F., Bracharz, S., and Marschalek, R. (2016). DDX6 transfers P-TEFb kinase to the AF4/AF4N (AFF1) super elongation complex. *Am. J. Blood Res.* 6, 28–45.

Narita, T., Ishida, T., Ito, A., Masaki, A., Kinoshita, S., Suzuki, S., et al. (2017). Cyclin-dependent kinase 9 is a novel specific molecular target in adult T-cell leukemia/lymphoma. *Blood* 130, 1114–1124. doi: 10.1182/blood-2016-09-741983

Peng, J., Zhu, Y., Milton, J. T., and Price, D. H. (1998). Identification of multiple cyclin subunits of human P-TEFb. *Genes Dev.* 12, 755–762. doi: 10.1101/gad.12.5.755

Ryan, A. F. (2003). The cell cycle and the development and regeneration of hair cells. *Curr. Top. Dev. Biol.* 57, 449–466.

Shi, F., Kempfle, J. S., and Edge, A. S. B. (2012). Wnt-responsive Lgr5-expressing stem cells are hair cell progenitors in the cochlea. *J. Neurosci.* 32, 9639–9648. doi: 10.1523/JNEUROSCI.1064-12.2012

Shilatifard, A., Conaway, R. C., and Conaway, J. W. (2003). The RNA polymerase II elongation complex. *Annu. Rev. Biochem.* 72, 693–715. doi: 10.1146/annurev.biochem.72.121801.161551

Smith, E., and Shilatifard, A. (2010). The chromatin signaling pathway: diverse mechanisms of recruitment of histone-modifying enzymes and varied biological outcomes. *Mol. Cell* 40, 689–701. doi: 10.1016/j.molcel.2010.11.031

Sun, W., Yang, S., Liu, K., and Salvi, R. J. (2017). Hearing loss and auditory plasticity. *Hear. Res.* 347, 1–2. doi: 10.1016/j.heares.2017.03.010

Warchol, M. E., Lambert, P. R., Goldstein, B. J., Forge, A., and Corwin, J. T. (1993). Regenerative proliferation in inner ear sensory epithelia from adult guinea pigs and humans. *Science* 259, 1619–1622.

Wiernik, P. H. (2016). Alvocidib (flavopiridol) for the treatment of chronic lymphocytic leukemia. *Expert Opin. Investig. Drugs* 25, 729–734. doi: 10.1517/13543784.2016.1169273

World Health Organization [WHO] (2019). *Fact Sheet. Deafness and Hearing Impairment.* Available online at http://www.who.int/mediacentre/factsheets/fs300/en/index.html (accessed March 20, 2019).

Xu, J., Ueno, H., Xu, C. Y., Chen, B., Weissman, I. L., and Xu, P.-X. (2017). Identification of mouse cochlear progenitors that develop hair and supporting cells in the organ of Corti. *Nat. Commun.* 8:15046. doi: 10.1038/ncomms 15046

Youm, I., and Li, W. (2018). Cochlear hair cell regeneration: an emerging opportunity to cure noise-induced sensorineural hearing loss. *Drug Discov. Today* 23, 1564–1569. doi: 10.1016/j.drudis.2018.05.001

Zeidner, J. F., and Karp, J. E. (2015). Clinical activity of alvocidib (flavopiridol) in acute myeloid leukemia. *Leuk. Res.* 39, 1312–1318. doi: 10.1016/j.leukres.2015. 10.010

Zhang, S., Zhang, Y., Dong, Y., Guo, L., Zhang, Z., Shao, B., et al. (2020). Knockdown of Foxg1 in supporting cells increases the trans-differentiation of supporting cells into hair cells in the neonatal mouse cochlea. *Cell Mol. Life Sci.* 77, 1401–1419. doi: 10.1007/s00018-019-03291-2

Zhou, C.-C., Xiong, Q.-C., Zhu, X.-X., Du, W., Deng, P., Li, X.-B., et al. (2017). AFF1 and AFF4 differentially regulate the osteogenic differentiation of human MSCs. *Bone Res.* 5:17044. doi: 10.1038/boneres. 2017.44

Zhu, Y., Pe'ery, T., Peng, J., Ramanathan, Y., Marshall, N., Marshall, T., et al. (1997). Transcription elongation factor P-TEFb is required for HIV-1 tat transactivation *in vitro. Genes Dev.* 11, 2622–2632. doi: 10.1101/gad.11.20.2622

15

Effects of Age, Cognition and Neural Encoding on the Perception of Temporal Speech Cues

Lindsey Roque[1], Hanin Karawani[1,2], Sandra Gordon-Salant[1] and Samira Anderson[1]*

[1] Department of Hearing and Speech Sciences, University of Maryland, College Park, College Park, MD, United States,
[2] Department of Communication Sciences and Disorders, University of Haifa, Haifa, Israel

*Correspondence:
Samira Anderson
sander22@umd.edu

Older adults commonly report difficulty understanding speech, particularly in adverse listening environments. These communication difficulties may exist in the absence of peripheral hearing loss. Older adults, both with normal hearing and with hearing loss, demonstrate temporal processing deficits that affect speech perception. The purpose of the present study is to investigate aging, cognition, and neural processing factors that may lead to deficits on perceptual tasks that rely on phoneme identification based on a temporal cue – vowel duration. A better understanding of the neural and cognitive impairments underlying temporal processing deficits could lead to more focused aural rehabilitation for improved speech understanding for older adults. This investigation was conducted in younger (YNH) and older normal-hearing (ONH) participants who completed three measures of cognitive functioning known to decline with age: working memory, processing speed, and inhibitory control. To evaluate perceptual and neural processing of auditory temporal contrasts, identification functions for the contrasting word-pair WHEAT and WEED were obtained on a nine-step continuum of vowel duration, and frequency-following responses (FFRs) and cortical auditory-evoked potentials (CAEPs) were recorded to the two endpoints of the continuum. Multiple linear regression analyses were conducted to determine the cognitive, peripheral, and/or central mechanisms that may contribute to perceptual performance. YNH participants demonstrated higher cognitive functioning on all three measures compared to ONH participants. The slope of the identification function was steeper in YNH than in ONH participants, suggesting a clearer distinction between the contrasting words in the YNH participants. FFRs revealed better response waveform morphology and more robust phase-locking in YNH compared to ONH participants. ONH participants also exhibited earlier latencies for CAEP components compared to the YNH participants. Linear regression analyses revealed that cortical processing significantly contributed to the variance in perceptual performance in the WHEAT/WEED identification functions. These results suggest that reduced neural precision contributes to age-related speech perception difficulties that arise from temporal processing deficits.

Keywords: aging, temporal processing, speech perception, cognition, frequency-following response, cortical auditory-evoked potentials

INTRODUCTION

Older adults often report difficulty understanding speech, particularly in adverse listening environments (CHABA, 1988). Such difficulty could be attributed to numerous listener factors associated with the natural aging process, including age-related hearing loss (Dubno et al., 1984; Helfer and Wilber, 1990), cognitive decline (McClearn et al., 1997; Lin, 2011; Lin et al., 2013) and reduced auditory temporal processing (Schneider et al., 1994; Pichora-Fuller and Singh, 2006). Previous studies have focused on peripheral hearing loss, and ensuing loss of frequency selectivity (Florentine et al., 1980), as a primary mechanism for older adults' speech understanding difficulties (Dubno et al., 1984; Koeritzer et al., 2018). Older adults with normal hearing, however, report similar difficulties understanding speech that may be attributed to temporal processing deficits as well as spectral deficits (Matschke, 1990). Füllgrabe et al. (2015) investigated the interplay and relative contributions of aging, cognition, and temporal processing on speech processing in younger and older normal-hearing (ONH) adults and found that sensitivity to temporal cues and cognitive ability were related to speech-in-noise identification scores. The present study aims to expand their research by including neural processing measures in a model that compares peripheral, central (midbrain and cortical processing) and cognitive contributions to perceptual performance on a perceptual task that relies on phoneme identification based on a temporal cue. In the following paragraphs, a brief overview of the role of cognition, temporal processing, and central processing in age-related speech perception deficits will be provided.

Aging affects multiple cognitive processes important for speech understanding, including working memory, processing speed and inhibitory control, which may contribute to reductions in speech understanding in older adults (Burke, 1997; Hedden and Gabrieli, 2004). Working memory is a higher-level cognitive process involving the temporary storage and processing of a limited amount of information, which is then either discarded or converted to long-term memory (Lunner, 2003; Lunner and Sundewall-Thoren, 2007). Individuals with limited working memory capacity have reduced speech recognition performance, possibly due to reduced ability to "fill in gaps" when parts of speech are inaudible or misunderstood (Lunner and Sundewall-Thoren, 2007; Gordon-Salant and Cole, 2016; Johns et al., 2018). Like working memory, reductions in speed of information processing may hinder speech perception, especially for artificially speeded (i.e., time-compressed) speech (Wingfield, 1996; Gordon-Salant and Fitzgibbons, 2001). Accuracy of speech recognition, especially in noise, is influenced by working memory capacity whereas speed of recognition is influenced by processing speed (Daneman and Hannon, 2007; Ronnberg et al., 2008, 2013; Genova et al., 2012). Inhibitory control is an individual's ability to disregard irrelevant stimuli in the presence of relevant incoming stimuli (Pichora-Fuller and Singh, 2006). Older adults also experience greater difficulty understanding words while simultaneously ignoring irrelevant or asynchronous stimuli presented through both auditory and visual media, thus demonstrating reduced inhibitory control compared to young adults (Dey and Sommers, 2015; Cohen and Gordon-Salant, 2017; Gordon-Salant et al., 2017). It is theorized that processing a degraded acoustic signal (as would occur with reduced audibility and/or imprecise auditory temporal processing) forces older adults to rely on cognition for speech understanding (Pichora-Fuller et al., 1995; Wingfield and Grossman, 2006). If so, an interplay between older adults' degraded auditory temporal processing and cognitive decline may exist and further exacerbate their speech perception difficulties.

Age-related degradation in auditory temporal processing may also contribute to older adults' difficulty understanding speech. Speech signals in everyday listening situations (i.e., rapid speech, reverberant environments, noisy environments) are characterized by temporal alterations relative to "clean" speech (Gordon-Salant and Fitzgibbons, 1993; Gordon-Salant et al., 2010). For example, older adults seem to use temporal cues less effectively than do young adults in distinguishing between contrasting word-pairs that differ on the basis of duration cues. Older adults require longer intervals of silence preceding the final fricative to differentiate DISH from DITCH compared to younger adults (Gordon-Salant et al., 2006; Roque et al., 2019). Poorer duration discrimination in older versus younger adults has been demonstrated for relatively simple stimuli (i.e., tone bursts) and more complex signals (i.e., silent gaps embedded in tonal sequences) (Fitzgibbons and Gordon-Salant, 1995). This poorer performance in older adults may arise from reduced temporal precision secondary to physiological changes throughout the central auditory system, even in the presence of normal audiometric thresholds (Anderson et al., 2012; Presacco et al., 2016).

Electrophysiological measurements of auditory brainstem and cortex can be used to examine the neurophysiological mechanisms underlying age-related reductions in auditory temporal processing as manifest on behavioral tasks. The frequency-following response (FFR) is a measure that primarily arises from the inferior colliculus (IC) for stimulus frequencies greater than 100 Hz and reflects the temporal and spectral characteristics of a presented stimulus (Moushegian et al., 1973; Smith et al., 1975; Bidelman, 2018). Because the FFR provides an indirect measure of neural response fidelity of the IC, it may provide a non-invasive means of revealing aging deficits that have previously been demonstrated in single-neuron studies in the IC. For example, using an aging-mouse model, Walton et al. (1998) found that older mice had fewer IC neurons that fired in response to short-duration gaps than did younger mice. In humans, the FFR has previously revealed reduced neural synchronization to speech and non-speech stimuli in older compared to younger adults, which may lead to disruptions in phase locking to presented auditory stimuli (Clinard et al., 2010; Presacco et al., 2016; Roque et al., 2019). Previous electrophysiological studies have demonstrated that older adults exhibit decreased encoding of sustained components of presented stimuli compared to dynamic components. For example, Presacco et al. (2015) recorded FFRs to 170-ms speech syllables /da/ and /a/

and observed that neural firing in response to the /a/ syllable (as represented by response amplitude) significantly decreased after approximately 110 ms in older adults, but this drop in amplitude was not observed in younger adults. Interestingly, no such difference was noted for the /da/ syllable, which contained a 60-ms transition. This inability of older adults to sustain neural firing suggests that reduced neural synchrony secondary to loss of auditory nerve fibers may contribute to age-related response decay (Schmiedt et al., 1996; Walton et al., 1998; Presacco et al., 2015). Presacco et al. (2015) recorded responses to synthesized stimuli; the present study will expand on the original study to determine if response decay is present in older adults for vowels in naturally produced words.

Cortical auditory-evoked potentials (CAEPs) can be used to examine age-related reductions in neural synchronization at the level of apical dendrites of pyramidal neurons located within auditory cortex (Tan et al., 2004; Kerr et al., 2008). Diminished efficiency of post-synaptic GABA neurotransmission in the ascending auditory pathway may contribute to age-related reductions in inhibitory neurotransmission in primary auditory cortex (Caspary et al., 2008). Reduced inhibitory neurotransmission may impede older individuals' auditory temporal processing, as observed in delayed cortical firing and CAEP latencies in older rats compared to younger rats (Juarez-Salinas et al., 2010). These age-related delays in cortical peak latencies have also been observed in human models (Tremblay et al., 2003; Maamor and Billings, 2017; Roque et al., 2019). The stimulus-locked activity recorded in the CAEP may consequently provide insight as to the cortical mechanisms underlying the timing and efficiency of speech processing.

The purpose of the present study is to investigate the interacting effects of aging, cognition, and neural encoding on the ability to identify phonemes based on vowel duration. To accomplish this objective, the same stimuli were used for both behavioral measures and FFR and CAEP electrophysiological measures. It was hypothesized that age-related temporal processing deficits, particularly a loss of neural synchrony to a sustained vowel, would hinder older adults' ability to discriminate between the contrasting word pair WHEAT and WEED. Specifically, it was posited that (1) reduced temporal precision would be reflected in older adults' reduced phase locking and poorer morphology in the FFR to a sustained vowel and in their prolonged peak latencies in the CAEP, relative to those of younger adults, (2) that cognitive performance, specifically processing speed, would correlate with precision of neural encoding and behavioral performance, and (3) that neural encoding, working memory, speed of information processing, and/or inhibitory control would contribute to the variance in speech perception based on a vowel duration contrast. A better understanding of the neural deficits underlying older adults' perception of temporal speech cues could lead to more focused aural rehabilitation for improved speech understanding and increased socialization among the aging population, including those with normal peripheral hearing.

MATERIALS AND METHODS

Participants

Participants comprised younger normal-hearing (YNH, $n = 30$, 22 Females, 18–24 years, mean age and standard deviation 21.01 ± 1.55) and ONH ($n = 30$, 22 Females, 55–76 years, mean age and standard deviation 63.78 ± 5.12) adults. Clinically normal hearing was defined as pure-tone thresholds ≤20 dB HL at octave frequencies from 125 to 4000 Hz and ≤30 dB HL at 6000 and 8000 Hz bilaterally, with no interaural asymmetries ≥15 dB HL at more than two adjacent frequencies (see **Figure 1**). Participants were screened with two cognitive measures: the Montreal Cognitive Assessment (MoCA; Nasreddine et al., 2005) and the Wechsler Abbreviated Scale of Intelligence (WASI; Zhu and Garcia, 1999). The screening criteria were scores ≥26 on the MoCA and IQs ≥85 on the WASI. MoCA mean scores and standard deviations were 27.83 ± 1.42 and 27.90 ± 1.40 for YNH and ONH participants, respectively. YNH and ONH participants obtained mean WASI scores and standard deviations of 108.90 ± 10.68 and 107.20 ± 15.70, respectively. There was no significant effect of age on MoCA score [$t_{(58)} = 0.18$, $p = 0.86$] or WASI score [$t_{(58)} = 0.49$, $p = 0.63$]. Inclusion criteria also included normal auditory brainstem response (ABR) wave V absolute latencies (≤6.8 ms) to click stimuli and no interaural asymmetry exceeding 0.2 ms. Participants with a history of neurological dysfunction or middle ear surgery were excluded from the study. All participants were monolingual, native English speakers recruited from the Maryland, Virginia, and Washington, DC areas. All procedures were reviewed and approved by the Institutional Review Board (IRB) at the University of Maryland, College Park. Participants provided informed consent and were compensated for their time.

Stimuli

Test stimuli comprised the contrasting word pair WHEAT (249 ms) and WEED (311 ms) that were first described in Gordon-Salant et al. (2006). This word-pair contrast depends on the single acoustic cue of vowel duration preceding the final plosive, ranging from 93 ms (WHEAT) to 155 ms (WEED). A continuum of vowel duration was created from isolated recordings of the two natural words produced by an adult American male. The endpoint stimulus perceived as WEED was a hybrid in which the final plosive /d/ was excised and replaced with a high-amplitude release from the final burst in the naturally produced WHEAT token. The continuum of vowel duration was subsequently created by removing 7–8 ms intervals of the steady-state vocalic region of WEED until it was 93 ms (the WHEAT endpoint). All stimuli were low-pass filtered at 4000 Hz at 12 dB/octave, to minimize the possible effects of high-frequency hearing threshold differences. For the perceptual identification functions, participants were presented with all nine tokens of the WHEAT/WEED continuum of vowel duration preceding the final plosive, ranging from 93 ms (WHEAT) to 155 ms (WEED). For the electrophysiology recordings, only the two endpoints of the WHEAT/WEED continuum were presented.

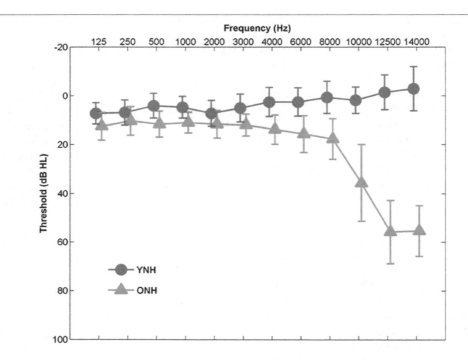

FIGURE 1 | Mean audiometric thresholds of younger normal-hearing (YNH, blue) and older normal-hearing (ONH, red) participants from 125 Hz to 14,000 Hz. Clinically normal hearing was defined as pure-tone thresholds ≤20 dB HL at octave frequencies from 125 to 4000 Hz and ≤30 dB HL from 6000 to 8000 Hz. Error bars: ± 1 standard deviation.

Procedures
Cognitive
Cognition was assessed using the National Institutes of Health (NIH) Toolbox Cognition Test Battery[1], which comprised the following: List Sorting Working Memory Test, Pattern Comparison Processing Speed Test, and Flanker Inhibitory Control and Attention Test. All three measures were administered on an iPad tablet. An experimenter assisted the participants in completing demographic questions asked on the iPad prior to testing.

List sorting working memory test
The List Sorting Test comprises a sequencing task in which a series of animals and/or foods were presented auditorily in the sound field and visually on the iPad screen. The participant then sorted the presented stimuli in a series and sequenced them in size order from smallest to largest (Tulsky et al., 2014). With each correct response, an additional item was added to the series, with a maximum of seven items in a series. With an incorrect response, the participant was given a second trial with a series of equal length. Testing was discontinued when the participant accurately responded to all the series or when the participant answered incorrectly during two consecutive trials. Each participant completed two versions of the test: the "1-list" version contained only names of animals, while the "2-list" version contained the names of both animals and foods. During the "2-list" version, the participant categorized the stimuli

in the series before sequencing them in size order. Responses were scored for total correct responses across the two versions (Tulsky et al., 2014).

Pattern comparison processing speed test
The Pattern Comparison Test is a timed task in which participants were visually presented with two images on the tablet screen and indicated whether the images were identical or not. The two images may differ in type, complexity, or number of stimuli (Weintraub et al., 2013). Responses were scored for number of correct responses completed in 90 s (Carlozzi et al., 2015).

Flanker inhibitory control and attention test
During the Flanker Test, the participant was visually presented with a row of arrows, with a target arrow located in the center of the row. The participant then identified the left or right orientation of the centrally located arrow while ignoring the surrounding arrows, which may be congruous or incongruous in their orientation. Participants completed 25 trials. Accuracy and response time to target arrows surrounded by incongruent arrows were recorded as measures of inhibitory control and executive attention (Zelazo et al., 2014).

Perceptual
Participants completed an identification task similar to that implemented in Gordon-Salant et al. (2006) using the entire WHEAT/WEED continuum. The experiment was controlled and responses recorded using MATLAB (MathWorks, version 2012a). During testing, participants were seated at a desktop

---

[1]www.nihtoolbox.org

computer in a sound-attenuated booth. Three boxes were displayed on the computer monitor: one that read "Begin Trial" and two boxes below that read "WHEAT" and "WEED." Participants initiated each trial by clicking the "Begin Trial" box, so testing was self-paced. Stimuli were presented monaurally to the right ear via an ER-2 insert earphone (Etymotic Research, Elk Grove Village, IL, United States) at 75 dB SPL. Following each stimulus presentation, participants indicated whether the stimulus was perceived as WHEAT or WEED by clicking on the corresponding box on the monitor. Prior to testing, participants completed a training run using only the endpoints of the WHEAT/WEED continuum and were provided feedback following each trial. Once participants achieved 90% accuracy during the training run, they completed five experimental runs, during which feedback was not be provided. Stimuli along the WHEAT/WEED continuum were each presented in quiet a total of ten times during the experimental run.

Electrophysiology (EEG)

EEG recordings took place during two test sessions: FFRs were recorded during one session, and ABR and CAEP recordings occurred during the other. During the recordings, participants were seated in a reclining chair in an electrically shielded, sound-attenuated booth and watched a silent, closed-captioned movie of their choice to facilitate a relaxed but wakeful state.

ABR

Auditory brainstem response testing to 100-μs click stimuli was performed on all participants using the Intelligent Hearing Systems Smart EP system (Intelligent Hearing Systems, Miami, FL, United States) to verify neural integrity and to provide a measure of peripheral hearing status. Clicks were presented monaurally to each ear via ER-3A insert earphone (Intelligent Hearing Systems, Miami, FL, United States) at 80 dB SPL, using a two-channel, four-electrode (Cz active, one forehead ground electrode, two earlobe reference electrodes) vertical montage. Two sets of 2000 sweeps were obtained at a presentation rate of 21.1 Hz for each ear.

FFR

Frequency-following responses were recorded to the two extrema of the WHEAT-WEED continuum using the Biosemi ActiABR-200 acquisition system (Biosemi B.V., Netherlands). The WHEAT and WEED stimulus waveforms were presented monaurally to the right ear via Presentation software through an ER-1 insert earphone (Etymotic Research, Elk Grove Village, IL, United States) at 75 dB SPL using alternating polarities. FFRs were recorded with a five-electrode vertical montage (Cz active, two forehead offset CMS/DRL electrodes, two earlobe reference electrodes) at a sampling rate of 16,384 Hz. A minimum of 3000 artifact-free sweeps were obtained from each participant at a rate of 2.06 Hz for WHEAT and 1.83 Hz for WEED.

CAEP

Cortical auditory-evoked potentials were also recorded to the two endpoints of the WHEAT-WEED continuum presented at 75 dB SPL at a rate of 0.83 Hz, with an interstimulus interval (ISI) of 0.96 s. The Biosemi Active Two system was used to record responses at a sampling rate of 2,048 Hz via a 32-channel electrode cap with earlobe electrodes (A1 and A2) serving as references. A minimum of 500 artifact-free sweeps were obtained for each stimulus from each participant.

Data Analysis
Cognitive

In the NIH Toolbox application, standard scores were obtained for each of the three subtests for each participant based on normative data, as described in Carlozzi et al. (2015). For each cognitive measure (working memory, processing speed, and inhibitory control), individual raw scores were ranked to create scaled scores. A normative transformation was then applied to the ranks to derive a standard normal distribution, which was then rescaled to have a mean of 100 and a standard deviation of 15. The individual scaled scores were averaged and subsequently re-normalized.

Perceptual

Identification functions were computed for each individual participant by calculating the percent identification of WHEAT responses for each step along the continuum. From each identification function, the 50% crossover point was obtained to indicate the boundary of stimulus categorization. Slope of the linear portion was also calculated to represent participant distinction between the contrasting speech tokens. The 50% perceptual crossover point was obtained from each identification function using the Wichmann and Hill (2001a,b) fitting procedure and the PSIGNIFIT software[2]. Slope values were not obtained using the PSIGNIFIT software, as it takes into account the entire identification function, and performance was equivalent between groups at the extrema of the WHEAT-WEED continuum. Slope was subsequently calculated by performing linear regression analysis on the linear portion of each identification function, which approximately fell between 20 and 80% identification of WHEAT.

Electrophysiology (EEG)
ABR

ABR data were offline bandpass filtered from 70–2000 Hz using a zero-phase, 6th order Butterworth filter. An average was taken of the total 4,000 sweeps collected for each ear. In MATLAB, an automated peak-picking algorithm identified latencies and amplitudes for Waves I, III, and V within 0.5 ms of expected peak latencies, which were based on average values obtained in Anderson et al. (2012). Peak identification was confirmed by a trained peak picker who made changes where appropriate. Wave I amplitude was calculated from each participant's average click response to verify neural integrity and serve as a peripheral measure of auditory processing. A derived horizontal montage was used to maximize Wave I amplitude. It was observed that Wave I amplitude was not normally distributed, so a square-root transformation was applied to the data. This transformed Wave I amplitude was used in subsequent statistical analyses.

---

[2]https://sourceforge.net/projects/psignifit/

FFR data reduction

Recorded data were analyzed in MATLAB (MathWorks, version R2011b) after being converted into MATLAB format using the pop_biosig function from EEGLAB (Delorme and Makeig, 2004). Sweeps with amplitude in the ± 30 μV range were retained. Accepted sweeps were offline bandpass filtered from 70 to 2000 Hz using a zero-phase, 4th order Butterworth filter and averaged over a 660-ms time window in MATLAB. To maximize the response of the temporal envelope, a final average response was created by averaging sweeps of both polarities.

Stimulus-to-response (STR) correlation

STR examines the fidelity of participants' response waveforms in approximating the stimulus waveforms and can be considered as a means to quantify response morphology. Stimulus envelopes were extracted and bandpass filtered with the same filter used for the response envelopes. STR r values were obtained in MATLAB by shifting stimulus waveforms in time relative to response waveforms until reaching a maximum correlation from 10–300 ms.

Phase locking factor (PLF)

PLF was calculated to assess each individual participant's phase tracking to the stimulus temporal envelope. PLF was obtained using an identical procedure to that implemented in previous studies (Jenkins et al., 2018; Roque et al., 2019). To calculate PLF values, Morlet wavelets (Tallon-Baudry et al., 1996) were used to decompose the signal from 80 to 800 Hz. Individual PLF values were calculated for the fundamental frequency (F_0) of the stimulus vowel /i/ (138 Hz) and averaged for each participant group. PLF values were calculated for the early (60–120 ms for both speech tokens) and late vowel regions (140–200 ms for WHEAT and 200–260 ms for WEED) to examine each participant's ability to initiate and sustain neural firing, respectively.

CAEP

Accepted sweeps were offline bandpass filtered from 1 to 30 Hz using a zero-phase, 4th order Butterworth filter. Eye movements were removed from the filtered data using a regression-based electrooculography reduction method (Romero et al., 2006; Schlögl et al., 2007). A 500 to 1000-ms time window was referenced to the stimulus onset for each sweep. A final response was averaged from the first 500 artifact-free sweeps. The denoising source separation (DSS) algorithm was used to remove noise/artifact from all 32 recorded channels (Särelä and Valpola, 2005; Cheveigné and Simon, 2008; Bellier et al., 2015), and to provide a measure of overall activity that is not biased toward activity from one electrode. Amplitude and latency were calculated for each prominent component of the P1-N1-P2 complex obtained from the DSS algorithm for each participant. A MATLAB automated peak-peaking algorithm was used to identify the latencies for P1, N1, and P2 in their expected time regions and to calculate area amplitudes under the curve that correspond to the designated time regions. The expected time regions were as follows: P1 (40–90 ms), N1 (90–140 ms), and P2 (140–240 ms). These expected latency regions were determined based on the average waveform for the Cz electrode, obtained for all participants.

Statistical Analysis

All statistics were conducted in SPSS version 23.0. Independent-samples t tests were performed for group comparisons on ABR Wave I amplitude, perceptual 50% crossover points, slope of the identification functions, and the NIH Toolbox Cognition Test Battery measures. Repeated-measures analyses of variance (RMANOVAs) were performed to examine between-subject effects of group (YNH vs. ONH) and within-subject effects of stimulus (WHEAT vs. WEED) on FFR variables (STR, early PLF, and late PLF) and CAEP variables (peak latency and amplitude). Within-subject effects of vowel region (early vs. late) were also examined on FFR PLF variables. Independent-samples t tests and paired-samples t tests were used to perform *post hoc* analyses when significant interactions were observed. Pearson's correlations were performed to examine relationships among cognitive, perceptual, FFR, and CAEP measures. Linear regression analyses were performed with slope of the identification functions entered as the dependent variable. Independent variables were chosen to represent different levels of the auditory system, including contributions from peripheral (Wave I amplitude), midbrain (WEED STR), and cortical variables (WEED P1 Latency). STR was chosen to represent midbrain contributions instead of PLF because a greater effect size for group differences was demonstrated for STR. We chose WEED instead of WHEAT because we expected that aging effects would be more pronounced for a longer duration vowel (Presacco et al., 2015). Cognitive variables (working memory, processing speed, and inhibitory control) were also included as independent variables. The "Stepwise" method of hierarchical regression, an automatic procedure for selecting statistical models, was performed to avoid the bias of order entry present for other methods of linear regression (i.e., hierarchical). Residuals for normality were examined to ensure that linear regression analysis was appropriate for the data. Collinearity diagnostics were completed with satisfactory variance inflation factor (highest = 1.20) and tolerance (lowest = 0.84) scores, ruling out strong correlations between predictor variables.

RESULTS

Cognitive

Figure 2 displays mean scores and standard deviations obtained for each participant group on the three subtests of the NIH Toolbox Cognition Test Battery. We noted that 9 of 30 YNH participants demonstrated standard scores greater than two standard deviations above the mean and removed their processing speed ($n = 8$) and inhibitory control scores ($n = 1$) from group comparison and linear regression analyses. Additionally, processing speed scores for 2 of the 30 ONH participants who exhibited standard scores greater than two standard deviations below the mean were similarly excluded from further analyses. A significant effect of group was observed on working memory [$t_{(58)} = 3.99$, $p < 0.01$], processing speed,

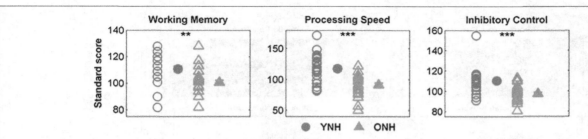

FIGURE 2 | Individual and mean standard scores for younger normal-hearing (YNH, blue) and older normal-hearing (ONH, red) participants on the List Sorting Working Memory Test, Pattern Comparison Processing Speed Test, and Flanker Inhibitory Control Test. YNH participants had higher scores than ONH participants on all three subtests of the NIH Toolbox Cognition Test Battery. Error bars: ± 1 standard error. **$p < 0.01$, ***$p < 0.001$.

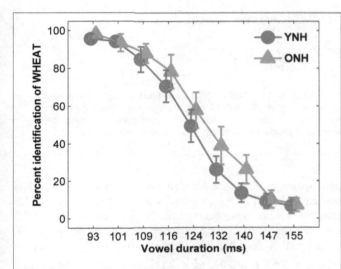

FIGURE 3 | Average identification functions for percentage of trials identified as WHEAT as a function of vowel duration for each participant group. Younger normal-hearing (YNH, red) participants exhibited sharper slopes for the identification functions than did older normal-hearing (ONH, blue) participants, indicating a clearer distinction between WHEAT and WEED. Error bars: ± 1 standard error.

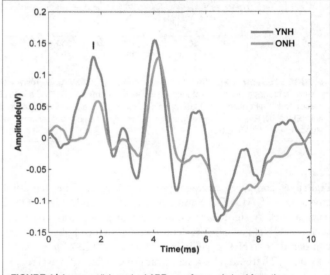

FIGURE 4 | Average click-evoked ABR waveforms, derived from the horizontal electrode montage, for YNH (blue), and ONH (red) participants.

$[t_{(48)} = 3.56, p < 0.01]$ and inhibitory control $[t_{(57)} = 5.86, p < 0.001]$. For each subtest, YNH participants demonstrated higher standard scores compared to ONH participants.

Perceptual

The average identification functions for YNH and ONH participants are displayed in **Figure 3**. An effect of group was observed for slope of the identification function $[t_{(58)} = 2.49, p = 0.02]$ but not for 50% crossover point $[t_{(58)} = 1.72, p = 0.09]$. YNH participants demonstrated steeper slopes compared to ONH participants, indicating clearer distinction between WHEAT and WEED.

Electrophysiology (EEG)
ABR

Figure 4 displays the average click-evoked ABR waveform derived from the horizontal electrode montage for each participant group. Average Wave I amplitude values were 0.38

and 0.25 μV for YNH and ONH participants, respectively. YNH participants demonstrated significantly higher Wave I amplitudes compared to ONH participants $[t_{(58)} = 5.66, p < 0.001]$.

FFR
STR

Figure 5 compares average YNH and ONH response waveforms (panel C) to stimulus spectra (panel A), and waveforms (panel B). Individual and average STR r values to WHEAT and WEED are displayed in panels D and E, respectively. There were significant main effects of group $[F_{(1,58)} = 16.42, p < 0.001, \eta_p^2 = 0.22]$ and stimulus on STR $[F_{(1,58)} = 6.19, p = 0.02, \eta_p^2 = 0.01]$, as well as a significant group × stimulus interaction $[F_{(1,58)} = 4.74, p = 0.03, \eta_p^2 = 0.08]$. YNH response waveforms better mirrored the WEED stimulus waveform than did ONH response waveforms $[t_{(58)} = 4.18, p < 0.001]$. However, no group difference was observed for the WHEAT stimulus waveform $[t_{(58)} = 1.44, p = 0.16]$. STR r values were higher for WEED than for WHEAT in the YNH participants $[t_{(29)} = 2.68, p = 0.01]$ but not in the ONH participants $[t_{(29)} = 0.32, p = 0.76]$.

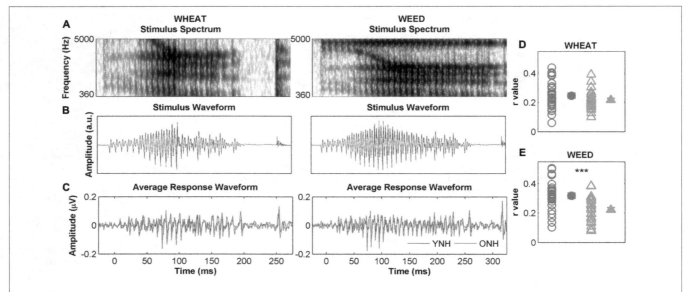

FIGURE 5 | Left panel: Spectra **(A)** and waveforms **(B)** for WHEAT (93-ms vowel duration; left column), and WEED (155-ms vowel duration; right column) speech tokens. Average response waveforms **(C)** in the time domain to WHEAT and WEED for younger normal-hearing (YNH, blue) and older normal-hearing (ONH, red) participants. Right panel: Individual (open symbol) and average (closed symbol) stimulus-to-response correlation *r* values for each participant group to **(D)** WHEAT and **(E)** WEED. Response waveforms of YNH participants more closely mirrored the stimulus waveforms than did those of ONH participants. Error bars: ± 1 standard error. ***$p < 0.001$.

PLF

Figure 6 compares average phase locking to the temporal envelopes of WHEAT and WEED for YNH and ONH participants. A significant main effect of group was observed, such that ONH participants demonstrated reduced phase locking compared to YNH participants [$F_{(1,58)} = 11.87$, $p = 0.001$, $\eta_p^2 = 0.17$]. There was also a significant main effect of vowel region (early vs. late) [$F_{(1,58)} = 15.64$, $p < 0.001$, $\eta_p^2 = 0.21$]. For both participant groups, phase locking declined from the early vowel region to the late vowel region. A significant stimulus × region interaction was observed [$F_{(1,58)} = 4.54$, $p = 0.04$, $\eta_p^2 = 0.07$], such that the decline in phase locking from the early to late vowel region was more pronounced to WEED than to WHEAT. No other significant main effects or interactions were noted.

CAEP

An omnibus RMANOVA was conducted to compare differences between YNH and ONH groups for the three cortical peak (P1, N1, P2) amplitudes and latencies across both stimuli (WHEAT vs. WEED).

Latency

Figure 7 displays average CAEP response waveforms obtained from the DSS analysis, as well as individual and average peak amplitudes and latencies for YNH and ONH participants. There was a significant main effect of group on CAEP peak latency [$F_{(1,58)} = 8.06$, $p < 0.01$, $\eta_p^2 = 0.12$] and a significant peak × group interaction [$F_{(2,57)} = 5.08$, $p = 0.01$, $\eta_p^2 = 0.16$]. RMANOVA models (within-group variable: stimulus, between-group variable: age group) were subsequently performed to examine differences for each peak individually. The ONH

participants exhibited earlier peak latencies compared to YNH participants for P1 [$F_{(1,58)} = 33.23$, $p < 0.001$, $\eta_p^2 = 0.36$]. No group difference was observed for N1 latency [$F_{(1,58)} = 0.12$, $p = 0.73$, $\eta_p^2 < 0.01$] or P2 latency [$F_{(1,58)} = 1.40$, $p = 0.24$, $\eta_p^2 = 0.02$]. A stimulus × peak interaction was also observed [$F_{(2,57)} = 3.63$, $p = 0.03$, $\eta_p^2 = 0.11$], such that P1 was earlier for WHEAT than for WEED [$t_{(59)} = 2.20$, $p = 0.03$]. No other significant interactions were observed [all *p* values > 0.05].

Amplitude

No significant effects of group [$F_{(1,58)} = 2.46$, $p = 0.12$, $\eta_p^2 = 0.04$] or stimulus [$F_{(1,58)} = 3.58$, $p = 0.06$, $\eta_p^2 = 0.06$] were observed on CAEP peak amplitudes. However, there was a peak × group interaction [$F_{(2,57)} = 6.21$, $p = 0.004$, $\eta_p^2 = 0.18$], and ANOVA models were subsequently performed for each peak individually. ONH participants exhibited larger P1 amplitudes than YNH participants [$F_{(1,58)} = 5.35$, $p = 0.02$, $\eta_p^2 = 0.08$]. No effect of group was observed for N1 or P2 amplitude to either stimulus [all *p* values > 0.05].

Multiple Linear Regression

Results of the multiple linear regression analyses indicated that cortical factors predicted variance in slope of the identification functions. **Table 1** displays Pearson's correlation coefficients (*r*) among the predictor variables entered in the linear regression analyses. **Table 2** displays the standardized coefficients and levels of significance for the independent variables for the one model created during the Stepwise linear regression analysis. Slope of the perceptual identification functions correlated with WEED P1 Latency [$r = -0.39$, $p < 0.01$]. All three cognitive measures significantly correlated with one another [all *p* values < 0.05],

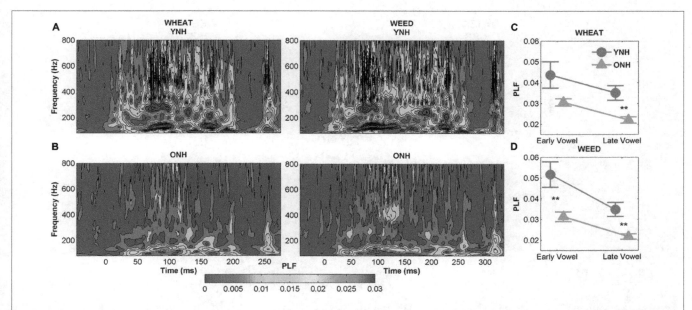

FIGURE 6 | Average phase-locking factor (PLF) to the temporal envelope of WHEAT (left column) and WEED (right column) stimuli represented in the time-frequency domain, with hotter (red) colors indicating increased phase locking in younger normal-hearing (YNH) **(A)** and older normal-hearing (ONH) **(B)** participants. Right panel: Average PLF values to the 138-Hz fundamental frequency in the early and late time regions corresponding to the vowel /i/ of WHEAT **(C)** and WEED **(D)**. ONH participants demonstrated reduced phase locking compared to YNH participants. For both participant groups, phase locking declined from the early vowel region to the late vowel region to both stimuli. Error bars: ± 1 standard error. **p < 0.01.

with the exception of working memory and processing speed, which did not correlate [$p = 0.32$]. Wave I amplitude significantly correlated with all other variables entered into the correlation matrix [all p values < 0.01], except for WEED STR [$p = 0.06$] and processing speed [$p = 0.45$]. During the linear regression analysis, predictor variables sampled were Wave I amplitude, WEED STR, WEED P1 Latency, working memory, processing speed, and inhibitory control. These predictor variables were chosen due to observed group differences and to represent potential peripheral, central, and cognitive contributions. In the final model only WEED P1 Latency significantly contributed to variance in slope. This model was a good fit for the data [$F_{(1, 48)} = 8.22$, $p < 0.01$], with an R^2 value of 0.15.

DISCUSSION

The purpose of the current study was to investigate the interplay between cognition, perception, and neural processing of temporal speech cues to gain a better understanding of the communication difficulties often experienced by older adults with normal hearing. To accomplish this objective, we investigated the effects of age on neural temporal encoding underlying phoneme identification based on vowel duration, as well as possible cognitive contributions to variability in perceptual performance on a phoneme identification task. The data support some, but not all, of our initial hypotheses. As expected, younger adults exhibited higher cognitive functioning in the domains of working memory, speed of information processing, and inhibitory control relative to older adults. Younger adults also demonstrated sharper slopes for the perceptual identification functions than did

older adults, suggesting a clearer distinction between WHEAT and WEED. Electrophysiological measurements revealed age-related deficits in neural encoding of the extrema of the WHEAT/WEED continuum of vowel duration at both the level of the auditory brainstem and cortex. FFRs revealed poorer morphology (reduced STR correlations) and reduced phase locking to the stimulus temporal envelopes (lower PLF values) in older adults compared to younger adults. In contrast to our initial hypothesis, CAEPs revealed earlier P1 latencies for older adults than for younger adults. Additionally, linear regression analyses revealed that only cortical factors significantly contributed to variance in slope of the perceptual identification functions.

Cognitive Functioning

Consistent with previous studies, older adults demonstrated decreased cognitive functioning in the domains of working memory (Salthouse and Babcock, 1991), processing speed (Salthouse, 1996), and inhibitory control (Salthouse, 2010). For individuals above 20 years of age, validity studies of the NIH Toolbox Cognition Battery have found significant negative correlations between age and performance on the List Sorting Working Memory Test, Pattern Comparison Processing Speed Test, and Flanker Inhibitory Control and Attention Test (Weintraub et al., 2013).

Perceptual

Although the procedure for the perceptual identification task stemmed from that implemented in Gordon-Salant et al. (2006), different patterns of results were observed

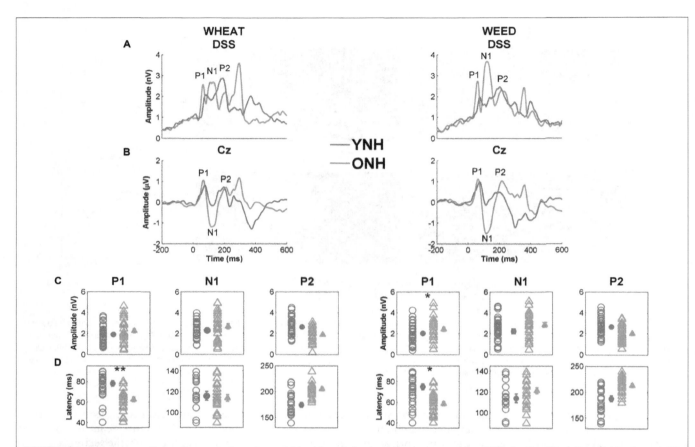

FIGURE 7 | Grand average cortical auditory-evoked waveforms obtained through the denoising source separation (DSS) algorithm **(A)** and from the Cz electrode **(B)** for younger normal-hearing (YNH, blue) and older normal-hearing (ONH, red) participants. Note that the time regions for latency and amplitude analyses were based on the Cz electrode waveforms. The waveforms with Individual (open symbol) and average (closed symbol) amplitudes **(C)** and latencies **(D)** for prominent cortical peaks to WHEAT (left column) and WEED (right column) obtained from the DSS algorithm. P1 latencies were earlier in the ONH compared to YNH participants for both stimuli. Error bars: ± 1 standard error. *$p < 0.05$, **$p < 0.01$.

TABLE 1 | Intercorrelations among slope and the independent peripheral, central, and cognitive variables.

Variables	1. Slope	2. Wave I AMP	3. WEED STR	4. WEED P1 LAT	5. WM	6. PS	7. IC
1. Slope							
2. Wave I AMP	−0.21						
3. WEED STR	0.13	0.27					
4. WEED P1 LAT	−0.39**	0.41**	0.02				
5. Working Memory (WM)	−0.13	0.46**	0.10	0.18			
6. Processing Speed (PS)	−0.08	0.11	0.30*	0.14	0.15		
7. Inhibitory Control (IC)	−0.21	0.31*	0.17	0.21	0.45**	0.58***	

*Results of Pearson's correlational analysis indicated that the slope is only correlated to WEED P1 LAT. All three cognitive variables are strongly correlated with one another, except for working memory, and processing speed. Wave I amplitude correlated with all other predictor variables, except for processing speed. *$p < 0.05$, **$p < 0.01$, ***$p < 0.001$. AMP, amplitude; STR, stimulus-to-response correlation; LAT, latency.*

between the original experiment and the current study. For the contrasting word-pair WHEAT and WEED, younger and older adults with normal hearing did not significantly differ in 50% crossover point or slope of the identification functions in Gordon-Salant et al. (2006). In the current study, performance between groups was equivalent for the 50% crossover point, but younger adults demonstrated steeper slopes than did older adults. The different result patterns may be attributed to differences in presentation level utilized in the two different studies. Gordon-Salant et al. (2006) utilized a presentation level of 85 dB SPL compared to the 75 dB SPL presentation level used in the current study. Audibility may consequently impact the clarity of older adults' distinction between WHEAT and WEED, with softer presentation levels obscuring their ability to distinguish between the contrasting word pair.

TABLE 2 | Summary of "Stepwise" regression analysis for variables contributing to slope of the perceptual identification functions.

Variable	R^2 change	β	p value
Model 1	0.15		0.006
WEED P1 LAT		−0.39	0.006

Standardized (β) coefficients in a model automatically generated by evaluating the significance of each variable's contribution to slope of the perceptual identification functions. Only one model was generated, in which WEED P1 LAT predicts significant variance in slope. All other variables were excluded from the model (Wave I AMP, WEED STR, working memory, processing speed, and inhibitory control). STR, stimulus-to-response correlation; LAT, latency.

Peripheral Function

The click-evoked ABR was used to evaluate peripheral function, as age-related reductions in Wave I amplitude have been previously documented (Psatta and Matei, 1988; Grose et al., 2019). While the association between aging and hearing loss is believed to drive these group differences, the present study demonstrates that older adults with clinically normal hearing can also exhibit reduced Wave I amplitude compared to younger adults. It has been suggested that noise exposure may contribute to reduced Wave I amplitudes in adults who simultaneously demonstrate normal pure-tone thresholds and cochlear outer hair cell function (Konrad-Martin et al., 2012; Bramhall et al., 2017). Most of the current literature supporting this noise-induced cochlear synaptopathy, however, exists among animal models; the evidence is mixed in humans (Bharadwaj et al., 2015; Liberman et al., 2016; Grose et al., 2017). It is possible, however, that Wave I may be decreased in amplitude due to age-related losses of auditory nerve fibers and cochlear synaptopathy that are independent of noise exposure history (Schmiedt et al., 1996; Sergeyenko et al., 2013). Elevated thresholds in the extended high-frequency range in the older listeners may also be a factor in the reduced Wave I amplitudes (Verhulst et al., 2016).

Subcortical Representation

Similar to the results observed in Roque et al. (2019), aging affected FFR response morphology. Older adults exhibited less accurate neural representations of stimulus waveforms than younger adults. Rat models have also demonstrated similar aging effects on neural representation of sinusoidally amplitude-modulated tones (Parthasarathy and Bartlett, 2011). Older rats' response fidelity was poorer than those of younger rats, suggesting that temporal processing deficits limit the older rats' ability to encode changing envelope shapes (as would also occur in speech). This degraded neural representation of speech stimuli in the aging midbrain may be attributed to reduced neural synchrony. Human studies have also suggested that desynchronization may inhibit older adults' ability to encode the rapidly changing temporal and spectral properties of speech (Anderson et al., 2012; Presacco et al., 2015, 2016).

In contrast to the results found in Roque et al. (2019), however, the present study observed aging effects on phase locking to the temporal envelope of WHEAT and WEED. The difference in findings between the two studies may be attributed to the fact that phase locking was examined to a vowel region

following the plosive /d/ in Roque et al. (2019), whereas the current study examined phase locking to a vowel region following a glide. Overall, reduced phase locking was observed to the glide-vowel region in WHEAT/WEED than to the plosive-vowel region in the DISH/DITCH contrast used in the Roque et al. (2019) study. This difference might be due to increased synchronous firing generated by the shorter stimulus length of the stop-constant burst in the DISH/DITCH contrast compared to that generated by the glide. Brief stimuli are most effective at generating synchronous firing (Durrant and Boston, 2007). Because deficits in temporal synchronization in the IC as shown in mice (Walton et al., 1998) may underlie older adults' reduced phase locking, age-related reductions in neural synchrony would be exacerbated for the processing of longer-duration signals (i.e., glides) compared to shorter-duration signals (i.e., plosives).

Presacco et al. (2015) compared aging effects on the encoding of the synthetic plosive-vowel syllable /da/ and vowel /a/. Younger participants exhibited more robust FFR encoding than older participants, but these group differences were more pronounced for the sustained vowel region, especially in the last 60 ms of the /a/ vowel during which an abrupt decrease in synchronization was seen in many of the older participants. Based on these results, we had hypothesized that older participants' phase locking would decline from the early vowel region to the late vowel region to a greater extent than in young participants due to an inability to sustain neural firing. Results of the current study, however, showed that both younger and older participants were unable to maintain phase locking over time. Neural adaptation at the levels of the auditory nerve and midbrain may limit the duration of neural firing, particularly in response to a static signal (Sumner and Palmer, 2012; Pérez-González and Malmierca, 2014), leading to a reduction in phase locking over time. Additionally, the older participants' phase locking did not decrease over time to the same degree as the younger participants. The older participants' phase locking was already reduced and close to the noise floor in the early vowel region; therefore, their phase locking cannot decrease to the same extent as in younger participants with sustained stimulation.

Cortical Representation

It has been suggested that prominent CAEP components correspond to different sub-conscious processes that precede the conscious percept of an incoming stimulus. P1 and N1 are earlier-occurring peaks that reflect the pre-perceptual detection and focusing of attention to presented stimuli, respectively (Näätänen and Winkler, 1999). P2 emerges later, around 200 ms, and may reflect auditory object identification of presented stimuli (Näätänen and Winkler, 1999). Earlier and larger early peak components have been observed in older adults compared to young adults using magnetoencephalography (MEG) (Brodbeck et al., 2018). This neural activity, occurring at ∼30 ms, was source-localized to left temporal lobe, in regions lateral and inferior to auditory cortex. Brodbeck et al. (2018) suggested that this increased engagement of neural activity during speech detection may reflect increased neural excitability due to an age-related imbalance of inhibitory and excitatory processes that has been shown in animal models (Caspary et al., 1995; Hughes et al.,

2010). This increased excitability may manifest as robust onset responses (i.e., larger and earlier) to a presented auditory signal (Alain et al., 2014).

In contrast to Roque et al. (2019), the present study did not observe group differences in P2 latency. The lack of difference in the current study may be due to greater low-frequency energy for the initial consonant in WHEAT/WEED (F1 starting frequency: 320 Hz, F2 starting frequency: 900 Hz) compared to that for DISH/DITCH (F1 starting frequency: 465 Hz, F2 starting frequency: 2080 Hz). Additionally, stricter audiometric criteria and lower age cutoffs were employed in the present study compared to Roque et al. (2019) for the older participants. Stimuli were also low-pass filtered at 4000 Hz to ensure audibility. Reduced audibility may affect the robustness of auditory object identification represented by the P2 peak component; therefore, these study design factors would all reduce audibility confounds for high-frequency stimuli, where we found the largest group differences. Finally, the previous studies that reported delayed P2 latencies in older compared to younger adults used different cortical analyses (Tremblay et al., 2003; Billings et al., 2015), either reporting on a single electrode (e.g., Cz) or reporting global field power, which yields the standard deviation across all electrodes over time (Skrandies, 2005). The DSS algorithm used in this study may minimize group differences by reducing noise that might be otherwise present in the older adults' responses.

Relationships Among Cognitive, Perceptual, and EEG Variables

Select cortical variables (peak latency) contributed to variance in perceptual performance. Cortical processing appears to be an important factor in perceptual performance in young adults (Billings et al., 2013). In older adults, Billings et al. (2015) found that N1 and P2 amplitudes and latencies predicted recognition of sentences presented at various signal-to-noise ratios. In contrast to the current study, they did not find correlations between the P1 components and behavioral performance. This difference in findings may be due to the nature of the behavioral task. Repeating sentences in noise would draw on cognitive processes to a greater extent than identifying words in quiet and may have increased engagement for the later cortical components. In our study, we included the FFR to evaluate processing at subcortical levels. The extent to which the cortex compensates for auditory degradation at earlier subcortical levels may determine successful behavioral performance. We noted that the regression analysis was driven by a correlation in the older participants ($r = -0.39$) that was not significant in the younger participants ($r = -0.27$). In the older adults, earlier latencies correlated with shallower slopes. This finding is consistent with a previous MEG study that found an increase in early activity for the more ambiguous stimuli on a perceptual identification function in young adults (Gwilliams et al., 2018). Therefore, earlier latencies (i.e., greater cortical activation) may suggest that the endpoints of the identification function are ambiguous, resulting in a shallower slope.

Although previous studies found that midbrain factors significantly contribute to the perception of temporal speech cues

(Roque et al., 2019), the current study only observed neural contributions from auditory cortex. It is possible that these results diverge from those previously documented due to the fact that Roque et al. (2019) examined contributing factors to 50% crossover point, whereas this study examined contributions to slope of the perceptual identification functions. Because slope corresponds to the listeners' subjective distinction of two words it is likely dependent on auditory object identification, which occurs at the level of the auditory cortex (Ross et al., 2013). Although precise representation of the speech signal in midbrain may impact auditory object representation in cortex, the degree to which the cortex compensates for age-related deterioration in phase locking may be the most important contributing factor to perception of temporal cues. No correlations were observed between subcortical and cortical variables in the present study when including both younger and older participants in the analysis and when performing the correlations separately for each group (all p values > 0.05). Bidelman et al. (2014) observed a correlation between magnitude of first formant representation in the brainstem and the CAEP N1- P2 amplitude in older adults. It should be noted that this association seems to be mediated by hearing loss. Bidelman et al. (2014) suggested that this relationship implied more redundancy along the ascending auditory system in older adults. In addition, Presacco et al. (2019) found that the reconstruction accuracy in cortex correlated with midbrain quiet-to-noise correlations in participants with hearing loss but not in participants with normal hearing. Presacco et al. (2019) suggested that hearing loss alters connectivity between midbrain and cortex, so perhaps correlations among these factors would have been observed if participants with hearing loss had been included in the present study.

Peripheral and cognitive variables did not contribute to variance in perceptual performance. The original purpose of the present study was to examine effects of aging independent of peripheral hearing loss. The stimuli used in the present study were low-pass filtered at 4000 Hz to reduce audibility confounds. Therefore, it is expected that peripheral factors would have played a larger role for unfiltered stimuli. Further, reduced auditory perception (i.e., peripheral hearing loss) may force listeners to employ cognitive processes for speech understanding (Pichora-Fuller et al., 1995; Wingfield and Grossman, 2006). We note that the perceptual identification task used in the present study was not cognitively demanding. Although the task likely employed short-term memory, we theorize that cognitive processing would have significantly contributed to variance in perceptual performance had our task employed sentence-level materials and/or speech stimuli presented in noise, all of which would increase the cognitive load required for the task and are known to be related to working memory (Akeroyd, 2008; Füllgrabe et al., 2015).

It should be noted that the present study did not employ a task that combines a cognitive task (e.g., working memory or response inhibition) with behavioral testing or EEG recording. The current study was primarily interested in the neural representation of a specific temporal speech cue, and we therefore needed to present stimuli for thousands (FFR) or hundreds (CAEP) of trials to obtain adequate noise-free recordings in the time domain. An alternate approach would be to record cortical responses during an active listening task that might task attention or memory. This approach has been used previously to document the differing effects of attention on cortical processing in younger versus older adults (Henry et al., 2017).

CONCLUSION

The current study showed that neural encoding of P1 latency in the auditory cortex contributed to older adults' less distinct perceptions of contrasting word pairs differing in vowel duration, compared to younger adults. The communication struggles resulting from reduced temporal precision may lead to older adults' misunderstanding of spoken language and subsequent frustration, especially among those with normal hearing who often state that they can hear a talker just fine but have difficulty understanding what was said. It remains an open question as to whether auditory training can improve temporal processing (Henshaw and Ferguson, 2013). In an aging rat model, auditory training was able to partially reverse age-related declines in myelination and improve temporal processing in the auditory cortex, possibly mediated by an increase in inhibitory neurotransmission (de Villers-Sidani et al., 2010). An imbalance of inhibitory/excitatory transmission may lead to more diffuse neural firing, decreased temporal processing, and poor perception (Caspary et al., 2008). Given that decreased inhibition may mediate overrepresentation in auditory cortex, auditory training and/or pharmacologic intervention may lead to restoration of the precise temporal processing needed for the discrimination of speech stimuli.

AUTHOR CONTRIBUTIONS

SA and LR designed the experiment. SG-S and HK provided inputs into the study design and theoretical framework. LR and HK collected and analyzed the data. LR, HK, SG-S, and SA wrote the manuscript.

ACKNOWLEDGMENTS

The authors wish to thank Alanna Schloss, Logan Fraser, and Abigail Anne Poe for their assistance in data collection and analysis.

REFERENCES

Akeroyd, M. A. (2008). Are individual differences in speech reception related to individual differences in cognitive ability? A survey of twenty experimental studies with normal and hearing-impaired adults. Int. J. Audiol. 47, 53–71. doi: 10.1080/14992020802301142

Alain, C., Roye, A., and Salloum, C. (2014). Effects of age-related hearing loss and background noise on neuromagnetic activity from auditory cortex. Front. Syst. Neurosci. 8:8. doi: 10.3389/fnsys.2014.00008

Anderson, S., Parbery-Clark, A., White-Schwoch, T., and Kraus, N. (2012). Aging affects neural precision of speech encoding. J. Neurosci. 32, 14156–14164. doi: 10.1523/jneurosci.2176-12.2012

Bellier, L., Bouchet, P., Jeanvoine, A., Valentin, O., Thai-Van, H., and Caclin, A. (2015). Topographic recordings of auditory evoked potentials to speech: subcortical and cortical responses. Psychophysiology 52, 594–599. doi: 10.1111/psyp.12369

Bharadwaj, H. M., Masud, S., Mehraei, G., Verhulst, S., and Shinn-Cunningham, B. G. (2015). Individual differences reveal correlates of hidden hearing deficits. J. Neurosci. 35, 2161–2172. doi: 10.1523/jneurosci.3915-14.2015

Bidelman, G. M. (2018). Subcortical sources dominate the neuroelectric auditory frequency-following response to speech. Neuroimage 175, 56–69. doi: 10.1016/j.neuroimage.2018.03.060

Bidelman, G. M., Villafuerte, J. W., Moreno, S., and Alain, C. (2014). Age-related changes in the subcortical-cortical encoding and categorical perception of speech. Neurobiol. Aging 35, 2526–2540. doi: 10.1016/j.neurobiolaging.2014.05.006

Billings, C. J., Mcmillan, G. P., Penman, T. M., and Gille, S. M. (2013). Predicting perception in noise using cortical auditory evoked potentials. J. Assoc. Res. Otolaryngol 14, 891–903. doi: 10.1007/s10162-013-0415-y

Billings, C. J., Penman, T. M., Mcmillan, G. P., and Ellis, E. M. (2015). Electrophysiology and perception of speech in noise in older listeners: Effects of hearing impairment and age. Ear Hear. 36, 710–722. doi: 10.1097/aud.0000000000000191

Bramhall, N. F., Konrad-Martin, D., Mcmillan, G. P., and Griest, S. E. (2017). Auditory brainstem response altered in humans with noise exposure despite normal outer hair cell function. Ear Hear 38, e1–e12. doi: 10.1097/aud.0000000000000370

Brodbeck, C., Presacco, A., and Simon, J. Z. (2018). Neural source dynamics of brain responses to continuous stimuli: speech processing from acoustics to comprehension. Neuroimage 172, 162–174. doi: 10.1016/j.neuroimage.2018.01.042

Burke, D. M. (1997). Language, aging, and inhibitory deficits: evaluation of a theory. J. Gerontol. 52B, 254–264. doi: 10.1093/geronb/52B.6.P254

Carlozzi, N. E., Beaumont, J. L., Tulsky, D. S., and Gershon, R. C. (2015). The NIH toolbox pattern comparison processing speed test: normative data. Arch. Clin. Neuropsychol. 30, 359–368. doi: 10.1093/arclin/acv031

Caspary, D. M., Ling, L., Turner, J. G., and Hughes, L. F. (2008). Inhibitory neurotransmission, plasticity and aging in the mammalian central auditory system. J. Exp. Biol. 211, 1781–1791. doi: 10.1242/jeb.013581

Caspary, D. M., Milbrandt, J. C., and Helfert, R. H. (1995). Central auditory aging: GABA changes in the inferior colliculus. Exp. Gerontol. 30, 349–360. doi: 10.1016/0531-5565(94)00052-5

CHABA (1988). Speech understanding and aging. J. Acoust. Soc. Am. 83, 859–895. doi: 10.1121/1.395965

Cheveigné, A. D., and Simon, J. Z. (2008). Denoising based on spatial filtering. J. Neurosci. Methods 171, 331–339. doi: 10.1016/j.jneumeth.2008.03.015

Clinard, C. G., Tremblay, K. L., and Krishnan, A. R. (2010). Aging alters the perception and physiological representation of frequency: evidence from human frequency-following response recordings. Hear. Res. 264, 48–55. doi: 10.1016/j.heares.2009.11.010

Cohen, J. I., and Gordon-Salant, S. (2017). The effect of visual distraction on auditory-visual speech perception by younger and older listeners. J. Acoust. Soc. Am. 141:El470. doi: 10.1121/1.4983399

Daneman, M., and Hannon, B. (2007). "What do working memory span tasks like reading span really measure?," in The Cognitive Neuroscience of Working Memory, eds N. Osaka, R. H. Logie, and M. D'esposito (New York: Oxford University Press), 21–42. doi: 10.1093/acprof:oso/9780198570394.003.0002

de Villers-Sidani, E., Alzghoul, L., Zhou, X., Simpson, K. L., Lin, R. C. S., and Merzenich, M. M. (2010). Recovery of functional and structural age-related changes in the rat primary auditory cortex with operant training. Proc. Natl. Acad. Sci. U.S.A. 107, 13900–13905. doi: 10.1073/pnas.1007885107

Delorme, A., and Makeig, S. (2004). EEGLAB: an open source toolbox for analysis of single-trial EEG dynamics including independent component analysis. J. Neurosci. Methods 134, 9–21. doi: 10.1016/j.jneumeth.2003.10.009

Dey, A., and Sommers, M. S. (2015). Age-related differences in inhibitory control predict audiovisual speech perception. *Psychol. Aging* 30, 634–646. doi: 10.1037/pag0000033

Dubno, J. R., Dirks, D., and Morgan, D. (1984). Effects of age and mild hearing loss on speech recognition in noise. *J. Acoust. Soc. Am.* 76, 87–96. doi: 10.1121/1.391011

Durrant, J. D., and Boston, J. R. (2007). "Stimuli for auditory evoked potential assessment," in *Auditory Evoked Potentials, Basic Principle and Clinical Application*, eds R. F. Burkard, M. Don, and J. J. Eggermont (Baltimore: Lippincott Williams and Wilkins).

Fitzgibbons, P. J., and Gordon-Salant, S. (1995). Age effects on duration discrimination with simple and complex stimuli. *J. Acoust. Soc. Am.* 98, 3140–3145. doi: 10.1121/1.413803

Florentine, M., Buus, S., Scharf, B., and Zwicker, E. (1980). Frequency selectivity in normally-hearing and hearing-impaired observers. *J. Speech Lang. Hear Res.* 23, 646–669. doi: 10.1044/jshr.2303.646

Füllgrabe, C., Moore, B. C. J., and Stone, M. A. (2015). Age-group differences in speech identification despite matched audiometrically normal hearing: contributions from auditory temporal processing and cognition. *Front. Aging Neurosci.* 6:347. doi: 10.3389/fnagi.2014.00347

Genova, H. M., Lengenfelder, J., Chiaravalloti, N. D., Moore, N. B., and Deluca, J. (2012). Processing speed versus working memory: Contributions to an information-processing task in multiple sclerosis. *Appl. Neuropsychol. Adult* 19, 132–140. doi: 10.1080/09084282.2011.643951

Gordon-Salant, S., and Cole, S. S. (2016). Effects of age and working memory capacity on speech recognition performance in noise among listeners with normal hearing. *Ear Hear* 37, 593–602. doi: 10.1097/aud.0000000000000316

Gordon-Salant, S., and Fitzgibbons, P. J. (2001). Sources of age-related recognition difficulty for time-compressed speech. *J. Speech Lang. Hear Res.* 44, 709–719. doi: 10.1044/1092-4388(2001/056)

Gordon-Salant, S., and Fitzgibbons, P. J. (1993). Temporal factors and speech recognition performance in young and elderly listeners. *J. Speech Hear. Res.* 36, 1276–1285. doi: 10.1044/jshr.3606.1276

Gordon-Salant, S., Yeni-Komshian, G. H., and Fitzgibbons, P. J. (2010). Recognition of accented English in quiet and noise by younger and older listeners. *J. Acoust. Soc. Am.* 128, 3152–3160. doi: 10.1121/1.3495940

Gordon-Salant, S., Yeni-Komshian, G. H., Fitzgibbons, P. J., and Barrett, J. (2006). Age-related differences in identification and discrimination of temporal cues in speech segments. *J. Acoust. Soc. Am.* 119, 2455–2466. doi: 10.1121/1.2171527

Gordon-Salant, S., Yeni-Komshian, G. H., Fitzgibbons, P. J., Willison, H. M., and Freund, M. S. (2017). Recognition of asynchronous auditory-visual speech by younger and older listeners: a preliminary study. *J. Acoust. Soc. Am.* 142:151. doi: 10.1121/1.4992026

Grose, J. H., Buss, E., and Elmore, H. (2019). Age-related changes in the auditory brainstem response and suprathreshold processing of temporal and spectral modulation. *Trends Hearing* 23:2331216519839615. doi: 10.1177/2331216519839615

Grose, J. H., Buss, E., and Hall, J. W. III (2017). Loud music exposure and cochlear synaptopathy in young adults: Isolated auditory brainstem response effects but no perceptual consequences. *Trends Hear.* 21:2331216517737417. doi: 10.1177/2331216517737417

Gwilliams, L., Linzen, T., Poeppel, D., and Marantz, A. (2018). In spoken word recognition, the future predicts the past. *J. Neurosci.* 38, 7585–7599. doi: 10.1523/JNEUROSCI.0065-18.2018

Hedden, T., and Gabrieli, J. D. (2004). Insights into the ageing mind: a view from cognitive neuroscience. *Nat. Rev. Neurosci.* 5, 87–96. doi: 10.1038/nrn1323

Helfer, K. S., and Wilber, L. A. (1990). Hearing loss, aging, and speech perception in reverberation and noise. *J. Speech Hear. Res.* 33, 149–155. doi: 10.1044/jshr.3301.149

Henry, M. J., Herrmann, B., Kunke, D., and Obleser, J. (2017). Aging affects the balance of neural entrainment and top-down neural modulation in the listening brain. *Nat. Commun.* 8:15801. doi: 10.1038/ncomms15801

Henshaw, H., and Ferguson, M. A. (2013). Efficacy of individual computer-based auditory training for people with hearing loss: a systematic review of the evidence. *PLoS One* 8:e62836. doi: 10.1371/journal.pone.0062836

Hughes, L. F., Turner, J. G., Parrish, J. L., and Caspary, D. M. (2010). Processing of broadband stimuli across A1 layers in young and aged rats. *Hear. Res.* 264, 79–85. doi: 10.1016/j.heares.2009.09.005

Jenkins, K. A., Fodor, C., Presacco, A., and Anderson, S. (2018). Effects of amplification on neural phase locking, amplitude, and latency to a speech syllable. *Ear Hear* 39, 810–824. doi: 10.1097/aud.0000000000000538

Johns, A. R., Myers, E. B., and Skoe, E. (2018). Sensory and cognitive contributions to age-related changes in spoken word recognition. *Lang. Linguist. Compass* 12:e12272. doi: 10.1111/lnc3.12272

Juarez-Salinas, D. L., Engle, J. R., Navarro, X. O., and Recanzone, G. H. (2010). Hierarchical and serial processing in the spatial auditory cortical pathway is degraded by natural aging. *J. Neurosci.* 30, 14795–14804. doi: 10.1523/jneurosci.3393-10.2010

Kerr, C. C., Rennie, C. J., and Robinson, P. A. (2008). Physiology-based modeling of cortical auditory evoked potentials. *Biol. Cybern.* 98, 171–184. doi: 10.1007/s00422-007-0201-1

Koeritzer, M. A., Rogers, C. S., Van Engen, K. J., and Peelle, J. E. (2018). The impact of age, background noise, semantic ambiguity, and hearing loss on recognition memory for spoken sentences. *J. Speech Lang. Hearing Res.* 61, 740–751. doi: 10.1044/2017_JSLHR-H-17-0077

Konrad-Martin, D., Dille, M. F., Mcmillan, G., Griest, S., Mcdermott, D., Fausti, S. A., et al. (2012). Age-related changes in the auditory brainstem response. *J. Am. Acad. Audiol.* 23, 18–35. doi: 10.3766/jaaa.23.1.3

Liberman, M. C., Epstein, M. J., Cleveland, S. S., Wang, H., and Maison, S. F. (2016). Toward a differential diagnosis of hidden hearing loss in humans. *PLoS One* 11:e0162726. doi: 10.1371/journal.pone.0162726

Lin, F., Yaffe, K., Xia, J., and Al, E. (2013). Hearing loss and cognitive decline in older adults. *J. Am. Med. Assoc. Inter. Med.* 173, 293–299. doi: 10.1001/jamainternmed.2013.1868

Lin, F. R. (2011). Hearing loss and cognition among older adults in the United States. *J. Gerontol. Ser. A Biol. Sci. Med. Sci.* 66, 1131–1136. doi: 10.1093/gerona/glr115

Lunner, T. (2003). Cognitive function in relation to hearing aid use. *Int. J. Audiol.* 42, S49–S58. doi: 10.3109/14992020309074624

Lunner, T., and Sundewall-Thoren, E. (2007). Interactions between cognition, compression, and listening conditions: Effects on speech-in-noise performance in a two-channel hearing aid. *J. Am. Acad. Audiol.* 18, 604–617. doi: 10.3766/jaaa.18.7.7

Maamor, N., and Billings, C. J. (2017). Cortical signal-in-noise coding varies by noise type, signal-to-noise ratio, age, and hearing status. *Neurosci. Lett.* 636, 258–264. doi: 10.1016/j.neulet.2016.11.020

Matschke, R. G. (1990). Frequency selectivity and psychoacoustic tuning curves in old age. *Acta Otolaryngol. Suppl.* 476, 114–119. doi: 10.3109/00016489109127264

McClearn, G. E., Johansson, B., Berg, S., Pedersen, N. L., Ahern, F., Petrill, S. A., et al. (1997). Substantial genetic influence on cognitive abilities in twins 80 or more years old. *Science* 276, 1560–1563. doi: 10.1126/science.276.5318.1560

Moushegian, G., Rupert, A. L., and Stillman, R. D. (1973). Scalp-recorded early responses in man to frequencies in the speech range. *Electroencephalogr. Clin. Neurophysiol.* 35, 665–667. doi: 10.1016/0013-4694(73)90223-X

Näätänen, R., and Winkler, I. (1999). The concept of auditory stimulus representation in cognitive neuroscience. *Psychol. Bull.* 125, 826–859. doi: 10.1037//0033-2909.125.6.826

Nasreddine, Z. S., Phillips, N. A., Bédirian, V., Charbonneau, S., Whitehead, V., Collin, I., et al. (2005). The montreal cognitive assessment, MoCA: a brief screening tool for mild cognitive impairment. *J. Am. Geriatr. Soc.* 53, 695–699. doi: 10.1111/j.1532-5415.2005.53221.x

Parthasarathy, A., and Bartlett, E. L. (2011). Age-related auditory deficits in temporal processing in F-344 rats. *Neuroscience* 192, 619–630. doi: 10.1016/j.neuroscience.2011.06.042

Pérez-González, D., and Malmierca, M. S. (2014). Adaptation in the auditory system: an overview. *Front. Integr. Neurosci.* 8:19. doi: 10.3389/fnint.2014.00019

Pichora-Fuller, M., Schneider, B., and Daneman, M. (1995). How young and old adults listen to and remember speech in noise. *J. Acoust. Soc. Am.* 97, 593–608. doi: 10.1121/1.412282

Pichora-Fuller, M. K., and Singh, G. (2006). Effects of age on auditory and cognitive processing: implications for hearing aid fitting and audiologic rehabilitation. *Trends Amplif.* 10, 29–59. doi: 10.1177/108471380601000103

Presacco, A., Jenkins, K., Lieberman, R., and Anderson, S. (2015). Effects of aging on the encoding of dynamic and static components of speech. *Ear Hear* 36, e352–e363. doi: 10.1097/aud.0000000000000193

Presacco, A., Simon, J. Z., and Anderson, S. (2016). Evidence of degraded representation of speech in noise, in the aging midbrain and cortex. *J. Neurophysiol.* 116, 2346–2355. doi: 10.1152/jn.00372.2016

Presacco, A., Simon, J. Z., and Anderson, S. (2019). Speech-in-noise representation in the aging midbrain and cortex: Effects of hearing loss. *PLoS One* 14:e0213899. doi: 10.1371/journal.pone.0213899

Psatta, D. M., and Matei, M. (1988). Age-dependent amplitude variation of brainstem auditory evoked potentials. *Electroencephalogr. Clin. Neurophysiol.* 71, 27–32. doi: 10.1016/0168-5597(88)90016-0

Romero, S., Mananas, M. A., and Barbanoj, M. J. (2006). Quantitative evaluation of automatic ocular removal from simulated EEG signals: regression vs. second order statistics methods. *Conf. Proc. IEEE Eng. Med. Biol. Soc.* 1, 5495–5498. doi: 10.1109/iembs.2006.260338

Ronnberg, J., Lunner, T., Zekveld, A., Sorqvist, P., Danielsson, H., Lyxell, B., et al. (2013). The ease of language understanding (ELU) model: theoretical, empirical, and clinical advances. *Front. Syst. Neurosci.* 7:31. doi: 10.3389/fnsys.2013.00031

Ronnberg, J., Rudner, M., Foo, C., and Lunner, T. (2008). Cognition counts: a working memory system for ease of language understanding (ELU). *Int. J. Audiol.* 47(Suppl. 2), S99–S105. doi: 10.1080/14992020802301167

Roque, L., Gaskins, C., Gordon-Salant, S., Goupell, M. J., and Anderson, S. (2019). Age effects on neural representation and perception of silence duration cues in speech. *J. Speech Lang. Hear. Res.* 62, 1099–1116. doi: 10.1044/2018_JSLHR-H-ASCC7-18-0076

Ross, B., Jamali, S., and Tremblay, K. L. (2013). Plasticity in neuromagnetic cortical responses suggests enhanced auditory object representation. *BMC Neurosci.* 14:151. doi: 10.1186/1471-2202-14-151

Salthouse, T. A. (1996). The processing-speed theory of adult age differences in cognition. *Psychol. Rev.* 103, 403–428. doi: 10.1037//0033-295x.103.3.403

Salthouse, T. A. (2010). Is flanker-based inhibition related to age? Identifying specific influences of individual differences on neurocognitive variables. *Brain Cogn.* 73, 51–61. doi: 10.1016/j.bandc.2010.02.003

Salthouse, T. A., and Babcock, R. L. (1991). Decomposing adult age differences in working memory. *Dev. Psychol.* 27:763. doi: 10.1037//0012-1649.27.5.763

Särelä, J., and Valpola, H. (2005). Denoising source separation. *J. Mach. Learn. Res.* 6, 233–272.

Schlögl, A., Keinrath, C., Zimmermann, D., Scherer, R., Leeb, R., and Pfurtscheller, G. (2007). A fully automated correction method of EOG artifacts in EEG recordings. *Clin. Neurophysiol.* 118, 98–104. doi: 10.1016/j.clinph.2006.09.003

Schmiedt, R. A., Mills, J. H., and Boettcher, F. A. (1996). Age-related loss of activity of auditory-nerve fibers. *J. Neurophysiol.* 76, 2799–2803. doi: 10.1152/jn.1996.76.4.2799

Schneider, B. A., Pichora-Fuller, M. K., Kowalchuk, D., and Lamb, M. (1994). Gap detection and the precedence effect in young and old adults. *J. Acoust. Soc. Am.* 95, 980–991. doi: 10.1121/1.408403

Sergeyenko, Y., Lall, K., Liberman, M. C., and Kujawa, S. G. (2013). Age-related cochlear synaptopathy: an early-onset contributor to auditory functional decline. *J. Neurosci.* 33, 13686–13694. doi: 10.1523/jneurosci.1783-13.2013

Skrandies, W. (2005). Brain mapping of visual evoked activity - topographical and functional components. *Acta Neurol. Taiwan.* 14, 164–178.

Smith, J. C., Marsh, J. T., and Brown, W. S. (1975). Far-field recorded frequency-following responses: evidence for the locus of brainstem sources. *Electroencephalogr. Clin. Neurophysiol.* 39, 465–472. doi: 10.1016/0013-4694(75)90047-4

Sumner, C. J., and Palmer, A. R. (2012). Auditory nerve fibre responses in the ferret. *Eur. J. Neurosci.* 36, 2428–2439. doi: 10.1111/j.1460-9568.2012.08151.x

Tallon-Baudry, C., Bertrand, O., Delpuech, C., and Pernier, J. (1996). Stimulus specificity of phase-locked and non-phase-locked 40 hz visual responses in human. *J. Neurosci.* 16, 4240–4249. doi: 10.1523/JNEUROSCI.16-13-04240.1996

Tan, A. Y., Zhang, L. I., Merzenich, M. M., and Schreiner, C. E. (2004). Tone-evoked excitatory and inhibitory synaptic conductances of primary auditory cortex neurons. *J. Neurophysiol.* 92, 630–643. doi: 10.1152/jn.01020.2003

Tremblay, K., Piskosz, M., and Souza, P. (2003). Effects of age and age-related hearing loss on the neural representation of speech cues. *Clin. Neurophysiol.* 114, 1332–1343. doi: 10.1016/S1388-2457(03)00114-7

Tulsky, D. S., Carlozzi, N., Chiaravalloti, N. D., Beaumont, J. L., Kisala, P. A., Mungas, D., et al. (2014). NIH Toolbox Cognition Battery (NIHTB-CB): List sorting test to measure working memory. *J. Int. Neuropsychol. Soc.* 20, 599–610. doi: 10.1017/s135561771400040x

Verhulst, S., Jagadeesh, A., Mauermann, M., and Ernst, F. (2016). Individual differences in auditory brainstem response wave characteristics. *Trends Hear.* 20:233121651667218. doi: 10.1177/2331216516672186

Walton, J. P., Frisina, R. D., and O'neill, W. E. (1998). Age-related alteration in processing of temporal sound features in the auditory midbrain of the CBA mouse. *J. Neurosci.* 18, 2764–2776. doi: 10.1523/JNEUROSCI.18-07-02764.1998

Weintraub, S., Dikmen, S. S., Heaton, R. K., Tulsky, D. S., Zelazo, P. D., Bauer, P. J., et al. (2013). Cognition assessment using the NIH toolbox. *Neurology* 80, S54–S64. doi: 10.1212/WNL.0b013e3182872ded

Wichmann, F. A., and Hill, N. J. (2001a). The psychometric function: I. Fitting, sampling, and goodness of fit. *Percept. Psychophys.* 63, 1293–1313. doi: 10.3758/BF03194544

Wichmann, F. A., and Hill, N. J. (2001b). The psychometric function: II. Bootstrap-based confidence intervals and sampling. *Percept. Psychophys.* 63, 1314–1329. doi: 10.3758/BF03194545

Wingfield, A. (1996). Cognitive factors in auditory performance: context, speed of processing, and constraints of memory. *J. Am. Acad. Audiol.* 7, 175–182.

Wingfield, A., and Grossman, M. (2006). Language and the aging brain: patterns of neural compensation revealed by functional brain imaging. *J. Neurophysiol.* 96, 2830–2839. doi: 10.1152/jn.00628.2006

Zelazo, P. D., Anderson, J. E., Richler, J., Wallner-Allen, K., Beaumont, J. L., Conway, K. P., et al. (2014). NIH Toolbox Cognition Battery (CB): validation of executive function measures in adults. *J. Int. Neuropsychol. Soc.* 20, 620–629. doi: 10.1017/s1355617714000472

Zhu, J., and Garcia, E. (1999). *The Wechsler Abbreviated Scale of Intelligence (WASI)*. New York, NY: Psychological Corporation.

16

mito-TEMPO Attenuates Oxidative Stress and Mitochondrial Dysfunction in Noise-Induced Hearing Loss *via* Maintaining TFAM-mtDNA Interaction and Mitochondrial Biogenesis

Jia-Wei Chen[1†], Peng-Wei Ma[1†], Hao Yuan[1†], Wei-Long Wang[1], Pei-Heng Lu[1], Xue-Rui Ding[1], Yu-Qiang Lun[1], Qian Yang[2]* and Lian-Jun Lu[1]*

[1]Department of Otolaryngology Head and Neck Surgery, Tangdu Hospital, Fourth Military Medical University, Xi'an, China,
[2]Department of Experimental Surgery, Tangdu Hospital, Fourth Military Medical University, Xi'an, China

*Correspondence:
Lian-Jun Lu
lulianj@fmmu.edu.cn
Qian Yang
qianyang@fmmu.edu.cn

†These authors have contributed equally to this work

The excessive generation of reactive oxygen species (ROS) and mitochondrial damage have been widely reported in noise-induced hearing loss (NIHL). However, the specific mechanism of noise-induced mitochondrial damage remains largely unclear. In this study, we showed that acoustic trauma caused oxidative damage to mitochondrial DNA (mtDNA), leading to the reduction of mtDNA content, mitochondrial gene expression and ATP level in rat cochleae. The expression level and mtDNA-binding function of mitochondrial transcription factor A (TFAM) were impaired following acoustic trauma without affecting the upstream PGC-1α and NRF-1. The mitochondria-target antioxidant mito-TEMPO (MT) was demonstrated to enter the inner ear after the systemic administration. MT treatment significantly alleviated noise-induced auditory threshold shifts 3d and 14d after noise exposure. Furthermore, MT significantly reduced outer hair cell (OHC) loss, cochlear ribbon synapse loss, and auditory nerve fiber (ANF) degeneration after the noise exposure. In addition, we found that MT treatment effectively attenuated noise-induced cochlear oxidative stress and mtDNA damage, as indicated by DHE, 4-HNE, and 8-OHdG. MT treatment also improved mitochondrial biogenesis, ATP generation, and TFAM-mtDNA interaction in the cochlea. These findings suggest that MT has protective effects against NIHL via maintaining TFAM-mtDNA interaction and mitochondrial biogenesis based on its ROS scavenging capacity.

Keywords: noise-induced hearing loss, reactive oxygen species, mitochondrial transcription factor A, mitochondrial biogenesis, sensory hair cells, rat model

INTRODUCTION

Hearing loss is the most prevalent sensory disorder and affects more than 1.5 billion people worldwide (WHO, 2021). Common causes of acquired sensorineural hearing loss include exposure to loud noise (Sha and Schacht, 2017), aminoglycosides (He et al., 2017), platinum-based chemotherapy (Fernandez et al., 2020), heavy metals (Ding et al., 2019), and aging (He et al., 2021a). With the rapid development of modern society, noise has become one of the most common environmental pollutants in industrial and recreational settings. Exposure to high-intensity or chronic noise leads to noise-induced hearing loss (NIHL).

Moderate noise leads to temporary threshold shift (TTS) that completely recovers to normal in 1–2 weeks. However, high-intensity or chronic noise can result in permanent threshold shift (PTS), i.e., irreversible hearing loss (Kurabi et al., 2017). According to WHO, about 10% of the world's population is exposed to noise, 5.3% of whom develop NIHL (WHO, 2021). Those who experience hearing loss have difficulties in social communication, which may cause potential mental and cognitive disorders such as anxiety, depression, and dementia (Loughrey et al., 2018; Blazer and Tucci, 2019).

The cochlea is a metabolically active auditory sensory organ. Loud noise causes a dramatic increase in energy consumption of the cochlea (Chen et al., 2012). Production of reactive oxygen species (ROS) was observed in the cochlea in a few minutes following noise exposure, including superoxide ($O_2\cdot-$), hydroxyl radical ($\cdot OH$), and hydrogen peroxide (H_2O_2). Moreover, ROS can be generated continuously for 7–10 days after cessation of the noise exposure (Ohlemiller et al., 1999; Yamashita et al., 2004). A lower level of ROS induced by moderate noise is reported to induce autophagy which protects against NIHL (Yuan et al., 2015). However, high-intensity noise induces excess ROS and activates 5' adenosine monophosphate-activated protein kinase (AMPK), leading to hair cell death and hearing loss (Wu et al., 2020). Oxidative stress has been considered as a key factor in the mechanism of NIHL (Fetoni et al., 2019). ROS in the cochlea mainly comes from the mitochondrial metabolism of various cells. Mitochondrial pathology and dysfunction are associated with hearing loss of various etiologies (Fischel-Ghodsian et al., 2004; Böttger and Schacht, 2013). Mitochondria are essential organelles with several vital functions including energy production, maintenance of calcium homeostasis, and regulation of apoptosis (Lin and Beal, 2006). Due to the proximity to ROS production, mitochondria are also the first organelles damaged by ROS. The phenomenon of mitochondrial damage has been reported to be involved in NIHL in previous studies (Coleman et al., 2007; Park et al., 2012). However, the underlying mechanism has not been fully elucidated yet.

The mitochondrial DNA (mtDNA) is a circular double-stranded DNA located in the matrix of mitochondria, encoding 13 essential subunits of the mitochondrial respiratory chain (MRC; Scarpulla, 2008). Due to the lack of the repair mechanism and histone proteins like genomic DNA, mtDNA is more susceptible to the damage by ROS (Tsutsui et al., 2009). Mitochondrial transcription factor A (TFAM), a nucleus-encoded protein, is essential for the stabilization and maintenance of mtDNA. TFAM can bind to mtDNA in a sequence-independent manner to compact and stabilize the genome. In addition, TFAM can also bind sequence-specifically to promoter regions of mtDNA, initiating transcription and replication of mtDNA (Kang et al., 2007; Chandrasekaran et al., 2015). Previous studies have reported mitochondrial disintegration and vacuolization in hair cells (HCs) after acoustic trauma (Coleman et al., 2007; Park et al., 2012). However, the specific mechanism of noise-induced mitochondrial damage remains unclear. There are few studies on the alterations of the cochlear mtDNA content and expression level after acoustic trauma. Whether TFAM

dysregulation is involved in the pathogenesis of NIHL is still unknown.

Recently, several novel antioxidants that specifically target mitochondria have been developed for the treatment of oxidative stress-related diseases (Zinovkin and Zamyatnin, 2019). 2-(2,2,6,6-tetramethylpiperidin-1-oxyl-4-ylamino)-2-oxoethyl (mito-TEMPO) is a mitochondria-target antioxidant with strong superoxide scavenging capacity and several hundred-fold accumulations in mitochondria (Shetty et al., 2019). A previous study demonstrated that mito-TEMPO (MT) can ameliorate renal fibrosis by reducing oxidative stress, mitochondrial dysfunction, and inflammation (Liu et al., 2018). In addition, recent studies have shown that MT has a protective effect against acetaminophen-induced hepatotoxicity with a wider therapeutic time window than N-acetyl-L-cysteine (NAC; Du et al., 2017; Abdullah-Al-Shoeb et al., 2020). Systemic administration of MT was able to alleviate ischemic brain damage in rats (Li et al., 2018). In addition, MT can pass through the blood-brain barrier (BBB) which is structurally similar to the blood-labyrinth barrier (BLB) in stria vascularis of the cochlea (Zhelev et al., 2013; Nyberg et al., 2019). However, whether MT has a protective effect on hearing has not been reported yet.

In the present study, we explored whether MT has a protective effect against NIHL and the underlying mechanism using an *in vivo* rat model. We first detected whether MT entered the inner ear after the systemic administration. Then we investigated the alleviation of noise-induced hearing loss, outer hair cell (OHC) loss, inner hair cell (IHC) ribbon synapse loss, and auditory nerve fiber (ANF) degeneration with systemic use of MT. We hypothesized that MT exerted the protective effect on hearing via reducing mtDNA oxidative damage, stabilizing the TFAM-mtDNA interaction, maintaining mitochondrial biogenesis and function.

MATERIALS AND METHODS

Animals

Sixty-two female adult Sprague-Dawley rats (200–250 g) were used in this study. Two rats were used for the determination of MT in the cochlea. Sixty Rats were randomly assigned to three groups ($n = 20$ for each group): control, noise + vehicle treatment, noise + MT treatment. All animals were kept at $22 \pm 1°C$ under a 12 h light/12 h dark cycle with free access to water and food. All procedures of the animal experiments were approved by the Institutional Animal Care and Use Committee of Fourth Military Medical University.

Auditory Brainstem Response (ABR) Measurements

The hearing function of 18 animals ($n = 6$ for each group) was evaluated by auditory brainstem response (ABR) at four frequencies of 8, 16, 24, and 32 kHz. ABR measurements were carried out 2 days before (−2d), 3 days after (+3d) and 14 days after (+14d) the noise exposure to evaluate the baseline hearing function and noise-induced auditory threshold shifts. Rats were anesthetized with an intraperitoneal injection of the cocktail anesthetic (chloral hydrate, pentobarbital sodium, and magnesium sulfate). Body temperature was maintained at near 37°C with a heating pad. Three subdermal electrodes were inserted at the vertex of the skull (active), the left mastoid (reference), and the right mastoid (ground). Tucker-Davis Technologies (TDT) RZ6 System was used to generate acoustic stimuli and record the responses. Tone pip stimuli at 8, 16, 24, and 32 kHz (5-ms-duration with 2.5-ms rise–fall time) were delivered monaurally with an earphone inserted into the external auditory canal of the left ear. Acoustic stimuli were generated from 90 dB and then attenuated in 10-dB and 5-dB steps until no ABR waves were recognizable. A total of 1,024 responses were averaged for each stimulus level. ABR wave II was used to determine ABR thresholds for each frequency. The thresholds were defined as the lowest intensity able to evoke repeatable response waves.

Drug Administration

MT (Sigma-Aldrich, SML0737) was dissolved in normal saline as a stock solution and stored at −20°C. The stock solution was diluted with normal saline at a concentration of 0.5 mg/ml before the injection. For animals in the MT treatment group, a dose of 1 mg/kg was selected based on the previous studies (Liu et al., 2018; Xing et al., 2021). For the animals to be sacrificed on day 1, MT was injected intraperitoneally (i.p.) 24 h before, 1 h before, and immediately after noise exposure. The Animals to be sacrificed on day 3 and 14 received three additional injections once daily for the following 3 days. The animals in the control group and the vehicle treatment group received three or six injections of normal saline with the same experimental procedure.

Perilymph Extraction and Sample Preparation

Two rats were injected intraperitoneally with 1 mg/kg MT. Fifteen minutes after the injection, rats were sacrificed and the cochleae were harvested. Then 2 μl of perilymph was sampled using a capillary tube from the round window of the cochlea. A total of 8 μl of perilymph was pooled and used for the determination of MT. Then 100 μl of methanol was added to the sample. After vortexing, the sample was centrifuged at 5,000×g for 10 min at 4°C. The supernatant was retained and used for liquid chromatography tandem mass spectrometry (LC-MS/MS) analysis.

Chromatographic Separation and MS/MS Detection

The LC-MS/MS analysis was performed with the Triple Quadrupole LC/MS (Agilent, 6470B, USA). Chromatographic separation was performed using an Agilent C18 column (100 × 2.1 mm i.d., 3 μm particle size). The sample injection volume was 10 μl. The column temperature was maintained at 35°C. Then a gradient of mobile phase A (0.1%(v/v) formic acid in 5 mM ammonium acetate) and mobile phase B (acetonitrile) was run at 0.3 ml/min as follows: 95% A and 5% B, 0–15 min; 20% A and 80% B, 15–17 min; 100% A, 17–20 min. The MS/MS analysis was performed in the positive electrospray ionization

(ESI+) mode. The source temperature was kept at 500°C. The ion spray voltage was 4,500 V, and the curtain gas was set to 35 psi. The detection of the ions was operated in the multiple reaction monitoring (MRM) mode, monitoring transitions of m/z 474.2 → 320.1 for MT. The quantification of the MT in the perilymph was analyzed by calculating the peak area ratios using the external standard.

Acoustic Trauma

The acoustic trauma was induced by continuous noise exposure. The rats were placed separately in wire cages located in a sound-proof room. The acoustic signal of 8–16 kHz octave band noise was generated by RZ6 Noise software. Then the signal was amplified and output by the power amplifier (Crown, XLi800, China) and four loudspeakers (CHUANGMU, CP-75A, China). The level of the noise was maintained at 112 ± 1 dB SPL confirmed by the Sound Level Meter. Animals were exposed to noise for 2 h.

Immunofluorescence Histochemistry for Surface Preparations and Frozen Sections of the Cochlea

Twelve animals used for the analyses of 4-HNE, DHE, 8-OHdG level, and TFAM-mtDNA interaction were sacrificed 1 h after the noise exposure. Eighteen animals used for analyses of OHC loss, IHC ribbon synapse loss, and ANF degeneration were sacrificed 14d after the noise exposure. Rat cochleae were quickly dissected from the temporal bones following rapid decapitation. The round and oval windows were opened after removing the stapes. Then the cochleae were gently perfused with 4% paraformaldehyde (PFA) in 0.1 M phosphate-buffered saline (PBS) via the round window, and kept in the fixative overnight at 4°C. After the fixation, the cochleae were rinsed three times with PBS for 5 min and then decalcified with 10% ethylenediaminetetraacetic acid (EDTA) for 5 days at room temperature with a daily solution change. After the decalcification, the cochleae were rinsed three times with PBS for 5 min. For cochlear surface preparations, the organ of Corti (OC) was dissected in PBS by carefully removing the lateral wall, Reissner's membrane, and the tectorial membrane of the cochlea using micro-dissecting forceps and scissors under a stereomicroscope (Olympus, SZ61, Japan). Then the specimens were transferred into a 96-well plate, followed by permeabilization using 1% Triton X-100 in PBS for 15 min at room temperature. The specimens were blocked with immunol staining blocking buffer (Leagene, IH0338) for 1 h at room temperature. Then the specimens were incubated overnight at 4°C with the following primary antibodies: Myosin VIIa (Proteus Biosciences, #25-6790, 1:1,000), TFAM (Abcam, ab252432, 1:500), dsDNA (Abcam, ab27156, 1:500). After being rinsed with PBS three times, the specimens were incubated for 2 h at room temperature in darkness with following secondary antibodies: donkey anti-rabbit IgG Alexa Fluor 594 (Invitrogen, A21207, 1:200), donkey anti-mouse IgG Alexa Fluor 488 (Invitrogen, A21202, 1:200). After being rinsed with PBS three times, the specimens were incubated with Acti-Stain 670 Phalloidin (Cytoskeleton, #PHDN1-A, 1:70) or

DAPI (Roche, #10236276001, 1 μg/ml) for 30 min at room temperature.

For immunolabeling of IHC ribbon synapses, the specimens were permeabilized with 3% Triton X-100 in PBS for 30 min at room temperature. After blocking for 1 h, the specimens were incubated overnight at 37°C with following primary antibodies: Myosin VIIa (Proteus Biosciences, #25-6790, 1:1,000), CtBP2 (BD Bioscience, #612044, 1:500), GluR2 (Alomone Labs, AGC-005, 1:1,000). After being rinsed with PBS three times, the specimens were incubated for 2 h at room temperature in darkness with following secondary antibodies: goat anti-rabbit IgG Alexa Fluor 568 (Invitrogen, A11036, 1:200), goat anti-mouse IgG1 Alexa Fluor 647 (Invitrogen, A21240, 1:200), goat anti-mouse IgG2a Alexa Fluor 488 (Invitrogen, A21131, 1:200). After the final rinse with PBS, each specimen was dissected into the apex, middle and base turns. Each cochlear turn was transferred to the slide and placed in the mounting medium (Vector, H-1000). Finally, the specimen was covered with a coverslip and the edge was sealed with transparent nail polish.

For the preparation of cochlear frozen sections, the decalcified cochleae were incubated in 10% sucrose and 20% sucrose for 4 h and 30% sucrose overnight at 4°C for dehydration. Then the specimens were embedded in an optimal cutting temperature (OCT) compound. The midmodiolar cryosections at a thickness of 8 μm were prepared using a Cryostat Microtome (Leica, CM1860, Germany). The sections were permeabilized with 0.5% Triton X-100 in PBS for 15 min at room temperature, followed by blocking with immunol staining blocking buffer for 1 h at room temperature. Then the sections were incubated overnight at 4°C with following primary antibodies: Myosin VIIa (Proteus Biosciences, #25-6790, 1:1,000), Tuj1 (GeneTex, GTX631836, 1:200), 4-HNE (GeneTex, GTX17571, 1:50), 8-OHdG (Abcam, ab48508, 1:200), Tuj1(ABclonal, A17913, 1:500). After being rinsed with PBS three times, the specimens were incubated with secondary antibodies for 2 h at room temperature in darkness. For DHE staining, the permeabilized sections were incubated with 1 μM DHE solution (Beyotime, S0063) for 30 min at 37°C in darkness. After being rinsed with PBS three times, a drop of mounting medium with DAPI (Vector, H-1200) was added onto the section. Finally, the section was covered with a coverslip and the edge was sealed with transparent nail polish. Images were obtained with the Confocal Laser Scanning Microscope (CLSM; Olympus, FV1000, Japan) under identical parameter settings in each experiment.

Quantitative or Semi-quantitative Analyses of the Fluorescence Signals

The quantitative or semi-quantitative analyses of the fluorescence signals were conducted with ImageJ software (version 1.53a, USA). For the OHC counting 14d after noise exposure, cochlear surface preparations labeled with Myosin VIIa and DAPI were used. The OHC counting was measured in apex, middle and base turns of surface preparations in 0.3-mm segments. The absence of both the nucleus (DAPI) and the cell body (Myosin VIIa) was considered as the OHC loss. The mean OHC survival in each group was calculated with four

specimens. The quantification of IHC ribbon synapses was analyzed in the 0.1-mm segment of the surface preparation (containing about 10 IHCs), corresponding to frequencies of 16–20 kHz. The juxtaposition of CtBP2 and GluA2 was considered as the paired synapse. The total number of paired fluorescent spots was counted and divided by the number of IHC within the image. For the analysis of ANF density, cochlear frozen sections immunolabelled with Tuj1 and Myosin VIIa were used. The intensity of Tuj1 fluorescent signals in nerve fibers in the upper-base turn of the cochlea was analyzed and considered as ANF density. For the semi-quantitative analyses of 8-OHdG and 4-HNE expression, the intensity of the fluorescent signals in SGNs, HCs, or SV region in the upper-base turn of the cochlea was analyzed. Briefly, the images were converted into 8-bit grayscale type. The intensity of the background signal was subtracted and the average grayscale intensity of SGNs, HCs or SV region was then measured. The relative grayscale values were calculated by normalizing the ratio to the control group. The quantification of TFAM-mtDNA interaction was analyzed in the 70-μm segment at the base turn of the surface preparation. Those green fluorescent spots (dsDNA) in the cytoplasm that were not colocalized with red ones (TFAM) were considered as naked mtDNA. The total naked mtDNA spots in OHCs were counted and divided by the number of OHC within the image. All quantitative and semi-quantitative analyses were performed in four specimens for each group.

Extraction of Cochlear DNA and RNA

Six animals were sacrificed on day 1 after the third injection and six animals were sacrificed on day 3 after the ABR testing. The cochleae were dissected in Hanks' balanced salt solution on ice and frozen in liquid nitrogen until use. Twelve cochleae ($n = 4$ for each group) of the animals sacrificed on day 1 were used for the extraction of total RNA. Twelve cochleae ($n = 4$ for each group) of the animals sacrificed on day 3 were used for genomic DNA (gDNA) extraction. The gDNA and total RNA were extracted using the Tissue DNA Extraction Kit (TIANGEN, DP304) and RNeasy Plus Mini Kit (QIAGEN, #74134) according to the manufacturer's instructions, respectively. The purity and concentration of the DNA and RNA products were analyzed using the microplate spectrophotometer (BioTek, Epoch, USA). Then the isolated RNA was reverse transcribed to cDNA using PrimeScript RT Master Mix (TaKaRa, RR036A). The gDNA and cDNA products were stored at −20°C until use.

Quantification of mtDNA Copy Number and Mitochondrial Nd6 mRNA Expression

The mtDNA copy number and mitochondrial Nd6 expression were quantified by real-time polymerase chain reaction (PCR) assay using Real-Time PCR Detection System (Bio-Rad, CFX96, USA). The real-time PCR reaction system was prepared using TB Green Premix Ex Taq II (TaKaRa, RR820A) according to the manufacturer's instructions. The nuclear gene β-actin was used as the internal control. For the quantification of mtDNA copy number, the gDNA was used for the template. The cycle threshold (Ct) values of 12S rRNA (mtDNA) and β-actin (nDNA) were used to determine the relative mtDNA copy number. The following primers were designed: β-actin Forward: CTACCTCGCTGCAGGATCG, β-actin Reverse: GTCTACACCGCGGGAATACG, 12S rRNA Forward: AAGGAGAGGGCATCAAGCAC, and 12S rRNA Reverse: TATCACTGCTGAGTCCCGTG.

For the measurement of mitochondrial Nd6 mRNA expression, the cDNA was used as a template. The relative mRNA expression was estimated by the Ct values of Nd6 (mtDNA expression) and β-actin (nDNA expression). The following primers were designed: β-actin Forward: GGAGATTA CTGCCCTGGCTCCTA, β-actin Reverse: GACTCATCGTAC TCCTGCTTGCTG, Nd6 Forward: ACCCTCAAGTCTCCGG GTA, and Nd6 Reverse: GTCTAGGGTTGGCGTTGAAG. The relative levels of mtDNA copy number and mRNA expression in each group were analyzed using the $2^{-\Delta\Delta Ct}$ method.

ATP Level Measurement

Twelve animals ($n = 4$ for each group) in each group were sacrificed for cochlear ATP level measurement 1 h after the noise exposure. Two cochleae of an animal were quickly harvested and pooled as one sample. ATP levels in the cochlea were measured based on spectrophotometry using ATP Detection Kit (Solarbio, BC0305) according to the manufacturer's instructions. The working principle of the Kit is briefly described as follows. The Glucose and ATP are catalyzed by hexokinase to produce glucose 6-phosphate, which is further catalytically dehydrogenated to produce NADPH. The NADPH shows a characteristic absorption peak at 340 nm. The content of ATP is proportional to that of NADPH.

Extraction of Cochlear Protein and Immunoblotting

Twelve cochleae ($n = 4$ for each group) of six animals sacrificed on day 1 were homogenized in ice-cold RIPA lysis buffer (Beyotime, P0013B) containing protease inhibitor cocktail (Roche, #04693159001, Switzerland) using the cryogenic grinder. The tissue homogenate was placed on ice for 30 min, and then centrifuged at $12,000 \times g$ for 10 min at 4°C. The supernatant was retained and the protein concentration was determined using the BCA Determination Kit. Then the supernatant added with loading buffer was boiled for 5 min and stored at −20°C.

The protein samples (30 μg) were separated by 10–12% sodium dodecyl sulfate polyacrylamide gel electrophoresis (SDS-PAGE) electrophoresis and transferred to polyvinylidene fluoride (PVDF) membranes (Millipore, IPVH00010). After being blocked with 5% skimmed milk in TBS-T, the membranes were incubated for 1 h at room temperature on shaker and then overnight at 4°C with following primary antibodies: PGC-1α (Abcam, ab191838, 1:1,000), NRF-1 (GeneTex, GTX103179, 1:1,000), TFAM (Abcam, ab131607, 1:1,000), SOD2(GeneTex, GTX116093, 1:1,000), Bax (GeneTex, GTX109683, 1:1,000), ACTB (GeneTex, GTX109639, 1:2,000). The membranes were rinsed three times with TBS-T for 5 min, followed by incubation with HRP-linked secondary antibody (CST, #7074, 1:2,000) for 1 h at room temperature on a shaker. After being rinsed with TBS-T three times, the blots were visualized with chemiluminescent HRP substrate (Millipore, WBKLS0100) and

scanned using the Chemiluminescence Imaging System (Fusion, Solo 6S, China). The band intensities were quantified using the ImageJ software (version 1.53a, USA) and normalized by using ACTB as the internal control.

Statistics

Statistical analyses were conducted using IBM SPSS software (version 25.0, USA) and GraphPad Prism software (version 8.0, USA). The group comparisons were performed using two-tailed, two-sample Student's t-test or one-way analysis of variance (ANOVA). When the difference was significant, the LSD *post hoc* test was used to identify the difference between the two groups. The p-value of <0.05 was considered statistical significance. All the data were presented as mean ± standard deviation (SD).

RESULTS

MT Entered Inner Ear After Systemic Administration

In order to investigate whether MT existed in the inner ear after the systemic administration, we analyzed the concentration of MT in the perilymph of the cochlea using LC-MS/MS. The perilymph was extracted 15 min after the injection and used for the detection and quantification of MT. As shown in **Supplementary Figures 1A–C**, the retention time of the MT in the perilymph was 3.302 min. The mass-to-charge ratio (m/z) of the parent ion was 474.2, which was consistent with the relative molecular mass of MT losing a chloride ion (**Supplementary Figure 1D**). The concentration of the MT in the perilymph of the cochlea was 18.541 μg/kg 15 min after the injection. These results indicated that MT could pass through the BLB and enter the inner ear.

Administration of MT Attenuated Noise-Induced Auditory Threshold Shift

To address whether systemic use of MT might prevent NIHL, we designed the experimental procedure as shown in **Figure 1**. The hearing function of the animals was evaluated via ABR testing 2 days before (−2d), 3 and 14 days after (+3d and +14d) noise exposure. There is no significant difference in baseline ABR threshold between groups (**Supplementary Figure 2**). Compared with saline-treated rats, MT-treated rats showed significantly decreased TTS on day 3 and PTS on day 14 at 8, 16, 24, and 32 kHz (**Figures 2A–D**). The 112dB noise exposure for 2 h resulted in about 30–40 dB threshold shift at all four frequencies on day 14 in the vehicle-treated group. However, in the MT-treated group, the threshold at 8 kHz was completely recovered and threshold shifts at 24 and 32 kHz were both within 10 dB on day 14 (**Figures 2E,F**). These data indicated that MT administration was able to attenuate noise-induced transient and permanent hearing loss.

MT Treatment Prevented OHC Loss Induced by Acoustic Trauma

We then asked if MT exhibits a protective effect on the OHC, which is one of the most vulnerable structures of the cochlea during acoustic trauma. We used the surface preparation

mito-TEMPO Attenuates Oxidative Stress and Mitochondrial Dysfunction in Noise-Induced Hearing Loss...

173

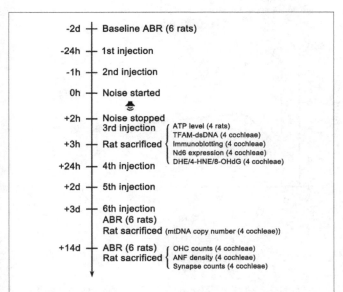

FIGURE 1 | Experimental timeline. The baseline hearing function of the rats was evaluated via ABR testing 2 days (2d) before the noise exposure. Rats were intraperitoneally injected with MT or vehicle (saline) 24 h and 1 h before the noise started. Then rats were exposed to 112dB SPL 8–16 kHz octave band noise for 2 h. The third shot was injected immediately after the noise stopped. One hour later, 12 animals in each group were sacrificed for analyses of oxidative stress level, mtDNA expression quantification, ATP measurement, immunoblotting and TFAM-mtDNA interaction. The rest of the animals received three additional injections once daily for the following 3 days. Then ABR testing were performed 3d after the noise exposure to evaluate TTS level. Then two animals in each group were sacrificed for the quantification of cochlear mtDNA copy number. After ABR testing 14d after the noise exposure for PTS level assessment, the remaining animals were sacrificed for analyses of OHC loss, IHC ribbon synapse loss and ANF degeneration. ABR, Auditory Brainstem Response.

technique to analyze the OHC loss 14 days after the noise exposure. The cochlea was divided into the apex, middle and base turns, which correspond to the low-, middle- and high-frequency regions of the cochlea. The loss of both the nucleus (DAPI) and the cell body (Myosin VIIa) was considered as the OHC loss. As shown in **Figures 3A,B**, noise overstimulation resulted in the most OHC loss at the base turn in the vehicle-treated group, showing 81.5% of the OHC survival. Compared with the vehicle-treated group, MT treatment significantly reduced noise-induced OHC loss at the base and middle turns of the cochlea. The OHC survival reached 95.2% at the base turn in the MT-treated group. These results indicated that MT was able to prevent OHC death after acoustic trauma.

MT Treatment Reduced IHC Ribbon Synapse Loss and ANF Degeneration Induced by Acoustic Trauma

Recent studies show that the loss of ribbon synapses between IHCs and spiral ganglion neurons (SGNs) is the primary pathology in NIHL, which is termed cochlear synaptopathy (Liberman and Kujawa, 2017). To explore the protective effect of MT against noise-induced IHC ribbon synapse loss, we quantified the number of paired ribbon synapses 14 days after

the noise exposure. The surface preparations of the cochlea at approximately 16–20 kHz region were immunolabelled with antibodies against CtBP2 and GluA2 to manifest the pre- and post-synaptic structures. The juxtaposition of CtBP2 and GluA2 represents the functional synapses. In the vehicle-treated group, a significant decrease in the number of paired synapses was observed after noise exposure. Compared with the vehicle-treated group, treatment with MT significantly reduced the noise-induced loss of the paired ribbon synapses (**Figures 4A,B**).

In addition, NIHL is associated with the degeneration of ANFs which extend from SGNs to IHC ribbon synapses (Kujawa and Liberman, 2009). We next explored the protective effect of MT against noise-induced ANF degeneration by measuring the density of the fiber 14 days after the noise exposure. Compared with the control group, there was more than 50% degeneration of ANF in the vehicle-treated group. The remaining nerve fibers were fragmented and in a disordered arrangement. However, treatment with MT significantly recovered the density of ANF after acoustic trauma. The integrity of nerve fibers was partially restored in the MT-treated group (**Figures 4C,D**). These results indicated the neuroprotective effect of the MT against IHC ribbon synapse loss and ANF degeneration in NIHL.

MT Treatment Mitigated Oxidative Stress in the Cochlea After the Noise Exposure

Excessive ROS production is a major causative factor in noise-induced cochlear injury and hearing loss. ROS oxidizes polyunsaturated fatty acids to produce cytotoxic aldehydes. Among these, 4-hydroxynonenal (4-HNE) represents one of the major products of lipid peroxidation (Di Domenico et al., 2017). Dihydroethidium (DHE) is a fluorescent dye for detecting the level of superoxide ion ($O_2\cdot^-$). In the presence of $O_2\cdot^-$, DHE is oxidized to 2-hydroxyethidium, the fluorescence of which can be measured at an excitation and emission wavelength of 480 nm and 567 nm (Fetoni et al., 2015). In the present study, the level of cochlear oxidative stress was analyzed by 4-HNE and DHE fluorescent staining. As shown in **Figure 5A**, noise overstimulation induced a substantial increase of 4-HNE generation in the cochlea. Increased 4-HNE was mainly observed in HCs, stria vascularis (SV), and SGNs of the cochlea (**Supplementary Figure 3**). Compared with the vehicle-treated group, MT treatment significantly attenuated 4-HNE generation after the noise exposure. The DHE assay showed similar results. MT treatment remarkably reduced the DHE fluorescence induced by the noise overstimulation (**Figure 5B**). These data indicated that MT alleviated noise-induced oxidative stress in the cochlea by reducing the level of lipid peroxidation and $O_2\cdot^-$ generation.

MT Treatment Alleviated mtDNA Oxidative Damage, and Maintained Mitochondrial Biogenesis and ATP Production After the Acoustic Trauma

The mitochondria are semi-autonomous organelles that contain their own circular genetic system. The mitochondrial genomes encode 13 essential protein subunits of the MRC complexes.

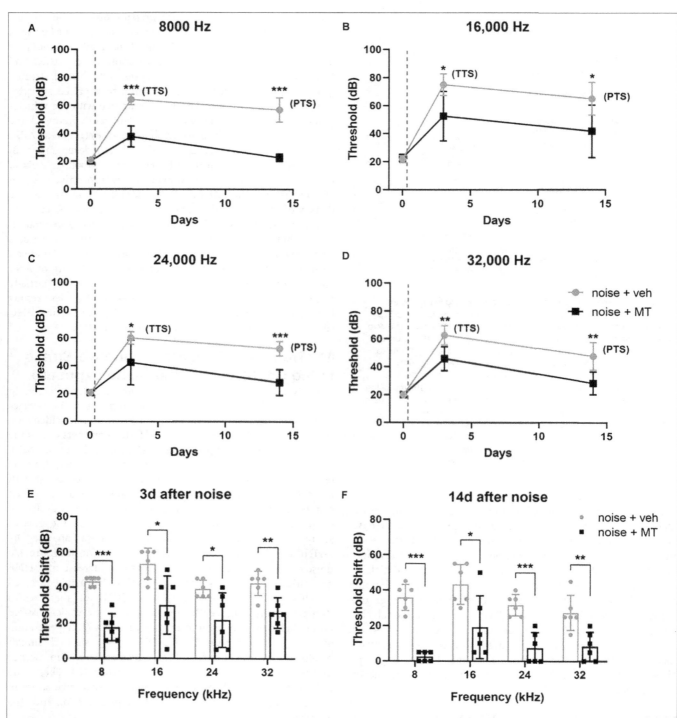

FIGURE 2 | MT treatment attenuated noise-induced auditory threshold shifts. **(A–D)** The auditory threshold alterations of the left ear of animals at 8, 16, 24 and 32 kHz over time. The baseline threshold, TTS, and PTS were evaluated before, 3d after and 14d after the noise exposure respectively. **(E,F)** The auditory threshold shifts over four frequencies on the day 3 and the day 14. The gray dotted lines indicate the time of acoustic trauma. Data are presented as means ± SD, n = 6 for each group, *p < 0.05, **p < 0.01, ***p < 0.001. MT, mito-TEMPO; TTS, temporary threshold shift; PTS, permanent threshold shift.

As is located close to the site of ROS generation, mtDNA molecules are easily damaged, resulting in decreased mtDNA content and mitochondrial dysfunction (Kang et al., 2007). 8-hydroxy-2'-deoxyguanosine (8-OHdG) is one of the most abundant oxidative adducts of DNA, reflecting the level of DNA oxidative damage (Han et al., 2020). In **Figures 6A,B**, a dramatic increase of 8-OHdG production was observed in the cytoplasm of SGNs following noise exposure. Since the DNA in cytoplasm

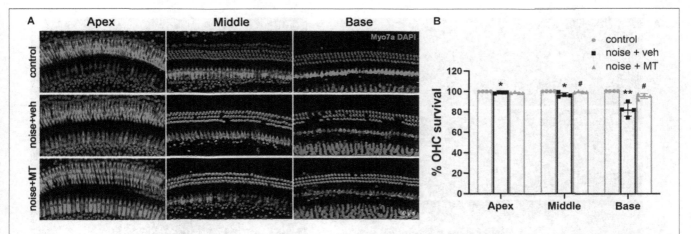

FIGURE 3 | MT treatment prevented noise-induced OHC loss. **(A)** Representative images of the apex, middle and base turn region of cochlear surface preparations 14 days after the noise exposure. HCs were indicated by Myosin VIIa (red) and DAPI (blue) fluorescent staining. **(B)** Quantification analysis of OHC survival in the apex, middle and base turn region of the cochlea 14 days after the noise exposure. Data are presented as means ± SD, $n = 4$ for each group, $^*p < 0.05$ vs. control group, $^{**}p < 0.01$ vs. control group, $^\#p < 0.05$ vs. vehicle-treated group. OHC, outer hair cell; HCs, hair cells.

refers to mtDNA, increased cytoplasmic 8-OHdG indicated that acoustic trauma-induced mtDNA oxidative damage in SGNs. Compared with the vehicle-treated group, treatment of MT significantly reduced noise-induced 8-OHdG production in SGNs.

Mitochondrial biogenesis relies on mtDNA replication and transcription to maintain mtDNA content and expression, and to produce new mitochondria. mtDNA is a multicopy genome and maintained at a relatively stable content (Scarpulla, 2008). Noise exposure resulted in a significant reduction of mtDNA content in the cochlea, reflected by the mtDNA copy number (**Figure 6C**). The mRNA level of MRC gene mt-Nd6 was also decreased after noise exposure, suggesting that the mtDNA expression in the cochlea was impaired by acoustic trauma (**Figure 6D**). In addition, ATP level in the cochlea was decreased following noise exposure, which indicated the dysfunction of the MRC (**Figure 6E**). However, treatment with MT significantly restored mtDNA content, mtDNA expression, and ATP level in the cochlea after noise exposure compared with the vehicle-treated group. These data indicated that MT was able to alleviate noise-induced mtDNA oxidative damage, maintain mitochondrial biogenesis and improve mitochondrial function of the cochlea.

MT Treatment Mitigated Noise-Induced Downregulation of TFAM and SOD2 Independent of the PGC-1α/NRF-1/TFAM Pathway

Mitochondrial biogenesis is a dynamic process of the generation of new mitochondria by synthesizing mitochondrial DNA and proteins. This activity requires several nucleus-encoded transcription factors, including peroxisome proliferator-activated receptor-gamma coactivator-1alpha (PGC-1α), nuclear respiratory factor 1 and 2 (NRF-1 and NRF-2), mitochondrial transcription factor A (TFAM), B1 (TFB1M), and B2 (TFB2M; Scarpulla, 2008). The PGC-1α/NRF-1/TFAM axis is the most studied pathway in regulating the replication and expression of

mtDNA and mitochondrial biogenesis (Zhao et al., 2013; Xiong et al., 2019). In the above experiment, we found that acoustic trauma led to the decline of mtDNA content and expression level. To further explore the underlying mechanism, we next investigated the expression of PGC-1α/NRF-1/TFAM after noise exposure. As shown in **Figures 7A–D**, the expression level of PGC-1α and NRF-1 did not change following noise exposure. However, noise overstimulation resulted in a significant decrease in TFAM expression in the cochlea (**Figures 7A,E**). These results indicated that noise-induced decline of mtDNA content and expression was associated with TFAM reduction independent of PGC-1α/NRF-1/TFAM pathway. Compared with the vehicle-treated group, MT treatment attenuated TFAM expression reduction after the noise exposure.

Of the family of superoxide dismutase (SODs), only SOD2 (Mn-SOD) is located in mitochondria (Gross et al., 2014). We observed that noise exposure induced a dramatic decrease in the expression of mitochondrial SOD2 (**Figures 7A,F**). MT treatment partially improved SOD2 expression compared with the vehicle-treated group. In addition, the expression of the pro-apoptotic protein Bax was slightly upregulated following acoustic trauma and alleviated by MT treatment (**Figures 7B,G**). These data suggested that MT prevented noise-induced disruption of the mitochondrial antioxidant defense, and inhibited apoptosis activation in the inner ear.

MT Treatment Improved the Disruption of TFAM-mtDNA Interaction in the Cochlea After the Noise Exposure

TFAM binds the D-loop region of the mitochondrial genome to initiate mtDNA transcription and replication. TFAM also maintains the stability of mtDNA in a sequence-independent binding manner. We investigated the mtDNA-binding ability of TFAM by immunofluorescence colocalization analysis of TFAM and the double-stranded DNA (dsDNA) in the cytoplasm. As shown in **Figure 8A**, most mtDNA molecules were bound

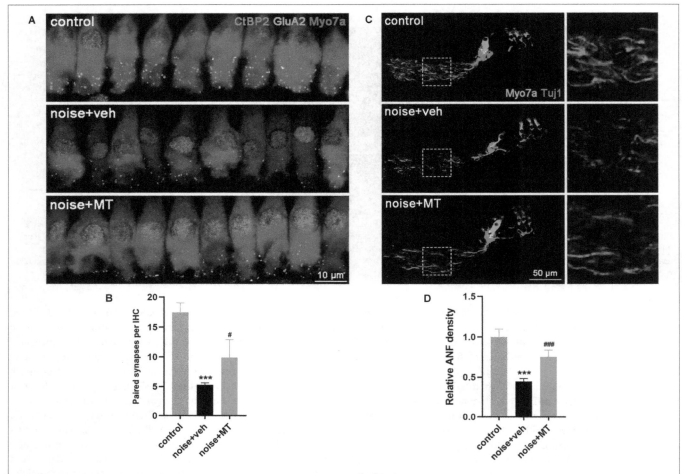

FIGURE 4 | MT treatment reduced IHC ribbon synapse loss and ANF degeneration induced by acoustic trauma. **(A)** Representative images of the IHC ribbon synapse at approximately 16–20 kHz region of the cochlea 14d after the noise exposure. Cochlear surface preparations were immunolabelled with CtBP2 (red), GluA2 (green) and Myosin VIIa (blue). **(B)** Quantification analysis of paired synapse per IHC, indicated by the juxtaposition of CtBP2 and GluA2. **(C)** Representative images of ANF and HCs in middle turn area of the midmodiolar sections 14d after the noise exposure. Cochlear sections were immunolabelled with Tuj1 (red) and Myosin VIIa (green). **(D)** Quantification analysis of ANF density 14d after the noise exposure. Data are presented as means ± SD, $n = 4$ for each group, ***$p < 0.001$ vs. control group, #$p < 0.05$ vs. vehicle-treated group, ###$p < 0.001$ vs. vehicle-treated group. IHC, inner hair cell; ANF, auditory nerve fiber.

to TFAM (yellow arrows) within sensory hair cells labeled by Phalloidin in the control group. However, noise exposure induced a reduction of TFAM-mtDNA interaction, leading to a significant increase of naked mtDNA (white arrows) in the cytoplasm of OHCs. MT treatment partially recovered the TFAM-mtDNA interaction and significantly alleviated the increase of naked mtDNA in OHCs (**Figures 8A,B**). These data indicated that the mtDNA-binding activity of TFAM was weakened in the cochlea following acoustic trauma. MT treatment could restore the binding function of TFAM.

DISCUSSION

MT is a novelly developed mitochondria-target antioxidant with the ability to pass through the phospholipid bilayer and accumulate in mitochondria. In the present study, we investigated the protective effect of MT against NIHL and the underlying mechanism in a rat model. We found that MT

reduced noise-induced threshold shift and prevented OHC loss, IHC ribbon synapse loss, and ANF degeneration after the noise exposure. We demonstrated that MT exerted its protective effect on hearing by reducing the level of oxidative stress and mtDNA damage, restoring TFAM-mtDNA interaction and mitochondrial function of the inner ear.

HCs and SGNs are two important cells responsible for the perception, mechanoelectrical transduction, and transmission of auditory signals. We found that acoustic trauma led to OHC loss while IHC remained intact. This differential vulnerability may be due to the difference in intrinsic antioxidant capacity between IHCs and OHCs (Sha et al., 2001; Rosenhall et al., 2019). However, the amount of paired ribbon synapses between IHCs and SGNs was significantly reduced after the noise exposure. ANFs are the peripheral neurites of SGNs. Noise-induced ANF degeneration was observed in our experiments. In addition, the damage of cochlear ribbon synapses and ANFs is also the pathologic change of noise-induced hidden hearing loss

mito-TEMPO Attenuates Oxidative Stress and Mitochondrial Dysfunction in Noise-Induced Hearing Loss...

177

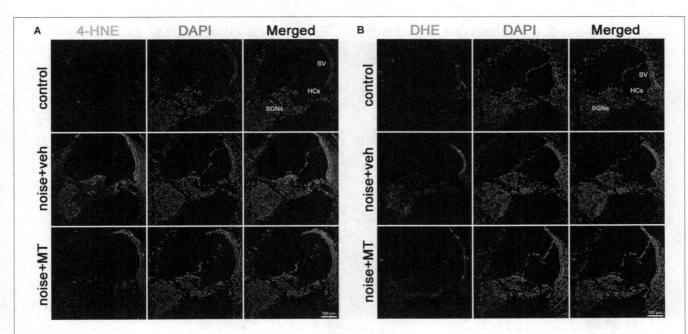

FIGURE 5 | MT treatment mitigated ROS generation in the cochlea. **(A)** Representative images of 4-HNE (green) and DAPI (blue) fluorescent staining in base turn area of the midmodiolar sections 1 h after the noise exposure. **(B)** Representative images of DHE (red) and DAPI (blue) fluorescent staining in base turn area of the midmodiolar sections 1 h after the noise exposure. Four cochleae form two animals were used in each group. HCs, hair cells; SV, stria vascularis; SGNs, spiral ganglion neurons; ROS, reactive oxygen species.

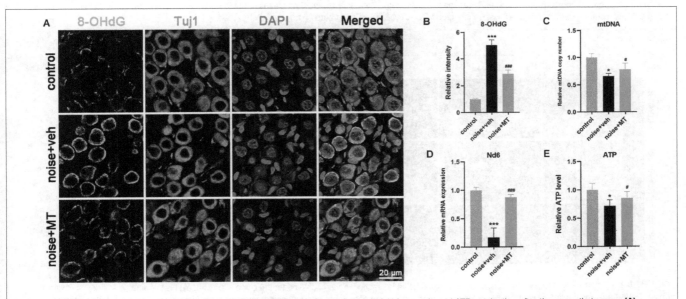

FIGURE 6 | MT treatment alleviated mtDNA oxidative damage, and maintained mitochondrial biogenesis and ATP production after the acoustic trauma. **(A)** Representative images of 8-OHdG (green), Tuj1 (red) and DAPI (blue) fluorescent staining in SGNs in frozen sections of the cochlea 1 h after the noise exposure. **(B)** Semi-quantitative analysis of the fluorescent intensity of 8-OHdG in SGNs 1 h after the noise exposure. **(C)** Real time-qPCR analysis of mtDNA copy number in the cochlea 3d after the noise exposure. **(D)** Real time-qPCR analysis of mitochondrial Nd6 expression level in the cochlear 1 h after the noise exposure. **(E)** The ATP level in the cochlea 1 h after the noise exposure. Data are presented as means ± SD, $n = 4$ for each group, $^{*}p < 0.05$ vs. control group, $^{***}p < 0.001$ vs. control group, $^{#}p < 0.05$ vs. vehicle-treated group, $^{###}p < 0.001$ vs. vehicle-treated group.

(NIHHL; Kujawa and Liberman, 2009; Liberman and Kujawa, 2017). The protective effect of MT on ribbon synapses and ANFs suggested its promising application to prevent NIHHL, which needs further investigations.

The present study showed increased oxidative stress indicated by cochlear 4-HNE and DHE level, which is consistent with previous studies (Park et al., 2014; Paciello et al., 2020; He et al., 2021b). We observed increased mtDNA oxidative damage

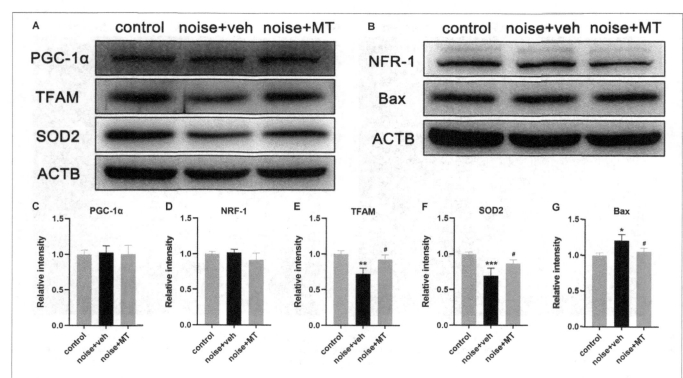

FIGURE 7 | MT treatment mitigated noise-induced downregulation of TFAM and SOD2 independent of the PGC-1α/NRF-1/TFAM pathway. **(A,B)** Immunoblotting of the PGC-1α, NRF-1, TFAM, SOD2, Bax, and ACTB protein in the cochlea 1 h after the noise exposure. **(C–G)** Quantification analysis of the optical density values of the immunoblot bands normalized by using ACTB as the internal control. Data are presented as means ± SD, $n = 4$ for each group, $*p < 0.05$ vs. control group, $**p < 0.01$ vs. control group, $***p < 0.001$ vs. control group, $\#p < 0.05$ vs. vehicle-treated group.

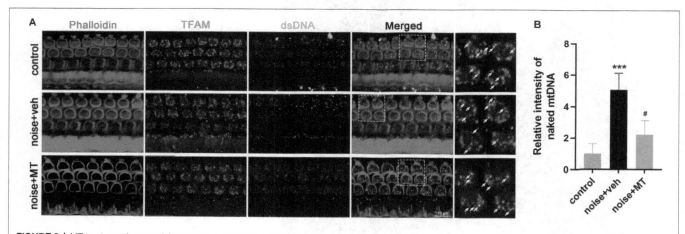

FIGURE 8 | MT treatment improved the disruption of TFAM-mtDNA interaction in the cochlea after the noise exposure. **(A)** Representative images of Phalloidin (blue), TFAM (red), and dsDNA (green) fluorescent staining in base turn area of the cochlear surface preparation 1 h after the noise exposure. Colocalized spots of TFAM and dsDNA were indicated in yellow arrows, while "orphan" dsDNA spots without colocalization of TFAM were indicated in the white arrows. **(B)** Quantification analysis of naked mtDNA in OHCs 1 h after the noise exposure. Data are presented as means ± SD, $n = 4$ for each group, $***p < 0.001$ vs. control group, $\#p < 0.05$ vs. vehicle-treated group.

indicated by 8-OHdG in SGNs 1 h after noise exposure. The cochlear mitochondrial function indicated by the ATP content was also impaired 1 h after the noise exposure, which is consistent with a previous study (Chen et al., 2012). Maintaining an adequate content of mtDNA copy number is important for cellular energy metabolism. Mitochondrial ROS induced by noise caused oxidative damage to mtDNA, resulting in mitochondrial dysfunction and energy insufficiency. SGNs are auditory neurons and consume a lot of energy in axoplasmic transport and electrical signal transmission. When the number and function of the mitochondria in SGNs are impaired, the transport of cellular cargos including neurotrophin might be disrupted, resulting in the degeneration of the neurites of SGNs. Mitochondrial biogenesis is an activity to generate new mitochondria from the existing ones. This process requires the coordination of mtDNA replication and expression and is regulated by several transcription factors. The present study showed that mtDNA content and expression level were both decreased after noise exposure, which indicated the impaired mitochondrial biogenesis in the inner ear after the acoustic trauma. Yu and colleagues found mtDNA common deletion induced by D-gal increased susceptibility to NIHL in rats (Yu et al., 2014), suggesting the correlation between mtDNA integrity and the pathogenesis of NIHL. Interestingly, we found that the mtDNA expression level decreased immediately following the acoustic trauma (1 h after the noise exposure). In contrast, mtDNA copy number did not reduce until the third day after the noise exposure. The possible explanation is that DNA is more stable and has a longer half-life than RNA. It takes time for mtDNA to be degraded after oxidative stress damage. Previous studies also showed that mtDNA copy numbers decrease several days after the environmental stress (Bagul et al., 2018; Sugasawa et al., 2021).

The PGC-1α/NRF-1/TFAM axis is one of the most important pathways in regulating mitochondrial biogenesis. However, there are few studies on the alteration of the PGC-1α/NRF-1/TFAM pathway during acoustic trauma. In order to further explore the mechanism by which mtDNA content and expression are impaired in NIHL, we analyzed the expression level of this pathway. We found that the expression level of TFAM significantly decreased after the noise exposure, while the expression level of PGC-1α and NRF-1 remained unchanged. In addition, the TFAM function, as indicated by the mtDNA-binding ability, was also disrupted in OHCs after the noise exposure. These results indicate that noise-induced ROS specifically impairs the expression and function of TFAM without affecting the upstream PGC-1α and NRF-1. OHCs exhibit electromotility and mechanically amplify sound-evoked vibrations, which is an energy-consuming process. The impaired TFAM-mtDNA interaction leads to an increase of naked mtDNA molecules, which are vulnerable to oxidative damage by ROS. The abnormal mtDNA hinders the expression of mitochondrial respiratory chain proteins and ATP synthesis and might contribute to OHC dysfunction and death. A previous study showed that the phosphorylation and acetylation of TFAM within its HMG-box 1 domain reduced the DNA binding affinity, leading to TFAM-mtDNA disassembly (King et al., 2018). In addition, phosphorylation at serine 55/56 facilitated rapid degradation of TFAM by the Lon protease in mitochondria (Lu et al., 2013). Since it has been reported that acoustic trauma activates the protein kinase such as AMPK and extracellular signal-regulated protein kinase (ERK) in the inner ear (Kurioka et al., 2015; Hill et al., 2016), phosphorylation regulation might play a relevant role in the impaired expression and binding function of TFAM after the noise exposure. This speculation deserves further exploration in future studies.

Since oxidative stress plays an important role in the pathogenesis of NIHL, the antioxidants have been extensively studied in attenuating NIHL (Pak et al., 2020). A number of antioxidants show protective effects against NIHL in animal models such as glutathione, N-acetylcysteine (NAC), D-methionine, vitamin C, water-soluble coenzyme Q10, ebselen, resveratrol, and HK-2 (Ohinata et al., 2000; Seidman, 2003; Duan et al., 2004; Lynch et al., 2004; McFadden et al., 2005; Fetoni et al., 2009; Ewert et al., 2012; Chen et al., 2020), some of which have entered clinical trials (Kopke et al., 2015; Kil et al., 2017; Rosenhall et al., 2019). However, conventional antioxidants cannot remove only excess ROS without suppressing physiological ROS which are important for signal transduction. Recently, mitochondria-target antioxidants have been developed for the treatment of oxidative stress-related disease for their capacity to scavenge ROS from the source (Fujimoto and Yamasoba, 2019). MT is the antioxidant TEMPOL conjugated to the lipophilic triphenylphosphonium (TPP) cation, which can easily pass through the phospholipid bilayer and accumulate several hundred-fold into mitochondria (Trnka et al., 2008). A previous study shows that MT is BBB-penetrating and can be used as the contrast media in enhanced-magnetic resonance imaging (MRI) of the brain (Zhelev et al., 2013). In the present study, we demonstrated the existent of MT in the inner ear after the systemic administration. The lipophilic property of MT makes it easy to pass through the BLB and exert the antioxidant effects in the inner ear. MT exhibited a protective effect on hearing and cochlear cells against acoustic trauma. MT treatment reduced mitochondrial ROS production induced by noise exposure and therefore alleviated mtDNA oxidative damage and mitochondrial dysfunction. These results are consistent with a recent study (Zhao et al., 2021) which showed that MT alleviated ischemic acute kidney injury via reducing mitochondrial ROS and promoting TFAM-mediated mtDNA maintenance.

This study has several limitations. First, the methods used for hearing function evaluation were relatively simple. Four tested frequencies of the ABR covered about 50% length of the cochlea (from 30% to 80%), and may not represent well the hearing status of the animal. In future studies, we will use distortion product otoacoustic emissions (DPOAE) and compound action potential (CAP) for a comprehensive assessment of hearing function. Secondly, due to the technical difficulties, the RNA of HCs and SGNs was unable to be separately isolated. The alterations of mRNA expression of HCs and SGNs could not be analyzed respectively. Other methods such as RNA fluorescence in situ hybridization (FISH) will be used in our future studies. Finally, electron microscopy analysis of mitochondria was not performed in the present studies. Since mitochondrial fusion and fission are crucial processes to maintain mitochondrial homeostasis (Chan, 2020), the morphological changes of cochlear mitochondria in NIHL will be further studied in the following work.

In summary, our results first show TFAM reduction and the disruption of TFAM-mtDNA interaction in NIHL. Noise-induced ROS lead to mtDNA oxidative damage, impairing mtDNA expression and mitochondrial biogenesis. MT treatment exhibits a protective effect on hearing, OHCs,

IHC synapses, and ANFs against acoustic trauma partially by maintaining TFAM-mtDNA interaction and mitochondrial biogenesis based on its strong capacity of mitochondrial ROS scavenging.

AUTHOR CONTRIBUTIONS

L-JL and QY designed the research. J-WC, P-WM, HY, W-LW, and P-HL performed the experiments. X-RD, Y-QL, and L-JL

analyzed the data. J-WC prepared the figures. J-WC, QY, and L-JL wrote the manuscript. All authors contributed to the article and approved the submitted version.

ACKNOWLEDGMENTS

We thank Xi-Wang Hu and Ren-Feng Wang for their valuable guidance in image acquisition and ABR measurement. We also thank Qian Huo for proofreading the manuscript.

REFERENCES

Abdullah-Al-Shoeb, M., Sasaki, K., Kikutani, S., Namba, N., Ueno, K., Kondo, Y., et al. (2020). The late-stage protective effect of mito-TEMPO against acetaminophen-induced hepatotoxicity in mouse and three-dimensional cell culture models. *Antioxidants (Basel)* 9:965. doi: 10.3390/antiox9100965

Bagul, P., Katare, P., Bugga, P., Dinda, A., and Banerjee, S. K. (2018). SIRT-3 modulation by resveratrol improves mitochondrial oxidative phosphorylation in diabetic heart through deacetylation of TFAM. *Cells* 7:235. doi: 10.3390/cells7120235

Blazer, D. G., and Tucci, D. L. (2019). Hearing loss and psychiatric disorders: a review. *Psychol. Med.* 49, 891–897. doi: 10.1017/S0033291718003409

Böttger, E. C., and Schacht, J. (2013). The mitochondrion: a perpetrator of acquired hearing loss. *Hear. Res.* 303, 12–19. doi: 10.1016/j.heares.2013.01.006

Chan, D. C. (2020). Mitochondrial dynamics and its involvement in disease. *Ann. Rev. Pathol.* 15, 235–259. doi: 10.1146/annurev-pathmechdis-012419-032711

Chandrasekaran, K., Anjaneyulu, M., Inoue, T., Choi, J., Sagi, A. R., Chen, C., et al. (2015). Mitochondrial transcription factor A regulation of mitochondrial degeneration in experimental diabetic neuropathy. *Am. J. Physiol. Endocrinol. Metab.* 309, E132–141. doi: 10.1152/ajpendo.00620.2014

Chen, G. D., Daszynski, D. M., Ding, D., Jiang, H., Woolman, T., Blessing, K., et al. (2020). Novel oral multifunctional antioxidant prevents noise-induced hearing loss and hair cell loss. *Hear. Res.* 388:107880. doi: 10.1016/j.heares.2019.107880

Chen, F. Q., Zheng, H. W., Hill, K., and Sha, S. H. (2012). Traumatic noise activates Rho-family GTPases through transient cellular energy depletion. *J. Neurosci.* 32, 12421–12430. doi: 10.1523/JNEUROSCI.6381-11.2012

Coleman, J. K. M., Kopke, R. D., Liu, J., Ge, X., Harper, E. A., Jones, G. E., et al. (2007). Pharmacological rescue of noise induced hearing loss using N-acetylcysteine and acetyl-l-carnitine. *Hear. Res.* 226, 104–113. doi: 10.1016/j.heares.2006.08.008

Di Domenico, F., Tramutola, A., and Butterfield, D. A. (2017). Role of 4-hydroxy-2-nonenal (HNE) in the pathogenesis of Alzheimer disease and other selected age-related neurodegenerative disorders. *Free Radic. Biol. Med.* 111, 253–261. doi: 10.1016/j.freeradbiomed.2016.10.490

Ding, X., Wang, W., Chen, J., Zhao, Q., Lu, P., and Lu, L. (2019). Salidroside protects inner ear hair cells and spiral ganglion neurons from manganese exposure by regulating ROS levels and inhibiting apoptosis. *Toxicol. Lett.* 310, 51–60. doi: 10.1016/j.toxlet.2019.04.016

Du, K., Farhood, A., and Jaeschke, H. (2017). Mitochondria-targeted antioxidant mito-tempo protects against acetaminophen hepatotoxicity. *Arch. Toxicol.* 91, 761–773. doi: 10.1007/s00204-016-1692-0

Duan, M., Qiu, J., Laurell, G., Olofsson, Å., Allen Counter, S., and Borg, E. (2004). Dose and time-dependent protection of the antioxidant N-l-acetylcysteine against impulse noise trauma. *Hear. Res.* 192, 1–9. doi: 10.1016/j.heares.2004.02.005

Ewert, D. L., Lu, J., Li, W., Du, X., Floyd, R., and Kopke, R. (2012). Antioxidant treatment reduces blast-induced cochlear damage and hearing loss. *Hear. Res.* 285, 29–39. doi: 10.1016/j.heares.2012.01.013

Fernandez, K., Spielbauer, K. K., Rusheen, A., Wang, L., Baker, T. G., Eyles, S., et al. (2020). Lovastatin protects against cisplatin-induced hearing loss in mice. *Hear. Res.* 389:107905. doi: 10.1016/j.heares.2020.107905

Fetoni, A. R., Paciello, F., Rolesi, R., Eramo, S. L., Mancuso, C., Troiani, D., et al. (2015). Rosmarinic acid up-regulates the noise-activated Nrf2/HO-1 pathway and protects against noise-induced injury in rat cochlea. *Free Radic. Biol. Med.* 85, 269–281. doi: 10.1016/j.freeradbiomed.2015.04.021

Fetoni, A. R., Paciello, F., Rolesi, R., Paludetti, G., and Troiani, D. (2019). Targeting dysregulation of redox homeostasis in noise-induced hearing loss: oxidative stress and ROS signaling. *Free Radic. Bio. Med.* 135, 46–59. doi: 10.1016/j.freeradbiomed.2019.02.022

Fetoni, A. R., Piacentini, R., Fiorita, A., Paludetti, G., and Troiani, D. (2009). Water-soluble Coenzyme Q10 formulation (Q-ter) promotes outer hair cell survival in a guinea pig model of noise induced hearing loss (NIHL). *Brain Res.* 1257, 108–116. doi: 10.1016/j.brainres.2008.12.027

Fischel-Ghodsian, N., Kopke, R. D., and Ge, X. (2004). Mitochondrial dysfunction in hearing loss. *Mitochondrion* 4, 675–694. doi: 10.1016/j.mito.2004.07.040

Fujimoto, C., and Yamasoba, T. (2019). Mitochondria-targeted antioxidants for treatment of hearing loss: a systematic review. *Antioxidants (Basel)* 8:109. doi: 10.3390/antiox8040109

Gross, J., Olze, H., and Mazurek, B. (2014). Differential expression of transcription factors and inflammation-, ROS- and cell death-related genes in organotypic cultures in the modiolus, the organ of corti and the stria vascularis of newborn rats. *Cell. Mol. Neurobiol.* 34, 523–538. doi: 10.1007/s10571-014-0036-y

Han, S., Du, Z., Liu, K., and Gong, S. (2020). Nicotinamide riboside protects noise-induced hearing loss by recovering the hair cell ribbon synapses. *Neurosci. Lett.* 725:134910. doi: 10.1016/j.neulet.2020.134910

He, Z., Guo, L., Shu, Y., Fang, Q., Zhou, H., Liu, Y., et al. (2017). Autophagy protects auditory hair cells against neomycin-induced damage. *Autophagy* 13, 1884–1904. doi: 10.1080/15548627.2017.1359449

He, Z., Li, M., Fang, Q., Liao, F., Zou, S., Wu, X., et al. (2021a). FOXG1 promotes aging inner ear hair cell survival through activation of the autophagy pathway. *Autophagy* 17, 4341–4362. doi: 10.1080/15548627.2021.1916194

He, Z., Pan, S., Zheng, H., Fang, Q., Hill, K., and Sha, S. (2021b). Treatment with calcineurin inhibitor FK506 attenuates noise-induced hearing loss. *Front. Cell Dev. Biol.* 9:648461. doi: 10.3389/fcell.2021.648461

Hill, K., Yuan, H., Wang, X., and Sha, S. H. (2016). Noise-induced loss of hair cells and cochlear synaptopathy are mediated by the activation of AMPK. *J. Neurosci.* 36, 7497–7510. doi: 10.1523/JNEUROSCI.0782-16.2016

Kang, D., Kim, S. H., and Hamasaki, N. (2007). Mitochondrial transcription factor A (TFAM): Roles in maintenance of mtDNA and cellular functions. *Mitochondrion* 7, 39–44. doi: 10.1016/j.mito.2006.11.017

Kil, J., Lobarinas, E., Spankovich, C., Griffiths, S. K., Antonelli, P. J., Lynch, E. D., et al. (2017). Safety and efficacy of ebselen for the prevention of noise-induced hearing loss: a randomised, double-blind, placebo-controlled, phase 2 trial. *Lancet* 390, 969–979. doi: 10.1016/S0140-6736(17)31791-9

King, G. A., Hashemi, S. M., Taris, K. H., Pandey, A. K., Venkatesh, S., Thilagavathi, J., et al. (2018). Acetylation and phosphorylation of human TFAM regulate TFAM-DNA interactions via contrasting mechanisms. *Nucleic Acids Res.* 46, 3633–3642. doi: 10.1093/nar/gky204

Kopke, R., Slade, M. D., Jackson, R., Hammill, T., Fausti, S., Lonsbury-Martin, B., et al. (2015). Efficacy and safety of N-acetylcysteine in prevention of noise induced hearing loss: a randomized clinical trial. *Hear. Res.* 323, 40–50. doi: 10.1016/j.heares.2015.01.002

Kujawa, S. G., and Liberman, M. C. (2009). Adding insult to injury: cochlear nerve degeneration after "temporary" noise-induced hearing loss. *J. Neurosci.* 29, 14077–14085. doi: 10.1523/JNEUROSCI.2845-09.2009

Kurabi, A., Keithley, E. M., Housley, G. D., Ryan, A. F., and Wong, A. C. Y. (2017). Cellular mechanisms of noise-induced hearing loss. *Hear. Res.* 349, 129–137. doi: 10.1016/j.heares.2016.11.013

Kurioka, T., Matsunobu, T., Satoh, Y., Niwa, K., Endo, S., Fujioka, M., et al. (2015). ERK2 mediates inner hair cell survival and decreases susceptibility to noise-induced hearing loss. *Sci. Rep.* 5:16839. doi: 10.1038/srep16839

Li, C., Sun, H., Xu, G., McCarter, K. D., Li, J., and Mayhan, W. G. (2018). Mito-tempo prevents nicotine-induced exacerbation of ischemic brain damage. *J. Appl. Physiol. (1985)* 125, 49–57. doi: 10.1152/japplphysiol.01084.2017

Liberman, M. C., and Kujawa, S. G. (2017). Cochlear synaptopathy in acquired sensorineural hearing loss: manifestations and mechanisms. *Hear. Res.* 349, 138–147. doi: 10.1016/j.heares.2017.01.003

Lin, M. T., and Beal, M. F. (2006). Mitochondrial dysfunction and oxidative stress in neurodegenerative diseases. *Nature* 443, 787–795. doi: 10.1038/nature05292

Liu, Y., Wang, Y., Ding, W., and Wang, Y. (2018). Mito-TEMPO alleviates renal fibrosis by reducing inflammation, mitochondrial dysfunction and endoplasmic reticulum stress. *Oxid. Med. Cell. Longev.* 2018:5828120. doi: 10.1155/2018/5828120

Loughrey, D. G., Kelly, M. E., Kelley, G. A., Brennan, S., and Lawlor, B. A. (2018). Association of age-related hearing loss with cognitive function, cognitive impairment and dementia: a systematic review and meta-analysis. *JAMA Otolaryngol. Head Neck Surg.* 144, 115–126. doi: 10.1001/jamaoto. 2017.2513

Lu, B., Lee, J., Nie, X., Li, M., Morozov, Y. I., Venkatesh, S., et al. (2013). Phosphorylation of human TFAM in mitochondria impairs DNA binding and promotes degradation by the AAA+ Lon protease. *Mol. Cell* 49, 121–132. doi: 10.1016/j.molcel.2012.10.023

Lynch, E. D., Gu, R., Pierce, C., and Kil, J. (2004). Ebselen-mediated protection from single and repeated noise exposure in rat. *Laryngoscope* 114, 333–337. doi: 10.1097/00005537-200402000-00029

McFadden, S. L., Woo, J. M., Michalak, N., and Ding, D. (2005). Dietary vitamin C supplementation reduces noise-induced hearing loss in guinea pigs. *Hear. Res.* 202, 200–208. doi: 10.1016/j.heares.2004.10.011

Nyberg, S., Abbott, N. J., Shi, X., Steyger, P. S., and Dabdoub, A. (2019). Delivery of therapeutics to the inner ear: the challenge of the blood-labyrinth barrier. *Sci. Transl. Med.* 11:eaao0935. doi: 10.1126/scitranslmed.aao0935

Ohinata, Y., Yamasoba, T., Schacht, J., and Miller, J. M. (2000). Glutathione limits noise-induced hearing loss. *Hear. Res.* 146, 28–34. doi: 10.1016/s0378-5955(00)00096-4

Ohlemiller, K. K., Wright, J. S., and Dugan, L. L. (1999). Early elevation of cochlear reactive oxygen species following noise exposure. *Audiol. Neurootol.* 4, 229–236. doi: 10.1159/000013846

Paciello, F., Di Pino, A., Rolesi, R., Troiani, D., Paludetti, G., Grassi, C., et al. (2020). Anti-oxidant and anti-inflammatory effects of caffeic acid: *in vivo* evidences in a model of noise-induced hearing loss. *Food Chem. Toxicol.* 143:111555. doi: 10.1016/j.fct.2020.111555

Pak, J. H., Kim, Y., Yi, J., and Chung, J. W. (2020). Antioxidant therapy against oxidative damage of the inner ear: protection and preconditioning. *Antioxidants (Basel)* 9:1076. doi: 10.3390/antiox 9111076

Park, J., Jou, I., and Park, S. M. (2014). Attenuation of noise-induced hearing loss using methylene blue. *Cell Death Dis.* 5:e1200. doi: 10.1038/cddis. 2014.170

Park, M., Lee, H. S., Song, J. J., Chang, S. O., and Oh, S. (2012). Increased activity of mitochondrial respiratory chain complex in noise-damaged rat cochlea. *Acta Otolaryngol.* 132, S134–S141. doi: 10.3109/00016489.2012. 659755

Rosenhall, U., Skoog, B., and Muhr, P. (2019). Treatment of military acoustic accidents with N-Acetyl-L-cysteine (NAC). *Int. J. Audiol.* 58, 151–157. doi: 10.1080/14992027.2018.1543961

Scarpulla, R. C. (2008). Transcriptional paradigms in mammalian mitochondrial biogenesis and function. *Physiol. Rev.* 88, 611–638. doi: 10.1152/physrev.00 025.2007

Seidman, M. (2003). Effects of resveratrol on acoustic trauma. *Otolaryngol. Head Neck Surg.* 129, 463–470. doi: 10.1016/s0194-5998(03)01586-9

Sha, S., and Schacht, J. (2017). Emerging therapeutic interventions against noise-induced hearing loss. *Expert Opin. Investig. Drugs.* 26, 85–96. doi: 10.1080/13543784.2017.1269171

Sha, S., Taylor, R., Forge, A., and Schacht, J. (2001). Differential vulnerability of basal and apical hair cells is based on intrinsic susceptibility to free radicals. *Hear. Res.* 155, 1–8. doi: 10.1016/s0378-5955(01)00224-6

Shetty, S., Kumar, R., and Bharati, S. (2019). Mito-TEMPO, a mitochondria-targeted antioxidant, prevents N-nitrosodiethylamine-induced hepatocarcinogenesis in mice. *Free Radic. Bio. Med.* 136, 76–86. doi: 10.1016/j. freeradbiomed.2019.03.037

Sugasawa, T., Ono, S., Yonamine, M., Fujita, S., Matsumoto, Y., Aoki, K., et al. (2021). One week of CDAHFD induces steatohepatitis and mitochondrial dysfunction with oxidative stress in liver. *Int. J. Mol. Sci.* 22:5851. doi: 10.3390/ijms22115851

Trnka, J., Blaikie, F. H., Smith, R. A. J., and Murphy, M. P. (2008). A mitochondria-targeted nitroxide is reduced to its hydroxylamine by ubiquinol in mitochondria. *Free Radic. Bio. Med.* 44, 1406–1419. doi: 10.1016/j. freeradbiomed.2007.12.036

Tsutsui, H., Kinugawa, S., and Matsushima, S. (2009). Mitochondrial oxidative stress and dysfunction in myocardial remodelling. *Cardiovasc. Res.* 81, 449–456. doi: 10.1093/cvr/cvn280

WHO. (2021). World report on hearing. Available online at: https://www.who.int/ publications/i/item/world-report-on-hearing.

Wu, F., Xiong, H., and Sha, S. (2020). Noise-induced loss of sensory hair cells is mediated by ROS/AMPKα pathway. *Redox. Biol.* 29:101406. doi: 10.1016/j. redox.2019.101406

Xing, H., Zhang, Z., Shi, G., He, Y., Song, Y., Liu, Y., et al. (2021). Chronic inhibition of mROS protects against coronary endothelial dysfunction in mice with diabetes. *Front. Cell Dev. Biol.* 9:643810. doi: 10.3389/fcell.2021. 643810

Xiong, H., Chen, S., Lai, L., Yang, H., Xu, Y., Pang, J., et al. (2019). Modulation of miR-34a/SIRT1 signaling protects cochlear hair cells against oxidative stress and delays age-related hearing loss through coordinated regulation of mitophagy and mitochondrial biogenesis. *Neurobiol. Aging* 79, 30–42. doi: 10.1016/j.neurobiolaging.2019.03.013

Yamashita, D., Jiang, H., Schacht, J., and Miller, J. M. (2004). Delayed production of free radicals following noise exposure. *Brain Res.* 1019, 201–209. doi: 10.1016/j.brainres.2004.05.104

Yu, J., Wang, Y., Liu, P., Li, Q., Sun, Y., and Kong, W. (2014). Mitochondrial DNA common deletion increases susceptibility to noise-induced hearing loss in a mimetic aging rat model. *Biochem. Biophys. Res. Commun.* 453, 515–520. doi: 10.1016/j.bbrc.2014.09.118

Yuan, H., Wang, X., Hill, K., Chen, J., Lemasters, J., Yang, S. M., et al. (2015). Autophagy attenuates noise-induced hearing loss by reducing oxidative stress. *Antioxid. Redox Signal.* 22, 1308–1324. doi: 10.1089/ars.2014.6004

Zhao, X., Sun, J., Hu, Y., Yang, Y., Zhang, W., Hu, Y., et al. (2013). The effect of overexpression of PGC-1α on the mtDNA4834 common deletion in a rat cochlear marginal cell senescence model. *Hear. Res.* 296, 13–24. doi: 10.1016/j. heares.2012.11.007

Zhao, M., Wang, Y., Li, L., Liu, S., Wang, C., Yuan, Y., et al. (2021). Mitochondrial ROS promote mitochondrial dysfunction and inflammation in ischemic acute kidney injury by disrupting TFAM-mediated mtDNA maintenance. *Theranostics* 11, 1845–1863. doi: 10.7150/thno.50905

Zhelev, Z., Bakalova, R., Aoki, I., Lazarova, D., and Saga, T. (2013). Imaging of superoxide generation in the dopaminergic area of the brain in Parkinson's disease, using Mito-TEMPO. *ACS Chem. Neurosci.* 4, 1439–1445. doi: 10.1021/cn400159h

Zinovkin, R. A., and Zamyatnin, A. A. (2019). Mitochondria-targeted drugs. *Curr. Mol. Pharmacol.* 12, 202–214. doi: 10.2174/1874467212666181127151059

17

Failure of Hearing Acquisition in Mice with Reduced Expression of Connexin 26 Correlates with the Abnormal Phasing of Apoptosis Relative to Autophagy and Defective ATP-Dependent Ca^{2+} Signaling in Kölliker's Organ

Lianhua Sun [1,2,3†], Dekun Gao [1,2,3†], Junmin Chen [1,2,3], Shule Hou [1,2,3], Yue Li [1,2,3], Yuyu Huang [1,2,3], Fabio Mammano [4,5*], Jianyong Chen [1,2,3*] and Jun Yang [1,2,3*]

[1]Department of Otorhinolaryngology-Head and Neck Surgery, Xinhua Hospital, Shanghai Jiaotong University School of Medicine, Shanghai, China, [2]Ear Institute, Shanghai Jiaotong University School of Medicine, Shanghai, China, [3]Shanghai Key Laboratory of Translational Medicine on Ear and Nose Diseases, Shanghai, China, [4]Department of Physics and Astronomy "G. Galilei", University of Padua, Padua, Italy, [5]Department of Biomedical Sciences, Institute of Biochemistry and Cell Biology, Italian National Research Council, Monterotondo, Italy

*Correspondence:
Jun Yang
yangjun@xinhuamed.com.cn
Jianyong Chen
chenjianyong@xinhuamed.com.cn
Fabio Mammano
fabio.mammano@unipd.it

†These authors have contributed equally to this work

Mutations in the *GJB2* gene that encodes connexin 26 (Cx26) are the predominant cause of prelingual hereditary deafness, and the most frequently encountered variants cause complete loss of protein function. To investigate how Cx26 deficiency induces deafness, we examined the levels of apoptosis and autophagy in *Gjb2*[loxP/loxP]; *ROSA26*[CreER] mice injected with tamoxifen on the day of birth. After weaning, these mice exhibited severe hearing impairment and reduced Cx26 expression in the cochlear duct. Terminal deoxynucleotidyl transferase dUTP nick end labeling (TUNEL) positive cells were observed in apical, middle, and basal turns of Kölliker's organ at postnatal (P) day 1 (P1), associated with increased expression levels of cleaved caspase 3, but decreased levels of autophagy-related proteins LC3-II, P62, and Beclin1. In Kölliker's organ cells with decreased Cx26 expression, we also found significantly reduced levels of intracellular ATP and hampered Ca^{2+} responses evoked by extracellular ATP application. These results offer novel insight into the mechanisms that prevent hearing acquisition in mouse models of non-syndromic hearing impairment due to Cx26 loss of function.

Keywords: apoptosis, ATP, autophagy, Ca^{2+}, development, deafness

Abbreviations: KO, Kölliker's organ; IHCs, inner hair cells; Cx26, gap junction protein beta-2; Cx30, gap junction protein beta-6.

INTRODUCTION

The sense of hearing originates in a portion of the cochlear sensory epithelium, the organ of Corti, which comprises two types of mechanosensory hair cells, the inner and outer hair cells (IHCs and OHCs), which do not express connexins, and at least six types of associated supporting cells, all of which express connexins. Connexin 26 (Cx26, encoded by the *GJB2* gene) and the closely related connexin 30 (Cx30, encoded by *GJB6*) are the prevailing isoforms expressed in non-sensory cells of both the epithelial and connective tissue of the developing and mature cochlea (Forge et al., 2003; Cohen-Salmon et al., 2005).

GJB2 mutations are a frequent cause of both syndromic and non-syndromic congenital deafness, with an unusually high carrier rate for truncating mutations among hearing-impaired individuals (Chan and Chang, 2014; Del Castillo and Del Castillo, 2017). Connexin proteins form large-pore hexameric plasma membrane channels, termed hemichannels, which may dock head-to-head in the extracellular space to form intercellular gap junction channels (Laird and Lampe, 2022). Interruption of the potassium ion recycling pathway *via* gap junction systems in the mammalian cochlea has been postulated as the cause of hereditary non-syndromic deafness (Kikuchi et al., 2000). However, this hypothesis lacks experimental proof and is contradicted by different studies (Beltramello et al., 2005; Jagger and Forge, 2015; Zhao, 2017). In contrast, the available evidence from mouse models points to a fundamental role played by connexins, particularly connexin hemichannels, during the crucial phases of postnatal cochlear development that lead to hearing acquisitions; reviewed in (Mammano, 2013, 2019).

In the developing rodent cochlea, the sensory epithelium is subdivided into a cellularly dense medial domain named Kölliker's organ and a less dense lateral domain, the lesser epithelial ridge (LER), separated by a central prosensory region that contains the precursors of the organ of Corti (Lim and Anniko, 1985; Lim and Rueda, 1992; Driver and Kelley, 2020). Kölliker's organ is one of the earliest structures in the inner ear, recognizable from embryonic (E) day 14 (E14) to postnatal (P) day 12–14 (P12–14, P0 indicates the day of birth), which marks the onset of hearing function that reaches adult-level auditory thresholds by the third postnatal week (Ehret, 1977).

In the pre-hearing phase of mouse cochlear development, Kölliker's organ cells release ATP periodically through connexin hemichannels (Schutz et al., 2010; Rodriguez et al., 2012; Xu et al., 2017; Zorzi et al., 2017; Mazzarda et al., 2020) to activate purinergic receptors in the surrounding cells, depolarize the hair cells and activate auditory nerve fibers (Tritsch et al., 2007; Wang and Bergles, 2015; Johnson et al., 2017; Eckrich et al., 2018; Ceriani et al., 2019). Spontaneous Ca^{2+} activity in the mouse postnatal cochlea wanes as the sensory epithelium and its innervation pattern mature, in parallel with intense remodeling which leads to the formation of the inner sulcus in place of the degenerated Kölliker's organ and outer sulcus in place of the LER (Lim and Anniko, 1985; Lim and Rueda, 1992; Driver and Kelley, 2020).

Ca^{2+} signaling, autophagic and apoptotic processes are key to this crucial remodeling phase (La Rovere et al., 2016; Bootman

et al., 2018; Mammano and Bortolozzi, 2018; Zhou et al., 2020; Soundarrajan et al., 2021). Recent work examined Kölliker's organ morphological changes with autophagy and apoptosis markers between P1 and P14 and showed that: (i) autophagy is present and associated closely with the remodeling that leads to Kölliker's organ degeneration; (ii) Kölliker's organ cells are digested and absorbed by autophagy before apoptosis occurs (Hou et al., 2019). Here, we extended those studies by investigating the complex interplay between apoptosis, autophagy, ATP, and Ca^{2+} signaling in connection with the failure of hearing acquisition induced by Cx26 deficiency in a mouse model of non-syndromic deafness.

MATERIALS AND METHODS

Animals

Gjb2^{loxP/loxP} mice (Cohen-Salmon et al., 2002) and ROSA26^{CreER} mice (Vooijs et al., 2001) used for this study were donated by Professor Weijia Kong of the Union Hospital Affiliated to Tongji Medical College, Huazhong University of Science and Technology. All experiments were performed on animals of both sexes following the guidelines approved by the Ethics Committee of Xinhua Hospital affiliated to Shanghai Jiaotong University School of Medicine.

Breeding and Tamoxifen Injection

To achieve time-conditional Cx26 deletion, we adopted a mating scheme previously used to generate mice with targeted ablation of Cx26 in the inner ear (Crispino et al., 2011; Fetoni et al., 2018). First, *Gjb2*^{loxP/loxP} mice were mated with ROSA26^{CreER} mice, yielding *Gjb2*^{loxP//wt}; ROSA26^{CreER} mice (wt = wild type *Gjb2* allele). Next, *Gjb2*^{loxP//wt}; ROSA26^{CreER} mice were mated with *Gjb2*^{loxP/loxP} mice to obtain *Gjb2*^{loxP/loxP}; ROSA26^{CreER} mice. Finally, to promote deletion of the floxed alleles, P0 offspring were given a single intraperitoneal (i.p.) injection of tamoxifen (TMX, T5648-1G, Sigma–Aldrich, USA), at a dose of 100 mg/kg of body weight, as previously reported (Sun et al., 2009; Chang et al., 2015).

Mouse Genotyping

Mouse genotyping was performed as previously described (Chen et al., 2018). The primer pairs used to detect the loxP sequences were as follows:

    forward 5'-CTTTCCAATGCTGGTGGAGTG-3';
    reverse 5'-ACAGAAATGTGTTGGTGATGG-3'.

Gjb2^{loxP/loxP} and wild-type mice generated a band of 322 bp and 288 bp, respectively.

Primer pairs used to detect the CreER sequences were as follows:

    forward   5'-TATCCAGGTTACGGATATAGTTCATG-3'; and

    reverse,   5'-AGCTAAACATGCTTCATCGTCGGTC-3', which generated a band of 700 bp.

Auditory Brainstem Response Test

Mice injected with tamoxifen at P0 were tested for auditory brainstem response (ABR) at P21 (Zhou et al., 2006). Six mice, three males, and three females were tested for each group. Animals were anesthetized with ketamine (120 mg/kg, i.p.) and chlorpromazine (20 mg/kg, i.p.) and placed in a sound-attenuating chamber on a heating pad to maintain body temperature. Tone burst stimuli were generated in the free field at frequencies of 4, 8, 16, and 32 kHz and amplitudes ranging from 0 to 100 dB sound pressure level (SPL) using a system equipped with the RZ6 hardware for data acquisition and sound production, Medusa4Z amplifier and MF1 multi-field magnetic speakers (TDT, Tucker-Davis Technologies, Alachua, FL, USA). Responses were amplified and averaged 512 times using the TDT BioSigRZ software.

Immunohistochemistry

Mice injected with tamoxifen at P0 were used to obtain cochlear tissue at P21 after rapid decapitation. The cochlea was fixed with 4% paraformaldehyde overnight, decalcified with 10% EDTA, embedded in paraffin and sectioned, stained for immunohistochemistry with primary antibodies selective for Cx26 (PA518618, Invitrogen, USA) and Cx30 (700258, Invitrogen, USA), followed by incubation with HRP labeled secondary antibody (donkey anti-goat IgG, goat anti-rabbit IgG, Servicebio). Finally, samples were incubated with a DAB reaction kit (G1212-200T, Servicebio, China), which is the chromogenic substrate of HRP, and images were collected using a Nikon E100 with Nikon DS-U3 imaging system.

Analyses of Cochlear Duct and Kölliker's Organ Tissues

Mice were injected with tamoxifen at P0 and sacrificed by decapitation after 24 h to obtain cochlear duct and Kölliker's organ tissues which were processed as described hereafter.

The cochlear duct was dissected in cold phosphate-buffered saline (PBS), fixed with 4% paraformaldehyde for 30 min, embedded in paraffin, and sectioned. A TUNEL detection kit (11684817910, Roche, Switzerland) was used to detect apoptosis in paraffin-embedded cochlear tissue sections following the manufacturer's protocols.

For immunofluorescence staining, paraffin sections were incubated with primary antibodies selective for c-cas3, LC3-II, P62 (GB11009-1, Servicebio; ab192890, Abcam; GB11239-1, Servicebio) and a secondary antibody (Cy3-sheep-anti-rabbit, GB21303, Servicebio) respectively. Processed samples were observed and imaged with a fluorescence microscope (Nikon ECLIPSE CI with Nikon DS-U3 imaging system) under uniform illumination and detection conditions. The excitation wavelength was 550 nm and the emission wavelength was 570 nm.

For Western blot analyses, tissues were dissected in cold PBS and frozen in liquid nitrogen immediately after decapitation. The total protein content of the cochlea was extracted in RIPA lysis buffer (Servicebio, Wuhan, China) and quantitated following the kit instructions (BCA Protein Assay Kit, Beyotime, Haimen, China). The same amount of protein (20 μg per lane) was electrophoresed in a 15% sodium dodecyl sulfate-polyacrylamide gel and transferred to polyvinylidene difluoride (PVDF) membranes. After blocking with TBST containing 5% skimmed milk for 1 h, the sample was incubated at 4°C overnight

with the primary antibodies selective for GAPDH (60004-1-lg, PTG), caspase 3 (66470-2-lg, PTG), Bcl-2 (GB13458, Servicebio), LC3 (GB11124, Servicebio), p62 (18420-1-AP, PTG), Beclin1 (GB112053, Servicebio). Next, samples were incubated at room temperature with horseradish peroxidase (HRP)-conjugated secondary antibody (GB23301, GB23303, Servicebio) for 1 h. The ECL reaction buffer (G2014, Servicebio) was added to detect the proteins in a Chemidoc XRS+ imaging system (BioRad, CA, USA).

For Luciferin–luciferase ATP bioluminescence assay, the cochlea was removed after rapid decapitation, the bony wall and the membranous labyrinth were separated from the apex to the base of the cochlea and the cochlear duct was dissected in cold phosphate-buffered saline (PBS). Next, the sensory epithelium was separated from the spiral ligament, Kölliker's organ was micro-dissected and placed in a lysis buffer (S0027, Beyotime, China) and lysed in a Polytron PT1200 homogenizer (Kinematica, Luzern, Switzerland). Finally, the total ATP concentration was measured with a luciferin-luciferase bioluminescence ATP assay kit (S0027, Beyotime, China) using the Chemidoc XRS+ imaging system. All measurements reported in this article fell within the linearity range of the ATP standard curve generated according to the manufacturer's instructions. All experiments were performed at room temperature (22–25°C).

Preparation of Kölliker's Organ Cultures From P0 Pups

For these experiments, we used pups from the same litter which was reserved for their tails for genotype identification during the experiment.

Kölliker's organ was micro-dissected in cold 1× Hank's balanced salt solution (HBSS, Thermo Fisher, 14025076, USA) as described above, transiently transferred to an Eppendorf tube containing DMEM/F12 mixed with 2% ampicillin (ST008, Beyotime, China) and then cultured as previously reported (Chen et al., 2018). Briefly, Kölliker's organ was divided into three fragments from apex to base and the fragments were placed in a 24-well plate containing a tissue culture-treated, round glass slide (14 mm diameter, WHB-24-CS, WHB) immersed in DMEM/F12 containing 1% ampicillin, 10% fetal bovine serum (10099-141, Gibco, Australia). Alternatively, for Ca^{2+} imaging experiments with fluo-4 (see below), Kölliker's organ fragments were placed on a tissue culture-treated glass-bottomed culture dish (801001, NEST, China). In either case, the culture medium was supplemented with 10 μM (Z)-4-hydroxytamoxifen (H7904, Sigma, Germany) to promote Cre recombinase-mediated *in vitro* excision of the floxed Cx26 alleles. Finally, samples were placed in an incubator (Thermo Scientific Forma Direct Heat CO_2 Incubators) and cultured at 37°C, 5% CO_2 for 12 h (Chen et al., 2018).

Visualization of ATP-Loaded Vesicles in Kölliker's Organ Cultures

Kölliker's organ cultures, prepared as described above from P0 pups, were treated with quinacrine dihydrochloride (5×10^{-6}

mol/L, orb320518, Biorbyt, UK) in $1\times$ PBS solution for 30 min in the dark, at room temperature, washed three times with PBS, fixed with 4% paraformaldehyde for 1 h, washed three more times with PBS, incubated with cell permeabilizing solution (0.1% Triton X-100 in PBS) for 20 min and blocking solution (10% donkey serum in PBS) for 1 h, washed three times with PBS for 5 min each, and incubated overnight with an anti-LAMP1 primary antibody—lysosome marker (ab208943, Abcam). The next day, Kölliker's organ cultures were removed from the primary antibody incubation solution, washed three times with PBS for 5 min each, and incubated with a secondary antibody (donkey anti-rabbit IgG, AlexaFluor 594, R37119, Invitrogen) at room temperature for 2 h, washed three times with PBS for 5 min each, and incubated with 4', 6-diamidino-2-phenylindole (DAPI, D9542, Sigma) nuclear staining solution for 8 min. Stained cultures were mounted in an antifade mounting medium (H-1200-10, Vectorlabs, USA) and imaged with a confocal microscope (TCS-SP8, Leica, Germany). Fluorescence images of quinacrine (green), DAPI (blue), and LAMP1 (red) were obtained with a $\times 63$ oil immersion objective (Leica) at excitation wavelengths of 488 nm, 405 nm, and 594 nm, respectively. The corresponding emission wavelengths were centered around 520 nm, 422 nm, and 617 nm, respectively.

Ca^{2+} Imaging With Fluo-4 in Kölliker's Organ Cultures

Kölliker's organ cultures, prepared as described above from P0 pups, were incubated for 20 min at 37°C in 4 μM fluo-4 AM loading solution (F14201, Thermo Fisher) containing 20% Pluronic F-127, mixed with five times volume of HBSS (14025076, Thermo Fisher) containing 1% fetal bovine serum, incubated for further 40 min at 37°C, washed with HEPES buffer (10 mM HEPES, 1 mM Na$_2$HPO$_4$, 137 mM NaCl, 5 mM KCl, 1 mM CaCl$_2$, 0.5 mM MgCl$_2$, 5 mM glucose, 0.1% BSA, pH 7.4) three times, resuspended in HEPES buffer, and incubated for another 10 min at 37°C to allow baseline Ca^{2+} levels to stabilize. Using a spinning-disk confocal microscope (Nikon CSU-W1, Japan) with excitation and emission wavelengths set at 494 nm and 516 nm, respectively, we first imaged the baseline fluorescence intensity of fluo-4 for 2 min. Thereafter, while continuing image collection, we replaced the incubation solution with a HEPES buffer supplemented with 30 μM ATP (A6559, Sigma–Aldrich, USA) to stimulate purinergic receptors of Kölliker's organ cells.

For off-line data analysis, single-pixel intensity values were background-subtracted and spatially averaged over regions of interest (ROIs) corresponding to individual cell bodies. Time-dependent fluctuations of intracellular Ca^{2+} levels were represented through the ratio F/F_0, where F is the ROI signal at time t and F_0 is the time-averaged pre-stimulus ROI intensity value (Mammano and Bortolozzi, 2010). F_{max} denotes the peak Ca^{2+}-dependent fluorescence intensity fluctuation within a given ROI during each recording period (7 min in total). Data were computed as mean $\pm$ standard deviation of $n = 30$–50 cells from three separate experiments.

Statistical Analysis

Statistical analysis of experimental data was performed with GraphPad Prism v8.0 (GraphPad Software, Inc., CA, USA) and Student's t-test. P = p-values less than 0.05 were considered statistically significant.

RESULTS

Severe Hearing Loss and Decreased Expression of Cx26 in the Cochlea of Gjb2$^{loxP/Loxp}$; ROSA26^{CreER} Mice Injected With Tamoxifen at P0

At P21, ABR results showed severe hearing loss in Gjb2$^{loxP/loxP}$; ROSA26^{CreER} mice that had been injected with tamoxifen at P0 (shortened as Cx26-cKD mice). Average hearing thresholds in these mice ($n = 6$) exceeded 80 dB at 4, 8, 16 and 32 kHz and were significantly more elevated ($P < 0.01$) than thresholds of other genotypes injected with TMX at P0 and used as controls (Gjb2$^{loxP/wt}$; ROSA26^{CreER}, $n = 5$; Gjb2$^{loxP/loxp}$, $n = 3$; Gjb2$^{loxP/wt}$, $n = 3$; Figure 1A). In addition, immunohistochemical staining revealed a collapsed organ of Corti with an almost invisible cochlear tunnel (Figure 1B) and a decreased expression of Cx26 in supporting cells of the organ of Corti, in epithelial cells of the inner sulcus and outer sulcus, in the spiral limbus, among fibrocytes of the lateral wall and in the basal cell region of the *stria vascularis* of Cx26-cKD mice (Figure 1C), whereas expression of Cx30 was increased (Figure 1D).

Abnormal Apoptosis and Autophagy in Kölliker's Organ of Cx26-cKD Mice

As mentioned in the introduction, prior work with mouse models indicate that Cx26 expression has a profound impact on the development of the cochlear sensory epithelium through a complex interplay between Ca^{2+} signaling, autophagy, and apoptosis; reviewed in Mammano and Bortolozzi (2018) and Mammano (2019). Therefore, we harvested the cochleae of Cx26-cKD mice at P1 and used a TUNEL assay to visualize apoptotic cells (Gorczyca et al., 1993) in 8 μm-thick transverse sections of the cochlear duct (Figures 2A,B). Positive cells (green) were observed exclusively in Kölliker's organ of the Cx26-cKD group, with 8 $\pm$ 1 positive cells (green) adjacent to the pro-sensory domain region in all cochlear turns, whereas no TUNEL positive cells were detected in the control group ($n = 3$). At this developmental stage, there was no sign of apoptosis in IHCs and OHCs of either Cx26-cKD or control groups.

Activated caspase-3 and -7 convert other procaspases to activated caspases, leading to the amplification of the apoptosis cascade (Slee et al., 1999; Logue and Martin, 2008). Thus, we quantified caspase 3 levels by immunofluorescence at P1 and detected significantly enhanced immunoreactivity in Kölliker's organ of all cochlear turns in the Cx26-cKD group compared to controls (Figures 2C,D, $P < 0.05$, $n = 3$).

LC3-II and p62 are widely used molecular markers of autophagy (Kabeya et al., 2000; Emanuele et al., 2020). At P1, we found diffused immunoreactivity against LC3-II in the sensory epithelium of the control group, with a peak in the pro-sensory

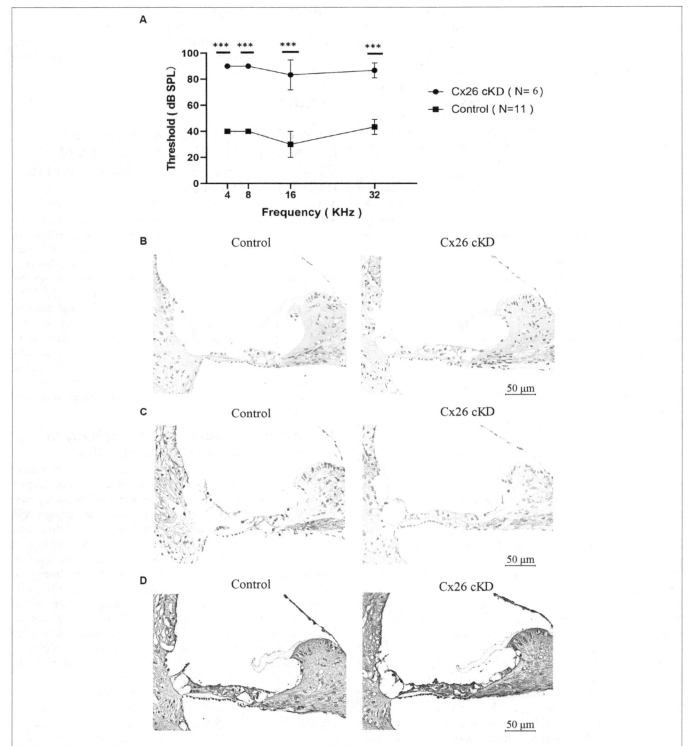

FIGURE 1 | Effect of tamoxifen injection at P0 on the auditory threshold and connexin expression at P21. **(A)** Auditory thresholds measured by pure tone ABRs vs. tone frequency; ***$p < 0.0001$. **(B–D)** Transverse sections of the cochlear duct stained with hematoxylin-eosin **(B)** or with antibodies selective for Cx26 **(C)** or Cx30 **(D)**. Scale bars = 50 μm.

region. In the Cx26-cKD group, immunoreactivity against LC3-II was significantly decreased in Kölliker's organ (**Figures 3A,B**, $P < 0.05$, $n = 3$). Likewise, we found decreased immunoreactivity against p62 in Kölliker's organ cells of the Cx26-cKD group compared to the control group (**Figures 3C,D**, $P < 0.001$, $n = 3$). Together, the results of **Figures 2**, **3** suggest that decreased

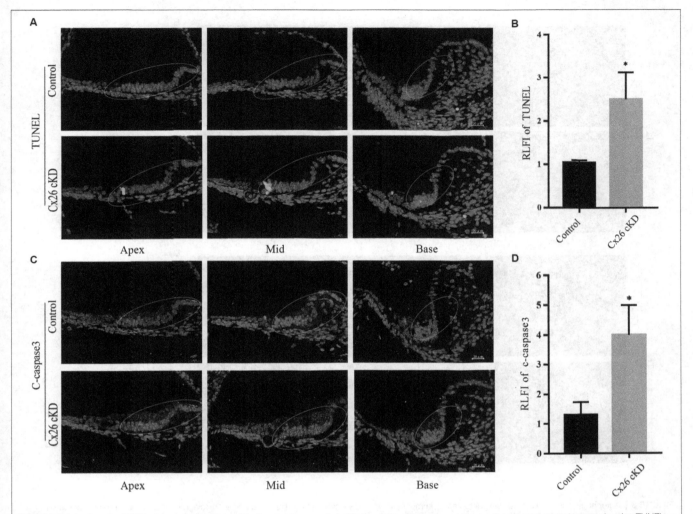

FIGURE 2 | Apoptosis of Kölliker's organ was detected by immunofluorescence staining at P1. **(A)** Representative confocal fluorescence images showing TUNEL positive cells (green) in Kölliker's organ of the Cx26-cKD group, but not in the control group. Blue signals correspond to cell nuclei stained with DAPI. Scale bars = 50 μm. **(B)** Average relative fluorescence intensity (RLFI) of TUNEL signals; * represent $p < 0.05$, $n = 3$. **(C)** Immunofluorescence staining of cleaved (c)-caspase 3 in the apical, middle, and basal turns of Kölliker's organ cells of Cx26-cKD group compared with the control group. Scale bars = 50 μm. **(D)** Average relative fluorescence intensity (RLFI) of the c-caspase 3 signal; * represents $P < 0.05$, $n = 3$.

expression of Cx26 leads to increased apoptosis and decreased autophagy in Kölliker's organ at P1.

To corroborate this conclusion, we investigated expression levels of apoptosis and autophagy markers by Western blotting (**Figure 4**). At P1, we confirmed that cleaved caspase-3 was upregulated in the Cx26-cKD group, with a significant difference compared with the control group ($P < 0.05$, $n = 5$; **Figures 4A,B**). However, these alterations did not involve the anti-apoptotic factor Bcl-2 (Vaux et al., 1992), which is expressed from the 15th day of embryonic development (E15) to P5 in the normal mouse cochlea (Ishii et al., 1996; Kamiya et al., 2001). Our Western blot analyses showed no statistically significant differences ($P > 0.05$, $n = 5$) in the expression level of Bcl-2 between the Cx26-cKD and control mice at P1 (**Figures 4A,B**).

In the normal mouse cochlea, beclin1 and other autophagy-related proteins start to be expressed in the late embryonic stage and continue to be upregulated after birth, until the inner

ear achieves functional maturity of the adult stage (de Iriarte Rodriguez et al., 2015). In the Cx26-cKD group, beclin1, LC3-II/I, and p62 were significantly downregulated compared with the control group ($P < 0.05$, $n = 5$; **Figures 4C,D**). Together, these results suggest that in Kölliker's organ of Cx26-cKD mice at P1, downregulation of autophagy is accompanied by the upregulation of apoptosis independent of Bcl-2 expression.

Decreased Total ATP Content in Kölliker's Organ of Cx26-cKD Mice

Prior work showed that decreased levels of Cx26 expression in the mouse postnatal cochlea reduce gap junction coupling, limiting the transfer of nutrients, and glucose in particular, from distant blood vessels to the avascular sensory epithelium (Fetoni et al., 2018). Upon glucose deprivation, autophagy is induced to supplement the metabolic pool and provide ATP through various mechanisms (Galluzzi et al., 2014). However, this process is

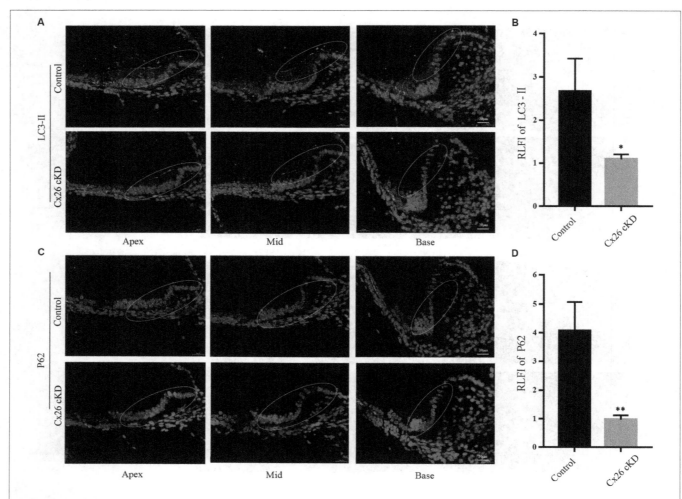

FIGURE 3 | Autophagy of Kölliker's organ was detected by immunofluorescence staining at P1. **(A)** In the apical, middle, and basal turns, immunoreactivity of LC3-II was intense in Kölliker's organ of the control group and markedly less intense in the Cx26-cKD group. Scale bars = 50 μm. **(B)** Average relative fluorescence intensity (RLFI) of LC3-II signal; * represents $P < 0.05$, $n = 3$. **(C)** Immunofluorescence staining of p62 was attenuated in Kölliker's organ cells of apical, middle, and basal turns in the Cx26-cKD group compared with the control group. Scale bars = 50 μm. **(D)** Average relative fluorescence intensity (RLFI) of p62; ** represents $P < 0.001$, $n = 3$.

hampered if autophagy is downregulated, therefore we predicted an overall reduced intracellular ATP concentration downstream of Cx26 knockdown.

To test this hypothesis, Cx26-cKD mice and their controls were sacrificed at P1. The micro-dissected Kölliker's organ was lysed and the total ATP concentration in the lysate was measured with a luciferin-luciferase bioluminescence ATP assay kit. To minimize the experimental changes, a standard curve was constructed for each experiment to estimate the corresponding ATP concentration (**Figure 5A**). ATP levels in the Cx26-cKD group were significantly reduced compared with the control group (**Figure 5B**; $P < 0.05$, $n = 4$), confirming our hypothesis.

Decreased Number of ATP-Loaded Vesicles in Kölliker's Organ of Cx26-cKD Mice

The vesicular nucleotide transporter, also known as solute carrier family 17 member 9 (SLC17A9), mediates lysosomal

ATP accumulation and plays an important role in lysosomal physiology and cell viability (Cao et al., 2014). Based on the results described above, we predicted that the overall reduced ATP availability should correspond to a lower amount of ATP in the lysosomes of Kölliker's organ cells, where prior work showed ATP is accumulated (Chen et al., 2019).

To test this hypothesis, we prepared Kölliker's organ cultures from untreated P0 pups of $Gjb2^{loxP/loxP}$; ROSA26^{CreER} mice, and control mice. To promote Cre recombinase-mediated *in vitro* excision of Cx26 floxed alleles, cultures were exposed to 10 μM (Z)-4-hydroxytamoxifen (HTMX) and thereafter inspected by transmitted light microscopy at 10, 20, and 40× magnification (**Figure 5C**). No visible differences were noted between the HTMX and control groups. Therefore, we proceeded to stain the cultures with DAPI (to label nuclei) and quinacrine, which functions as an ATP-binding agent and acridine derivative with a very high affinity to ATP and has been used to label ATP-containing vesicles (White et al., 1995; Chen et al., 2019).

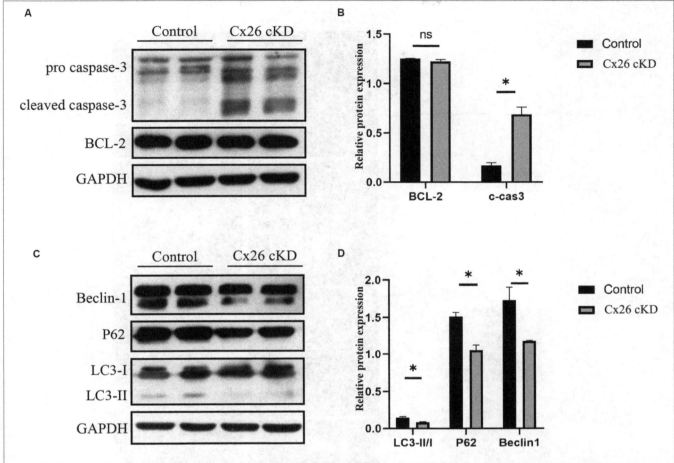

FIGURE 4 | Western blot analysis of apoptosis- and autophagy-related proteins in Kölliker's organ at P1. **(A)** Representative western blots for apoptosis-related proteins Bcl-2 and c-caspase 3. **(B)** Corresponding relative optical density; * represents $P < 0.05$, $n = 5$. **(C)** Representative western blots for autophagy-related proteins LC3-II, P62 and Beclin1. **(D)** Corresponding relative optical density; * represents $P < 0.05$, $n = 5$.

Samples were also immuno-stained with an anti-LAMP1 primary antibody (a lysosome marker) and a suitable secondary antibody (see "Materials and Methods" Section). The quinacrine signal (green) in the HTMX group was lower than in the control group, whereas LAMP1 immunoreactivity (red) was not significantly different between the two groups (**Figure 5D**). These qualitative results accord with the quantitative results of **Figure 5B** and suggest that, as a consequence of Cx26 knockdown, less ATP was accumulated in lysosomal vesicles of the Cx26-cKD group compared with the control group.

Decreased ATP-Evoked Intracellular Ca²⁺ Responses in Cx26-cKD Cochlear Cultures

To determine whether the alterations described above affect also Ca^{2+} signaling, HTMX-treated Kölliker's organ cultures were loaded with the selective Ca^{2+} indicator fluo-4 and challenged by the application of saturating amounts of exogenous ATP (30 μM, see "Materials and Methods" Section), expected to cause massive Ca^{2+} release from the ER. Ca^{2+} imaging revealed peak responses (F_{max}/F_0) in the $Gjb2^{loxP/loxP}$; $ROSA26^{CreER}$ group that were significantly downregulated compared with

the control group (1.86 ± 0.37 vs. 3.13 ± 0.77, $P < 0.05$, $n = 3$; **Figure 5F**). In addition, we noted that Ca^{2+} oscillations appeared during the declining phase of the responses in the control group but were absent in the $Gjb2^{loxP/loxP}$; $ROSA26^{CreER}$ group (see "Discussion" Section, for a possible explanation). Together, the results in **Figure 5**, show that the knockdown of Cx26 affects a major ATP-dependent Ca^{2+} signaling pathway in Kölliker's organ, which is crucial for organ development and hearing acquisition as summarized in the introduction.

DISCUSSION

The organ of Corti is the core part of the auditory system, composed of hair cells and supporting cells. The hair cells function in transducing the sound mechanical stimulation into the primary acoustic signals (Liu et al., 2019), while the spiral ganglions transmit primary acoustic information from hair cells in the organ of Corti to the higher auditory centers of the central nervous system (Wei et al., 2021). Hair cells are easily injured by excessive noise exposure (Guo et al., 2021;

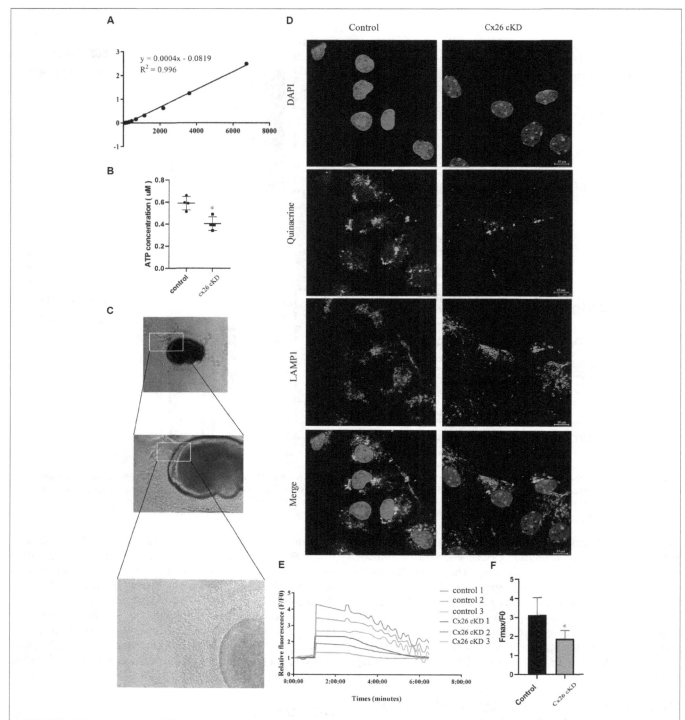

FIGURE 5 | ATP concentration and ATP-evoked Ca^{2+} signaling. **(A)** Representative standard curve used to calibrate bioluminescence signals: $Y = 0.0004X - 0.0819$, $R^2 = 0.996$. **(B)** ATP concentration estimated from luciferin-luciferase bioluminescence assay. $P < 0.05$, $n = 4$. **(C)** Representative transmitted light microscopy image of a Kölliker's organ culture viewed at 10×, 20×, and 40× magnification (from top to bottom). **(D)** Representative confocal fluorescence images of Kölliker's organ cultures labeled with quinacrine, anti-LAMP1 antibodies, and DAPI; scale bars = 10 μm. **(E)** Representative ATP-evoked Ca^{2+} responses of individual cells in Kölliker's organ cultures. **(F)** Quantification of F_{max}/F_0 signals; * represents $P < 0.05$, $n = 3$.

He et al., 2021), ototoxic drugs (He et al., 2017), aging (He et al., 2020), genetic factors (Fu et al., 2021), and infections (He et al., 2020).

Mouse models continue to provide critical insight into the functioning of the auditory system and deafness-associated genes (Bowl et al., 2017). Among these, it has long been known that Cx26 (*Gjb2*) biallelic deletion in mice is embryonically lethal due to impaired transplacental uptake of glucose (Gabriel et al., 1998). The *Gjb2*$^{loxP/loxP}$ mice used in this study (Cohen-Salmon et al., 2002), can overcome embryonic lethality if crossed with a suitable Cre-expressing strain to achieve tissue- and/or time-conditional deletion of the floxed alleles (Orban et al., 1992; Vooijs et al., 2001). Crossing *Gjb2*$^{loxP/loxP}$ mice with the Otog-Cre strain (Cohen-Salmon et al., 2002), or the Sox10-Cre strain (Anselmi et al., 2008) resulted in mice with severe hearing loss and developmental defects in the cochlear sensory epithelium (Cohen-Salmon et al., 2002; Crispino et al., 2011). Both *Gjb2*$^{loxP/loxP}$; Otog-Cre and *Gjb2*$^{loxP/loxP}$; Sox10-Cre mice are considered models of human DFNB1 non-syndromic hearing impairment, which is frequently associated with truncating mutations that yield non-functional Cx26 proteins (Chan and Chang, 2014; Del Castillo and Del Castillo, 2017).

Results obtained from time-dependent knockdown of Cx26 in tamoxifen-induced *Gjb2*$^{loxP/loxP}$; ROSA26^{CreER} mice (Chang et al., 2015; Chen et al., 2018) lend further support to the notion that Cx26 intercellular gap junction channels and hemichannels with normal permeability to nutrients and other metabolites and signaling molecules are essential for normal development of the cochlea and normal hearing acquisition (Mammano, 2019).

Here, using tamoxifen-induced knockdown of Cx26 in *Gjb2*$^{loxP/loxP}$; ROSA26^{CreER} mice, we found decreased levels of autophagy-related proteins beclin1, LC3-II, and p62 in the cochlea, indicating that autophagy was downregulated. These alterations were accompanied by increased apoptosis in the Kölliker's organ cells, which became apoptotic as early as P1 based on TUNEL assays and upregulation of c-caspase 3 expressions. The p62 marker is particularly interesting because increasing evidence points to the N-terminal arginylated BiP (R-BiP)/Beclin-1/p62 complex as having an important role in the crosstalk between apoptosis and autophagy, which greatly affects cell death (Song et al., 2018). Recent work examined this interplay in the normal developing cochlea and concluded that autophagy precedes apoptosis in the natural postnatal degeneration of Kölliker's organ cells and their regulated replacement by cuboidal cells of the inner sulcus (Hou et al., 2019).

The accelerated apoptosis described in this article is easily explained in the light of a recent study that linked decreased Cx26 expression to apoptosis *via* impaired nutrient delivery to the sensory epithelium through gap junction channels, the reduced release of the key antioxidant glutathione through connexin hemichannels, and deregulated expression of several genes under the transcriptional control of Nrf2, a redox-sensitive transcription factor that plays a pivotal role in oxidative stress regulation (Fetoni et al., 2018; Ding et al., 2020). Thus, we conclude that impairment of Cx26 function subverts the critically timed phasing of autophagy and apoptosis in the mouse postnatal cochlea, hijacks the hearing acquisition program, and dooms animals to deafness through increased oxidative stress. This conclusion is also supported by prior studies showing that Kölliker's organ cells did not completely degenerate until 2 weeks after birth in caspase 3 knockout mice, resulting in hyperplasia of supporting cells, degeneration of hair cells, and severe hearing loss (Takahashi et al., 2001),

strengthening the notion that a correctly executed postnatal apoptotic program is key to hearing acquisition in mice (Chen et al., 2020).

In non-sensory cells of the cochlear sensory epithelium, ATP binding to G protein-coupled P2Y receptors activates the production of IP$_3$ *via* phospholipase C (PLC), promoting Ca^{2+} release from the endoplasmic reticulum (ER) through IP$_3$ receptors (IP$_3$R) and consequent increase of the cytoplasmic free Ca^{2+} concentration (Mammano, 2013). Our Ca^{2+} imaging experiments show that the ATP/P2Y/PLC/IP$_3$ signal transduction cascade, which fuels Ca^{2+} signaling in Kölliker's organ, is downregulated by the knockdown of Cx26. To interpret these results, it is imperative to consider that: (i) all else held equal, the amount of Ca^{2+} released from the ER depends on the Ca^{2+} concentration in the ER; (ii) increased oxidative stress is associated with Cx26 downregulation in the developing cochlea (Fetoni et al., 2018; He et al., 2019). Thus, in our experimental conditions, SERCA pumps activity was lowered not only by the reduced availability of cytosolic ATP (this article) but also by the effect of oxidative stress (Kaplan et al., 2003). In addition, alterations in the redox state of critical thiols in the IP$_3$R lead to sensitization of IP$_3$R-mediated Ca^{2+} release associated with oxidative stress (Joseph et al., 2018), which may increase the steady-state Ca^{2+} leakage from the ER. The predicted net effect is a reduced Ca^{2+} content in the ER, hence a reduced driving force for Ca^{2+} transfer from the ER to cytosol driven by the signal transduction cascade mentioned above. This explains the reduced F_{max}/F_0 signals evoked by supramaximal exogenous ATP stimuli in Kölliker's organ cultures exposed to HTMX.

As for the issue of Ca^{2+} oscillations, data-driven computational modeling shows that they are governed by Hopf-type bifurcation and arise only within a limited range of extracellular ATP concentration through the interplay of IP$_3$R-mediated Ca^{2+} release from the ER and SERCA pump-mediated Ca^{2+} re-uptake into the ER (Ceriani et al., 2016). In control Kölliker's organ cultures, oscillations arose during the recovery phase from supramaximal stimulation, while the extracellular ATP concentration lowered due to diffusion and ATP hydrolysis mediated by ectonucleotidases expressed at the surface of the epithelium (Ceriani et al., 2016). As both SERCA pump activity and IP$_3$R are affected by oxidative stress, it comes as no surprise that Ca^{2+} oscillations were absent in Kölliker's organ cultures exposed to HTMX. This conclusion is supported also by experiments and mathematical modeling of the effects of oxidative stress on Ca^{2+} oscillation in other cellular systems (Antonucci et al., 2015).

In conclusion, our results provide further evidence for abnormal cochlear development in mice with reduced expression of Cx26, expound possible mechanisms of hearing acquisition failure, and produce novel insight, from a new perspective, for *GJB2*-related hereditary deafness.

AUTHOR CONTRIBUTIONS

LS and DG wrote the article. JuC, SH, YL, and YH analyzed the data. FM, JiC, and JY designed the study. All authors contributed to the article and approved the submitted version.

REFERENCES

Anselmi, F., Hernandez, V. H., Crispino, G., Seydel, A., Ortolano, S., Roper, S. D., et al. (2008). ATP release through connexin hemichannels and gap junction transfer of second messengers propagate Ca2+ signals across the inner ear. *Proc. Natl. Acad. Sci. U S A* 105, 18770–18775. doi: 10.1073/pnas.0800793105

Antonucci, S., Tagliavini, A., and Pedersen, M. G. (2015). Reactive oxygen and nitrogen species disturb Ca(2+) oscillations in insulin-secreting MIN6 beta-cells. *Islets* 7:e1107255. doi: 10.1080/19382014.2015.1107255

Beltramello, M., Piazza, V., Bukauskas, F. F., Pozzan, T., and Mammano, F. (2005). Impaired permeability to Ins(1,4,5)P3 in a mutant connexin underlies recessive hereditary deafness. *Nat. Cell Biol.* 7, 63–69. doi: 10.1038/ncb1205

Bootman, M. D., Chehab, T., Bultynck, G., Parys, J. B., and Rietdorf, K. (2018). The regulation of autophagy by calcium signals: do we have a consensus? *Cell Calcium* 70, 32–46. doi: 10.1016/j.ceca.2017.08.005

Bowl, M. R., Simon, M. M., Ingham, N. J., Greenaway, S., Santos, L., Cater, H., et al. (2017). A large-scale hearing loss screen reveals an extensive unexplored genetic landscape for auditory dysfunction. *Nat. Commun.* 8:886. doi: 10.1038/s41467-017-00595-4

Cao, Q., Zhao, K., Zhong, X. Z., Zou, Y., Yu, H., Huang, P., et al. (2014). SLC17A9 protein functions as a lysosomal ATP transporter and regulates cell viability. *J. Biol. Chem.* 289, 23189–23199. doi: 10.1074/jbc.M114.567107

Ceriani, F., Hendry, A., Jeng, J. Y., Johnson, S. L., Stephani, F., Olt, J., et al. (2019). Coordinated calcium signaling in cochlear sensory and non-sensory cells refines afferent innervation of outer hair cells. *EMBO J.* 38:e99839. doi: 10.15252/embj.201899839

Ceriani, F., Pozzan, T., and Mammano, F. (2016). The critical role of ATP-induced ATP release for Ca2+ signaling in nonsensory cell networks of the developing cochlea. *Proc. Natl. Acad. Sci. U S A* 113, E7194–E7201. doi: 10.1073/pnas.1616061113

Chan, D. K., and Chang, K. W. (2014). GJB2-associated hearing loss: systematic review of worldwide prevalence, genotype and auditory phenotype. *Laryngoscope* 124, E34–E53. doi: 10.1002/lary.24332

Chang, Q., Tang, W., Kim, Y., and Lin, X. (2015). Timed conditional null of connexin26 in mice reveals temporary requirements of connexin26 in key cochlear developmental events before the onset of hearing. *Neurobiol. Dis.* 73, 418–427. doi: 10.1016/j.nbd.2014.09.005

Chen, J., Hou, S., and Yang, J. (2019). ATP is stored in lysosomes of greater epithelial ridge supporting cells in newborn rat cochleae. *J. Cell. Biochem.* 120, 19469–19481. doi: 10.1002/jcb.29251

Chen, S., Xie, L., Xu, K., Cao, H.-Y., Wu, X., Xu, X.-X., et al. (2018). Developmental abnormalities in supporting cell phalangeal processes and cytoskeleton in the Gjb2 knockdown mouse model. *Dis. Model. Mech.* 11:dmm033019. doi: 10.1242/dmm.033019

Chen, B., Xu, H., Mi, Y., Jiang, W., Guo, D., Zhang, J., et al. (2020). Mechanisms of hearing loss and cell death in the cochlea of connexin mutant mice. *Am. J. Physiol. Cell Physiol.* 319, C569–C578. doi: 10.1152/ajpcell.00483.2019

Cohen-Salmon, M., del Castillo, F. J., and Petit, C. (2005). "Connexins responsiblbe for hereditary deafness - the tale unfolds," in *Gap Junctions in Development and Disease*, ed E. Winterhager (Berlin: Springer-Verlag), 111–134.

Cohen-Salmon, M., Ott, T., Michel, V., Hardelin, J. P., Perfettini, I., Eybalin, M., et al. (2002). Targeted ablation of connexin26 in the inner ear epithelial gap junction network causes hearing impairment and cell death. *Curr. Biol.* 12, 1106–1111. doi: 10.1016/s0960-9822(02)00904-1

Crispino, G., Di Pasquale, G., Scimemi, P., Rodriguez, L., Galindo Ramirez, F., De Siati, R. D., et al. (2011). BAAV mediated GJB2 gene transfer restores gap junction coupling in cochlear organotypic cultures from deaf Cx26Sox10Cre mice. *PLoS One* 6:e23279. doi: 10.1371/journal.pone.0023279

de Iriarte Rodriguez, R., Pulido, S., Rodriguez-de la Rosa, L., Magarinos, M., and Varela-Nieto, I. (2015). Age-regulated function of autophagy in the mouse inner ear. *Hear. Res.* 330, 39–50. doi: 10.1016/j.heares.2015.07.020

Del Castillo, F. J., and Del Castillo, I. (2017). DFNB1 non-syndromic hearing impairment: diversity of mutations and associated phenotypes. *Front. Mol. Neurosci.* 10:428. doi: 10.3389/fnmol.2017.00428

Ding, Y., Meng, W., Kong, W., He, Z., and Chai, R. (2020). The role of FoxG1 in the inner ear. *Front. Cell Dev. Biol.* 8:614954. doi: 10.3389/fcell.2020.614954

Driver, E. C., and Kelley, M. W. (2020). Development of the cochlea. *Development* 147:dev162263. doi: 10.1242/dev.162263

Eckrich, T., Blum, K., Milenkovic, I., and Engel, J. (2018). Fast Ca2+ transients of inner hair cells arise coupled and uncoupled to Ca2+ waves of inner supporting cells in the developing mouse cochlea. *Front. Mol. Neurosci.* 11:264. doi: 10.3389/fnmol.2018.00264

Ehret, G. (1977). Postnatal development in the acoustic system of the house mouse in the light of developing masked thresholds. *J. Acoust. Soc. Am.* 62, 143–148. doi: 10.1121/1.381496

Emanuele, S., Lauricella, M., D'Anneo, A., Carlisi, D., De Blasio, A., Di Liberto, D., et al. (2020). p62: friend or foe? Evidences for oncojanus and neurojanus roles. *Int. J. Mol. Sci.* 21:5029. doi: 10.3390/ijms21145029

Fetoni, A. R., Zorzi, V., Paciello, F., Ziraldo, G., Peres, C., Raspa, M., et al. (2018). Cx26 partial loss causes accelerated presbycusis by redox imbalance and dysregulation of Nfr2 pathway. *Redox Biol.* 19, 301–317. doi: 10.1016/j.redox.2018.08.002

Forge, A., Becker, D., Casalotti, S., Edwards, J., Marziano, N., and Nevill, G. (2003). Gap junctions in the inner ear: comparison of distribution patterns in different vertebrates and assessement of connexin composition in mammals. *J. Comp. Neurol.* 467, 207–231. doi: 10.1002/cne.10916

Fu, X., An, Y., Wang, H., Li, P., Lin, J., Yuan, J., et al. (2021). Deficiency of Klc2 induces low-frequency sensorineural hearing loss in C57BL/6J mice and human. *Mol. Neurobiol.* 58, 4376–4391. doi: 10.1007/s12035-021-02422-w

Gabriel, H. D., Jung, D., Butzler, C., Temme, A., Traub, O., Winterhager, E., et al. (1998). Transplacental uptake of glucose is decreased in embryonic lethal connexin26-deficient mice. *J. Cell Biol.* 140, 1453–1461. doi: 10.1083/jcb.140.6.1453

Galluzzi, L., Pietrocola, F., Levine, B., and Kroemer, G. (2014). Metabolic control of autophagy. *Cell* 159, 1263–1276. doi: 10.1016/j.cell.2014.11.006

Gorczyca, W., Traganos, F., Jesionowska, H., and Darzynkiewicz, Z. (1993). Presence of DNA strand breaks and increased sensitivity of DNA in situ to denaturation in abnormal human sperm cells: analogy to apoptosis of somatic cells. *Exp. Cell Res.* 207, 202–205. doi: 10.1006/excr.1993.1182

Guo, L., Cao, W., Niu, Y., He, S., Chai, R., and Yang, J. (2021). Autophagy regulates the survival of hair cells and spiral ganglion neurons in cases of noise, ototoxic drug and age-induced sensorineural hearing loss. *Front. Cell. Neurosci.* 15:760422. doi: 10.3389/fncel.2021.760422

He, Z., Fang, Q., Li, H., Shao, B., Zhang, Y., Zhang, Y., et al. (2019). The role of FOXG1 in the postnatal development and survival of mouse cochlear hair cells. *Neuropharmacology* 144, 43–57. doi: 10.1016/j.neuropharm.2018.10.021

He, Z., Guo, L., Shu, Y., Fang, Q., Zhou, H., Liu, Y., et al. (2017). Autophagy protects auditory hair cells against neomycin-induced damage. *Autophagy* 13, 1884–1904. doi: 10.1080/15548627.2017.1359449

He, Z.-H., Li, M., Fang, Q.-J., Liao, F.-L., Zou, S.-Y., Wu, X., et al. (2021). FOXG1 promotes aging inner ear hair cell survival through activation of the autophagy pathway. *Autophagy* 17, 4341–4362. doi: 10.1080/15548627.2021.1916194

He, Z.-H., Zou, S.-Y., Li, M., Liao, F.-L., Wu, X., Sun, H.-Y., et al. (2020). The nuclear transcription factor FoxG1 affects the sensitivity of mimetic aging hair cells to inflammation by regulating autophagy pathways. *Redox Biol.* 28:101364. doi: 10.1016/j.redox.2019.101364

Hou, S., Chen, J., and Yang, J. (2019). Autophagy precedes apoptosis during degeneration of the Kolliker's organ in the development of rat cochlea. *Eur. J. Histochem.* 63:3025. doi: 10.4081/ejh.2019.3025

Ishii, N., Wanaka, A., Ohno, K., Matsumoto, K., Eguchi, Y., Mori, T., et al. (1996). Localization of bcl-2, bax and bcl-x mRNAs in the developing inner ear of the mouse. *Brain Res.* 726, 123–128.

Jagger, D. J., and Forge, A. (2015). Connexins and gap junctions in the inner ear--it's not just about K(+) recycling. *Cell Tissue Res.* 360, 633–644. doi: 10.1007/s00441-014-2029-z

Johnson, S. L., Ceriani, F., Houston, O., Polishchuk, R., Polishchuk, E., Crispino, G., et al. (2017). Connexin-mediated signaling in nonsensory cells is crucial for the development of sensory inner hair cells in the mouse cochlea. *J. Neurosci.* 37, 258–268. doi: 10.1523/JNEUROSCI.2251-16.2016

Joseph, S. K., Young, M. P., Alzayady, K., Yule, D. I., Ali, M., Booth, D. M., et al. (2018). Redox regulation of type-I inositol trisphosphate receptors in intact mammalian cells. *J. Biol. Chem.* 293, 17464–17476. doi: 10.1074/jbc.RA118.005624

Kabeya, Y., Mizushima, N., Ueno, T., Yamamoto, A., Kirisako, T., Noda, T., et al. (2000). LC3, a mammalian homologue of yeast Apg8p, is localized in autophagosome membranes after processing. *EMBO J.* 19, 5720–5728. doi: 10.1093/emboj/19.21.5720

Kamiya, K., Takahashi, K., Kitamura, K., Momoi, T., and Yoshikawa, Y. (2001). Mitosis and apoptosis in postnatal auditory system of the C3H/He strain. *Brain Res.* 901, 296–302. doi: 10.1016/s0006-8993(01)02300-9

Kaplan, P., Babusikova, E., Lehotsky, J., and Dobrota, D. (2003). Free radical-induced protein modification and inhibition of Ca2+-ATPase of cardiac sarcoplasmic reticulum. *Mol. Cell. Biochem.* 248, 41–47. doi: 10.1023/a:1024145212616

Kikuchi, T., Adams, J. C., Miyabe, Y., So, E., and Kobayashi, T. (2000). Potassium ion recycling pathway *via* gap junction systems in the mammalian cochlea and its interruption in hereditary nonsyndromic deafness. *Med. Electron Microsc.* 33, 51–56. doi: 10.1007/s007950070001

La Rovere, R. M., Roest, G., Bultynck, G., and Parys, J. B. (2016). Intracellular Ca²⁺ signaling and Ca²⁺ microdomains in the control of cell survival, apoptosis and autophagy. *Cell Calcium* 60, 74–87. doi: 10.1016/j.ceca.2016.04.005

Laird, D. W., and Lampe, P. D. (2022). Cellular mechanisms of connexin-based inherited diseases. *Trends Cell Biol.* 32, 58–69. doi: 10.1016/j.tcb.2021.07.007

Lim, D. J., and Anniko, M. (1985). Developmental morphology of the mouse inner ear. A scanning electron microscopic observation. *Acta Otolaryngol. Suppl.* 422, 1–69.

Lim, D., and Rueda, J. (1992). "Structural development of the cochlea," in *Development of Auditory and Vestibular Systems - 2 (1st Edition)*, ed R. Romand (New York: Elsevier Science Publishing Co.), 33–58.

Liu, Y., Qi, J., Chen, X., Tang, M., Chu, C., Zhu, W., et al. (2019). Critical role of spectrin in hearing development and deafness. *Sci. Adv.* 5:eaav7803. doi: 10.1126/sciadv.aav7803

Logue, S. E., and Martin, S. J. (2008). Caspase activation cascades in apoptosis. *Biochem. Soc. Trans.* 36, 1–9. doi: 10.1042/BST0360001

Mammano, F. (2013). ATP-dependent intercellular Ca²⁺ signaling in the developing cochlea: facts, fantasies and perspectives. *Semin. Cell Dev. Biol.* 24, 31–39. doi: 10.1016/j.semcdb.2012.09.004

Mammano, F. (2019). Inner ear connexin channels: roles in development and maintenance of cochlear function. *Cold Spring Harb. Perspect. Med.* 9:a033233. doi: 10.1101/cshperspect.a033233

Mammano, F., and Bortolozzi, M. (2010). "Ca²⁺ imaging: principles of analysis and enhancement," in *Calcium Measurement Methods*, eds A. Verkhratsky and O. Petersen (New York: Humana Press), 57–80.

Mammano, F., and Bortolozzi, M. (2018). Ca(2+) signaling, apoptosis and autophagy in the developing cochlea: Milestones to hearing acquisition. *Cell Calcium* 70, 117–126. doi: 10.1016/j.ceca.2017.05.006

Mazzarda, F., D'Elia, A., Massari, R., De Ninno, A., Bertani, F. R., Businaro, L., et al. (2020). Organ-on-chip model shows that ATP release through connexin hemichannels drives spontaneous Ca²⁺ signaling in non-sensory cells of the greater epithelial ridge in the developing cochlea. *Lab Chip* 20, 3011–3023. doi: 10.1039/d0lc00427h

Orban, P. C., Chui, D., and Marth, J. D. (1992). Tissue- and site-specific DNA recombination in transgenic mice. *Proc. Natl. Acad. Sci. U S A* 89, 6861–6865. doi: 10.1073/pnas.89.15.6861

Rodriguez, L., Simeonato, E., Scimemi, P., Anselmi, F., Cali, B., Crispino, G., et al. (2012). Reduced phosphatidylinositol 4,5-bisphosphate synthesis impairs inner ear Ca²⁺ signaling and high-frequency hearing acquisition. *Proc. Natl. Acad. Sci. U S A* 109, 14013–14018. doi: 10.1073/pnas.1211869109

Schutz, M., Scimemi, P., Majumder, P., De Siati, R. D., Crispino, G., Rodriguez, L., et al. (2010). The human deafness-associated connexin 30 T5M mutation causes mild hearing loss and reduces biochemical coupling among cochlear non-sensory cells in knock-in mice. *Hum. Mol. Genet.* 19, 4759–4773. doi: 10.1093/hmg/ddq402

Slee, E. A., Harte, M. T., Kluck, R. M., Wolf, B. B., Casiano, C. A., Newmeyer, D. D., et al. (1999). Ordering the cytochrome c-initiated caspase cascade: hierarchical activation of caspases-2, -3, -6, -7, -8 and -10 in a caspase-9-dependent manner. *J.Cell Biol.* 144, 281–292. doi: 10.1083/jcb.144.2.281

Song, X., Lee, D. H., Dilly, A. K., Lee, Y. S., Choudry, H. A., Kwon, Y. T., et al. (2018). Crosstalk between apoptosis and autophagy is regulated by the arginylated BiP/Beclin-1/p62 complex. *Mol. Cancer Res.* 16, 1077–1091. doi: 10.1158/1541-7786.MCR-17-0685

Soundarrajan, D. K., Huizar, F. J., Paravitorghabeh, R., Robinett, T., and Zartman, J. J. (2021). From spikes to intercellular waves: tuning intercellular calcium signaling dynamics modulates organ size control. *PLoS Comput. Biol.* 17:e1009543. doi: 10.1371/journal.pcbi.1009543

Sun, Y., Tang, W., Chang, Q., Wang, Y., Kong, W., and Lin, X. (2009). Connexin30 null and conditional connexin26 null mice display distinct pattern and time course of cellular degeneration in the cochlea. *J. Comp. Neurol.* 516, 569–579. doi: 10.1002/cne.22117

Takahashi, K., Kamiya, K., Urase, K., Suga, M., Takizawa, T., Mori, H., et al. (2001). Caspase-3-deficiency induces hyperplasia of supporting cells and degeneration of sensory cells resulting in the hearing loss. *Brain Res.* 894, 359–367. doi: 10.1016/s0006-8993(01)02123-0

Tritsch, N. X., Yi, E., Gale, J. E., Glowatzki, E., and Bergles, D. E. (2007). The origin of spontaneous activity in the developing auditory system. *Nature* 450, 50–55. doi: 10.1038/nature06233

Vaux, D. L., Weissman, I. L., and Kim, S. K. (1992). Prevention of programmed cell death in Caenorhabditis elegans by human bcl-2. *Science* 258, 1955–1957. doi: 10.1126/science.1470921

Vooijs, M., Jonkers, J., and Berns, A. (2001). A highly efficient ligand-regulated Cre recombinase mouse line shows that LoxP recombination is position dependent. *EMBO Rep.* 2, 292–297. doi: 10.1093/embo-reports/kve064

Wang, H. C., and Bergles, D. E. (2015). Spontaneous activity in the developing auditory system. *Cell Tissue Res.* 361, 65–75. doi: 10.1007/s00441-014-2007-5

Wei, H., Chen, Z., Hu, Y., Cao, W., Ma, X., Zhang, C., et al. (2021). Topographically conductive butterfly wing substrates for directed spiral ganglion neuron growth. *Small* 17:2102062. doi: 10.1002/smll.202102062

White, P. N., Thorne, P. R., Housley, G. D., Mockett, B., Billett, T. E., and Burnstock, G. (1995). Quinacrine staining of marginal cells in the stria vascularis of the guinea-pig cochlea: a possible source of extracellular ATP? *Hear. Res.* 90, 97–105. doi: 10.1016/0378-5955(95)00151-1

Xu, L., Carrer, A., Zonta, F., Qu, Z., Ma, P., Li, S., et al. (2017). Design and characterization of a human monoclonal antibody that modulates mutant connexin 26 hemichannels implicated in deafness and skin disorders. *Front. Mol. Neurosci.* 10:298. doi: 10.3389/fnmol.2017.00298

Zhao, H. B. (2017). Hypothesis of K(+)-recycling defect is not a primary deafness mechanism for Cx26 (GJB2) Deficiency. *Front. Mol. Neurosci.* 10:162. doi: 10.3389/fnmol.2017.00162

Zhou, X., Jen, P. H., Seburn, K. L., Frankel, W. N., and Zheng, Q. Y. (2006). Auditory brainstem responses in 10 inbred strains of mice. *Brain Res.* 1091, 16–26. doi: 10.1016/j.brainres.2006.01.107

Zhou, H., Qian, X., Xu, N., Zhang, S., Zhu, G., Zhang, Y., et al. (2020). Disruption of Atg7-dependent autophagy causes electromotility disturbances, outer hair cell loss and deafness in mice. *Cell Death Dis.* 11:913. doi: 10.1038/s41419-020-03110-8

Zorzi, V., Paciello, F., Ziraldo, G., Peres, C., Mazzarda, F., Nardin, C., et al. (2017). Mouse Panx1 is dispensable for hearing acquisition and auditory function. *Front. Mol. Neurosci.* 10:379. doi: 10.3389/fnmol.2017.00379

18

Visual Rhyme Judgment in Adults with Mild-to-Severe Hearing Loss

Mary Rudner[1]*, Henrik Danielsson[1], Björn Lyxell[1,2], Thomas Lunner[3] and Jerker Rönnberg[1]

[1] Linnaeus Centre HEAD, Swedish Institute for Disability Research, Department of Behavioural Sciences and Learning, Linköping University, Linköping, Sweden, [2] Department of Special Needs Education, University of Oslo, Oslo, Norway, [3] Eriksholm Research Centre, Oticon A/S, Snekkersten, Denmark

*Correspondence:
Mary Rudner
mary.rudner@liu.se

Adults with poorer peripheral hearing have slower phonological processing speed measured using visual rhyme tasks, and it has been suggested that this is due to fading of phonological representations stored in long-term memory. Representations of both vowels and consonants are likely to be important for determining whether or not two printed words rhyme. However, it is not known whether the relation between phonological processing speed and hearing loss is specific to the lower frequency ranges which characterize vowels or higher frequency ranges that characterize consonants. We tested the visual rhyme ability of 212 adults with hearing loss. As in previous studies, we found that rhyme judgments were slower and less accurate when there was a mismatch between phonological and orthographic information. A substantial portion of the variance in the speed of making correct rhyme judgment decisions was explained by lexical access speed. Reading span, a measure of working memory, explained further variance in match but not mismatch conditions, but no additional variance was explained by auditory variables. This pattern of findings suggests possible reliance on a lexico-semantic word-matching strategy for solving the rhyme judgment task. Future work should investigate the relation between adoption of a lexico-semantic strategy during phonological processing tasks and hearing aid outcome.

Keywords: phonology, frequency, hearing impairment, working memory, lexico-semantic strategy

INTRODUCTION

Hearing impairment is a highly prevalent neurological condition that is associated with changes in brain organization, i.e., neural plasticity (Jayakody et al., 2018). This applies not only to pre-lingual hearing impairment and profound deafness (Lomber et al., 2010; Rudner, 2018) but also to acquired hearing loss (Ito et al., 1993; Cardin, 2016; Jayakody et al., 2018). Even mild hearing loss leads to neural plasticity (Campbell and Sharma, 2014) and recently we showed hearing-related variation in regional brain volume in a large middle-aged non-clinical cohort (Rudner et al., 2019).

Plasticity associated with hearing loss is found not only in the auditory pathway, including primary auditory cortex (Peelle et al., 2011; Eckert et al., 2012) and auditory processing regions in the superior temporal gyrus (Husain et al., 2011; Boyen et al., 2013; Yang et al., 2014; Rudner et al., 2019), but also in brain regions involved in higher order cognitive processing (Husain et al., 2011; Yang et al., 2014; Rudner et al., 2019), including phonological processing (Lazard et al., 2010;

Classon et al., 2013b; Rudner et al., 2013; Andin et al., 2018). This may reflect investment of cognitive resources in listening, especially under adverse conditions (Peelle and Wingfield, 2016; Rudner et al., 2019). Indeed, differences in functional hearing even in a non-clinical cohort are associated with differences in the volume of cognitive processing regions, including the hippocampus (Rudner et al., 2019), a subcortical structure that mediates long-term memory encoding and retrieval.

Long-term memory underpins language processing. To achieve understanding of a spoken message, the incoming speech signal has to be mapped onto knowledge representations stored in long-term memory (Rönnberg et al., 2013, 2019). Phonological representations of the sounds of words, which are dissociable from their lexical representations (Cutler, 2008), are fundamental to this process (Marslen-Wilson, 1987; Luce and Pisoni, 1998), and their importance increases when contextual or lexical information is impoverished (Mattys et al., 2005; Signoret and Rudner, 2019). When conditions for speech perception are optimal (Mattys et al., 2012), the process of matching the speech signal to phonological representations stored in long-term memory is seamless. However, when speech perception conditions are suboptimal, this automatic process may become conscious and effortful, as well as less sensitive to phonological detail (Mattys et al., 2014), and demand the engagement of working memory (Rönnberg et al., 2013, 2019). Although speech perception is relatively robust to minor matching failures, especially when rich context guides lexical selection (Mattys et al., 2012), major mismatch may disrupt processing of the speech signal. The role of working memory in speech understanding under adverse listening conditions includes the piecing together of fragments of target speech along with the suppression of unwanted sounds such as competing speech (Rönnberg et al., 2013, 2019).

Hearing impairment contributes to adverse listening conditions by making the speech signal weaker and reducing its spectral and temporal fidelity (Pichora-Fuller and Singh, 2006). Although hearing aids can amplify sound, their ability to selectively amplify target speech and suppress unwanted sounds is limited (Lunner et al., 2009). There is some evidence that hearing aids may reduce listening effort after a period of familiarization (Rudner et al., 2009; Giroud et al., 2017), improve working memory (Karawani et al., 2018) and slow cognitive decline in later life (Maharani et al., 2018). Hearing impairment may keep working memory in trim by demanding cognitive engagement during speech communication. Long-term memory, however, including the mental lexicon with its set of phonological representations, may decline through disuse (Rönnberg et al., 2011; Classon et al., 2013a).

Considering the key role of phonology in speech understanding, it is not surprising that hearing impairment is associated with changes in phonological processing ability. This applies both to individuals with severe hearing impairment (Andersson, 2002; Lazard et al., 2010; Classon et al., 2013a,c; Lazard and Giraud, 2017). and to individuals with undiagnosed hearing loss (Molander et al., 2013). Andersson (2002) suggested that post-lingual hearing loss leads to degradation of the phonological representations established through use of oral language, and that the mechanism behind this deterioration is the fading of phonological representations that are no longer regularly refreshed by optimal auditory perception.

Phonological processing ability is typically measured using a rhyme judgment task in which participants are asked to compare the sound of different words (Andersson, 2002; Lazard et al., 2010; Classon et al., 2013c). Visual administration circumvents the issue of differences in hearing ability for individuals with hearing impairment. Further, because the sound of words is not directly available in the written word, the participant must actively retrieve phonological representations from long-term memory to make the necessary comparison. This requirement is most obvious in languages that lack a one-to-one mapping between orthography and phonology. For example, in English the non-rhyming words "mint" and "pint" are orthographically similar and thus look as though they might rhyme in the same way as do "mint" and "lint." In order to determine that "mint" and "pint" do not actually rhyme, the sounds of those words have to be activated and compared. Conversely, "bough" and "cow" do rhyme despite orthographic indication to the contrary. Swedish, the language used in the current investigation, has a more regular mapping of orthography to phonology than English, but there are still examples of mismatch that can be exploited in a visual rhyme task (Andersson, 2002; Classon et al., 2013c). Andersson (2002) argued that the time it takes to determine whether two words rhyme (phonological processing speed) is associated with the quality of phonological representations, such that faster processing indicates better preserved phonological representations. However, Lazard and Giraud (2017) showed that acquired deafness can, in some cases, lead to faster phonological processing, although this phenomenon is associated with maladaptive cross-modal plasticity.

Using a visual rhyme judgment task, Classon et al. (2013c) studied phonological processing in adults with acquired severe hearing impairment. Like Andersson (2002), they found that mean phonological processing speed on trials in which phonology did not match orthography was lower than for adults with normal hearing. However, participants with hearing impairment who had good working memory capacity performed on a par with participants with normal hearing. Classon et al. (2013c) suggested that good working memory capacity facilitates good performance, possibly by allowing repeated double-checking of spelling and sound. Intriguingly, Classon et al. (2013c) also found that those same individuals had poorer subsequent recognition of items from mismatch conditions than their hearing-impaired peers with poorer working memory. Therefore, they suggested that when explicit processing resources are engaged during the overtly phonological strategy of repeated double-checking of spelling and sound, they become unavailable for deeper processing of the lexicosemantic characteristics of the stimuli which is required for long-term memory encoding (Craik and Tulving, 1975). A phonological strategy, involving grapheme to phoneme matching and related to good working memory capacity (Classon et al., 2013c), seems to be more predictive of successful auditory rehabilitation in persons with severe hearing impairment than a lexico-semantic strategy, involving whole-word matching (Lazard et al., 2010; Classon et al., 2013c) and it has been suggested that it may be appropriate to include phonological training in hearing rehabilitation (Moberly et al., 2017).

Rhyme judgment requires the activation of phonological representations relating to the final syllables of the relevant words. These representations reflect the sublexical patterning of phonemes including consonants and vowels. A double dissociation of the processing of consonants and vowels in neuropsychological patients shows that these are distinct categories of speech sounds (Caramazza et al., 2000). Vowels seem to provide more information than consonants when it comes to word segmentation (Mehler et al., 2006) while consonants seem to be more important than vowels for lexical access (Owren and Cardillo, 2006). Both functions are likely to be important for visual rhyme judgment. Vowels are distinguished by their relative formant frequency patterns that occupy a relatively low frequency range while consonants are generally distinguished by their higher frequency characteristics, although there is a large overlap in frequency (Ladefoged, 1993). Thus, based on the notion that hearing loss leads to degradation of phonological representations (Andersson, 2002), hearing loss in the low frequency range is likely to degrade phonological representations of vowel sounds and affect vowel processing while high frequency hearing loss is likely to degrade phonological representations of consonant sounds and affect consonant processing. Indeed, hearing loss seems to have a differential impact on the use of vowel and consonant cues during processing of auditorily gated speech (Fogerty et al., 2012). Further, persons with bilateral, symmetrical, mild-to-severe sensorineural hearing impairment belonging to the same cohort as the participants in the present study showed differences in consonant and vowel processing (Moradi et al., 2017).

The purpose of the present study is to investigate the relationship between phonological processing skills and low and high frequency hearing loss in adults with mild-to-severe hearing impairment. We predict that better phonological processing ability will be associated with better thresholds in both low and high frequency ranges reflecting the relative preservation of both vowel and consonant representations. Different impact of consonant and vowel cues during phonological processing will be indicated by a differential contribution of low and high frequency ranges. We also predict that speed of access to representations in long-term memory will account for additional variance in phonological processing skills along with working memory capacity, especially under mismatch conditions.

MATERIALS AND METHODS

The data for the current study were obtained from the N200 database (Rönnberg et al., 2016) under a data transfer agreement. The study was approved by the Regional Ethics Review Board (reference no. 55-09 T122-09) and all participants gave their informed consent.

Participants

212 individuals (91 female) with a mean age of 60.7 years (SD = 8.6 years) were included in the present study. They were all experienced hearing aids users with bilateral, symmetrical sensorineural hearing loss in the range mild-to-severe and were recruited to the longitudinal N200 study from the patient population at the Linköping University Hospital. They all had normal or corrected-to-normal vision and were native Swedish speakers. Data for all participants who had completed the rhyme judgment task at the first time point of the longitudinal N200 study are included in the present study.

Audiometric Tests

Pure tone audiometry (air-conduction thresholds) was performed in accordance with ISO/IEC 8253 (2010) on all participants in both ears at the frequencies 250, 500, 1000, 2000, 3000, 4000, 6000, and 8000 Hz. We were interested in the contribution of hearing acuity in the vowel and consonant frequency ranges. Vowels are identified most accurately by their first two formant frequencies, with F2 being the more important. Back vowels are likely to have second formant frequencies below 1,000 Hz while front vowels have second formant frequencies above 1,000 Hz, with some above 2,000 Hz. Swedish also has some rounded vowels which rely on third formant frequencies above 2,000 Hz. This means that there is an overlap between the lower frequencies that distinguish vowels and the higher frequencies in the range of 2,000 to 4,000 Hz which distinguish consonants. In order to optimize separation of frequencies distinguishing vowels and consonants while keeping constant the number of data points used, we calculated the better ear pure tone average (PTA) dB across 250, 500 and 1000 Hz for vowel frequency (M = 25.31, SD = 13.36) and the better ear PTA dB across 2000, 3000, and 4000 Hz for consonant frequency (M = 47.95, SD = 12.64). We acknowledge that the chosen vowel frequencies do not include the higher formant frequencies for front or rounded vowels. As the frequencies 6000 and 8000 may also contribute to the ability to distinguish consonants, we calculated a third better ear PTA dB across these two high frequencies (M = 58.12, SD = 16.75). Mean better ear PTA in the three frequency ranges is reported in **Table 1**.

Participants also reported number of years with hearing problems (M = 14.71, SD = 12.11) and how many years they had used hearing aids (M = 6.66, SD = 6.48). See **Table 1**.

Cognitive Tests

Participants performed a battery of cognitive tests described in detail in Rönnberg et al. (2016). In the current study we focus on rhyme judgment. However, we also take into account performance on tests of working memory (reading span), cognitive processing speed (physical matching) and lexical access (lexical decision) all of which are described below. These variables are included as the theoretical constructs they tap into may all influence phonological processing ability and thus rhyme judgment performance.

TABLE 1 | Means, standard deviations, and uncorrected correlations with confidence intervals.

Variable	M	SD	1	2	3	4	5	6	7	8	9	10
(1) Rhyme judgment Mismatch, ms	1891.36	478.96										
(2) Rhyme judgment Match, ms	1449.71	341.30	0.81** [0.75, 0.85]									
(3) Age, yrs	60.68	8.65	0.01 [-0.13, 0.14]	0.07 [-0.07, 0.20]								
(4) Reading span	15.94	3.91	-0.21** [-0.33, -0.08]	-0.28** [-0.40, -0.15]	-0.35** [-0.47, -0.23]							
(5) Vowel freq. dB	25.31	13.36	0.11 [-0.03, 0.24]	0.10 [-0.03, 0.24]	-0.05 [-0.18, 0.08]	0.10 [-0.04, 0.23]						
(6) Consonant freq. dB	47.95	12.64	0.09 [-0.05, 0.22]	0.12 [-0.01, 0.25]	0.23** [0.10, 0.36]	-0.02 [-0.16, 0.11]	0.29** [0.16, 0.41]					
(7) High freq. dB	58.12	16.75	0.14 [-0.00, 0.27]	0.17* [0.04, 0.30]	0.41** [0.29, 0.52]	-0.16* [-0.29, -0.03]	-0.08 [-0.21, 0.06]	0.53** [0.42, 0.62]				
(8) Lexical access speed, ms	977.18	202.24	0.65** [0.56, 0.72]	0.69** [0.61, 0.75]	0.07 [-0.06, 0.20]	-0.26** [-0.38, -0.13]	0.14* [0.01, 0.27]	0.22** [0.09, 0.35]	0.18** [0.05, 0.31]			
(9) Physical matching, ms	976.72	206.46	0.39** [0.27, 0.50]	0.40** [0.28, 0.51]	0.37** [0.25, 0.48]	-0.26** [-0.39, -0.13]	0.15* [0.01, 0.28]	0.19** [0.05, 0.31]	0.22** [0.09, 0.35]	0.56** [0.46, 0.65]		
(10) Hearing problems, yrs	14.71	12.11	0.03 [-0.10, 0.17]	0.07 [-0.07, 0.20]	-0.04 [-0.18, 0.09]	0.03 [-0.11, 0.17]	0.32** [0.19, 0.44]	0.40** [0.27, 0.50]	0.20** [0.07, 0.33]	0.07 [-0.06, 0.21]	0.06 [-0.07, 0.20]	
(11) Hearing aid use, yrs	6.66	6.48	0.08 [-0.06, 0.22]	0.04 [-0.10, 0.18]	0.16* [0.02, 0.29]	0.11 [-0.03, 0.25]	0.42** [0.30, 0.53]	0.49** [0.38, 0.59]	0.19** [0.05, 0.33]	0.05 [-0.09, 0.19]	0.05 [-0.09,. 019]	0.54** [0.43, 0.63]

M and SD are used to represent mean and standard deviation, respectively. Values in square brackets indicate the 95% confidence interval for each correlation. The confidence interval is a plausible range of population correlations that could have caused the sample correlation (Cumming, 2014). * indicates p < 0.05. ** indicates p < 0.01.

Rhyme Judgment

In the rhyme judgment task, two printed words are presented on a computer screen and the participant's task is to judge whether or not they rhyme with each other. There are equal numbers of rhyming and non-rhyming pairs and within both categories there are equal numbers of orthographically similar and orthographically diverse pairs. This means that there are four different kinds of trials:

(1) R+O+. Words that rhyme and are orthographically similar, e.g., FRITT/VITT (i.e., free/white).
(2) R+O−. Words that rhyme but are not orthographically similar, e.g., KURS/DUSCH (i.e., course/shower in Swedish pronounced [kuʃ/duʃ]).
(3) R-O+. Words that do not rhyme but are orthographically similar, e.g., TAGG/TUGG (i.e., thorn/chew).
(4) R−O−. Words that neither rhyme nor are orthographically similar, e.g., HÄST/TORN (i.e., horse/tower).

There are eight trials in each category. Button-press responses are given and the dependent variable is the mean response time for correct decisions for each of the four different trial types. Previous work has shown that it is harder to solve mismatching (i.e., R+O− and R-O+) than matching (i.e., R+O+ and R−O−) trials (Andersson, 2002; Classon et al., 2013c) and thus we expected longer response times for mismatch than match trials.

Physical Matching

In the physical matching test, two printed letters are presented simultaneously on a computer screen and the participant's task is to determine whether or not they are identical. Button press responses are given. There are 16 trials equally divided between true and false, and the dependent variable is the mean response time for correct trials. This is a measure of cognitive processing speed.

Lexical Decision

In the lexical decision task, strings of three letters (two consonants and one vowel) are presented on a computer screen and the participant's task is to determine whether or not the string constitutes a Swedish word. The strings are Swedish words, Swedish pseudowords (non-lexicalized but phonologically acceptable) or Swedish non-words (neither lexicalized nor phonologically acceptable). Button press responses are given. There are forty trials evenly distributed between true and false with pseudowords and non-words occurring equally often across false trials. The dependent variable is the mean response time for correct trials. This is a measure of lexical access speed.

Reading Span

The reading span test (Daneman and Carpenter, 1980; Baddeley et al., 1985; Rönnberg et al., 1989) is a test of simultaneous working memory maintenance and processing. Three-word sentences are presented word-by-word in blocks of 2–5 sentences and the participant's task is to first determine whether each sentence makes sense or not as it is presented and then at the end of each block recall either the first or the final word (as cued after the block) of each of the sentences included in the block in order of presentation (Lunner, 2003). The sentences are presented on a computer screen at a rate of one word per 800 msec. Half of the sentences make sense and the other half do not. There are two trials per block length, giving a total of 28 trials. The dependent variable was the total number of words correctly recalled.

Procedure

The data for the present study were collected at one and the same session lasting between 2 and 3 h. This was the first of three testing sessions, constituting the first time point of the longitudinal N200 study (see Rönnberg et al., 2016 for further details). Tests were administered in a fixed order for all participants. The order of the tests included in the present study was: pure tone audiometry, physical matching, lexical decision, rhyme judgment and reading span. Additional tests, not reported in the present study, were interleaved with these tests (for further details see Rönnberg et al., 2016).

Data Analysis

All analyses were done using R (Version 3.5.1; R Core Team, 2018). There were missing values for 25 data points. These were mainly due to technical problems with the testing equipment and therefore the missing data was considered to be missing completely at random. Imputation of data was done with multivariate imputation by chained equations using the MICE r package (van Buuren and Groothuis-Oudshoorn, 2011). Following the package recommendations, we obtained five different imputed datasets. The descriptive data presented in the article are based on the original data and the analyses are performed on the imputed data.

First, two repeated measures ANOVAs were performed to establish whether rhyme judgment performance in terms of both accuracy and latency was indeed poorer on mismatch conditions where the information provided by the orthography was misleading as regards the phonological similarity of the presented word pair than on match conditions where orthography agreed with phonology. Because we were interested in phonological processing differences under match and mismatch conditions (Classon et al., 2013c), data were collapsed over the two matching conditions R+O+ (Words that rhyme and are orthographically similar) and R−O− (Words that neither rhyme nor are orthographically similar) and over the two mismatching conditions R+O− (words that rhyme but are not orthographically similar) and R−O+ (words that do not rhyme but are orthographically similar). Response time for match conditions and mismatch conditions was then correlated (Pearson) with age, auditory and cognitive variables. Finally, regression analyses were performed to determine the relative contribution of auditory and cognitive variables to phonological processing ability. The assumptions for multiple regression was assessed with the gvlma r package (Pena and Slate, 2014), and were not met regarding skewness and kurtosis. Therefore, robust regression using the lmrob function in the robustbase r package (Maechler et al., 2018) was used. Variable selection in the regression was done using a stepwise forward method based on p-values with a cut-off of 0.1. In regression analysis, there is a growing consensus based on simulation studies (Steyerberg et al., 2001) and reviews (Moons et al., 2015) that a higher cut-off value than the standard 0.05 be used so that potentially important variables are not omitted.

RESULTS

There were no missing values on the rhyme judgment variables, and so it was not necessary to use the five imputed datasets in this analysis. Means, standard deviations and uncorrected correlations for match and mismatch conditions of the rhyme judgment task and other variables are shown in **Table 1**.

The ANOVA of rhyme judgment accuracy (proportion correct) scores showed a main effect of condition, $F(1,209) = 498.53$, $MSE = 41,119.68$, $p < 0.001$, $\eta^2 = 0.221$, where accuracy, as expected, was greater under match compared to mismatch conditions ($M_{match} = 0.98$, $M_{mismatch} = 0.77$). As rhyme judgment accuracy approached 100% in the match conditions, meaning that variance was skewed, response time was used as an index of phonological processing ability in the correlation and regression analyses. The response time ANOVA also showed a main effect of condition $F(1,209) = 236.12$, $MSE = 0.02$, $p < 0.001$, $\eta^2 = 0.332$, where responses, again as expected, were faster under match compared to mismatch conditions ($M_{match} = 1450$, $M_{mismatch} = 1891$). Together, these two ANOVAs confirm that the rhyme judgment task was solved more accurately and faster under match compared to mismatch conditions.

Correlations

Correlations are shown in **Table 1**. In the rhyme judgment data there was a strong positive correlation between match and mismatch conditions, showing that individuals who were faster on mismatch trials were also faster on match trials. Rhyme judgment performance did not correlate significantly with age but it correlated with the cognitive measures under both mismatch and match conditions. These significant correlations were strong regarding lexical access speed and cognitive processing speed, and moderate regarding reading span. Rhyme judgment performance correlated very weakly with audiometric measures. The only correlation that reached significance was between rhyme judgment under match conditions with high frequency hearing thresholds. Previous studies have examined the relation between rhyme judgment and average hearing thresholds across vowel and consonant ranges. To check that the lack of correlation with hearing thresholds in the present study was not due to separation of vowel and consonant frequencies, we calculated correlations for better ear PTA across the four frequencies 500, 1000, 2000, 4000 Hz. Neither of these correlations reached significance, Mismatch: $r = 0.12$, $p = 0.09$; Match $r = 0.13$, $p = 0.06$. To determine the relative contribution of age, auditory and cognitive variables to variance in rhyme judgment performance under match and mismatch conditions regression analyses were performed.

Regression

Robust regression analysis with stepwise elimination was performed separately for rhyme judgment performance under match and mismatch conditions. Mean response time was the dependent variable. The variables included in the regression were age; hearing thresholds at vowel, consonant and high frequencies, duration of hearing problems and hearing aid use as well as cognitive variables including reading span, lexical access speed and cognitive processing speed. The same remaining variables were found on all five imputed datasets. Therefore, pooled estimates over all datasets are presented. For the mismatch condition, only lexical access speed was a significant predictor, and that model had an adjusted R^2 of 0.45. For the match condition, lexical access speed and reading span both contributed to the model with adjusted R^2 of 0.55. The final models are presented in **Table 2**. There was no contribution of any auditory variable in either condition.

DISCUSSION

In the present study, we tested the phonological processing abilities of 212 individuals with varying degrees of hearing impairment in the range mild-to-severe taking part in the N200 study (Rönnberg et al., 2016). We did this by administering a visual rhyme task, and investigated whether variance in latency could be explained by hearing ability across the frequencies 250, 500, and 1000 Hz or across the frequencies 2000, 3000, and 4000 Hz or both ranges. The main finding in the regression analyses was that a substantial amount of the variance in rhyme judgment performance was explained by lexical access speed but that no additional variance was explained by auditory variables. In match but not mismatch conditions, reading span explained additional variance.

The visual rhyme judgment task used in the present study included four different types of trials that fall into two categories: mismatch (R+O−, R−O+) and match (R+O+, R−O−). There were 16 trials in each category. This is fewer than in some previous studies. For example, the study by Andersson (2002) included 25 trials in each category and the study by Classon et al. (2013c) included 96 trials in each category. Fewer trials means fewer word pairs compared for their phonological characteristics,

TABLE 2 | Table of estimates from robust regression for mismatch at the top and match conditions at the bottom.

Condition	Predictor	b	se	t	P
Mismatch					
	Intercept	317.112	119.009	2.665	0.008
	Lexical access speed	1.592	0.128	12.477	< 0.001
Match					
	Intercept	496.214	103.775	4.782	< 0.001
	Lexical access speed	1.070	0.080	13.397	< 0.001
	Reading span	−7.823	3.653	−2.141	0.033

These are the final models after variable selection, pooled over all five imputed data sets.

which in turn means that fewer phonemic contrasts are tested for each individual. Thus, the weakness of the association between hearing impairment and phonological processing in the current study may be partly due to the limited number of trials in the visual rhyme judgment task. This limitation is only partly compensated for by the substantial number of data points generated by the large number of participants. It is probably also due to the frequency ranges chosen to represent consonant and vowel perception. A different choice of frequencies may have shown that the auditory factors did correlate with rhyme judgment.

In line with previous work studying individuals with severe hearing impairment (Andersson, 2002; Classon et al., 2013c), results of the current study showed that performance was statistically significantly poorer on mismatch compared to the match trials. This applied both to the proportion correct and to latency. In match conditions, because the phonology matches the orthography, the correct answer can be obtained simply from the visible orthography relating to the two words presented for comparison without activating their phonology. However, because 50% of the trials are mismatches an orthographic strategy only will lead to poor overall performance. To achieve good performance overall, the phonology of the words must be accessed on the basis of the orthography presumably by individual grapheme/phoneme matching.

In the present study, the associations between phonological processing speed and variables of interest including lexical access speed, hearing thresholds and reading span were tested separately for match and mismatch conditions using Pearson's correlations. Phonological processing speed was strongly associated with lexical access speed and cognitive processing speed. Both these associations were positive showing that individuals with faster lexical access and cognitive processing speed also have faster phonological processing. Associations between phonological processing speed and hearing thresholds were surprisingly weak, considering our predictions, suggesting that phonological representations do not contribute to performance on the rhyme judgment task above and beyond lexical access speed. This is only likely to be the case if a non-phonological strategy is adopted. There was a moderate negative association with reading span (a measure of working memory capacity) showing that faster phonological processing is associated with greater working memory capacity, in line with our prediction.

Regression analysis resulted in two models explaining variance in phonological processing speed. One model related to mismatch conditions and showed that variance was largely explained by lexical access speed, but that there was no contribution of auditory measures; this was not surprising, considering the pattern of correlations. Importantly, although both lexical access speed and cognitive speed correlated with phonological processing speed, cognitive speed was not retained in the final regression model relating to mismatch. This suggests that lexical access speed specifically, rather than cognitive processing speed in general, is important for phonological processing in the sample studied here, in line with our prediction. Surprisingly, reading span did not contribute above and beyond

lexical access speed to the model pertaining to mismatch conditions. The other model related to match conditions and showed that variance was, again, largely explained by lexical access speed, but that reading span also contributed. Classon et al. (2013c) showed that individuals with severe hearing impairment but good working memory capacity could make up for their phonological processing deficit in the mismatch conditions of a visual rhyme task by intensifying their efforts at phonological recoding of orthographic information. Thus, we expected that reading span would contribute specifically to phonological processing under mismatch conditions in the present study. However, we found that working memory capacity indexed by reading span only explained variance under match conditions. This suggests that working memory is being employed to support processing in trials in which the orthography directly indicates whether the words rhyme or not rather than in trials that require repeated checking of sound and spelling (Classon et al., 2013c) and thus explicit engagement of phonological processing skills. Classon et al. (2013c) argued that individuals with severe hearing impairment but poor working memory seemed to adopt a lexico-semantic strategy involving whole-word matching to solve the visual rhyme judgment task (Lazard et al., 2010; Classon et al., 2013c). Such a strategy would be consistent with the results obtained in the present study.

Recently, Lazard and Giraud (2017) reported that adults with severe hearing impairment who adopted a lexico-semantic strategy during visual rhyme judgment responded faster but showed right occipito-temporal reorganization in the brain and poor rehabilitation prognosis with cochlear implants. They suggested that accurate but faster-than-average performance on a visual rhyme task may be a marker of maladaptive plasticity in adults with severe acquired hearing impairment. The brain reorganizes even with mild hearing impairment (Campbell and Sharma, 2014), and it is possible that use of a lexico-semantic strategy during visual rhyme judgment may be a marker of maladaptive plasticity even in early-stage hearing impairment. Indeed, we showed that even in a non-clinical cohort, poorer hearing is associated with smaller brain volume in auditory cortex and regions involved in cognitive processing (Rudner et al., 2019). It is important to establish whether phonological processing abilities are reduced even in early stage hearing impairment as indicated by Molander et al. (2013) and whether this is associated with neural reorganization.

Brain plasticity in connection with hearing impairment is both a threat and an opportunity, and auditory rehabilitation should target neural organization associated with good hearing health (Glick and Sharma, 2017). Activation of left lateralized phonological processing networks during visual rhyme judgment in individuals with severe hearing impairment is associated with successful outcome of cochlear implantation (Lazard and Giraud, 2017). The organization of phonological processing networks in individuals with early stage hearing impairment should be investigated to determine possible brain reorganization and its association with rehabilitation outcomes.

One way of maintaining a phonological strategy in preference to a lexico-semantic strategy during word processing may be targeted phonological training (Moberly et al., 2017). Ferguson and Henshaw (2015) proposed that training programs in which cognitive enhancement is embedded in auditory tasks may benefit the real-world listening abilities of adults with hearing impairment and Nakeva von Mentzer et al. (2013) reported evidence of training effects on phonological processing in children with hearing impairment. Future work should investigate whether training can help maintain left-lateralized phonological processing in adults with hearing impairment.

In conclusion, in a group of 212 adults with hearing impairment, we found evidence that auditory measures tested were only very weakly correlated with performance on a visual rhyme judgment task and once lexical access speed was accounted for, auditory measures did not explain additional variance in visual rhyme judgment performance. We tentatively propose that this finding may be explained by reliance on a lexico-semantic word-matching strategy during visual rhyme judgment, making phonological representations redundant or even a source of confusion. Future work should investigate possible neural plasticity in left-hemisphere phonological processing networks

of individuals with early-stage hearing impairment and how it can be shaped to promote good hearing health. It would also be beneficial to retest the original prediction that auditory factors would correlate with better performance in rhyme judgment tasks by using a more appropriate set of frequencies to test for consonant and vowel perception.

AUTHOR CONTRIBUTIONS

MR conceived the article and wrote the first draft. MR, HD, BL, TL, and JR designed the study and contributed to the final version of the article. HD performed the statistical analyses.

ACKNOWLEDGMENTS

The authors wish to thank Tomas Bjuvmar, Rina Blomberg, Elaine Ng, Carine Signoret, Victoria Stenbäck, Helena Torlofson, and Wycliffe Yumba for help with data collection.

REFERENCES

Andersson, U. (2002). Deterioration of the phonological processing skills in adults with an acquired severe hearing loss. *Eur. J. Cogn. Psychol.* 14, 335–352. doi: 10.1080/09541440143000096

Andin, J., Fransson, P., Rönnberg, J., and Rudner, M. (2018). fMRI evidence of magnitude manipulation during numerical order processing in congenitally deaf signers. *Neural Plast.* 2018:2576047. doi: 10.1155/2018/2576047

Baddeley, A., Logie, R. H., Nimmo-Smith, I., and Brereton, N. (1985). Components of fluent reading. *J. Mem. Lang.* 24, 119–131. doi: 10.1016/0749-596x(85)90019-1

Boyen, K., Langers, D. R. M., de Kleine, E., and van Dijk, P. (2013). Gray matter in the brain: differences associated with tinnitus and hearing loss. *Hear. Res.* 295, 67–78. doi: 10.1016/j.heares.2012.02.010

Campbell, J., and Sharma, A. (2014). Cross-modal re-organization in adults with early stage hearing loss. *PLoS One* 9:e90594. doi: 10.1371/journal.pone.0090594

Caramazza, A., Chialant, D., Capasso, R., and Miceli, G. (2000). Separable processing of consonants and vowels. *Nature* 403, 428–430. doi: 10.1038/35000206

Cardin, V. (2016). Effects of aging and adult-onset hearing loss on cortical auditory regions. *Front. Neurosci.* 10:199. doi: 10.3389/fnins.2016.00199

Classon, E., Löfkvist, U., Rudner, M., and Rönnberg, J. (2013a). Verbal fluency in adults with postlingually acquired hearing impairment. *Speech Lang. Hear.* 17, 88–100. doi: 10.1179/2050572813Y.0000000019

Classon, E., Rudner, M., Johansson, M., and Rönnberg, J. (2013b). Early ERP signature of hearing impairment in visual rhyme judgment. *Front. Aud. Cogn. Neurosci.* 4:241. doi: 10.3389/fpsyg.2013.00241

Classon, E., Rudner, M., and Rönnberg, J. (2013c). Working memory compensates for hearing related phonological processing deficit. *J. Commun. Disord.* 46, 17–29. doi: 10.1016/j.jcomdis.2012.10.001

Craik, F. I. M., and Tulving, E. (1975). Depth of processing and the retention of words in episodic memory. *J. Exp. Psychol. Gen.* 10, 268–294. doi: 10.1037//0096-3445.104.3.268

Cumming, G. (2014). The new statistics. *Psychol. Sci.* 25, 7–29. doi: 10.1177/0956797613504966

Cutler, A. (2008). The abstract representations in speech processing. *Q. J. Exp. Psychol.* 61, 1601–1619. doi: 10.1080/13803390802218542

Daneman, M., and Carpenter, P. A. (1980). Individual differences in working memory and reading. *J. Verbal Learn. Verbal Behav.* 19, 450–466.

Eckert, M. A., Cute, S. L., Vaden, K. I. Jr., Kuchinsky, S. E., and Dubno, J. R. (2012). Auditory cortex signs of age-related hearing loss. *J. Assoc. Res. Otolaryngol.* 13, 703–713. doi: 10.1007/s10162-012-0332-5

Ferguson, M. A., and Henshaw, H. (2015). Auditory training can improve working memory, attention, and communication in adverse conditions for adults with hearing loss. *Front. Psychol.* 6:556. doi: 10.3389/fpsyg.2015.00556

Fogerty, D., Kewley-Port, D., and Humes, L. E. (2012). The relative importance of consonant and vowel segments to the recognition of words and sentences: effects of age and hearing loss. *J. Acoust. Soc. Am.* 132, 1667–1678. doi: 10.1121/1.4739463

Giroud, N., Lemke, U., Reich, P., Matthes, K., and Meyer, M. (2017). The impact of hearing aids and age-related hearing loss on auditory plasticity across three months – an electrical neuroimaging study. *Hear. Res.* 353, 162–175. doi: 10.1016/j.heares.2017.06.012

Glick, H., and Sharma, A. (2017). Cross-modal plasticity in developmental and age-related hearing loss: clinical implications. *Hear. Res.* 343, 191–201. doi: 10.1016/j.heares.2016.08.012

Husain, F. T., Medina, R. E., Davis, C. W., Szymko-Bennett, Y., Simonyan, K., Pajor, N. M., et al. (2011). Neuroanatomical changes due to hearing loss and chronic tinnitus: a combined VBM and DTI study. *Brain Res.* 1369, 74–88. doi: 10.1016/j.brainres.2010.10.095

Ito, J., Sakakibara, J., Iwasaki, Y., and Yonekura, Y. (1993). Positron emission tomography of auditory sensation in deaf patients and patients with cochlear implants. *Ann. Otol. Rhinol. Laryngol.* 102, 797–801. doi: 10.1177/000348949310201011

Jayakody, D. M. P., Friedland, P. L., Martins, R. N., and Sohrabi, H. R. (2018). Impact of aging on the auditory system and related cognitive functions: a narrative review. *Front. Neurosci.* 12:125. doi: 10.3389/fnins.2018.00125

Karawani, H., Jenkins, K., and Anderson, S. (2018). Restoration of sensory input may improve cognitive and neural function. *Neuropsychologia* 114, 203–213. doi: 10.1016/j.neuropsychologia.2018.04.041

Ladefoged, P. (1993). *A Course in Phonetics*, 3rd Edn. New York, NY: Harcourt Brace Jovanovich.

Lazard, D. S., and Giraud, A. L. (2017). Faster phonological processing and right occipito-temporal coupling in deaf adults signal poor cochlear implant outcome. *Nat. Commun.* 8:14872. doi: 10.1038/ncomms14872

Lazard, D. S., Lee, H. J., Gaebler, M., Kell, C. A., Truy, E., and Giraud, A. L. (2010). Phonological processing in post-lingual deafness and cochlear implant outcome. *Neuroimage* 49, 3443–3451. doi: 10.1016/j.neuroimage.2009.11.013

Lomber, S. G., Meredith, M. A., and Kral, A. (2010). Cross-modal plasticity in specific auditory cortices underlies visual compensations in the deaf. *Nat. Neurosci.* 13, 1421–1427. doi: 10.1038/nn.2653

Luce, P. A., and Pisoni, D. A. (1998). Recognizing spoken words: the neighborhood activation model. *Ear Hear.* 19, 1–36. doi: 10.1097/00003446-199802000-00001

Lunner, T. (2003). Cognitive function in relation to hearing aid use. *Int. J. Audiol.* 42, S49–S58.

Lunner, T., Rudner, M., and Rönnberg, J. (2009). Cognition and hearing aids. *Scand. J. Psychol.* 50, 395–403. doi: 10.1111/j.1467-9450.2009.00742.x

Maechler, M., Rousseeuw, P., Croux, C., Todorov, V., Ruckstuhl, A., Salibian-Barrera, M., et al. (2018). *robustbase: Basic Robust Statistics R Package Version 0.93-3.* Available at: http://CRAN.R-project.org/package=robustbase (accessed May 17, 2019).

Maharani, A., Dawes, P., Nazroo, J., Tampubolon, G., Pendleton, N., and Sense-Cog WP1 group. (2018). Longitudinal relationship between hearing aid use and cognitive function in older americans. *J. Am. Geriatr. Soc.* 66, 1130–1136. doi: 10.1111/jgs.15363

Marslen-Wilson, W. (1987). Functional parallelism in spoken word recognition. *Cognition* 25, 71–103.

Mattys, S. L., Barden, K., and Samuel, A. G. (2014). Extrinsic cognitive load impairs low-level speech perception. *Psychon. Bull. Rev.* 21, 748–754. doi: 10.3758/s13423-013-0544-7

Mattys, S. L., Davis, M. H., Bradlow, A. R., and Scott, S. K. (2012). Speech recognition in adverse conditions: a review. *Lang. Cogn. Process.* 27, 953–978. doi: 10.1080/01690965.2012.705006

Mattys, S. L., White, L., and Melhorn, J. F. (2005). Integration of multiple speech segmentation cues: a hierarchical framework. *J. Exp. Psychol. Gen.* 134, 477–500. doi: 10.1037/0096-3445.134.4.477

Mehler, J., Peña, M., Nespor, M., and Bonatti, L. (2006). The "soul" of language does not use statistics: reflections on vowels and consonants. *Cortex* 42, 846–854. doi: 10.1016/s0010-9452(08)70427-1

Moberly, A. C., Harris, M. S., Boyce, L., and Nittrouer, S. (2017). Speech recognition in adults with cochlear implants: the effects of working memory, phonological sensitivity, and aging. *J. Speech Lang. Hear. Res.* 60, 1046–1061. doi: 10.1044/2016_JSLHR-H-16-0119

Molander, P., Nordqvist, P., Öberg, M., Lunner, T., Lyxell, B., and Andersson, G. (2013). Internet-based hearing screening using speech-in noise: validation and comparisons of self-reported hearing problems, quality of life and phonological representation. *BMJ Open* 3:e003223. doi: 10.1136/bmjopen-2013-003223

Moons, K. G. M., Altman, D. G., Reitsma, J. B., Ioannidis, J. P. A., Macaskill, P., Steyerberg, E. W., et al. (2015). Transparent reporting of a multivariable prediction model for individual prognosis Or diagnosis (TRIPOD): explanation and elaboration. *Ann. Int. Med.* 162, W1–W73. doi: 10.7326/M14-0698

Moradi, S., Lidestam, B., Danielsson, H., Ng, E. H. N., and Rönnberg, J. (2017). Visual cues contribute differentially to audiovisual perception of consonants and vowels in improving recognition and reducing cognitive demands in listeners with hearing impairment using hearing aids. *J. Speech Lang. Hear. Res.* 60, 2687–2703. doi: 10.1044/2016_JSLHR-H-16-0160

Nakeva von Mentzer, C., Lyxell, B., Sahlén, B., Wass, M., Lindgren, M., Ors, M., et al. (2013). Computer-assisted training of phoneme-grapheme correspondence for children who are deaf and hard of hearing: effects on phonological processing skills. *Int. J. Pediatr. Otorhinolaryngol.* 77, 2049–2057. doi: 10.1016/j.ijporl.2013.10.007

Owren, M. J., and Cardillo, G. C. (2006). The relative roles of vowels and consonants in discriminating talker identity versus word meaning. *J. Acoust. Soc. Am.* 119, 1727–1739. doi: 10.1121/1.2161431

Peelle, J. E., Troiani, V., Grossman, M., and Wingfield, A. (2011). Hearing loss in older adults affects neural systems supporting speech comprehension. *J. Neurosci.* 31, 12638–12643. doi: 10.1523/JNEUROSCI.2559-11.2011

Peelle, J. E., and Wingfield, A. (2016). The neural consequences of age-related hearing loss. *Trends Neurosci.* 39, 487–497. doi: 10.1016/j.tins.2016.05.001

Pena, E. A., and Slate, E. H. (2014). *Gvlma: Global Validation of Linear Models Assumptions.* Available at: https://CRAN.R-project.org/package=gvlma (accessed May 17, 2019).

Pichora-Fuller, M. K., and Singh, G. (2006). Effects of age on auditory and cognitive processing: implications for hearing aid fitting and audiologic rehabilitation. *Trends Amplif.* 10, 29–59. doi: 10.1177/108471380601000103

R Core Team (2018). *R: A Language and Environment for Statistical Computing.* Vienna: R Foundation for Statistical Computing.

Rönnberg, J., Arlinger, S., Lyxell, B., and Kinnefors, C. (1989). Visual evoked potentials: relation to adult speechreading and cognitive function. *J. Speech Hear. Res.* 32, 725–735. doi: 10.1044/jshr.3204.725

Rönnberg, J., Danielsson, H., Rudner, M., Arlinger, S., Sternäng, O., Wahlin, A., et al. (2011). Hearing loss is negatively related to episodic and semantic longterm memory but not to short-term memory. *J. Speech Lang. Hear. Res.* 54, 705–726. doi: 10.1044/1092-4388(2010/09-0088)

Rönnberg, J., Holmer, E., and Rudner, M. (2019). Cognitive hearing science and ease of language understanding. *Int. J. Audiol.* 58, 247–261. doi: 10.1080/14992027.2018.1551631

Rönnberg, J., Lunner, T., Ng, E. H. N., Lidestam, B., Zekveld, A. A., Sörqvist, P., et al. (2016). Hearing impairment, cognition and speech understanding: exploratory factor analyses of a comprehensive test battery for a group of hearing aid users, the n200 study. *Int. J. Audiol.* 55, 623–642. doi: 10.1080/14992027.2016.1219775

Rönnberg, J., Lunner, T., Zekveld, A., Sörqvist, P., Danielsson, H., Lyxell, B., et al. (2013). The ease of language understanding (ELU) model: theoretical, empirical, and clinical advances. *Front. Syst. Neurosci.* 7:31. doi: 10.3389/fnsys.2013.00031

Rudner, M. (2018). Working memory for linguistic and non-linguistic manual gestures: evidence, theory, and application. *Front. Psychol.* 9:679. doi: 10.3389/fpsyg.2018.00679

Rudner, M., Foo, C., Rönnberg, J., and Lunner, T. (2009). Cognition and aided speech recognition in noise: specific role for cognitive factors following nine-week experience with adjusted compression settings in hearing aids. *Scand. J. Psychol.* 50, 405–418. doi: 10.1111/j.1467-9450.2009.00745.x

Rudner, M., Karlsson, T., Gunnarsson, J., and Rönnberg, J. (2013). Levels of processing and language modality specificity in working memory. *Neuropsychologia* 51, 656–666. doi: 10.1016/j.neuropsychologia.2012.12.011

Rudner, M., Seeto, M., Keidser, G., Johnson, B., and Rönnberg, J. (2019). Poorer speech reception threshold in noise is associated with lower brain volume in auditory and cognitive processing regions. *J. Speech Lang. Hear. Res.* 62, 1117–1130. doi: 10.1044/2018_JSLHR-H-ASCC7-18-0142

Signoret, C., and Rudner, M. (2019). Hearing impairment and perceived clarity of predictable speech. *Ear Hear.* doi: 10.1097/AUD.0000000000000689 [Epub ahead of print].

Steyerberg, E. W., Eijkemans, M. J. C., Harrell, F. E., and Habbema, J. D. F. (2001). Prognostic modeling with logistic regression analysis. *Med. Decis. Making* 21, 45–56. doi: 10.1177/0272989X0102100106

van Buuren, S., and Groothuis-Oudshoorn, K. (2011). mice: multivariate imputation by chained equations in R. *J. Stat. Softw.* 45, 1–67.

Yang, M., Chen, H. J., Liu, B., Huang, Z. C., Feng, Y., Li, J., et al. (2014). Brain structural and functional alterations in patients with unilateral hearing loss. *Hear. Res.* 316, 37–43. doi: 10.1016/j.heares.2014.07.006

19

The Age-Related Central Auditory Processing Disorder: Silent Impairment of the Cognitive Ear

Rodolfo Sardone[1†], Petronilla Battista[2†], Francesco Panza[1,3*], Madia Lozupone[3,4], Chiara Griseta[1], Fabio Castellana[1], Rosa Capozzo[5], Maria Ruccia[2], Emanuela Resta[6,7], Davide Seripa[3], Giancarlo Logroscino[4,5*] and Nicola Quaranta[8]

[1] Unit of Epidemiological Research on Aging "Great Age Study," National Institute of Gastroenterology-Research Hospital, IRCCS "S. De Bellis," Bari, Italy, [2] Istituti Clinici Scientifici Maugeri I.R.C.C.S., Institute of Cassano Murge, Bari, Italy, [3] Geriatric Unit, Fondazione IRCCS "Casa Sollievo della Sofferenza," Foggia, Italy, [4] Department of Basic Medical Sciences, Neuroscience, and Sense Organs, University of Bari Aldo Moro, Bari, Italy, [5] Department of Clinical Research in Neurology, Center for Neurodegenerative Diseases and the Aging Brain, University of Bari Aldo Moro, "Pia Fondazione Cardinale G. Panico," Tricase, Italy, [6] Department of Cardiac, Thoracic, and Vascular Science, Institute of Respiratory Disease, University of Bari Aldo Moro, Bari, Italy, [7] Translational Medicine and Management of Health Systems, University of Foggia, Foggia, Italy, [8] Otolaryngology Unit, Department of Basic Medicine, Neuroscience, and Sense Organs, University of Bari Aldo Moro, Bari, Italy

*Correspondence:
Francesco Panza
geriat.dot@geriatria.uniba.it;
f_panza@hotmail.com
Giancarlo Logroscino
giancarlo.logroscino@uniba.it

† These authors have contributed equally to this work

Age-related hearing loss (ARHL), also called presbycusis, is a progressive disorder affecting hearing functions and among the elderly has been recognized as the third most frequent condition. Among ARHL components, the age-related central auditory processing disorder (CAPD) refers to changes in the auditory network, negatively impacting auditory perception and/or the speech communication performance. The relationship between auditory-perception and speech communication difficulties in age-related CAPD is difficult to establish, mainly because many older subjects have concomitant peripheral ARHL and age-related cognitive changes. In the last two decades, the association between cognitive impairment and ARHL has received great attention. Peripheral ARHL has recently been defined as the modifiable risk factor with the greatest impact on the development of dementia. Even if very few studies have analyzed the relationship between cognitive decline and age-related CAPD, a strong association was highlighted. Therefore, age-related CAPD could be a specific process related to neurodegeneration. Since these two disorders can be concomitant, drawing causal inferences is difficult. The assumption that ARHL, particularly age-related CAPD, may increase the risk of cognitive impairment in the elderly remains unchallenged. This review aims to summarize the evidence of associations between age-related CAPD and cognitive disorders and to define the diagnostic procedure of CAPD in the elderly. Finally, we highlight the importance of tailoring the rehabilitation strategy to this relationship. Future longitudinal studies with larger sample sizes and the use of adequate assessment tools that can disentangle cognitive dysfunction from sensory impairments are warranted.

Keywords: age-related hearing loss, central auditory processing disorder, cognitive function, rehabilitation, dementia, MCI, lifestyle, sensorial frailty

INTRODUCTION

Age-related hearing loss (ARHL), known as presbycusis as well, is a progressive disorder that affects hearing functions. It primarily consists of a high-frequency (4 to 8 kHz) increase of the hearing threshold (Gates and Mills, 2005). ARHL is a well-recognized condition in older age with a high prevalence in the general population, being about 20% over 65 years old but increasing to 65% over 85 years (Lin et al., 2011). Among ARHL components, the age-related central auditory processing disorder (CAPD) is defined as a peculiar deficit in the processing of auditory signals along the central auditory nervous system, including one or more areas of auditory discrimination, binaural and temporal processing, clinically featured in the elderly by the inability of understanding speech in a noisy environment (American Academy of Audiology, 2010). Two forms of CAPD are currently classified in the ICD-10 as H93.25, specifically acquired and congenital forms (World Health Organization [WHO], 2017). This disorder may be classified as developmental, acquired (i.e., as a consequence of infections, neurological diseases, stroke, or noise exposure), or secondary CAPD (British Society of Audiology [BSA], 2017). However, this classification does not include presentations like age-related CAPD, also called central presbycusis, which may affect specifically older adults (Iliadou et al., 2017). This last presentation is distinguished from the other CAPD because aging is probably the main cause. Indeed, many longitudinal and cross-sectional studies showed that the occurrence of CAPD in the elderly increases with age (Gates et al., 1996; Quaranta et al., 2014). For this reason, it has also been defined as central presbycusis (Gates, 2012).

Age-related CAPD presents specific characteristics: poor speech understanding in noisy environments, or with competing speech, or any other alteration in terms of acoustics features of speech perception (Gates, 2012). These problems can be related to degeneration of the central neural auditory pathways and are the direct consequence of the degeneration of linguistic abilities in the elderly (Rönnberg et al., 2013). However, speech perception impairment is also linked to other cognitive functions (i.e., executive and attentive functions). A clear example of this link is when listeners should match rapid acoustic input with memorized word representations and phonemes to successfully extract the proper meaning of the message. This process requires cognitive-linguistic abilities, specifically working memory (Craik, 2007; Rönnberg et al., 2013). Moreover, some longitudinal studies also suggested that age-related CAPD may be fundamental in determining an increased occurrence of incident cognitive decline and dementia such as Alzheimer's disease (AD) (Panza et al., 2018a). This association seems to be stronger when comparing CAPD with peripheral ARHL (Yuan et al., 2018). Recently, this CAPD-cognition link has been summarized by the provocative term "the cognitive ear," suggesting that hearing functions are not only processed by the ear and by the auditory cortex but also by other associative cortical areas (Peelle and Wingfield, 2016; Panza et al., 2018b).

The aim of the present brief review is twofold. Firstly, to summarize the evidence of associations between age-related CAPD and cognitive disorders, illustrating the usefulness of the cognitive ear construct. Secondly, to define the procedure for diagnosing CAPD in older subjects, because CAPD can be masked by the peripheral hearing deficit which is very frequent in the elderly. Indeed, the incidence of CAPD may therefore be underestimated.

CENTRAL AUDITORY FUNCTIONS: FROM THE PHYSIOLOGY OF AUDITORY PROCESSING TO THE CLINICAL DIAGNOSIS OF THE DISORDER

Aging causes profound physiologic changes in both the peripheral and central auditory systems (Willott, 1991). The most prominent age-related hearing changes occur in the cochlea. Schuknecht and Gacek (1993) have described 4 forms of peripheral ARHL, namely sensory, neural, strial, and conductive that lead to hearing loss, and poor speech understanding. The cochlear changes responsible for peripheral ARHL have a causal role in reducing gray matter volume in the auditory cortex (Eckert et al., 2012). In particular, Lin et al. (2014) showed that ARHL is associated with shrinking of the total brain volume and, specifically, of the right temporal lobe volume. The functional consequences of ARHL are related to speech understanding which becomes more difficult (Fitzgibbons and Gordon-Salant, 2010; Humes and Dubno, 2010). Using functional MRI, Peelle and Wingfield (2016), have demonstrated that poor hearing may cause reduced language processing in primary auditory pathways and an increased compensatory language activity in other neocortical areas, not usually involved in this process, such as the prefrontal areas, the premotor cortex, and the cingulo-opercular network. This extended network, supporting language processing in presbycusis patients, has been found also by other authors, who attributed particular relevance to the cingulo-opercular cortex, involved not only in speech comprehension in normal hearing subjects but also in patients presenting with mild hearing loss (i.e., Campbell and Sharma, 2013; Sharma and Glick, 2016). Recently, the cingulo-opercular cortex has been found atrophied in a group of patients with presbycusis who also had episodic memory dysfunctions (Belkhiria et al., 2019) suggesting that cochlear dysfunction is related to cortical damage and episodic memory impairments could reflect an impairment of the Papez circuit in presbycusis patients. Overall, all these studies demonstrate that ARHL is associated with an alteration of central auditory pathways. Interestingly, the cortical areas associated with ARHL are similar to those involved in subjects with mild cognitive impairment (MCI). Thus far, cingulate cortex hypoperfusion has been found in subjects with a high risk of conversion to AD dementia (Huang et al., 2002). Several cognitive functions are processed by the cingulate cortex, one of the most important being episodic memory, which has been found as a specific neuropsychological marker in subjects with early AD (i.e., Gainotti et al., 2014 Battista et al., 2017).

Concerning CAPD, two hypotheses have been proposed to explain the origin of the disorder: the mechanistic and the neurodegeneration models (Lindenberger et al., 2001;

Panza et al., 2018a). CAPD is generally defined as a peculiar impairment in the processing and analysis of auditory signals along the central auditory nervous system, referring also to the bottom-up and top-down neural connectivity (American Academy of Audiology, 2010). The former hypothesis suggests that CAPD can be the consequence of sensorial deprivation due to peripheral/cochlear damage (bottom-up theory). The neural pathways activity declines and connections are lost while the sensorial deprivation continues (Panza et al., 2018b). The other theory takes into account the strong association between CAPD and cognitive impairment, assuming the origin of CAPD to be an independent form of neurodegeneration (Humes et al., 2012). Regardless of what the correct theory may be, the causal pattern behind the alte Panza et al. (2018a) ration of central auditory pathways is still unknown (Jayakody et al., 2018). A new anatomical resource could be used, in the near future, to solve this dilemma: the human connectome, which has been developed from functional neuroimaging of thousands of healthy persons and provides a map of these brain connections. With the use of the connectome, lesions in different locations (e.g., cochlear nuclei and temporal cortex), that originated at different times, can be linked to common networks in a way that was not previously possible to identify, adding new variables to define causal inferences about the onset of age-related CAPD in normal hearing subjects (Fox, 2018).

Cortical Auditory Functions in Aging and Cognitive Effort in Understanding Degraded Speech

At a neural level, hearing impairment leads to a reduced activation of central auditory pathways, resulting in a compensatory increased activation of the cognitive control network, as well as dysfunctional auditory–limbic connectivity, and deafferentation-induced reduction in volume of the frontal brain regions. These pathologic changes decrease cognitive performance and increase the risk of depression by reducing cognitive reserve, increasing executive dysfunction, and disrupting normative emotion reactivity and regulation (Rutherford et al., 2018).

Since the term age-related CAPD refers to the difficulty in the processing of perception of auditory information in the central nervous system, it is a neurobiological activity which underlies that processing and gives rise to the electrophysiological auditory potentials (American Speech-Language-Hearing Association, 2005). This definition matches the typical cognitive, behavioral and electrophysiological auditory outcomes associated with the aging brain.

The main cognitive tasks processed by the prefrontal cortex are executive functions, and working memory abilities seem to be specifically involved when listeners match the rapid incoming sound to the memorized representations of words and phonemes in order to successfully extract the intended meaning (Rönnberg et al., 2013). Therefore, extracting information from a degraded signal requires a greater effort, contributing to increase the cognitive effort and hence interfering with other cognitive-linguistic operations. An intuitive way to understand the role of working memory is that if an incoming signal cannot be understood, it must be maintained for a longer time to allow other cognitive systems to process it in the time it takes to function (Peelle, 2018).

Clinical Assessment of Age-Related Central Auditory Processing Disorder

The most consistent clinical approach to detect age-related CAPD is by auditory behavioral assessment. At present, audiological tests have been validated primarily in subjects with a specific and well-determined impairment in the area associated with a particular auditory function (e.g., brainstem or temporal lobe tumors) (Bocca et al., 1954, 1955). In view of the many tests used in audiological practice for the definition of age-related CAPD, we have considered only those most commonly used in epidemiological studies to measure the association with cognitive impairment, as shown in **Figure 1**.

Speech in Noise Processing

Understanding words in background noise becomes more challenging with the passing of years, and the elderly have significantly more difficulties with respect to younger adults (Pronk et al., 2013). Auditory processing and cognition play an important role in the intelligibility of speech in noisy environments in older age. The effect of aging is evident in understanding words in competing situations (Gates et al., 2008), time-compressed speech (Vaughan et al., 2008), and binaural speech perception (Golding et al., 2006). Anatomical pathways involved in distinguishing useful signal from noise lie in the medial olivary complex. The modulation of the medial olivary complex on the outer hair cells, to reduce the gain of noisy signals, is primarily activated in the area of attentive-executive functions (dorsolateral prefrontal cortex) (Della Penna et al., 2007).

In an observational study of about 5000 subjects aged between 40 and 60 years a drop-in speech perception against noise was observed in both sexes as from 50 years old (Moore et al., 2014). This decline was higher in subjects with lower cognitive abilities (processing speed, memory, and reasoning).

Dichotic Processing

Dichotic listening can be defined as the contextual stimulation of both ears, with different signals reaching each ear. The role of the corpus callosum in dichotic processing has been exploited by several authors in the literature. For example, patients which present the language function lateralized in the left hemisphere, and with a clinical history of split-brain surgery, despite preoperatively normal dichotic processing abilities, presented a total inability to perform dichotic tests on left ear (Musiek et al., 1989). Jerger and Martin (2006) studied 172 older participants which present, at the Dichotic Sentence Identification test, for 58% of them, an impaired performance for the divided attention task (response required for both ears), while no alterations were found for the directed attention (response required for one ear while ignoring the other). The authors concluded that the pattern could underlying a cognitive in nature in 58% of cases and could

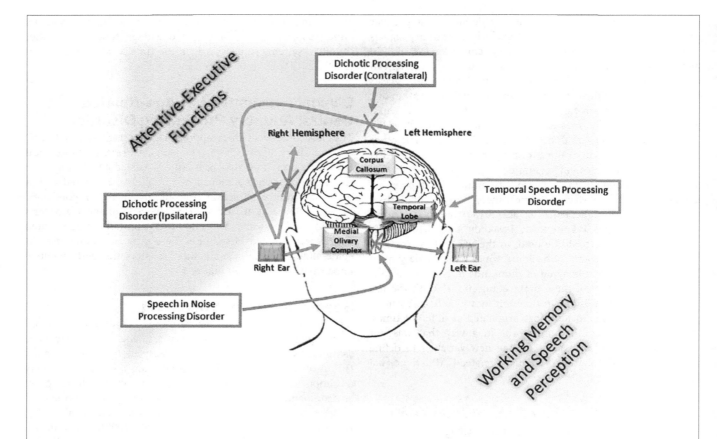

FIGURE 1 | Different pathophysiological pathways of the age-related central auditory processing disorder (CAPD). The figure illustrates the myriad deficits [i.e., dichotic processing (ipsilateral and contralateral), speech recognition in noise, and temporal speech processing involved in age-related CAPD]. Each of these disorders has a particular location along the auditory pathways, i.e., superior olivary complex and corpus callosum, medial olivary complex, and temporal lobe, respectively. Moreover, each of these auditory functions is associated with a cognitive process that is susceptible to the neurodegeneration. Specifically, executive and attentive functions are associated with speech in noise processing, dichotic ipsi and contralateral processing, which are highlighted in orange in the figure, while working memory and speech perception are associated with temporal speech processing which is displayed in pink in the figure.

be suggestive of structural abnormalities in the central nervous system for the 23% of cases.

A widely standardized dichotic test is by Synthetic Sentence Identification with Ipsilateral Competing Message (SSI-ICM) or a Contralateral Competing Message (SSI-CCM) (Jerger, 1973). The patient listens to an average narrative and is asked to identify 10 sentences superimposed on the narrative by the same speaker. Each sentence has no meaning even though each series of three words makes syntactical sense. The signal and the message are presented at the same intensity level, usually 40 dB above the hearing threshold. Since audibility is not an issue, the test requires the listener to attend to the message and ignore the narrative.

Temporal Processing

Temporal processing refers to the hearing ability to individuate short changes in stimulus duration (Boettcher, 2002). Detecting and discriminating timing differences in speech is important in competitive listening or noisy environments (Schneider, 1997). Detecting gaps in continuous signals (noise or sound) is the main feature of these processes and many tests have been proposed to assess it (Phillips et al., 2000; John et al., 2012). However, temporal

processes are heavily influenced by the hearing threshold and cognitive abilities such as working memory and attentive-executive functions, making it difficult to draw meaningful inferences about the effect of aging and cognitive impairment on them (Humes and Dubno, 2010). Cognitive functions such as working memory and attention decline with age, and this has a significant consequence on words understanding regardless of hearing status (Schneider et al., 2010).

Electrophysiological Assessment

Electrophysiological measures are widely used for the evaluation of the central auditory deficits. Most studies applied highly standardized electrophysiological evaluation methods. These are subdivided topographically according to the most probable location of the bioelectric signal derivation. Auditory Brainstem Response (ABR) is an evoked potential, which is primarily free of higher-order influences via the effect of quiet, conscious rest or sleep with closed eyes. Several age-related changes of ABR have been described (Boettcher, 2002). There is little evidence regarding the influence of temporal functions on the ABR. Temporal processing can be defined as the ability to resolve rapid changes in stimulus duration and a few studies have demonstrated, introducing gap in noise stimuli, that ABRs are modified in terms of latency and amplitude (Poth et al., 2001; Goll et al., 2011). In addition to the pathological changes in auditory pathways, mouse models and AD patients also showed increased ABR thresholds, and that a greater hearing loss was related to higher adjusted relative odds for dementia (Uhlmann et al., 1989; O'Leary et al., 2017). Cortical Event-Related Potentials include a wide range of electrophysiological tests aimed at the definition of several electrical patterns of age-related auditory impairment (Jerger and Lew, 2004). The P300 seems to be a sensitive electrophysiological test for CAPD, that is thought to reflect the speed of processing of auditory information. The P300 in clinical studies often use 1,000 and 2,000 Hz tone bursts as frequent and target (oddball) stimuli, respectively, although speech signals can also be used (Polich, 2004). The comparison of P300 in terms of latency of presentation was age-dependent, while insufficient evidence was found about electrophysiological features in the link between central auditory processing and cognition (Cintra et al., 2015).

Diagnosis of Age-Related Central Auditory Processing Disorder

There is currently no reference standard for diagnosing age-related CAPD (Vermiglio, 2016). The diagnosis is met when an alteration of the central auditory processes related to the effect of age occurs and no other cerebral pathologies can explain those alterations (Humes et al., 2012). The diagnosis of CAPD can be made if at least one of the above-described central auditory tests results impaired, as established by the corresponding cut-off scores and procedures (Humes et al., 2012).

According to Gates (2012), one of the most sensitive and widely used diagnostic tests to define age-related CAPD is the SSI test by Jerger (1973). The diagnosis made by this test is based on three criteria. Firstly, an unimpaired peripheral auditory function (<40 dB HL in the better ear) and a word recognition score in the quiet of 70% or better. Secondly, the patient must have adequate visual acuity to see the list of sentences (used to test for CAPD). Thirdly, the procedures are first administered in a "training" mode with the signal 10 dB louder than the message to ensure the patient understands the method. After that, the actual test is done at a 0-dB message-to-competition ratio; correct selection of 8 of the 10 presentations is considered normal (Gates, 2012). Moreover, the SSI-ICM appears to be more sensitive to detect dementia than the contralateral form (SSI-CCM) (Gates et al., 1995). In our clinical and research experience, we have found that the use of SSI-ICM seems to be a good standard for the diagnosis of CAPD in terms of accuracy and efficiency, and for the prediction of cognitive impairment in the elderly (Quaranta et al., 2014; Sardone et al., 2018).

In the elderly, peripheral ARHL is very common, but older individuals with impaired peripheral auditory function (>40 dB HL of pure tone average in the better ear) are not diagnosed with age-related CAPD. For this reason, nowadays the age-related CAPD component cannot be evaluated in older individuals with impaired peripheral auditory function. Possibly, the only way to solve this issue is with the use of advanced diagnostic methods that are able to bypass the cochlear input (i.e., neuroimaging methods). Consequently, the comorbidity between CAPD and peripheral ARHL could lead to underestimating the burden of the phenomenon and its consequences (Gates, 2012).

ASSOCIATION BETWEEN AGE-RELATED CENTRAL AUDITORY PROCESSING DISORDER AND COGNITIVE IMPAIRMENT

In the past 2 years, in cohorts studies an increasing body of meta-analytic evidence has demonstrated an increased risk of cognitive decline in peripheral ARHL (Panza et al., 2018a). Concerning age-related CAPD, few studies have investigated the relationship between this component of ARHL and cognitive impairment (Yuan et al., 2018). Specifically, this association has been found in some small-scale clinically based studies (Kurylo et al., 1993; Idrizbegovic et al., 2011, 2013; Edwards et al., 2017), two large-scale observational studies (Gates et al., 2010, 2011), one cross-sectional (Quaranta et al., 2014) and one longitudinal population-based study (Gates et al., 2002). Moreover, in the population-based Framingham cohort, Gates et al. (1996) observed that the risk of developing AD in age-related CAPD was 6.07 higher than in subjects of the same age with normal hearing. Another Italian population-based study, the Great Age Study, found an odds ratio of 11.2 in a cross-sectional survey, using the SSI-ICM test (Sardone et al., 2018).

The central component of ARHL could be the consequence of a peripheral auditory deficit, but on the other hand, central changes may be independent from peripheral ones, may be a combination of both auditory components, or, finally, a result of cognitive dysfunction. For this reason, the association between age-related CAPD and cognitive decline is usually considered only in subjects with normal hearing (Humes et al., 2012). So far, the most plausible hypothesis is that age-related CAPD and cognitive decline, particularly of executive functions, are associated (Craik, 2007).

Another way to define a pathophysiological association between age-related CAPD and cognitive decline could be to focus on the prodromal stages of dementia defined as MCI. The link between cognition and central auditory process has been demonstrated by the association between a diagnosis of MCI due to AD and poorer performance on tests of central auditory processing (i.e., Idrizbegovic et al., 2011). Furthermore, Iliadou and Kaprinis (2003) reviewed the literature and concluded that CAPD may be a precursor of AD, preceding the clinical diagnosis by 5 to 10 years. However, even if most of these clinical and epidemiological studies suggest a link between central auditory dysfunction and cognitive decline, the causal mechanisms underlying this link are still unknown (Wayne and Johnsrude, 2015). Moreover, although an association has been observed, no consistent data with longitudinal evidence are still available (Idrizbegovic et al., 2011, 2013; Quaranta et al., 2014; Edwards et al., 2017).

A seminal neuropathological study supported the hypothesis that age-related CAPD may result from a degenerative pathway other than cognitive decline, showing that brain amyloid-βββ, believed to be the initial event of AD, was uncommon in central auditory pathways early in the clinical course of the disease. By contrast, there was early formation of neurofibrillary tangles, mainly consisting of hyperphosphorylated tau protein, suggesting that neurodegeneration in the auditory system may be an ongoing process throughout the AD course (Sinha et al., 1993).

Therefore, further research is needed in order to disentangle the real causal association between pathological correlates of presbycusis (including cochlear receptor cell loss, stria vascularis atrophy, and auditory-nerve neuron loss) and the atrophy of specific brain regions, and consequently the related cognitive domains involved in subjects with CAPD (Shen et al., 2018). The only way to observe whether the neurodegenerative process starts from the frontal lobe (executive functions) or from the central auditory pathways could be through further longitudinal studies on a generalizable population with dynamic neuroimaging features.

CLINICAL IMPLICATIONS AND REHABILITATION

It is very difficult to devise rehabilitation strategies for a silent deficit like age-related CAPD, especially if associated with an initial cognitive impairment. One of the most logic approaches is to increase the listener's signal/noise ratio, controlling the acoustic environment in order to decrease listening difficulties. Reducing noise and reverberation and increasing the direct sound field (lower ceilings, less reverberating materials, and more preferential seating). This is also a top-down strategy aimed at reducing the cognitive load (Baran, 2002). Another strategy, this time bottom-up, in subjects with hearing aids could be to increase the gain of the near field signal, using a frequency-modulation system: listening skill may be further enhanced by frequency-modulation systems (Kricos, 2006) and using binaural stimulation in the hearing aids (increasing the loudness summation and localization of the sound source) (Walden and Walden, 2005).

Since age related central auditory dysfunction may be involved in the continuum from preclinical to advanced stages of dementia (Jayakody et al., 2018), it is very important to implement holistic and structured intervention for these subjects. Specifically, this intervention should combine auditory and cognitive functions, increasing sensorial input and decreasing the cognitive effort/working memory ability, respectively (see **Figure 1**).

Caregivers together with patients who are experiencing contextually age-related CAPD and cognitive impairment should undergo counseling with audiologists and neuropsychologists to start awareness training that includes instruction in the use of meaningful gestures and beneficial conversational techniques such as speaking more clearly, with long intervals, and with more enunciation (Kiessling et al., 2003). A rehabilitation protocol that includes both hearing training and a cognitive

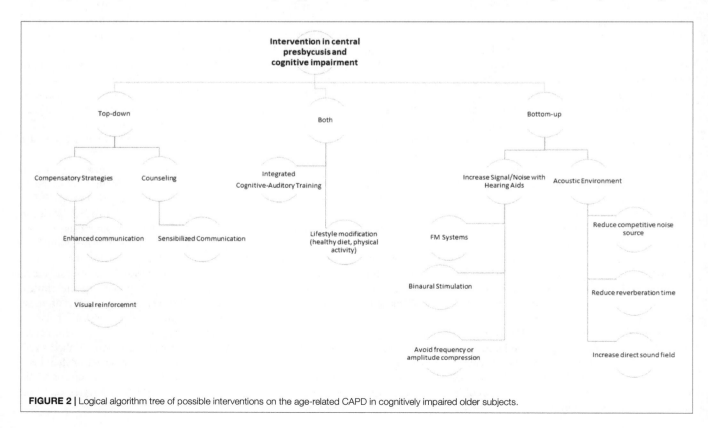

FIGURE 2 | Logical algorithm tree of possible interventions on the age-related CAPD in cognitively impaired older subjects.

rehabilitation may be useful to delay the synergic effect of both deficits. Additionally, individuals with age-related CAPD may improve the subjective impairment participating in individual and/or group training sessions (**Figure 2**; Heine and Browning, 2002). Therefore, it is evident that intervention on all risk factors that cause both cognitive impairment and hearing loss may, in some way, slow down the vicious circle of reverse causality, i.e., intervening on lifestyle factors. A diet fulfilling the Mediterranean-type dietary pattern with a high presence of antioxidant-rich foods and an anaerobic physical activity for at least 20 minutes 5 days a week could be recommended as a useful adjuvant to the combined rehabilitation therapy for hearing loss and cognitive impairment (**Figure 2**; Solfrizzi et al., 2018). However, the evidence supporting the effectiveness of any particular intervention approach is relatively weak due to the lack of good quality interventional studies.

FUTURE DIRECTIONS AND CONCLUSION

The central auditory deficit is a silent impairment because it does not have an immediate impact on daily functions. As consequences, two fundamental problems arise. The first is that the subject is usually not aware of his/her deficits and tends to minimize the handicap, often avoiding situations that could trigger it, such as avoiding noisy or crowded places. This predisposes patients to a social isolation that has been shown to have an important effect on cognitive status (Lozupone et al., 2018). The second point is that age-related CAPD is often associated with a deficit of some cognitive domains, in particular executive functions. This could mask the coexistence of the two conditions and delay the institution of rehabilitative and preventive interventions.

When the clinical suspicion of age-related CAPD and cognitive impairment is confirmed, clinicians should be sufficiently aware to be able to address patients to rehabilitation programs. The first target of future research should be to improve the diagnosis of CAPD in the elderly, when cognitive disorders are present, relying on the identification of specific psychoacoustic, clinical, or objective auditory markers (core measures) to guide focused management provision. Finally, fundamental pathways to radically change the trajectories of the degeneration of the "cognitive ear" lie in two future directions. The first direction will involve high quality audiological assessment supported by a targeted use of next generation neuroimaging. The second direction lies in demonstrating the benefits of next generation hearing restoration devices (cochlear implants and hearing aids) empowered with artificial intelligence algorithms in order to reduce competitive acoustic signals. The rehabilitative outcomes of these devices need to be tested by means of well-designed controlled clinical trials, during tailored intervention on cognitive impairment and CAPD." (Jayakody et al., 2018; Panza et al., 2018a).

AUTHOR CONTRIBUTIONS

RS, PB, FP, GL, and NQ contributed substantially to the conception and design of the work, drafting and revising the manuscript for important intellectual content, approved the final version to be published, and agreed to be accountable for all aspects of the work. CG, FC, RC, ML, MR, ER, and DS drafted corresponding sections of the manuscript. All authors approved the final version to be published and agreed to be accountable for all aspects of the work.

ACKNOWLEDGMENTS

We thank Dr. Tiziana Lozupone for her useful comments on the manuscript. We also thank all the "Great Age" Research Team. This manuscript is the result of the research work on frailty undertaken by the "Italia Longeva: Research Network on Aging" team, supported by the resources of the Italian Ministry of Health – Research Networks of National Health Institutes.

REFERENCES

American Academy of Audiology (2010). *Diagnosis, Treatment and Management of Children and Adults with Central Auditory Processing Disorder*. Available at: https://audiology-web.s3.amazonaws.com/migrated/CAPD%20Guidelines% 208-2010.pdf_539952af956c79.73897613.pdf (accessed May 31, 2019).

American Speech-Language-Hearing Association (2005). *(Central) Auditory Processing Disorders [Technical Report]*. Available at: http://www.asha.org/ policy/TR2005-00043/ (accessed May 31, 2019).

Baran, J. (2002). Managing auditory processing disorders in adolescents and adults. *Semin. Hear.* 23, 327–336. doi: 10.1055/s-2002-35881

Battista, P., Salvatore, C., and Castiglioni, I. (2017). Optimizing neuropsychological assessments for cognitive, behavioral, and functional impairment classification: a machine learning study. *Behav. Neurol.* 2017:1850909. doi: 10.1155/2017/ 1850909

Belkhiria, C., Vergara, R. C., San Martin, S., Leiva, A., Marcenaro, B., Martinez, M., et al. (2019). Cingulate cortex atrophy is associated with hearing loss in presbycusis with cochlear amplifier dysfunction. *Front. Aging Neurosci.* 11:97. doi: 10.3389/fnagi.2019.00097

Bocca, E., Calearo, C., and Cassinari, V. (1954). A new method for testing hearing in temporal lobe tumours; preliminary report. *Acta Otolaryngol.* 44, 219–221. doi: 10.3109/00016485409128700

Bocca, E., Calearo, C., Cassinari, V., and Migliavacca, F. (1955). Testing "cortical" hearing in temporal lobe tumours. *Acta Otolaryngol.* 45, 289–304. doi: 10.3109/ 00016485509124282

Boettcher, F. A. (2002). Presbycusis and the auditory brainstem response. *J. Speech Lang. Hear. Res.* 45, 1249–1261.

British Society of Audiology [BSA] (2017). *Position Statement and Practice Guidance, Auditory Processing Disorder (APD)*. Available at: http://www.thebsa.org.uk/wp-content/uploads/2017/04/APD-Position- Statement-Practice-Guidance-APD-2017.pdf (accessed May 31, 2019).

Campbell, J., and Sharma, A. (2013). Compensatory changes in cortical resource allocation in adults with hearing loss. *Front. Syst. Neurosci.* 7:71. doi: 10.3389/ fnsys.2013.00071

Cintra, M. T. G., Tavares, M. S., Gomes, S. A., de Oliveira Gonçalves, T., Matos da Cunha, L. C., Utsch Gonçalves, D., et al. (2015). P300 evoked potential and risk of mild cognitive impairment progression to Alzheimer's dementia: a literature review. *J. Neurol. Neurophysiol.* 6:322.

Craik, F. I. (2007). The role of cognition in age-related hearing loss. *J. Am. Acad. Audiol.* 18, 539–547. doi: 10.3766/jaaa.18.7.2

Della Penna, S., Brancucci, A., Babiloni, C., Franciotti, R., Pizzella, V., Rossi, D., et al. (2007). Lateralization of dichotic speech stimuli is based on specific auditory pathway interactions. *Cereb. Cortex* 17, 2303–2311. doi: 10.1093/cercor/bhl139

Eckert, M. A., Cute, S. L., Vaden, K. I., Kuchinsky, S. E., and Dubno, J. R. (2012). Auditory cortex signs of age-related hearing loss. *J. Assoc. Res. Otolaryngol.* 13, 703–713. doi: 10.1007/s10162-012-0332-5

Edwards, J. D., Lister, J. J., Elias, M. N., Tetlow, A. M., Sardina, A. L., Sadeq, N. A., et al. (2017). Auditory processing of older adults with probable mild cognitive impairment. *J. Speech Lang. Hear. Res.* 60, 1427–1435. doi: 10.1044/2016_JSLHR-H-16-0066

Fitzgibbons, P. J., and Gordon-Salant, S. (2010). *Behavioral Studies with Aging Humans: Hearing Sensitivity and Psychoacoustics.* New York, NY: Springer, 111–134.

Fox, M. D. (2018). Mapping symptoms to brain networks with the human connectome. *N. Engl. J. Med.* 379, 2237–2245. doi: 10.1056/nejmra1706158

Gainotti, G., Quaranta, D., Vita, M. G., and Marra, C. (2014). Neuropsychological predictors of conversion from mild cognitive impairment to Alzheimer's disease. *J. Alzheimers Dis.* 38, 481–495. doi: 10.3233/jad-130881

Gates, G. A. (2012). Central presbycusis: an emerging view. *Otolaryngol. Head Neck Surg.* 147, 1–2. doi: 10.1177/0194599812446282

Gates, G. A., Anderson, M. L., McCurry, S. M., Feeney, M. P., and Larson, E. B. (2011). Central auditory dysfunction as a harbinger of Alzheimer dementia. *Arch. Otolaryngol. Head Neck Surg.* 137, 390–395. doi: 10.1001/archoto.2011.28

Gates, G. A., Beiser, A., Rees, T. S., D'Agostino, R. B., and Wolf, P. A. (2002). Central auditory dysfunction may precede the onset of clinical dementia in people with probable Alzheimer's disease. *J. Am. Geriatr. Soc.* 50, 482–488. doi: 10.1046/j.1532-5415.2002.50114.x

Gates, G. A., Cobb, J. L., Linn, R. T., Rees, T., Wolf, P. A., and D'Agostino, R. B. (1996). Central auditory dysfunction, cognitive dysfunction, and dementia in older people. *Arch. Otolaryngol. Head Neck Surg.* 122, 161–167. doi: 10.1001/archotol.1996.01890140047010

Gates, G. A., Feeney, M. P., and Mills, D. (2008). Cross-sectional age-changes of hearing in the elderly. *Ear Hear.* 29, 865–874. doi: 10.1097/aud.0b013e318181adb5

Gates, G. A., Gibbons, L. E., McCurry, S. M., Crane, P. K., Feeney, M. P., and Larson, E. B. (2010). Executive dysfunction and presbycusis in older persons with and without memory loss and dementia. *Cogn. Behav. Neurol.* 23, 218–223. doi: 10.1097/WNN.0b013e3181d748d7

Gates, G. A., Karzon, R. K., Garcia, P., Peterein, J., Storandt, M., Morris, J. C., et al. (1995). Auditory dysfunction in aging and senile dementia of the Alzheimer's type. *Arch. Neurol.* 52, 626–634.

Gates, G. A., and Mills, J. H. (2005). Presbycusis. *Lancet* 366, 1111–1120.

Golding, M., Taylor, A., Cupples, L., and Mitchell, P. (2006). Odds of demonstrating auditory processing abnormality in the average older adult: the blue mountains hearing study. *Ear Hear.* 27, 129–138. doi: 10.1097/01.aud.0000202328.19037.ff

Goll, J. C., Kim, L. G., Hailstone, J. C., Lehmann, M., Buckley, A., Crutch, S. J., et al. (2011). Auditory object cognition in dementia. *Neuropsychologia* 49, 2755–2765. doi: 10.1016/j.neuropsychologia.2011.06.004

Heine, C., and Browning, C. J. (2002). Communication and psychosocial consequences of sensory loss in older adults: overview and rehabilitation directions. *Disabil. Rehabil.* 24, 763–773. doi: 10.1080/09638280210129162

Huang, C., Wahlund, L. O., Svensson, L., Winblad, B., and Julin, P. (2002). Cingulate cortex hypoperfusion predicts Alzheimer's disease in mild cognitive impairment. *BMC Neurol.* 2:9. doi: 10.1186/1471-2377-2-9

Humes, L. E., and Dubno, J. R. (2010). *Factors Affecting Speech Understanding in Older Adults.* New York, NY: Springer, 211–257.

Humes, L. E., Dubno, J. R., Gordon-Salant, S., Lister, J. J., Cacace, A. T., Cruickshanks, K. J., et al. (2012). Central presbycusis: a review and evaluation of the evidence. *J. Am. Acad. Audiol.* 23, 635–666. doi: 10.3766/jaaa.23.8.5

Idrizbegovic, E., Hederstierna, C., Dahlquist, M., Nordström, C. K., Jelic, V., and Rosenhall, U. (2011). Central auditory function in early Alzheimer's disease and in mild cognitive impairment. *Age Ageing* 40, 249–254. doi: 10.1093/ageing/afq168

Idrizbegovic, E., Hederstierna, C., Dahlquist, M., and Rosenhall, U. (2013). Short-term longitudinal study of central auditory function in Alzheimer's disease and mild cognitive impairment. *Dement. Geriatr. Cogn. Dis. Extra* 3, 468–471. doi: 10.1159/000355371

Iliadou, V., and Kaprinis, S. (2003). Clinical psychoacoustics in Alzheimer's disease central auditory processing disorders and speech deterioration. *Ann. Gen. Hosp. Psychiatry* 2:12.

Iliadou, V. V., Ptok, M., Grech, H., Pedersen, E. R., Brechmann, A., Deggouj, N., et al. (2017). A european perspective on auditory processing disorder-current knowledge and future research focus. *Front. Neurol.* 8:622. doi: 10.3389/fneur.2017.00622

Jayakody, D. M., Friedland, P. L., Martins, R. N., and Sohrabi, H. R. (2018). Impact of aging on the auditory system and related cognitive functions: a narrative review. *Front. Neurosci.* 12:125. doi: 10.3389/fnins.2018.00125

Jerger, J. (1973). Audiological findings in aging. *Adv. Otorhinolaryngol.* 20, 115–124.

Jerger, J., and Lew, H. L. (2004). Principles and clinical applications of auditory evoked potentials in the geriatric population. *Phys. Med. Rehabil. Clin. N. Am.* 151, 235–250. doi: 10.1016/s1047-9651(03)00099-8

Jerger, J., and Martin, J. (2006). Dichotic listening tests in the audiological assessment of auditory processing disorders. *Audiol. Med.* 4, 25–34. doi: 10.1080/16513860600567823

John, A. B., Hall, J. W., and Kreisman, B. M. (2012). Effects of advancing age and hearing loss on gaps-in-noise test performance. *Am. J. Audiol.* 21, 242–250. doi: 10.1044/1059-0889(2012/11-0023)

Kiessling, J., Pichora-Fuller, M. K., Gatehouse, S., Stephens, D., Arlinger, S., and Chisolm, T. (2003). Candidature for and delivery of audiological services: special needs of older people. *Int. J. Audiol.* 42(Suppl. 2), S92–S101.

Kricos, P. B. (2006). Audiologic management of older adults with hearing loss and compromised cognitive/psychoacoustic auditory processing capabilities. *Trends Amplif.* 10, 1–28. doi: 10.1177/10847138060100010

Kurylo, D. D., Corkin, S., Allard, T., Zatorre, R. J., and Growdon, J. H. (1993). Auditory function in Alzheimer's disease. *Neurology* 43, 1893–1899.

Lin, F. R., Ferrucci, L., An, Y., Goh, J. O., Doshi, J., Metter, E. J., et al. (2014). Association of hearing impairment with brain volume changes in older adults. *Neuroimage* 90, 84–92. doi: 10.1016/j.neuroimage.2013.12.059

Lin, F. R., Thorpe, R., Gordon-Salant, S., and Ferrucci, L. (2011). Hearing loss prevalence and risk factors among older adults in the United States. *J. Gerontol. A Biol. Sci. Med. Sci.* 66, 582–590. doi: 10.1093/gerona/glr002

Lindenberger, U., Scherer, H., and Baltes, P. B. (2001). The strong connection between sensory and cognitive performance in old age: not due to sensory acuity reductions operating during cognitive assessment. *Psychol. Aging* 16, 196–205. doi: 10.1037/0882-7974.16.2.196

Lozupone, M., Panza, F., Piccininni, M., Copetti, M., Sardone, R., Imbimbo, B. P., et al. (2018). Social dysfunction in older age and relationships with cognition, depression, and apathy: the GreatAGE study. *J. Alzheimers Dis.* 65, 989–1000. doi: 10.3233/JAD-180466

Moore, D. R., Edmondson-Jones, M., Dawes, P., Fortnum, H., McCormack, A., Pierzycki, R. H., et al. (2014). Relation between speech-in-noise threshold, hearing loss and cognition from 40–69 years of age. *PLoS One* 9:e107720. doi: 10.1371/journal.pone.0107720

Musiek, F. E., Kurdziel-Schwan, S., Kibbe, K. S., Gollegly, K. M., Baran, J. A., and Rintelmann, W. F. (1989). The dichotic rhyme task: results in split-brain patients. *Ear Hear.* 10, 33–39. doi: 10.1097/00003446-198902000-00006

O'Leary, T. P., Shin, S., Fertan, E., Dingle, R. N., Almuklass, A., Gunn, R. K., et al. (2017). Reduced acoustic startle response and peripheral hearing loss in the 5xFAD mouse model of Alzheimer's disease. *Genes Brain Behav.* 16, 554–563. doi: 10.1111/gbb.12370

Panza, F., Lozupone, M., Sardone, R., Battista, P., Piccininni, M., Dibello, V., et al. (2018a). Sensorial frailty: age-related hearing loss and the risk of cognitive impairment and dementia in later life. *Ther. Adv. Chronic Dis.* doi: 10.1177/2040622318811000 [Epub ahead of print].

Panza, F., Quaranta, N., and Logroscino, G. (2018b). Sensory changes and the hearing loss–cognition link: the cognitive ear. *JAMA Otolaryngol. Head Neck Surg.* 144, 127–128.

Peelle, J. E. (2018). Listening effort: how the cognitive consequences of acoustic challenge are reflected in brain and behavior. *Ear Hear.* 39, 204–214. doi: 10.1097/AUD.0000000000000494

Peelle, J. E., and Wingfield, A. (2016). The neural consequences of age-related hearing loss. *Trends Neurosci.* 39, 486–497. doi: 10.1016/j.tins.2016.05.001

Phillips, S. L., Gordon-Salant, S., Fitzgibbons, P. J., and Yeni-Komshian, G. (2000). Frequency and temporal resolution in elderly listeners with good and poor word recognition. *J. Speech Lang. Hear. Res.* 43, 217–228. doi: 10.1044/jslhr. 4301.217

Polich, J. (2004). Clinical application of the P300 event-related brain potential. *Phys. Med. Rehabil. Clin. N. Am.* 15, 133–161. doi: 10.1016/s1047-9651(03) 00109-8

Poth, E. A., Boettcher, F. A., Mills, J. H., and Dubno, J. R. (2001). Auditory brainstem responses in younger and older adults for broadband noises separated by a silent gap. *Hear. Res.* 161, 81–86. doi: 10.1016/s0378-5955(01) 00352-5

Pronk, M., Deeg, D. J., Festen, J. M., Twisk, J. W., Smits, C., Comijs, H. C., et al. (2013). Decline in older persons' ability to recognize speech in noise: the influence of demographic, health-related, environmental, and cognitive factors. *Ear Hear.* 34, 722–732. doi: 10.1097/AUD.0b013e3182994eee

Quaranta, N., Coppola, F., Casulli, M., Barulli, M. R., Panza, F., Tortelli, R., et al. (2014). The prevalence of peripheral and central hearing impairment and its relation to cognition in older adults. *Audiol. Neurootol.* 19(Suppl. 1), 10–14. doi: 10.1159/000371597

Rönnberg, J., Lunner, T., Zekveld, A., Sörqvist, P., Danielsson, H., Lyxell, B., et al. (2013). The ease of language understanding (ELU) model: theoretical, empirical, and clinical advances. *Front. Syst. Neurosci.* 7:31. doi: 10.3389/fnsys. 2013.00031

Rutherford, B. R., Brewster, K., Golub, J. S., Kim, A. H., and Roose, S. P. (2018). Sensation and psychiatry: linking age-related hearing loss to late-life depression and cognitive decline. *Am. J. Psychiatry* 175, 215–224. doi: 10.1176/appi.ajp. 2017.17040423

Sardone, R., Battista, P., Tortelli, R., Piccininni, M., Coppola, F., Guerra, V., et al. (2018). Relationship between central and peripheral presbycusis and mild cognitive impairment in a population-based study of Southern Italy: the "Great Age Study". *Neurology* 90(15 Suppl.):P1.131.

Schneider, B. (1997). Psychoacoustics and aging: implications for everyday listening. *J. Speech Lang. Pathol. Audiol.* 21, 111–124.

Schneider, B. A., Pichora-Fuller, K., and Daneman, M. (2010). *Effects of Senescent Changes in Audition and Cognition on Spoken Language Comprehension.* New York, NY: Springer, 167–210.

Schuknecht, H. F., and Gacek, M. R. (1993). Cochlear pathology in presbycusis. *Ann. Otol. Rhinol. Laryngol.* 102(1 Pt 2), 1–16. doi: 10.1177/00034894931020s101

Sharma, A., and Glick, H. (2016). Cross-modal re-organization in clinical populations with hearing loss. *Brain Sci.* 6:4. doi: 10.3390/brainsci6010004

Shen, Y., Ye, B., Chen, P., Wang, Q., Fan, C., Shu, Y., et al. (2018). Cognitive decline, dementia, alzheimer's disease and presbycusis: examination of the possible molecular mechanism. *Front. Neurosci.* 12:394. doi: 10.3389/fnins.2018. 00394

Sinha, U. K., Hollen, K. M., Rodriguez, R., and Miller, C. A. (1993). Auditory system degeneration in Alzheimer's disease. *Neurology* 43, 779–785.

Solfrizzi, V., Agosti, P., Lozupone, M., Custodero, C., Schilardi, A., Valiani, V., et al. (2018). Nutritional interventions and cognitive-related outcomes in patients with late-life cognitive disorders: a systematic review. *Neurosci. Biobehav. Rev.* 95, 480–498. doi: 10.1016/j.neubiorev.2018.10.022

Uhlmann, R. F., Larson, E. B., Rees, T. S., Koepsell, T. D., and Duckert, L. G. (1989). Relationship of hearing impairment to dementia and cognitive dysfunction in older adults. *JAMA* 261, 1916–1919. doi: 10.1001/jama.261.13.1916

Vaughan, N., Storzbach, D., and Furukawa, I. (2008). Investigation of potential cognitive tests for use with older adults in audiology clinics. *J. Am. Acad. Audiol.* 197, 533–541. doi: 10.3766/jaaa.19.7.2

Vermiglio, A. J. (2016). On diagnostic accuracy in audiology: central site of lesion and central auditory processing disorder studies. *J. Am. Acad. Audiol.* 27, 141–156. doi: 10.3766/jaaa.15079

Walden, T. C., and Walden, B. E. (2005). Unilateral versus bilateral amplification for adults with impaired hearing. *J. Am. Acad. Audiol.* 16, 574–584. doi: 10. 3766/jaaa.16.8.6

Wayne, R. V., and Johnsrude, I. S. (2015). A review of causal mechanisms underlying the link between age-related hearing loss and cognitive decline. *Ageing Res. Rev.* 23, 154–166. doi: 10.1016/j.arr.2015.06.002

Willott, J. F. (1991). *Aging and the Auditory System: Anatomy, Physiology, and Psychophysics.* San Diego, CA: Singular Publishing Group.

World Health Organization [WHO] (2017). *Deafness and Hearing Loss, Fact Sheet.* Available at: http://www.who.int/mediacentre/factsheets/fs300/en/ (accessed May 31, 2019).

Yuan, J., Sun, Y., Sang, S., Pham, J. H., and Kong, W. J. (2018). The risk of cognitive impairment associated with hearing function in older adults: a pooled analysis of data from eleven studies. *Sci. Rep.* 8:2137. doi: 10.1038/s41598-018-20496-w

20

The Acute Effects of Furosemide on Na-K-Cl Cotransporter-1, Fetuin-A and Pigment Epithelium-Derived Factor in the Guinea Pig Cochlea

Jesper Edvardsson Rasmussen*, Patrik Lundström, Per Olof Eriksson,
Helge Rask-Andersen, Wei Liu[†] and Göran Laurell[†]

Otorhinolaryngology and Head and Neck Surgery, Department of Surgical Sciences, Uppsala University, Uppsala, Sweden

*Correspondence:
Jesper Edvardsson Rasmussen
jesper.rasmussen@surgsci.uu.se

[†]These authors share senior
authorship

Background: Furosemide is a loop diuretic used to treat edema; however, it also targets the Na-K-Cl cotransporter-1 (NKCC1) in the inner ear. In very high doses, furosemide abolishes the endocochlear potential (EP). The aim of the study was to gain a deeper understanding of the temporal course of the acute effects of furosemide in the inner ear, including the protein localization of Fetuin-A and PEDF in guinea pig cochleae.

Material and Method: Adult guinea pigs were given an intravenous injection of furosemide in a dose of 100 mg per kg of body weight. The cochleae were studied using immunohistochemistry in controls and at four intervals: 3 min, 30 min, 60 min and 120 min. Also, cochleae of untreated guinea pigs were tested for Fetuin-A and PEDF mRNA using RNAscope® technology.

Results: At 3 min, NKCC1 staining was abolished in the type II fibrocytes in the spiral ligament, followed by a recovery period of up to 120 min. In the stria vascularis, the lowest staining intensity of NKCC1 presented after 30 min. The spiral ganglion showed a stable staining intensity for the full 120 min. Fetuin-A protein and mRNA were detected in the spiral ganglion type I neurons, inner and outer hair cells, pillar cells, Deiters cells and the stria vascularis. Furosemide induced an increased staining intensity of Fetuin-A at 120 min. PEDF protein and mRNA were found in the spiral ganglia type I neurons, the stria vascularis, and in type I and type II fibrocytes of the spiral ligament. PEDF protein staining intensity was high in the pillar cells in the organ of Corti. Furosemide induced an increased staining intensity of PEDF in type I neurons and pillar cells after 120 min.

Conclusion: The results indicate rapid furosemide-induced changes of NKCC1 in the type II fibrocytes. This could be part of the mechanism that causes reduction of the EP within minutes after high dose furosemide injection. Fetuin-A and PEDF are present in many cells of the cochlea and probably increase after furosemide exposure, possibly as an otoprotective response.

Keywords: furosemide (frusemide), NKCC1 = Na^+-K^+-$2Cl^-$ cotransporter, type II fibrocyte, fetuin-A, PEDF, stria vascularis, organ of corti (OoC), spiral ganglion neurons

INTRODUCTION

Furosemide is a loopdiuretic widely used in the treatment of edema in patients with congestive heart failure, liver failure, or kidney disease. It has an ototoxic effect if used in high doses (Schwartz et al., 1970; Santos and Nadol, 2017; Robertson et al., 2019). Loopdiuretics cause diuresis and lower blood pressure by inhibiting Na^+-K^+-$2Cl^-$ cotransporters 1 and 2 (NKCC1, NKCC2) in the loop of Henle in the kidney, thus increasing the loss of Na^+, K^+, and water in the urine. NKCC1 is expressed in many tissues in the body and is also present in the inner ear (Crouch et al., 1997), while NKCC2 is kidney-specific (Delpire and Gagnon, 2018). In the inner ear, furosemide is reported to inhibit NKCC1 in the stria vascularis (Shindo et al., 1992).

Due to the greatly increased risk of synergistic damage to the cochlea, furosemide is not suitable for use with other ototoxic drugs such as aminoglycosides and cisplatin (Laurell and Engström, 1989; Alam et al., 1998; Hirose and Sato, 2011; Li et al., 2011). Furosemide reduces the endocochlear DC potential (EP) generated in the stria vascularis (Kusakari et al., 1978; Asakuma and Snow, 1980; Sewell, 1984). EP is the driving force that allows K^+ to swiftly enter the hair cells in response to sound stimulus (Tasaki and Spyropoulos, 1959) initiating the first step of otoacoustic neurotransmission. The prolonged treatment of experimental animals with furosemide induces edema and intercellular vacuoles in the marginal cells of the stria vascularis and eventually hair cell loss in the organ of Corti (Forge, 1976; Pike and Bosher, 1980; Forge and Brown, 1982; Rarey and Ross, 1982; Naito and Watanabe, 1997). Postmortem studies have reported similar changes in the human cochlea (Arnold et al., 1981; Santos and Nadol, 2017). EP decreases in experimental animals within a few min of a high dose of furosemide, and recovers almost completely after 120 min (Kusakari et al., 1978; Asakuma and Snow, 1980; Sewell, 1984). The morphological changes in the stria vascularis induced by furosemide are observed much later. The exact mechanism behind the initial rapid EP loss is not known. Vasoconstriction and anoxia have been proposed as mechanisms involved in the initial loss of EP in experiments using another loop diuretic (Ding et al., 2002, 2016).

Fetuin-A, also known as alpha-2-HS-glycoprotein (AHSG), is a protein belonging to the cystatin super family synthesized in the liver and adipose tissue. Its best-known functions are the regulation of bone mineralization and protection against extra osseous calcium phosphate deposits by binding calcium phosphates (Jahnen-Dechent et al., 1997). Fetuin-A also plays a part in the anti-acute phase response (Lebreton et al., 1979; Wang and Sama, 2012), plaque formation in arteriosclerosis (Westenfeld et al., 2009; Trepanowski et al., 2015) and insulin resistance (Trepanowski et al., 2015).

Pigment epithelium-derived factor (PEDF), also known as Serpin-F1 (SERPINF1), is a neuroprotective, neurotrophic, and anti-angiogenetic protein first identified in the retinal pigment epithelia (Tombran-Tink et al., 1991). It is also reported to have regulating functions in osteogenesis, to promote stem cell renewal and inhibit tumor angiogenesis (Brook et al., 2020). PEDF has been identified in the stria vascularis, spiral ganglion,

neurons, and basilar membrane in the rat inner ear (Gleich and Piña, 2008).

We previously reported that Fetuin-A and PEDF are part of the human perilymph (Edvardsson Rasmussen et al., 2018) and the endolymphatic sac endolymph proteome (Ölander et al., 2021). It is not known whether Fetuin-A is expressed in any cells of the inner ear or if it only appears extracellularly in the perilymph and endolymph.

The aim of the study was to gain a deeper understanding of the temporal course of the acute effects of furosemide in the inner ear, including the protein localization of Fetuin-A and PEDF in guinea pig cochleae.

MATERIAL AND METHODS

Experimental Design

Using a guinea pig animal model, protein localization and staining intensity in the cochlea was studied after an intravenous (IV) injection of 100 mg/kg body weight of furosemide. This dose is previously known to abolish the EP (Kusakari et al., 1978). The following intervals were used: 3 min, 30 min, 60 min and 120 min. Three guinea pigs were used for each interval and as controls. The guinea pigs were anesthetized, intravenously injected with furosemide and then decapitated at the desired point in time. The cochleae were quickly dissected from the temporal bone and fixated. The cochleae were cryosectioned, stained using the immunofluorescence technique and photographed with a confocal microscope. Sections from three guinea pigs without furosemide exposure were also examined using RNAscope® technology. Image analysis densitometry was performed in ImageJ to semi-quantify the protein staining intensity.

Animals

Adult (age 6–9 weeks) albino guinea pigs of both sexes (body weight 262–310 g) were used in the experiment, 15 guinea pigs for immunohistochemistry and three for RNAscope examination. The animals were housed in an enriched environment with 12/12-h day and night cycle and a temperature of 21°C and 60% humidity. They had free access to food and water. All animal procedures were performed in accordance with local ethical guidelines at Uppsala University and national legislation and regulation concerning the care and use of laboratory animals.

Furosemide Administration

The animals were deeply anesthetized using ketamine (40 mg/kg, intramuscularly; Pfizer AB, Sweden) and xylazine (10 mg/kg, intramuscularly; Bayer, Denmark). Ophthalmic ointment was applied to the eyes to prevent corneal ulceration. The animals were given a local anesthetic by subcutaneous injection of bupivacaine hydrochloride (2.5 mg/ml) before exposure of the internal jugular vein, which was used for the IV injection. In total 12 guinea pigs were injected with 100 mg/kg of furosemide IV and were sacrificed by decapitation at four different intervals. Three control animals received the same anesthesia but were not given the furosemide injection.

Sample Preparation

After decapitation, the temporal bone was removed and the bulla opened to expose the cochlea. Small fenestrations were performed in the apex and the round window (RW) within minutes and the cochlea was gently flushed with a 4% formaldehyde solution stabilized with phosphate buffer. The cochlea was immersed in 4% formaldehyde for 24 h and then in 0.5% formaldehyde until decalcification in 0.1 M Na-ethylenediaminetetraacetic acid (EDTA). After decalcification the cochlea was rinsed and placed in a 15% sucrose solution for 24 h followed by a gradual infiltration of 15% sucrose and Tissue-Tek Optimal Cutting Temperature (OCT) Cryomount (Histolab, Sweden) for 4 days. Finalized by infusion of pure OCT overnight, after which the cochlea was embedded in OCT. The cochlea was cryosectioned with a microtome into 8 μm thick sections throughout the cochlea and mounted on Super Frost Plus slides (Menzel-Gläser, Braunschweig, Germany), and stored in a freezer at −70°C prior to immunohistochemistry (IHC) preparation.

Immunohistochemistry

Cochlear sections were stained according to the following protocol. Sections were rinsed three times in a glass slide staining jar with 0.01 M Phosphate Buffer Saline (PBS) with pH7.4 (Medicago) for 5 min (3 × 5 min). They were then incubated in 0.4% triton X-100 diluted in PBS at room temperature (RT) for 30 min and rinsed in PBS (3 × 5 min). The sections were incubated with primary antibodies diluted in 2% bovine serum albumin (BSA) in a humidified atmosphere at 4°C for 20 h. A negative control section was at the same time incubated with 2% BSA without primary antibody (Burry, 2011). Surplus primary antibody solution was carefully removed, and the slides were rinsed with PBS (3 × 5 min). All the sections, including negative control, were incubated with secondary antibody conjugated to Alexa Fluor 405, 488, 555, and 670 (Thermo Fisher Scientific, Sweden) for 2 h under RT. Slides were rinsed with PBS (3 × 5 min). Counterstaining was performed with the nuclear dye DAPI (4′,6-diamidino-2-phenylindole dihydrochloride) for 5–7 min at RT, after which slides were rinsed with PBS (3 × 5 min). Mounting was done with ProLong® Gold or ProLong® Glass Antifading Mountant and cover slipped with the specified cover glass (0.17 ± 0.005 mm) for optically matching confocal and super-resolution (SIM) microscopes. At least one representative section from each animal was selected for analysis of immunohistochemistry after all the confocal images were assessed. Images from basal or mid turn were selected since the protein localization and intensity were uniform in between

the turns. Antibodies used for immunohistochemistry are listed in **Table 1**.

RNAscope Protocol

RNA *in situ* hybridization (ISH) trials were performed using RNAscope®. The frozen fixed (4% paraformaldehyde) cochlear tissue sections were prepared according to the manufacturer's instructions with the RNAscope® Reagent Kit (Bio-Techne, Minneapolis, USA) (kit version 2). Sections were briefly pretreated with H_2O_2 (10 min, RT) and protease III (30 min, 40°C). After protease III incubation, the sections were subjected to RNAscope hybridization assay. The paired double-Z oligonucleotide probes were designed and produced by Bio-Techne based on the targets' gene ID. To start the hybridization, the RNA probe fluid was added to the slide with sections. Incubation continued in a HybEZ™ Oven (Bio-Techne) for 2 h at 40°C. After hybridization incubation, the slides were washed using 1× RNAscope® Wash Buffer. Sections were then incubated with RNAscope® Multiplex FL v2 Amp 1, Amp 2, and Amp 3 (for 30, 30, and 15 min respectively) sequentially at 40°C to amplify the signal. For signal development, RNAscope® Multiplex FL v2 hP-C1, HRP-C2 and HRP-C3 were added to the sections sequentially (incubation time 15 min each). For detecting signals, TSA-diluted Opal™ 520, 570, and 690 fluorophores were added to sections after HRP-C1, C2, and C3, incubating the sections for 30 min at 40°C for each HRP-fluorophore pare. Each of the three fluorophore incubations was followed by washing with 1× RNAscope® Wash Buffer. Multiplex FL v2 hP blocker, specific for each channel, was added and incubated in the oven at 40°C for 15 min. Finally, the sections were counterstained with DAPI and the slides cover slipped with ProLong® Glass Antifade Mountant (Thermo Fisher Scientific). RNAscope ISH produces puncta of signal that represent a single mRNA transcript (Grabinski et al., 2015).

A DapB probe was used for negative control. DapB is only present in a very rare strain of soil bacteria and should not produce any signal in the tissue, hence it's utility as a negative control. Our RNAscope negative control result was consistent with the RNAscope technical protocol. The probes used for RNAscope are listed in **Table 2**.

Imaging and Photography

Confocal laser scanning microscopy was performed using a Nikon TE2000 inverted fluorescence microscope equipped with a three-channel laser emission system with three emission spectra filters (maxima 358, 461, and 555 nm). Confocal images were acquired using a Nikon EZ-C1 (ver. 3.80) software, with all

TABLE 1 | Immunohistochemistry antibodies.

Antibody	Type	Species reactivity	Dilution	Host	Catalogue number	Producer
Fetuin-A	P	GP	1:100	Rabbit	ABIN2778140	Antibodies-online.com
PEDF	P	H, M	1:50	Rabbit	NBP2-19767	Novus biological
NKCC1	P	H, M, R	1:100	Rabbit	Ab59791	Abcam
Parvalbumin	M	H, M, R, P	1:200	Mouse	MAB1572	Merck
Tubulin β3	M	H, M, R, P etc.	1:200	Mouse	MAB1637	Merck

List of antibodies used for imunohistochemistry. Type: Polyclonal (P); monoclonal (M). Species reactivty: guinea pig (GP); human (H); mouse (M); rat (R); porcine (P).

TABLE 2 | RNAscope probes.

Protein	Species	Gene	Gene ID	Probe	Producer
PEDF	Guinea pig	SerpinF1	100216362	874151	BioTechne
Fetuin-A	Guinea pig	AHSG	100135479	897851-C2	BioTechne

List of probes used for RNAscope®.

acquisition settings kept equal within each figure, except for the blue (DAPI) channel which was optimized for illustration of the morphology. The Nikon EZ-C1 was also used for reconstructions of z-stacks to 3D-images. The confocal images were saved as tag image file format red-green-blue (TIFF-RGB) with a resolution of 512 × 512 pixels and transferred to Fiji ImageJ 1.53C (Schindelin et al., 2012). Fiji ImageJ was used to perform densitometry. The image was split into channels for red, green, and blue immunostaining. The channel of interest was isolated and converted into a grayscale image in which each pixel was assigned a value between 0 and 65,535 depending on the intensity of immunofluorescence, where 0 is black and 65,535 is white. The grayscale image was used for intensity measurement. A region of interest was manually drawn to exclude areas of the sample that were not subject to examination. The threshold for minimum intensity required of a pixel to be included was set according to "Li" to remove background pixels (Li and Lee, 1993; Li and Tam, 1998). Fiji ImageJ measured the histogram of the remaining pixels and their intensity value. The mean intensity value of the remaining pixels was calculated. All immunohistochemistry images selected for analysis in controls and at 120 min were included in densitometry analysis. Densitometry values were calculated for one representative confocal image from each animal in the controls and 120 min group, and presented as mean values with error bars for standard deviation. Counting and rating of the nuclei staining of Fetuin-A was done in one representative confocal image from each animal in the five groups. The staining of the nuclei of the marginal cells of the stria vascularis and the type I neurons of the spiral ganglia were rated as no, weak or strong intensity. Mean and standard deviation was calculated.

RESULTS

Longitudinal Pattern of Immunostaining

Patterns of immunohistochemistry were studied at the four intervals and compared to control. Densitometry was calculated for 0 and 120 min for Fetuin-A and PEDF immunohistochemistry and Fetuin-A nuclei staining was rated and counted. The presence of Fetuin-A mRNA and PEDF mRNA in guinea pigs not exposed to furosemide were analyzed using RNAscope. The protein localization and signal intensity as well as mRNA detection were uniform in the different turns of the cochlea when the sections were studied visually. The results are presented below for the different compartments of the cochlea.

The Lateral Cochlear Wall

NKCC1 is known to be localized to the baso-lateral wall of the marginal cells in the stria vascularis (Crouch et al., 1997) and

the type II fibrocytes of the spiral ligament (Spicer and Schulte, 1991). The control animals showed strong NKCC1 staining intensity in the marginal cells of the stria vascularis and type II fibrocytes in the spiral prominence region. Confocal microscopy revealed a drastic reduction of NKCC1 staining intensity in the type II fibrocytes at 3 min compared to the control. A progressive increase of NKCC1 staining intensity followed at the subsequent intervals in the type II fibrocytes until 120 min when NKCC1 staining intensity had nearly recovered to control levels (**Figure 1**).

The marginal cells of the stria vascularis had stronger NKCC1 staining intensity in the controls and at all intervals following furosemide injection compared to the type II fibrocytes. The staining intensity of NKCC1 in the stria vascularis was decreased at 3 min, but was prominently lower at 30 min. Thereafter the staining intensity of NKCC1 gradually recovered in the stria vascularis (**Figure 2**).

Fetuin-A protein was detected with a low and consistent staining intensity in the stria vascularis, spiral ligament and bone surrounding the cochlear structures in the controls. The stria vascularis had the strongest staining intensity of the different compartments in the lateral wall, and some of the marginal cells' nuclei showed Fetuin-A staining (**Figure 3**). The percentage of marginal cell nuclei with strong Fetuin-A staining increased between 30 min and 120 min after furosemide injection. In the control group had 35% of the marginal cells' nuclei a strong staining intensity, which was in the 120 min group increased to 63%. However, the mean staining intensity of stria vascularis did not change (**Figure 4**).

PEDF protein was detected in the stria vascularis, spiral prominence epithelia and type I and type II fibrocytes, while the type III, IV, and V fibrocytes were negative. The stria vascularis was positive for PEDF in all cell layers. PEDF staining intensity was similar in the spiral prominence and in the stria vascularis (**Figure 5**). There were no visual differences in PEDF protein localization or staining intensity in the lateral wall after furosemide exposure compared to the controls (**Figure 6**).

The Spiral Ganglion

NKCC1 was detected in the cell membrane of the spiral ganglion neurons in all controls and furosemide exposed animals, with no difference during the studied period of 120 min.

Fetuin-A protein was seen in the cytoplasm and nuclei of the spiral ganglion type I neurons (**Figure 7**). The mean percent of type I neuron cell nuclei with strong Fetuin-A staining was 26% in the controls. This was increased to 49% at 60 min, and 53% at 120 min (**Figure 4**). The mean intensity of the total staining in the spiral ganglion measured with densitometry in controls and at 120 min was presented in **Figure 6**.

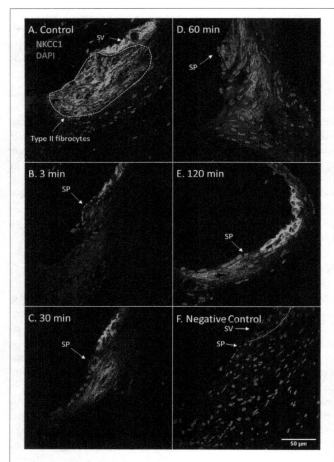

FIGURE 1 | NKCC1 in type II fibrocytes following furosemide injection. **(A–F)** Staining intensity of NKCC1 in the type II fibrocyte following administration of furosemide with DAPI staining of cell nuclei. Focus was set on the type II fibrocytes. Spiral prominence (SP); Stria vascularis (SV). **(A)** Normal NKCC1 staining in type II fibrocytes in a control guinea pig. **(B)** At 3 min after injection there was almost no staining of NKCC1 in the type II fibrocytes. **(C)** At 30 min the staining intensity of NKCC1 in the type II fibrocytes had returned to a low level. **(D)** At 60 min staining intensity was still decreased compared to control. **(E)** After 120 min the signal intensity had returned to near initial levels. **(F)** Negative control section with DAPI.

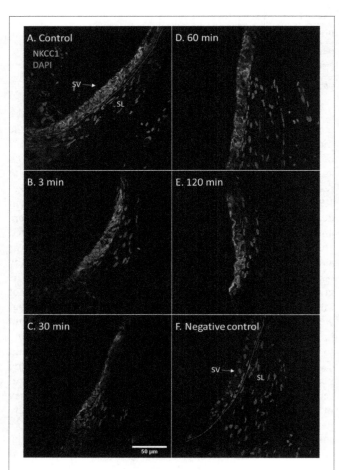

FIGURE 2 | NKCC1 in the stria vascularis following furosemide injection. **(A–F)** Staining intensity of NKCC1 in the marginal cells of the stria vascularis following furosemide injection with DAPI staining of nuclei. Focus was set on the stria vascularis. Spiral ligament (SL); Stria vascularis (SV). **(A)** Normal NKCC1 staining in the stria vascularis in a control animal. **(B)** Intensity had decreased after 3 min. **(C)** The lowest intensity was seen at 30 min. **(D)** It then recovers partially at 60 min. **(E)** Further recovery at 120 min. **(F)** Negative control with DAPI.

PEDF protein was detected in the cytoplasm of the type I neurons in the spiral ganglion in the control and at all intervals after furosemide administration (**Figure 8**). The signal was stable over time and densitometry indicates a minor increase in the type I neurons at 120 min (**Figure 6**).

The Organ of Corti

Fetuin-A protein was detected with a strong staining intensity in the pillar cells of the control animals. The inner and outer hair cells (IHCs and OHCs) and Deiters cells had a low staining in the control and was judged negative. However, after furosemide exposure, the signal intensity increased markedly in the pillar cells, and after 120 min also in IHCs, OHCs, and Deiters cells (**Figure 9**). Densitometry measurement showed an increased mean value of the signal intensity in the organ of Corti at 120 min (**Figure 4**).

Immunohistochemistry detected PEDF protein in the pillar cells and Deiters cells in the controls. After 120 min PEDF protein were also detected in the IHCs, OHCs, and Deiter cells in the organ of Corti. The staining intensity increased most in the pillar cells. No immunostaining was observed in the basilar membrane in the guinea pig's organ of Corti (**Figure 10**). Densitometry showed that the mean staining intensity of PEDF in organ of Corti had increased by 120 min and the highest staining intensity in the organ of Corti was observed in the pillar cells (**Figure 6**).

RNAscope

The RNAscope technique was used in untreated guinea pigs with consistent results compared to the protein localization detected with immunohistochemistry in all cochlear compartments, except for PEDF in the organ of Corti.

In the cochlear lateral wall, Fetuin-A mRNA transcripts were detected in the whole stria vascularis and spiral ligament. In the

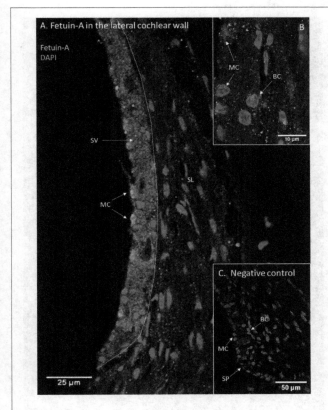

FIGURE 3 | Fetuin-A in the lateral cochlear wall. Protein localization of Fetuin-A in the lateral cochlear wall of a control guinea pig. Spiral ligament (SL); Stria vascularis (SV); Spiral prominence (SP); Marginal cell (MC); Basal cell (BC). **(A)** Fetuin-A protein in the spiral ligament, spiral prominence, and stria vascularis. **(B)** Inset of higher magnification of stria vascularis. Marginal cells (MC) and also basal cells (BC) have Fetuin-A protein. **(C)** Negative control of lateral wall with stria vascularis, spiral prominence and spiral ligament. Vessels have a weak unspecific staining.

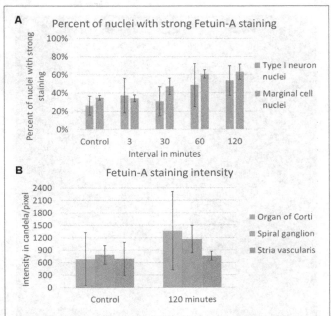

FIGURE 4 | Rating of Fetuin-A nuclei staining and densitometry. **(A)** Rating of Fetuin-A staining intensity in type I neuron nuclei (orange) and marginal cell nuclei (gray). Result presented as the mean value of each group, with error bars showing standard deviation. **(B)** Densitometry of Fetuin-A staining intensity. Result presented as mean value of the control and 120 min group, with error bars showing standard deviation. Intensity increased in the organ of Corti (blue) and the spiral ganglion (orange), with no change in the stria vascularis (gray).

spiral ganglion, Fetuin-A transcripts were detected in the type I neurons. In the organ of Corti Fetuin-A mRNA transcripts were detected in the IHCs, OHCs, pillar cells, and Deiters cells as well as Hensen's cells and Boetcher's cells in accordance with the findings in the furosemide groups (**Figure 11**).

PEDF mRNA transcripts were found in the basal cells of the stria vascularis and in type I and type II fibrocytes. In the lateral wall, transcripts were most abundant in type II fibrocytes. In the spiral ganglion, type I neurons had abundant transcripts. No PEDF mRNA was found in the organ of Corti in the control guinea pig, despite positive protein immunohistochemistry (**Figure 12**).

DISCUSSION

Furosemide-Induced Changes to NKCC1 Staining

This explorative study has identified a new important target and possible mechanisms of furosemide ototoxicity. Many previous experimental studies have shown that a high dose of furosemide, either alone or in combination with other ototoxic drugs,

causes a rapid reduction in the endocochlear potential (EP) (Kusakari et al., 1978; Asakuma and Snow, 1980; Sewell, 1984). In the guinea pig cochleae, we observed that furosemide targets NKCC1 in type II fibrocytes in the spiral ligament almost immediately after an IV administration. The spiral ligament fibrocytes are classified into types I to V (Spicer and Schulte, 1991). The classification is based on the expression of specific ion pumps or channels and the location in the spiral ligament. The function of the spiral ligament fibrocytes is believed to be active recirculation of K+ from the hair cells and perilymph back to the stria vascularis (Spicer and Schulte, 1996). Disruption of the spiral ligament is known to decrease the EP and increase the threshold of the auditory brainstem response (ABR) in experimental animals (Kikuchi et al., 2000; Marcus et al., 2002; Takiguchi et al., 2013; Yoshida et al., 2015; Kitao et al., 2016). The major transporting mechanisms of K+ are thought to be through gap junctions and connexin channels, inward rectifying potassium channel Kir4.1 and the ion pumps NKCC1 and Na-K-ATPase (Spicer and Schulte, 1991, 1996; Weber et al., 2001; Liu et al., 2017). The type II fibrocytes are recognized by expression of Na-K-ATPase and NKCC1 (Spicer and Schulte, 1991; Crouch et al., 1997) and they are located in the spiral prominence area and outer sulcus inferior to stria vascularis. Observations in a mouse model after acute cochlear energy trauma revealed that hearing recovery was linked to re-expression of Na-K-ATPase and connexin26 (Kitao et al., 2016). Furthermore, reductions in NKCC1 and NK-K-ATPase in type II fibrocytes in addition to

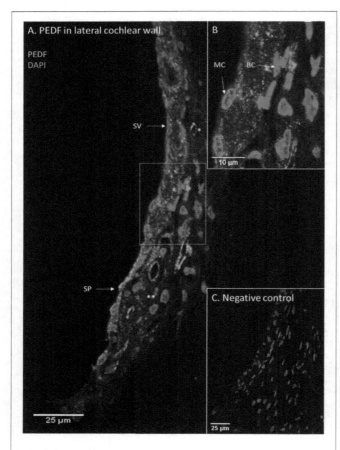

FIGURE 5 | PEDF in the lateral cochlear wall. PEDF protein localization in the lateral cochlear wall. Stria vascularis (SV); Spiral prominence (SP); Marginal cell (MC); Basal cell (BC); type I fibrocytes (*); type II fibrocytes (**). (A) PEDF was localized to the spiral ligament, the stria vascularis and the spiral prominence. In the spiral ligament were type I and II fibrocytes PEDF positive. (B) Inset of higher magnification of marked area in (A). The distribution of PEDF in sub-cellular level of stria vascularis and spiral ligament. (C) Negative control of the immunohistochemistry.

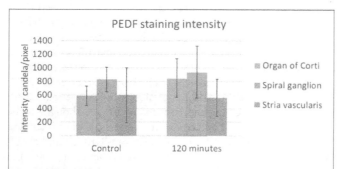

FIGURE 6 | PEDF in the stria vascularis following furosemide injection. Densitometry of PEDF staining intensity. Result presented as mean values of the control and 120 min group, with error bars showing standard deviation. The organ of Corti (blue) showed a large increase and in the spiral ganglion (orange) a marginal increase, while the stria vascularis (gray) had no change.

age-related hearing loss have been reported in Sprague-Dawley rats (Takiguchi et al., 2013). Another experiment, in which the

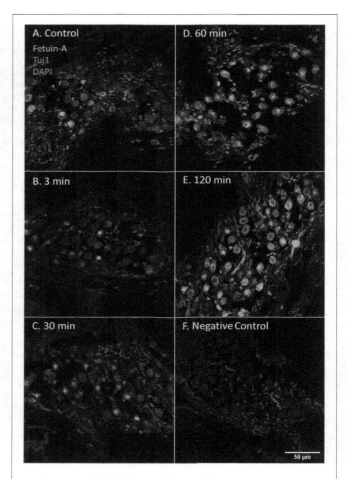

FIGURE 7 | Fetuin-A in the spiral ganglion following furosemide injection. (A–F) Fetuin-A protein staining of guinea pig spiral ganglion following IV furosemide injection. (A) Fetuin-A protein was localized to the type I neurons cytoplasm and nuclei in the control. (B–E) The staining intensity after furosemide at different intervals. (F) Negative control.

perilymph compartment was perfused with the loop diuretic bumetanide, showed a decrease in EP at the same time as an increase in the intrastrial space, K$^+$, indicating a blockade of NKCC1 in the lateral wall and marginal cells (Yoshida et al., 2015). This is in line with the present finding of immediate reduction in NKCC1 staining in type II fibrocytes, and this loss of function may be the first target of the loop diuretic effect on EP.

Previous research has shown that NKCC1 is located in the basolateral surface of marginal cells in the stria vascularis (Shindo et al., 1992; Crouch et al., 1997) and in type II fibrocyte (Spicer and Schulte, 1991). While NKCC1 staining intensity reached the lowest point in type II fibrocytes at 3 min after furosemide administration, the stria vascularis was most inhibited at 30 min after furosemide administration. This time difference might be explained by the vascular structure of the lateral wall of the cochlea. The concept of a barrier system between the blood compartment and inner ear structures is widely accepted. In analyzing the barrier systems between the blood compartment and inner ear structures, it is anatomically and functionally

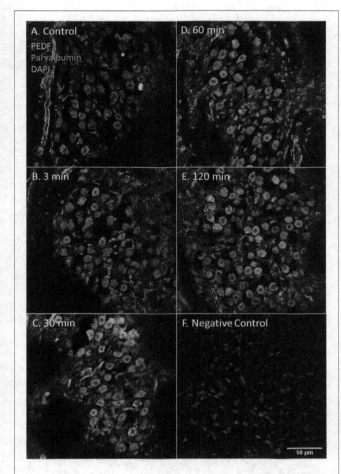

FIGURE 8 | PEDF in the spiral ganglion following furosemide injection. **(A–F)** PEDF protein staining of guinea pig spiral ganglion following IV furosemide injection. **(A)** In the control was PEDF localized in the cytoplasm of the spiral ganglion type I neurons. **(B–E)** The staining intensity after furosemide at the different intervals. **(F)** Negative control.

relevant to separate the blood-labyrinth barrier into the blood-perilymph barrier and the intrastrial fluid-blood barrier (Juhn and Rybak, 1981; Cohen-Salmon et al., 2007). The intrastrial fluid-barrier in the stria vascularis is formed by endothelial cells connected to each other by tight junctions and surrounded by a basal membrane. The next layer is formed by pericytes and perivascular resident macrophage-like melanocytes (PVM/M) around the capillaries (Juhn and Rybak, 1981; Cohen-Salmon et al., 2007; Liu et al., 2016; Shi, 2016). This barrier protects the stria vascularis and the endolymphatic compartment from exogenous substances in the circulatory system. The other parts of the spiral ligament, including the type II fibrocytes, are protected by the more permeable blood-perilymph barrier. This barrier consists of endothelial cells connected to each other by tight junctions but with a few fenestrations (Jahnke, 1980). It is known that the blood-perilymph barrier is more permeable than the intrastrial fluid-blood barrier (Sterkers et al., 1987; Juhn et al., 2001; Counter et al., 2017). Experiments on the permeability of the blood-perilymph barrier in the chinchilla

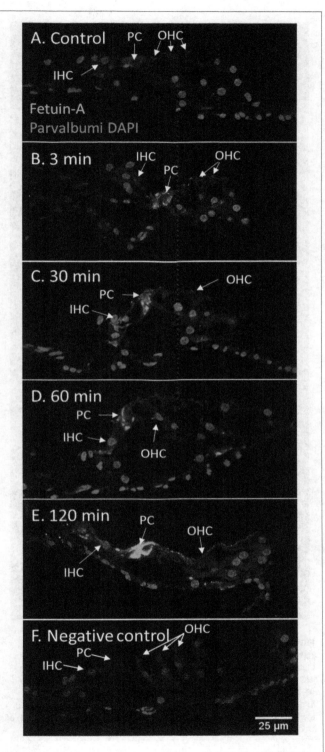

FIGURE 9 | Fetuin-A in the organ of Corti following furosemide injection. **(A–F)** Fetuin-A protein localization and staining intensity in the guinea pig's organ of Corti following IV furosemide injection. Parvalbumin stains the IHC red. **(A)** In the control was Fetuin-A detected in the pillar cells. **(B–E)** Staining intensity in the guinea pig's organ of Corti following IV furosemide injection. Fetuin-A staining was greatly increased in the pillar cells, and the IHCs, OHCs, and Deiters were positive after 120 min. **(F)** Negative control of organ of Corti.

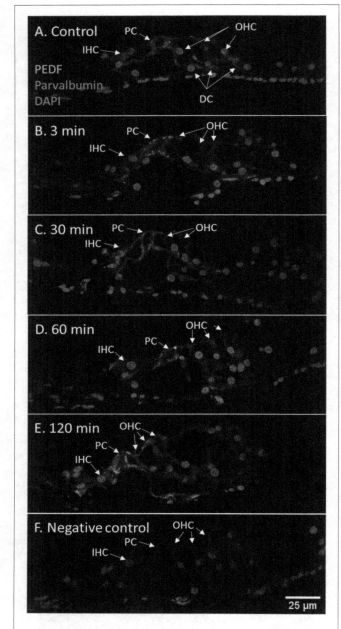

FIGURE 10 | PEDF in guinea pig organ of Corti following furosemide injection. **(A–F)** PEDF protein localization and staining intensity in the guinea pig's organ of Corti following IV furosemide injection. Parvalbumin stains the IHC red. **(A)** PEDF was in the control detected in pillar cells and Deiters cells. **(B–E)** Staining intensity in the guinea pig's organ of Corti following IV furosemide injection. **(E)** At 120 min staining increased in the pillar cells and the IHCs and OHCs stained for PEDF protein. **(F)** Negative control of organ of Corti.

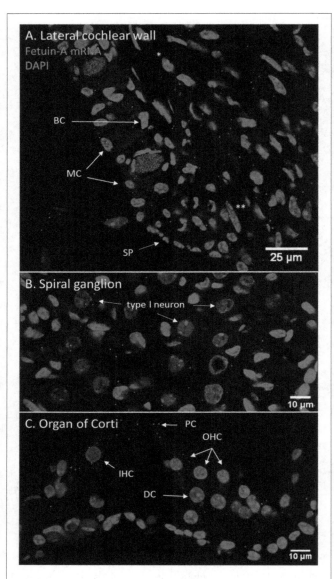

FIGURE 11 | Fetuin-A m-RNA in the guinea pig cochlea. **(A–C)** RNAscope of Fetuin-A mRNA in the control guinea pig cochlea. Red dots indicate mRNA transcripts. DAPI staining of nuclei. Spiral prominence (SP); Marginal cell (MC); Basal cell (BC); type I fibrocytes (*); type II fibrocytes (**). **(A)** Fetuin-A mRNA was detected in all cell layers of stria vascularis, spiral ligament, and prominence. **(B)** The spiral ganglion type I neurons had Fetuin-A mRNA transcripts, but in small numbers. **(C)** In the guinea pig organ of Corti was Fetuin-A mRNA transcripts detected in the IHCs, OHCs, Deiters cells (DC), and pillar cells (PC). PEDF mRNA in the guinea pig cochlea.

demonstrate that EP loss after furosemide administration is correlated to the concentration of the drug in perilymph (Juhn and Rybak, 1981). More recent findings in an MRI study showed a much slower opening of the intrastrial fluid-barrier after the administration of a high dose of furosemide (Videhult Pierre et al., 2020) than the expected loss of EP. We, therefore, consider the observation of a more rapid loss of NKCC1 in type II fibrocytes than in marginal cells, to be consistent with previous experiments on inner ear barriers and the differences in the permeability of the barriers might be a mechanism behind the more rapid effect on the type II fibrocytes of furosemide.

The changes seen in NKCC1 staining intensity of the type II fibrocytes were very rapid and might therefore not be related to change in the gene expression (Ding et al., 2014). Regulation of NKCC1 activity has been studied in

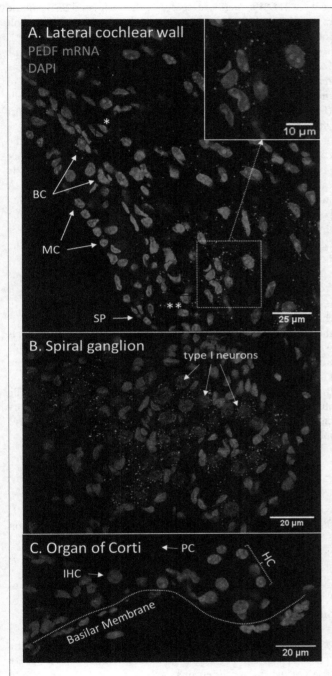

FIGURE 12 | (A–C) RNAscope of PEDF mRNA in the normal guinea pig cochlea. Red dots indicate mRNA transcripts. DAPI staining of nuclei. Spiral prominence (SP); Marginal cell (MC); Basal cell (BC); Hensen's cells (HC); type I fibrocytes (*); type II fibrocytes (**). **(A)** PEDF mRNA transcripts were found in the stria vascularis, spiral ligament, and spiral prominence. The type II fibrocytes had the most abundant transcripts. Transcripts were detected in type I fibrocytes in the basal layer of the stria vascularis. **(B)** The spiral ganglion type I neurons demonstrate high numbers of PEDF mRNA transcripts. **(C)** No PEDF mRNA were found in the organ of Corti.

2020). Examples of posttranslational mechanisms contributing to the regulation of NKCC1 are glycosylation and phosphorylation. Glycosylation of the N-terminal increases membrane trafficking (Singh et al., 2015) and ion transportation (Ye et al., 2012) of NKCC1. Phosphorylation of NKCC1 by Serine/threonine-protein kinase WNK3 activates NKCC1 ion transportation and de-phosphorylationby protein phosphatase 1 inhibits ion transportation (Kahle et al., 2005). If these mechanisms can also be influenced by a high dose of furosemide has not been reported earlier. Studies on the structural molecular interaction of furosemide and NKCC1 are few. Furosemide has been reported to bind transiently to the Cl⁻ transporting site of NKCC1 (Somasekharan et al., 2012). If the binding of furosemide to the NKCC1 protein interferes with the binding of the immunohistochemistry antibody against NKCC1 or if posttranslational modifications of NKCC1 could explain the loss of signal intensity has yet to be elucidated.

Longitudinal Fetuin-A Response

The vulnerability of the cochlea to insults induced by various ototoxic drugs has been known for decades. The combination of an aminoglycoside antibiotic and furosemide has been shown to induce an inflammatory response in the cochlea (García-Alcántara et al., 2018; Kaur et al., 2018). Whether an immune response in the cochlea can be activated by a single high dose of furosemide as used in the present study remains open to question. There has been no previous mapping of Fetuin-A in either human cochlear structures or in experimental research. In the cochleae of our control guinea pigs, Fetuin-A was present in the neurons of the spiral ganglion, pillar cells of the organ of Corti and marginal cells of the stria vascularis. Following furosemide administration, a clear temporal staining pattern for Fetuin-A was observed in the cochlea, with an increase of the protein staining intensity in all the Fetuin-A-positive cells after 60–120 min. After 120 min Fetuin-A protein was also detected in IHCs, OHCs, and Deiters cells. To further explore the Fetuin-A expression, we analyzed control guinea pig cochleae for Fetuin-A mRNA using the RNAscope method. The presence of Fetuin-A mRNA in the cells of the cochleae where Fetuin-A protein was detected, verified the results obtained by immunohistochemistry, and indicates that the Fetuin-A gene was expressed. Presence of Fetuin mRNA suggest that the observation of a time-dependent increase of Fetuin-A staining intensity in these cochlear structures may be a manifestation of local cellular activation due to furosemide ototoxicity, in contrast to an increased uptake from the systemic circulation.

Fetuin-A is a multifunctional protein known to be primarily secreted from the liver and reported to be mainly involved in anti-inflammatory mechanisms (Lebreton et al., 1979; Wang and Sama, 2012). In the early phase of an acute inflammation, Fetuin-A concentration in plasma is lowered by pro-inflammatory cytokines and increased by the late inflammation response (Wang and Sama, 2012). Fetuin-A does, however, protect against peripheral artery disease in patients with chronic kidney disease (Westenfeld et al., 2009; Jirak et al., 2019). On the other hand, Fetuin-A is shown to increase insulin resistance and arteriosclerosis in patients

brain tissue and posttranslational mechanisms are reported to contribute to homeostatic regulation (Watanabe and Fukuda,

with metabolic syndrome (Trepanowski et al., 2015). Fetuin-A function can, therefore, be considered to be dualistic. In our earlier assessment of perilymph proteome in patients with vestibular schwannoma, Fetuin-A was found to be positively correlated with preserved hearing (Edvardsson Rasmussen et al., 2018). We therefore interpret the finding of increased Fetuin-A after injection with furosemide as a possible otoprotective function after acute insults to the cochlea.

Longitudinal PEDF Response

PEDF protein was detected with immunohistochemistry in the lateral cochlear wall, spiral ganglion and organ of Corti in control guinea pigs. The protein was most evident in type II fibrocytes, the basal and marginal cells of the stria vascularis, the type I neurons of the spiral ganglion and in the pillar cells in the organ of Corti. After 120 min of IV furosemide administration, PEDF had increased in the type I neurons and in the pillar cells. IHCs, OHCs, and Deiters cells were also PEDF-positive after 120 min. PEDF was not detected in the basilar membrane in guinea pigs, which has been reported in rats (Gleich and Piña, 2008). PEDF gene expression was further analyzed using RNAscope in the cochleae of normal guinea pigs and we found mRNA transcripts in spiral ganglion type 1 neurons, type I and type II fibrocytes, marginal cells, and basal cells of the stria vascularis. The finding of mRNA transcripts was a first validation of the detected protein localization and indicate that PEDF gene expression was active in these cells. We could not confirm PEDF mRNA in the organ of Corti, although the immunohistochemistry protein localization was consistent in the experiment. Based on these results, we speculate that PEDF could be produced by cells in the lateral cochlear wall and can reach the organ of Corti from the endolymph. An alternative possible explanation could be that PEDF was transported by axonal transportation from the type I neurons to the organ of Corti. However, it cannot fully be ruled out that PEDF gene transcription could be very low in the organ of Corti in the normal situation and could be increased from cellular stress induced by furosemide.

PEDF has been reported in the perivascular melanocyte-like macrophages (PVM/M) (Zhang et al., 2012), part of the second layer in the intrastrial fluid-blood barrier. Further, the PEDF signaling pathway was reported to be important for the formation of tight junctions between endothelial cells to maintain the integrity of the intrastrial fluid-blood barrier after acoustic trauma (Zhang et al., 2013). The timing of the increase of PEDF staining intensity in our experiment was similar to that observed after acoustic trauma by Zhang et al. (2013). Stimulation of PEDF production was reported to increase the survival of PVM/M in cell culture and stimulate the formation of tight junctions (Zhang et al., 2021). It could therefore be part of a counter mechanism to the increased permeability of the intrastrial fluid-blood barrier caused by furosemide (Videhult Pierre et al., 2020).

Increased staining intensity of PEDF protein were observed in the organ of Corti in the pillar cells, IHCs, OHCs, and Deiters cells after 120 min. PEDF is known to promote the survival of photoreceptors and retinal ganglion cells (Barnstable and Tombran-Tink, 2004; Polato and Becerra, 2016; Zwanzig et al., 2021) and the suppression of pro-inflammatory cytokines (Ma

et al., 2021). We, therefore, speculate that increased PEDF in the organ of Corti also promotes cell survival after the cochlear insult induced by furosemide.

We detected PEDF in the cytoplasm of the spiral ganglion type I neurons, and an increase in PEDF over time reaching a maximum at 60–120 min. The PEDF increase was similar to the known neuroprotective response in retinal ganglion cells (Unterlauft et al., 2012) and probably a mechanism to protect type I neurons from undergoing apoptosis.

The finding of increased Fetuin-A and PEDF in the cochlea after furosemide exposure and the information of their anti-inflammatory and protective functions suggest a possible causal effect behind the observed correlation of high Fetuin-A in perilymph and preserved hearing in vestibular schwannoma patients (Edvardsson Rasmussen et al., 2018). Given the reported links between PEDF-gene mutations and hereditary otosclerosis (Ziff et al., 2016), it is relevant to further explore PEDF in the inner ear.

It may be argued that it is difficult to draw conclusions from a longitudinal study using immunohistochemistry, as it is not possible to follow immunohistochemically changes in the inner ear over time in the same experimental animal. We, therefore, created a timeline comparing different individuals with carefully minimized experimental differences. This immunohistochemistry study was designed to gain more knowledge of time-dependent changes induced by furosemide in the cochlea. However, the number of animals used in the study did not allow for statistical analysis of the signal intensity changes. One further limitation of the study was that no in vivo measurements of ABRs or EP were taken.

CONCLUSION

NKCC1 staining was found to be greatly reduced in type II fibrocytes of the spiral ligament 3 min after the administration of a high dose of furosemide. The NKCC1 signal followed the temporal course previously reported for EP recovery. This suggests that one underlying mechanism of EP decrease following furosemide administration could be the disruption of K^+ recirculation via the type II fibrocytes into the syncytium of the stria vascularis.

PEDF and Fetuin-A protein were both present in the stria vascularis, spiral ganglion and organ of Corti in controls. The cells with high staining of both proteins were marginal cells of the stria vascularis, type I neurons and pillar cells. The presence of Fetuin-A mRNA and PEDF mRNA shows a local gene expression in the cochlea. There was a temporal pattern with increase in both Fetuin-A and PEDF 120 min after furosemide administration, indicating that these proteins may play a role in the cellular response to cochlear insults.

AUTHOR CONTRIBUTIONS

GL, PE, and JE conceived the study design and primary hypothesis. WL and JE performed the immunohistochemical staining and microscopy. WL also performed the RNAscope and microscopy. PL was responsible for the densitometry analysis. HR-A and JE interpreted the morphological results. All authors discussed the results and thereafter JE wrote the manuscript. All authors contributed to the article and approved the submitted version.

ACKNOWLEDGMENTS

We would like to specially thank Anette Fransson PhD for excellent technical work in the laboratory.

REFERENCES

Alam, S. A., Ikeda, K., Kawase, T., Kikuchi, T., Katori, Y., Watanabe, K., et al. (1998). Acute effects of combined administration of kanamycin and furosemide on the stria vascularis studied by distortion product otoacoustic emission and transmission electron microscopy. *Tohoku J. Exp. Med.* 186, 79–86. doi: 10.1620/tjem.186.79

Arnold, W., Nadol, J. B., and Weidauer, H. (1981). Ultrastructural histopathology in a case of human ototoxicity due to loop diuretics. *Acta Otolaryngol.* 91, 399–414. doi: 10.3109/00016488109138521

Asakuma, S., and Snow, J. B. (1980). Effects of furosemide and ethacrynic acid on the endocochlear direct current potential in normal and kanamycin sulfate-treated guinea pigs. *Otolaryngol. Head Neck Surg.* 88, 188–193.

Barnstable, C. J., and Tombran-Tink, J. (2004). Neuroprotective and antiangiogenic actions of PEDF in the eye: molecular targets and therapeutic potential. *Prog. Retin. Eye Res.* 23, 561–577. doi: 10.1016/j.preteyeres.2004.05.002

Brook, N., Brook, E., Dharmarajan, A., Chan, A., and Dass, C. R. (2020). Pigment epithelium-derived factor regulation of neuronal and stem cell fate. *Exp. Cell Res.* 389:111891. doi: 10.1016/j.yexcr.2020.11 1891

Burry, R. W. (2011). Controls for immunocytochemistry. *J. Histochem. Cytochem.* 59, 6–12. doi: 10.1369/jhc.2010.956920

Cohen-Salmon, M., Regnault, B., Cayet, N., Caille, D., Demuth, K., Hardelin, J.-P., et al. (2007). Connexin30 deficiency causes instrastrial fluid-blood barrier disruption within the cochlear stria vascularis. *Proc. Natl. Acad. Sci. U S A* 104, 6229–6234. doi: 10.1073/pnas.0605108104

Counter, S. A., Nikkhou-Aski, S., Damberg, P., Berglin, C. E., and Laurell, G. (2017). Ultra-high-field (9.4 T) MRI analysis of contrast agent transport across the blood-perilymph barrier and intrastrial fluid-blood barrier in the mouse inner ear. *Otol. Neurotol.* 38, 1052–1059. doi: 10.1097/MAO. 0000000000001458

Crouch, J. J., Sakaguchi, N., Lytle, C., and Schulte, B. A. (1997). Immunohistochemical localization of the Na-K-Cl co-transporter (NKCC1) in the gerbil inner ear. *J. Histochem. Cytochem.* 45, 773–778. doi: 10.1177/002215549704500601

Delpire, E., and Gagnon, K. B. (2018). Na$^+$-K$^+$-2Cl$^-$ cotransporter (NKCC) physiological function in nonpolarized cells and transporting epithelia. *Compr. Physiol.* 8, 871–901. doi: 10.1002/cphy.c17 0018

Ding, B., Frisina, R. D., Zhu, X., Sakai, Y., Sokolowski, B., and Walton, J. P. (2014). Direct control of Na$^+$-K$^+$-2Cl$^-$-cotransport protein (NKCC1) expression with aldosterone. *Am. J. Physiol. Cell Physiol.* 306, C66–C75. doi: 10.1152/ajpcell.00096.2013

Ding, D., Liu, H., Qi, W., Jiang, H., Li, Y., Wu, X., et al. (2016). Ototoxic effects and mechanisms of loop diuretics. *J. Otol.* 11, 145–156. doi: 10.1016/j.joto.2016. 10.001

Ding, D., McFadden, S. L., Woo, J. M., and Salvi, R. J. (2002). Ethacrynic acid rapidly and selectively abolishes blood flow in vessels supplying the lateral wall of the cochlea. *Hear. Res.* 173, 1–9. doi: 10.1016/s0378-5955(02)00585-3

Edvardsson Rasmussen, J., Laurell, G., Rask-Andersen, H., Bergquist, J., and Eriksson, P. O. (2018). The proteome of perilymph in patients with vestibular schwannoma. A possibility to identify biomarkers for tumor associated hearing loss. *PLoS One* 13:e0198442. doi: 10.1371/journal.pone.0198442

Forge, A. (1976). Observations on the stria vascularis of the guinea pig cochlea and the changes resulting from the administration of the diuretic furosemide. *Clin. Otolaryngol. Allied Sci.* 1, 211–219. doi: 10.1111/j.1365-2273.1976.tb00879.x

Forge, A., and Brown, A. M. (1982). Ultrastructural and electrophysiological studies of acute ototoxic effects of furosemide. *Br. J. Audiol.* 16, 109–116. doi: 10.3109/03005368209081455

García-Alcántara, F., Murillo-Cuesta, S., Pulido, S., Bermúdez-Muñoz, J. M., Martínez-Vega, R., Milo, M., et al. (2018). The expression of oxidative stress response genes is modulated by a combination of resveratrol and N-acetylcysteine to ameliorate ototoxicity in the rat cochlea. *Hear. Res.* 358, 10–21. doi: 10.1016/j.heares.2017.12.004

Gleich, O., and Piña, A. L. (2008). Protein expression of pigment-epithelium-derived factor in rat cochlea. *Cell Tissue Res.* 332, 565–571. doi: 10.1007/s00441-008-0608-6

Grabinski, T. M., Kneynsberg, A., Manfredsson, F. P., and Kanaan, N. M. (2015). A method for combining rnascope *in situ* hybridization with immunohistochemistry in thick free-floating brain sections and primary neuronal cultures. *PLoS One* 10:e0120120. doi: 10.1371/journal.pone.01 20120

Hirose, K., and Sato, E. (2011). Comparative analysis of combination kanamycin-furosemide versus kanamycin alone in the mouse cochlea. *Hear. Res.* 272, 108–116. doi: 10.1016/j.heares.2010.10.011

Jahnen-Dechent, W., Schinke, T., Trindl, A., Müller-Esterl, W., Sablitzky, F., Kaiser, S., et al. (1997). Cloning and targeted deletion of the mouse fetuin gene*. *J. Biol. Chem.* 272, 31496–31503. doi: 10.1074/jbc.272.50.31496

Jahnke, K. (1980). The blood-perilymph barrier. *Arch. Otorhinolaryngol.* 228, 29–34. doi: 10.1007/BF00455891

Jirak, P., Stechemesser, L., Moré, E., Franzen, M., Topf, A., Mirna, M., et al. (2019). Clinical implications of fetuin-A. *Adv. Clin. Chem.* 89, 79–130. doi: 10.1016/bs. acc.2018.12.003

Juhn, S. K., Hunter, B. A., and Odland, R. M. (2001). Blood-labyrinth barrier and fluid dynamics of the inner ear. *Int. Tinnitus J.* 7, 72–83.

Juhn, S. K., and Rybak, L. P. (1981). Labyrinthine barriers and cochlear homeostasis. *Acta Otolaryngol.* 91, 529–534. doi: 10.3109/00016488109138538

Kahle, K. T., Rinehart, J., de los Heros, P., Louvi, A., Meade, P., Vazquez, N., et al. (2005). WNK3 modulates transport of Cl- in and out of cells: implications for control of cell volume and neuronal excitability. *Proc. Nat. Acad. Sci. U S A* 102, 16783–16788. doi: 10.1073/pnas.0508307102

Kaur, T., Ohlemiller, K. K., and Warchol, M. E. (2018). Genetic disruption of fractalkine signaling leads to enhanced loss of cochlear afferents following ototoxic or acoustic injury. *J. Comp. Neurol.* 526, 824–835. doi: 10.1002/cne. 24369

Kikuchi, T., Adams, J. C., Miyabe, Y., So, E., and Kobayashi, T. (2000). Potassium ion recycling pathway *via* gap junction systems in the mammalian cochlea and its interruption in hereditary nonsyndromic deafness. *Med. Electron Microsc.* 33, 51–56. doi: 10.1007/s007950070001

Kitao, K., Mizutari, K., Nakagawa, S., Matsunaga, T., Fukuda, S., and Fujii, M. (2016). Recovery of endocochlear potential after severe damage to lateral wall fibrocytes following acute cochlear energy failure. *Neuroreport* 27, 1159–1166. doi: 10.1097/WNR.0000000000000673

Kusakari, J., Ise, I., Comegys, T. H., Thalmann, I., and Thalmann, R. (1978). Effect of ethacrynic acid, furosemide and ouabain upon the endolymphatic potential and upon high energy phosphates of the stria vascularis. *Laryngoscope* 88, 12–37. doi: 10.1002/lary.1978.88.1.12

Laurell, G., and Engström, B. (1989). The combined effect of cisplatin and furosemide on hearing function in guinea pigs. *Hear. Res.* 38, 19–26. doi: 10.1016/0378-5955(89)90124-x

Lebreton, J. P., Joisel, F., Raoult, J. P., Lannuzel, B., Rogez, J. P., and Humbert, G. (1979). Serum concentration of human alpha 2 HS glycoprotein during the inflammatory process: evidence that alpha 2 HS glycoprotein is a negative acute-phase reactant. *J. Clin. Invest.* 64, 1118–1129. doi: 10.1172/JCI109551

Li, Y., Ding, D., Jiang, H., Fu, Y., and Salvi, R. (2011). Co-administration of cisplatin and furosemide causes rapid and massive loss of cochlear hair cells in mice. *Neurotox. Res.* 20:307. doi: 10.1007/s12640-011-9244-0

Li, C. H., and Lee, C. K. (1993). Minimum cross entropy thresholding. *Pattern Recognit.* 26, 617–625. doi: 10.1016/0031-3203(93)90115-D

Li, C. H., and Tam, P. K. S. (1998). An iterative algorithm for minimum cross entropy thresholding. *Pattern Recognit. Lett.* 19, 771–776. doi: 10.1016/S0167-8655(98)00057-9

Liu, W., Edin, F., Blom, H., Magnusson, P., Schrott-Fischer, A., Glueckert, R., et al. (2016). Super-resolution structured illumination fluorescence microscopy of the lateral wall of the cochlea: the connexin26/30 proteins are separately expressed in man. *Cell Tissue Res.* 365, 13–27. doi: 10.1007/s00441-016-2359-0

Liu, W., Schrott-Fischer, A., Glueckert, R., Benav, H., and Rask-Andersen, H. (2017). The human "cochlear battery" – claudin-11 barrier and ion transport proteins in the lateral wall of the cochlea. *Front. Mol. Neurosci.* 10:239. doi: 10.3389/fnmol.2017.00239

Ma, B., Zhou, Y., Liu, R., Zhang, K., Yang, T., Hu, C., et al. (2021). Pigment epithelium-derived factor (PEDF) plays anti-inflammatory roles in the pathogenesis of dry eye disease. *Ocul. Surf.* 20, 70–85. doi: 10.1016/j.jtos.2020.12.007

Marcus, D. C., Wu, T., Wangemann, P., and Kofuji, P. (2002). KCNJ10 (Kir4.1) potassium channel knockout abolishes endocochlear potential. *Am. J. Physiol. Cell Physiol.* 282, C403–C407. doi: 10.1152/ajpcell.00312.2001

Naito, H., and Watanabe, K. (1997). Alteration in capillary permeability of horseradish peroxidase in the stria vascularis and movement of leaked horseradish peroxidase after administration of furosemide. *ORL J. Otorhinolaryngol. Relat. Spec.* 59, 248–257. doi: 10.1159/000276948

Ölander, C., Edvardsson Rasmussen, J., Eriksson, P. O., Laurell, G., Rask-Andersen, H., and Bergquist, J. (2021). The proteome of the human endolymphatic sac endolymph. *Sci Rep.* 11:11850. doi: 10.1038/s41598-021-89597-3

Pike, D. A., and Bosher, S. K. (1980). The time course of the strial changes produced by intravenous furosemide. *Hear. Res.* 3, 79–89. doi: 10.1016/0378-5955(80)90009-x

Polato, F., and Becerra, S. P. (2016). Pigment epithelium-derived factor, a protective factor for photoreceptors *in vivo*. *Adv. Exp. Med. Biol.* 854, 699–706. doi: 10.1007/978-3-319-17121-0_93

Rarey, K. E., and Ross, M. D. (1982). A survey of the effects of loop diuretics on the zonulae occludentes of the perilymph-endolymph barrier by freeze fracture. *Acta Otolaryngol.* 94, 307–316. doi: 10.3109/00016488209128918

Robertson, C. M. T., Bork, K. T., Tawfik, G., Bond, G. Y., Hendson, L., Dinu, I. A., et al. (2019). Avoiding furosemide ototoxicity associated with single-ventricle repair in young infants*. *Pediatr. Crit. Care Med.* 20:350. doi: 10.1097/PCC.0000000000001807

Santos, F., and Nadol, J. B. (2017). Temporal bone histopathology of furosemide ototoxicity. *Laryngoscope Investig. Otolaryngol.* 2, 204–207. doi: 10.1002/lio2.108

Schindelin, J., Arganda-Carreras, I., Frise, E., Kaynig, V., Longair, M., Pietzsch, T., et al. (2012). Fiji: an open-source platform for biological-image analysis. *Nat. Methods* 9, 676–682. doi: 10.1038/nmeth.2019

Schwartz, G. H., David, D. S., Riggio, R. R., Stenzel, K. H., and Rubin, A. L. (1970). Ototoxicity induced by furosemide. *N Engl. J. Med.* 282, 1413–1414. doi: 10.1056/NEJM197006182822506

Sewell, W. F. (1984). The effects of furosemide on the endocochlear potential and auditory-nerve fiber tuning curves in cats. *Hear. Res.* 14, 305–314. doi: 10.1016/0378-5955(84)90057-1

Shi, X. (2016). Pathophysiology of the cochlear intrastrial fluid-blood barrier (review). *Hear. Res.* 338, 52–63. doi: 10.1016/j.heares.2016.01.010

Shindo, M., Miyamoto, M., Abe, N., Shida, S., Murakami, Y., and Imai, Y. (1992). Dependence of endocochlear potential on basolateral Na+ and Cl-concentration: a study using vascular and perilymph perfusion. *Jpn. J. Physiol.* 42, 617–630. doi: 10.2170/jjphysiol.42.617

Singh, R., Almutairi, M. M., Pacheco-Andrade, R., Almiahuob, M. Y. M., and Di Fulvio, M. (2015). Impact of hybrid and complex N-Glycans on cell surface targeting of the endogenous chloride cotransporter Slc12a2. *Int. J. Cell Biol.* 2015, 1–20. doi: 10.1155/2015/505294

Somasekharan, S., Tanis, J., and Forbush, B. (2012). Loop diuretic and ion-binding residues revealed by scanning mutagenesis of transmembrane helix 3 (TM3) of Na-K-Cl cotransporter (NKCC1). *J. Biol. Chem.* 287, 17308–17317. doi: 10.1074/jbc.M112.356014

Spicer, S. S., and Schulte, B. A. (1991). Differentiation of inner ear fibrocytes according to their ion transport related activity. *Hear. Res.* 56, 53–64. doi: 10.1016/0378-5955(91)90153-z

Spicer, S. S., and Schulte, B. A. (1996). The fine structure of spiral ligament cells relates to ion return to the stria and varies with place-frequency. *Hear. Res.* 100, 80–100. doi: 10.1016/0378-5955(96)00106-2

Sterkers, O., Ferrary, E., Saumon, G., and Amiel, C. (1987). Na and nonelectrolyte entry into inner ear fluids of the rat. *Am. J. Physiol.* 253, F50–F58. doi: 10.1152/ajprenal.1987.253.1.F50

Takiguchi, Y., Sun, G., Ogawa, K., and Matsunaga, T. (2013). Long-lasting changes in the cochlear K^+ recycling structures after acute energy failure. *Neurosci. Res.* 77, 33–41. doi: 10.1016/j.neures.2013.06.003

Tasaki, I., and Spyropoulos, C. S. (1959). Stria vascularis as source of endocochlear potential. *J. Neurophysiol.* 22, 149–155. doi: 10.1152/jn.1959.22.2.149

Tombran-Tink, J., Chader, G. G., and Johnson, L. V. (1991). PEDF: a pigment epithelium-derived factor with potent neuronal differentiative activity. *Exp. Eye Res.* 53, 411–414. doi: 10.1016/0014-4835(91)90248-d

Trepanowski, J. F., Mey, J., and Varady, K. A. (2015). Fetuin-A: a novel link between obesity and related complications. *Int. J. Obes. (Lond)* 39, 734–741. doi: 10.1038/ijo.2014.203

Unterlauft, J. D., Eichler, W., Kuhne, K., Yang, X. M., Yafai, Y., Wiedemann, P., et al. (2012). pigment epithelium-derived factor released by Müller glial cells exerts neuroprotective effects on retinal ganglion cells. *Neurochem. Res.* 37, 1524–1533. doi: 10.1007/s11064-012-0747-8

Videhult Pierre, P., Edvardsson Rasmussen, J., Nikkhou Aski, S., Damberg, P., and Laurell, G. (2020). High-dose furosemide enhances the magnetic resonance signal of systemic gadolinium in the mammalian cochlea. *Otol. Neurotol.* 41, 545–553. doi: 10.1097/MAO.0000000000002571

Wang, H., and Sama, A. E. (2012). Anti-inflammatory role of Fetuin-A in Injury and Infection. *Curr. Mol. Med.* 12, 625–633. doi: 10.2174/156652412800620039

Watanabe, M., and Fukuda, A. (2020). "Post-translational modification of neuronal chloride transporters," in *Neuronal Chloride Transporters in Health and Disease*, ed Xin Tang (Academic Press Elsevier), 243–255. Available online at: https://linkinghub.elsevier.com/retrieve/pii/B97801281531850 0011X.

Weber, P. C., Cunningham III, C. D., and Schulte, B. A. (2001). Potassium recycling pathways in the human cochlea. *Laryngoscope* 111, 1156–1165. doi: 10.1097/00005537-200107000-00006

Westenfeld, R., Schäfer, C., Krüger, T., Haarmann, C., Schurgers, L. J., Reutelingsperger, C., et al. (2009). Fetuin-A protects against atherosclerotic calcification in CKD. *J. Am. Soc. Nephrol.* 20, 1264–1274. doi: 10.1681/ASN.2008060572

Ye, Z.-Y., Li, D.-P., Byun, H. S., Li, L., and Pan, H.-L. (2012). NKCC1 upregulation disrupts chloride homeostasis in the hypothalamus and increases neuronal activity-sympathetic drive in hypertension. *J. Neurosci.* 32, 8560–8568. doi: 10.1523/JNEUROSCI.1346-12.2012

Yoshida, T., Nin, F., Ogata, G., Uetsuka, S., Kitahara, T., Inohara, H., et al. (2015). NKCCs in the fibrocytes of the spiral ligament are silent on the unidirectional K^+ transport that controls the electrochemical properties in the mammalian cochlea. *Pflugers Arch.* 467, 1577–1589. doi: 10.1007/s00424-014-1597-9

Zhang, W., Dai, M., Fridberger, A., Hassan, A., DeGagne, J., Neng, L., et al. (2012). Perivascular-resident macrophage-like melanocytes in the inner ear are essential for the integrity of the intrastrial fluid-blood barrier. *Proc. Nat. Acad. Sci. U S A* 109:10388. doi: 10.1073/pnas.1205210109

Zhang, F., Dai, M., Neng, L., Zhang, J. H., Zhi, Z., Fridberger, A., et al. (2013). Perivascular macrophage-like melanocyte responsiveness to acoustic trauma—a salient feature of strial barrier associated hearing loss. *FASEB J.* 27, 3730–3740. doi: 10.1096/fj.13-232892

Zhang, J., Fan, W., Neng, L., Chen, B., Zuo, B., and Lu, W. (2021). Long non-coding RNA Rian promotes the expression of tight junction proteins in endothelial cells by regulating perivascular-resident macrophage-like melanocytes and PEDF secretion. *Hum. Cell* 34, 1093–1102. doi: 10.1007/s13577-021-00521-3

Ziff, J. L., Crompton, M., Powell, H. R. F., Lavy, J. A., Aldren, C. P., Steel, K. P., et al. (2016). Mutations and altered expression of SERPINF1 in patients with familial otosclerosis. *Hum. Mol. Genet.* 25, 2393–2403. doi: 10.1093/hmg/ddw106

Zwanzig, A., Meng, J., Müller, H., Bürger, S., Schmidt, M., Pankonin, M., et al. (2021). Neuroprotective effects of glial mediators in interactions between retinal neurons and Müller cells. *Exp. Eye Res.* 209:108689. doi: 10.1016/j.exer.2021.108689

21

On the Possible Overestimation of Cognitive Decline: The Impact of Age-Related Hearing Loss on Cognitive-Test Performance

Christian Füllgrabe*

School of Sport, Exercise and Health Sciences, Loughborough University, Loughborough, United Kingdom

Correspondence:
Christian Füllgrabe
c.fullgrabe@lboro.ac.uk

Individual differences and age-related normal and pathological changes in mental abilities require the use of cognitive screening and assessment tools. However, simultaneously occurring deficits in sensory processing, whose prevalence increases especially in old age, may negatively impact cognitive-test performance and thus result in an overestimation of cognitive decline. This hypothesis was tested using an impairment-simulation approach. Young normal-hearing university students performed three memory tasks, using auditorily presented speech stimuli that were either unprocessed or processed to mimic some of the perceptual consequences of age-related hearing loss (ARHL). Both short-term-memory and working-memory capacities were significantly lower in the simulated-hearing-loss condition, despite good intelligibility of the test stimuli. The findings are consistent with the notion that, in case of ARHL, the perceptual processing of auditory stimuli used in cognitive assessments requires additional (cognitive) resources that cannot be used toward the execution of the cognitive task itself. Researchers and clinicians would be well advised to consider sensory impairments as a confounding variable when administering cognitive tasks and interpreting their results.

Keywords: age-related hearing loss, hearing-loss simulation, cognitive performance, short-term memory, working memory, young normal hearing

INTRODUCTION

Over the past decades, there has been increasing interest in the role of cognition in (the decline of) speech processing across the adult lifespan (see **Figure 1** in Füllgrabe and Rosen, 2016b). Indeed, even after controlling for factors affecting hearing thresholds and suprathreshold auditory processes (e.g., Humes et al., 1994; Füllgrabe et al., 2015; Johannesen et al., 2016), speech-in-noise perception remains largely variable among listeners. Idiosyncratic variability and ontogenetic declines in cognitive functioning (e.g., Salthouse, 2004) are likely to explain at least some of the unaccounted variance. Consequently, many studies in hearing science nowadays use inclusion or exclusion criteria based on performance in cognitive screening tests, and/or assess cognitive abilities as covariates when trying to explain speech-processing abilities. In clinical audiology, it is being debated (e.g., Shen et al., 2016) whether cognitive screening should be part of the standard assessment for a more individualized rehabilitation (American Speech-Language-Hearing Association, 2018). Finally, it is important to remember that cognitive testing constitutes the very basis of the study of the lifespan trajectory of cognitive abilities in healthy and pathological aging.

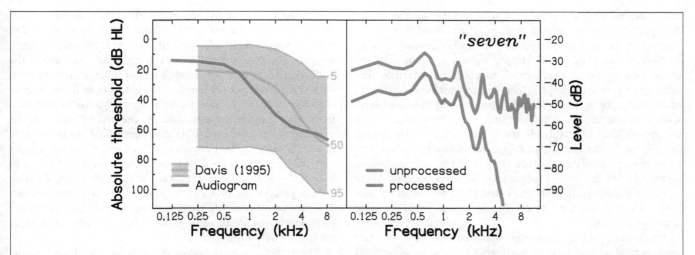

FIGURE 1 | (Left panel) Extrapolated audiometric thresholds for an average 75-year-old listener (audiogram), used for the simulation of age-related hearing loss. For comparison, mean audiometric thresholds for 70- to 79-year-olds from a population-representative sample (Davis, 1995) are shown in the form of audiograms corresponding to the 5th, 50th, and 95th percentiles (light-gray lines). (Right panel) Average power spectra of the unprocessed (blue line; used with the NH group) and processed (purple line; used with the SHL group) spoken word "seven".

Presumably for reasons of convenience and universal usability, most cognitive tests require the administrator to provide verbal instructions, and a substantial number use at least some auditorily presented stimuli (e.g., Mini Mental State Examination, Folstein et al., 1975; California Verbal Learning Test, Delis et al., 1987; auditory Stroop tasks, MacLeod, 1991). One such test is the Digit Span (DS) test, which, as part of well-established psychological test and screening batteries, such as the Wechsler Adult Intelligence Scales (Wechsler, 2008), the Wechsler Memory Scale (Wechsler, 2009), the Clinical Evaluation of Language Fundamentals (Semel et al., 2003), and the Montreal Cognitive Assessment (Nasreddine et al., 2005), is widely used by clinicians and researchers alike. The DS test comes in two versions: In the Forward DS (FDS) test, digit sequences spoken by the test administrator must be recalled in the order in which they were heard; performance on this test assesses short-term memory, i.e., the ability to temporarily store information. In the Backward DS (BDS) test, sequences of spoken digits must be recalled in reverse order; common wisdom assumes that performance on this test assesses working memory (WM), i.e., the ability to simultaneously store and process information (Baddeley, 1992), but empirical evidence indicates that the reordering of digits might require relatively little additional WM processing (Engle et al., 1999; Bopp and Verhaeghen, 2005). In contrast, complex span tests, such as the Sentence Span test developed by Daneman and Carpenter (1980), are designed to assess the key properties of the limited-capacity WM system, namely, memory storage and information processing. In the auditory version of this task, the so-called Listening Span (LS) test (e.g., Wingfield et al., 1988; Salthouse and Babcock, 1991; Lindenberger et al., 2001; Smith and Pichora-Fuller, 2015), lists of auditorily presented sentences must be processed (e.g., by judging the plausibility of the sentence), and information, provided during the presentation of the list (e.g., the sentence-final words), must be recalled at the end of the list.

A considerable number of hearing studies and most cognitive-aging studies include older participants, generally defined as over the age of 65 years (Erber, 2010). It is well known that sensory processing declines across adulthood, with one third of the over-65-year-olds being affected by disabling hearing loss (World Health Organization, 2019). However, hearing abilities of the study participants are either not assessed (as is the case in most cognitive-aging studies) or, if known (as is the case in most hearing studies), not necessarily considered when interpreting cognitive performance. Indeed, when the possibility of age-related hearing loss (ARHL) in the test sample is acknowledged by the authors, its impact on cognitive-test performance is either minimized (on the basis that "the experimenter raised their voice," "the participants judged the used volume as adequate," "the participants were asked to choose their preferred volume," or "the participants wore their hearing aids") or simply dismissed as warranting further investigation in future studies. Such methodological laxness is astonishing given the converging evidence that hearing impairment in older participants is associated with poorer cognitive performance (e.g., Rabbitt, 1991; McCoy et al., 2005; for a review, see Wingfield et al., 2005).

To further demonstrate the assessment-related impact of hearing loss on cognitive performance, the present study simulated audiometric and suprathreshold auditory processing deficits associated with ARHL in young normal-hearing participants and quantified their combined effect on memory span in several auditory-based memory tasks.

METHODS

Participants

Fifty-six young (aged 18–22 years) native-English-speaking volunteers were recruited from the undergraduate student population of Loughborough University (United Kingdom), and received course credit for participating in the study. All participants completed the internet version of the hearing-screening test offered by the British hearing charity "Action on Hearing Loss" (https://www.actiononhearingloss. org.uk/hearing-health/check-your-hearing/) to establish that none had any hearing impairment. The test consists of listening to diotically presented triple digits (e.g., 6–2–5) in a fixed-level speech-shaped background noise (Smits et al., 2004) and varying the speech level to adaptively track the level for 50% correct identification. The test shows a high specificity (0.93) and test performance correlates strongly ($r \sim 0.8$) with the pure-tone average (PTA) for octave frequencies between 0.5 and 4 kHz (Smits et al., 2004). It is assumed that those who pass the test have a PTA of less than 23 dB HL, reflecting "good" hearing (Smits et al., 2006).

Participants were randomly assigned to one of two experimental groups: (i) 30 participants (77% females) with a mean age of 19.1 years [standard deviation (SD) = 1.1] formed the "normal-hearing" (NH) group that listened to unprocessed stimuli, and (ii) 26 participants (86% females) with a mean age of 19.3 years ($SD = 1.3$) formed the "simulated hearing loss" (SHL) group that listened to degraded speech. The small age difference between groups was not significant (Mann-Whitney U-test, $p = 0.394$, 2-tailed).

Stimuli and Procedure

For the NH group, the stimuli were presented at 70 dB Sound Pressure Level. For the SHL group, the same sound-level settings were used, but the audio signals were processed using an algorithm developed by Nejime and Moore (1997) to simulate the following perceptual consequences of ARHL: (i) elevated hearing thresholds (by attenuating the frequency components in several frequency bands according to the threshold values given as an input); (ii) reduced frequency selectivity (by spectrally smearing the speech signal; Baer and Moore, 1994); and (iii) loudness recruitment (by expanding the range of the signal's envelope; Moore and Glasberg, 1993). The algorithm was implemented in a custom-written MATLAB program and received as its input the audiometric thresholds of an average 75-year-old listener (see left panel of **Figure 1**), as extrapolated by Fontan et al. (2017) from epidemiological audiometric data (Cruickshanks et al., 1998). The reason for choosing this particular age was that it falls centrally within the age range explored in many previous studies assessing older persons. The effect of the simulation on the power spectrum of the word "seven" is illustrated in the right panel of **Figure 1**.

The digit sequences for the two DS tests were taken from the Wechsler Adult Intelligence Scale - Third Edition (WAIS-III UK; Wechsler, 1997). In the FDS test, digit sequences of increasing length (from two to nine digits) were presented auditorily for immediate verbal recall. There were two trials for each sequence length. The final FDS score corresponded to the sum of recalled digits for all entirely correctly reported sequences; the maximum possible total score was 88. In the BDS test, digit sequences of increasing length (containing two to eight digits) had to be recalled in reverse order. The final BDS score was computed in the same way as the FDS score; the maximum possible total score was 70. An initial practice trial was given for each test.

For the LS test, short, grammatically correct sentences (e.g., "The ball bounced away"), taken from Rönnberg et al. (1989), were presented auditorily. Half of the sentences were sensible, whereas the others were absurd (e.g., "The pear drove the bus"). Sentences were arranged in sets of three to six sentences, with three trials per set length. The task was to listen to each sentence and then to indicate by a verbal "yes/no" response if the sentence made sense or not. At the end of each set, the participant was instructed to recall either the first or the last word of each sentence. The position (first or last) of the word to be remembered varied pseudo-randomly (with first-word recalls in half of the sets) but was identical for all participants. Prior to testing, practice was given in the form of one three-sentence set. The number of correctly recalled words in any order out of the total number of words to be recalled (i.e., 54) was taken as an estimate of WM capacity.

The timings used in the memory tasks were based on the rate of stimulus presentation recommended by the WAIS-III UK (Wechsler, 1997) for the two DS tests, or used by Rönnberg et al. (1989). The order of the tests was counterbalanced in the NH group and nearly counterbalanced in the SHL group. General test instructions were provided verbally by the experimenter at the start of each test. The test stimuli were recorded from an adult male native-British speaker with a standard British accent prior to the study, using a 44.1-kHz sampling rate with 32-bit quantization, and played diotically to the participant using the open-source audio software Audacity. All testing and the hearing screening took place in a quiet experimental room of the Sleep Laboratory of the School of Sport, Exercise and Health Sciences at Loughborough University, and used an HP (Palo Alto, CA) 250 G4 laptop, an external RME (Haimhausen, Germany) Babyface soundcard, and Sennheiser (Wedemark, Germany) HD580 headphones.

To investigate whether the simulation of hearing loss affected the intelligibility of the speech tokens, and thereby directly affected performance on the memory tasks, the SHL participants were asked, once the memory tests were completed, to listen to all digits and sentences once again and to repeat back what they had heard (in the case of sentences, only the first or last word of each sentence, which had to be recalled during the LS test, was scored).

RESULTS

The results for the three cognitive tests are given in **Table 1**. On average, raw scores for the SHL group were lower than those for the NH group, by 8, 10, and 10 percentage points for the FDS, BDS, and LS tests, respectively.

To allow for the comparison across tests, the data were transformed into z scores, using the mean and the SD of the entire group (i.e., NH and SHL groups combined), prior to statistical analyses, and are shown in **Figure 2**. The effect size, expressed as Cohen's d^{1}, was medium ($0.5 \leq d < 0.8$) for the two DS tests and large ($d \geq 0.8$) for the LS test (see bottom of each

---

[1] Given the unequal sample size of the two listener groups, Cohen's d was calculated using the square root of the pooled variance rather than the mean variance (Howell, 2002).

TABLE 1 | Group-mean raw scores on the three cognitive tests for the normal-hearing (NH) and simulated-hearing-loss (SHL) groups, and statistical results from independent-samples t-tests (degrees of freedom, df; t-value, t; p-value, p) for z score–transformed performance on each of the three memory tests.

Cognitive measures	Listener group		Statistical results		
	NH	SHL	df	t	p
Forward digit span (out of 88)	43.3	36.5	54	2.143	0.019
Backward digit span (out of 70)	32.3	25.6	54	2.652	0.005
Listening span (out of 54)	28.6	23.4	54	4.104	<0.001

The maximum score is given in parentheses next to the name of the test.

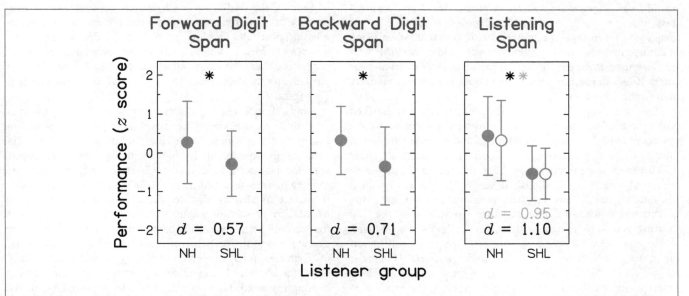

FIGURE 2 | Group-mean performance (in z scores) between participants with normal hearing (NH; blue symbols) and participants with simulated hearing loss (SHL; purple symbols) for the three cognitive tasks. Error bars represent ±1 SD. The effect size is given by Cohen's d at the bottom of each panel. The asterisk indicates a significant group difference at $p < 0.05$. For the Listening-Span test, Cohen's d in light gray and the open symbols pertain to results obtained after excluding six SHL participants who did not show perfect intelligibility for the target speech.

panel in **Figure 2**). For all tests, performance differed significantly between the two listener groups, as indicated by independent-samples t-tests (all $p \leq 0.019$, 1-tailed; for full results, see the three rightmost columns in **Table 1**).

The two listener groups also differed significantly in the number of errors on the semantic-judgment task of the LS test (Mann–Whitney U-test, $p < 0.001$, 2-tailed; data not shown), with the SHL group producing, on average, five times more errors (mean = 7.4) than the NH group (mean = 1.5).

All SHL participants correctly recognized the nine digits, but six of them (23%) failed to recognize two to four target words, representing 4 to 7% of the total number of words to be remembered in the LS test. Hence, all results of the LS test were reanalyzed, excluding those participants (see information in gray in the right panel of **Figure 2**). Although the value of the effect size was smaller compared to that observed when all SHL participants were considered, the effect size remained large (Cohen's $d = 0.95$). The group difference was still highly significant [$t(48) = 3.30$, $p = 0.001$, 1-tailed].

DISCUSSION AND CONCLUSIONS

The observed results are consistent with the "effortfulness hypothesis" originally proposed by Rabbitt (1968, 1991)[2] that suggests that, in suboptimal listening conditions (e.g., due to the presence of background noise or hearing impairment), the early stages of speech processing require additional efforts, thereby limiting the remaining cognitive resources available for the encoding in memory what was heard. Indeed, the present study found that the simulation of ARHL had an acute deleterious effect on the cognitive-test performance of young normal-hearing undergraduate university students, presumably free of cognitive impairment. For the here simulated level of ARHL, the reduction in forward and backward digit spans was not due to impaired intelligibility, as all participants

---

[2]More recently, this notion has been discussed under the name of the "information-degradation hypothesis of aging" (Schneider and Pichora-Fuller, 2000; Wingfield et al., 2005; Wayne and Johnsrude, 2015).

in the SHL group were able to identify the processed test tokens. This observation could be interpreted as evidence that suprathreshold auditory processing deficits associated with ARHL alone cause a decline in memory performance. In the LS task, some participants of the SHL group were unable to recognize all to-be-remembered target words. Audibility or intelligibility of the other words of the carrier sentence could also have been suboptimal (but was not assessed in the present study). The higher number of errors in the simple semantic-judgment task found in the SHL group could be explained by such partial intelligibility of the sentences and/or insufficient cognitive resources available for the judgment task due to words being unintelligible or intelligible but degraded. Taken together, the results suggest that, when using auditory material to cognitively assess older persons who (un)beknown to the experimenter experience audiometric and/or suprathreshold auditory processing deficits, performance is likely to be underestimated.

The simulation used in the present study mimicked only some of the perceptual consequences associated with a moderate ARHL, namely, elevation of audiometric thresholds, loss of frequency selectivity, and loudness recruitment. There is currently no consensus on how to simulate changes in temporal processing abilities (Brian C. J. Moore, personal communication). However, there is converging evidence that sensitivity to temporal fine structure worsens with age and hearing loss (for a meta-analysis, see Füllgrabe and Moore, 2018) and that it plays a role in speech identification in quiet (Lorenzi et al., 2006) and in noise (Füllgrabe et al., 2015), possibly mediated via cognitive abilities such as selective auditory attention (Ruggles et al., 2012) and WM capacity (Füllgrabe and Rosen, 2016a). In addition, audiometric sensitivity further declines with age in the old-old and oldest-old, possibly at an accelerated rate (Göthberg et al., 2019). Both aforementioned caveats suggest that the present study underestimates the actual detrimental effect of auditory deficits on cognitive-test performance, especially in the oldest members of the population.

Qualitatively, the trends observed in the present study are in line with previous results, showing that signal attenuation (Lindenberger et al., 2001; Jorgensen et al., 2016), and background noise or other types of signal distortion (e.g., Rabbitt, 1968; Heinrich et al., 2008; Heinrich and Schneider, 2011) reduce the size of the memory span for auditorily presented speech tokens. Also, compared to age-matched normal-hearing controls, hearing-impaired persons perform lower on a variety of other auditory-based cognitive tasks (Rabbitt, 1991; van Boxtel et al., 2000; Dupuis et al., 2015), but it is unclear if this is due to auditory impairment affecting acutely the perceptual processing of test stimuli during cognitive assessment, or altering long-lastingly cognitive processing *per se*. Using an ARHL-simulation approach and young normal-hearing participants, the present study demonstrated that the former hypothesis is a possible, at least partial explanation for the apparently age-related cognitive decline that is observed when performance is assessed using auditory stimuli.

The reported findings have implications for the interpretation of previous and the design of future studies, assessing cognitive performance in unscreened older participants:

First, published reports of a worsening of performance on FDS and BDS tasks with age (e.g., Grégoire and Van der Linden, 1997; Myerson et al., 2003; Bopp and Verhaeghen, 2005) might at least partially reflect the consequences of ARHL on memory capacity, and less an age-related decline in the "true" ability to retain and process information. Consequently, models of cognitive aging, based on these data, probably overestimate the loss in memory capacity across the adult lifespan.

Second, the finding of a correlation between performance on auditory-based cognitive tests and performance on speech-identification tests in older people should not be interpreted as clear evidence for a cognitive involvement in speech processing, as this association could be caused, at least partially, by the deleterious effect of ARHL on performance in both tasks.

Third, future research assessing cognitive abilities should take into consideration the possible impact of ARHL on cognitive-test performance. This could be done by (ia) controlling experimentally (by including only participants with normal hearing functions) or (ib) statistically (by measuring sensory performance and using this information as a covariate) the effect of sensory decline, (ii) compensating for sensory deficits (by presenting stimuli at clearly suprathreshold levels, for example, by increasing the presentation level or by providing hearing aids to the participants), and (iii) using a visual version of cognitive tests originally including auditory-based tasks (e.g., the Montreal Cognitive Assessment for the severely hearing impaired, Lin et al., 2017). However, these alternative approaches come with their own limitations: (ia) as age-related sensory decline is ubiquitous, older persons with young-like sensory processing are hard to find, and their results are not representative of the general older population; (ib) statistically controlling for sensory deficits does not account for their effects over time in more central processing stations (Willott, 1996) that might negatively affect cognitive performance; (ii) the rehabilitative effect of amplification of the test material on cognitive performance has yet to be demonstrated (Saunders et al., 2018; Shen et al., 2020), as intelligibility of the test stimuli is not necessarily an issue (as shown in the present study), and high presentation levels (causing the broadening of the auditory filters and spectral smearing; Glasberg and Moore, 2000) and the use of hearing aids (resulting in the distortion of the speech signal; Moore, 2008) might impair speech processing and thus affect cognitive performance; and (iii) delivering instructions and test stimuli in the visual domain could still result in compromised cognitive performance as visual acuity also declines with increasing age (Gittings and Fozard, 1986; Klein et al., 1991).

Finally, as regards the clinical use of auditory-based screening and assessment tools (e.g., when diagnosing neurological disorders such as dementia, using the Hopkins Verbal Learning Test; Brandt, 1991), clinicians should be made aware of the risk of misdiagnosis associated with hearing impairment (Gates et al., 1996). For example, clinical-test manuals (e.g., Wechsler, 2008) could caution against the high prevalence of age-related auditory (and also visual) deficits in older test participants and their negative impact on cognitive-test performance. Routine assessment of sensory processing abilities in patients and participants would confirm the presence and severity of sensory impairments, but it is presently unclear how such additional information could be used to obtain a pure estimate of cognitive functioning [see issues discussed under (ib), (ii), and (iii) in the previous paragraph].

In conclusion, for older persons with sensory impairments, the perceptual processing of degraded internal representations of the test stimuli might require additional cognitive resources (Pichora-Fuller et al., 2016) that are unavailable for the execution of the cognitive task itself and, thus, compromise performance because of the limited nature of cognitive resources (Kahneman, 1973). This bias in cognitive-test performance might not be an issue when the aim of the cognitive assessment is to predict a person's real-life difficulties, as sensory deficits also play a role in everyday functioning (e.g., Brennan et al., 2005; Heyl and Wahl, 2012). However, establishing the relative contributions of sensory and cognitive factors to cognitive-test performance is crucial for the accurate diagnosis of the etiology of these difficulties and, thus, for their effective rehabilitation.

AUTHOR CONTRIBUTIONS

CF designed the study, analyzed and plotted the data, and wrote the manuscript.

ACKNOWLEDGMENTS

The author is grateful to Lionel Fontan and Maxime Le Coz for providing the hearing-loss simulation, and to Lucas Ward for collecting the data. The author also thanks Patrick M. A. Rabbitt, Tom Baer, Brian C. J. Moore, and the two reviewers for insightful comments on earlier versions of the manuscript.

REFERENCES

American Speech-Language-Hearing Association (2018). *Scope of Practice in Audiology.* Available online at: https://www.asha.org/policy/sp2018-00353/ (accessed January 16, 2020).

Baddeley, A. (1992). Working memory. *Science* 255, 556–559. doi: 10.1126/science.1736359

Baer, T., and Moore, B. C. J. (1994). Effects of spectral smearing on the intelligibility of sentences in the presence of interfering speech. *J. Acoust. Soc. Am.* 95, 2277–2280. doi: 10.1121/1.408640

Bopp, K. L., and Verhaeghen, P. (2005). Aging and verbal memory span: a meta-analysis. *J. Gerontol. B Psychol. Sci. Soc. Sci.* 60, P223–233. doi: 10.1093/geronb/60.5.P223

Brandt, J. F. (1991). The Hopkins Verbal Learning Test: development of a new memory test with six equivalent forms. *Clin. Neuropsychol.* 5, 125–142. doi: 10.1080/13854049108403297

Brennan, M., Horowitz, A., and Su, Y. (2005). Dual sensory loss and its impact on everyday competence. *Gerontol.* 45, 337–346. doi: 10.1093/geront/45.3.337

Cruickshanks, K. J., Wiley, T. L., Tweed, T. S., Klein, B. E., Klein, R., Mares-Perlman, J. A., et al. (1998). Prevalence of hearing loss in older adults in Beaver Dam, Wisconsin. The epidemiology of hearing loss study. *Am. J. Epidemiol.* 148, 879–886. doi: 10.1093/oxfordjournals.aje.a009713

Daneman, M., and Carpenter, P. A. (1980). Individual-differences in working memory and reading. *J. Verbal Learn. Verbal Behav.* 19, 450–466. doi: 10.1016/S0022-5371(80)90312-6

Davis, A. (1995). *Hearing in Adults.* London: Whurr.

Delis, D. C., Kramer, J. H., Kaplan, E., and Ober, B. A. (1987). *California Verbal Learning Test - Research Edition.* San Antonio: The Psychological Corporation. doi: 10.1037/t15072-000

Dupuis, K., Pichora-Fuller, M. K., Chasteen, A. L., Marchuk, V., Singh, G., and Smith, S. L. (2015). Effects of hearing and vision impairments on the Montreal Cognitive Assessment. *Aging Neuropsychol. Cogn.* 22, 413–437. doi: 10.1080/13825585.2014.968084

Engle, R. W., Tuholski, S. W., Laughlin, J. E., and Conway, A. R. (1999). Working memory, short-term memory, and general fluid intelligence: a latent-variable approach. *J. Exp. Psychol. Gen.* 128, 309–331. doi: 10.1037/0096-3445.128.3.309

Erber, J. T. (2010). *Aging and Older Adulthood.* New York, NY: Wiley-Blackwell.

Folstein, M. F., Folstein, S. E., and McHugh, P. R. (1975). Mini-mental state. A practical method for grading the cognitive state of patients for the clinician. *J. Psychiatr. Res.* 12, 189–198. doi: 10.1016/0022-3956(75)90026-6

Fontan, L., Ferrané, I., Farinas, J., Pinquier, J., Tardieu, J., Magnen, C., et al. (2017). Automatic speech recognition predicts speech intelligibility and comprehension for listeners with simulated age-related hearing loss. *J. Speech Lang. Hear. Res.* 60, 2394–2405. doi: 10.1044/2017_JSLHR-S-16-0269

Füllgrabe, C., and Moore, B. C. J. (2018). The association between the processing of binaural temporal-fine-structure information and audiometric threshold and age: a meta-analysis. *Trends Hear.* 22:2331216518797259. doi: 10.1177/2331216518797259

Füllgrabe, C., Moore, B. C. J., and Stone, M. A. (2015). Age-group differences in speech identification despite matched audiometrically normal hearing: contributions from auditory temporal processing and cognition. *Front. Aging Neurosci.* 6:347. doi: 10.3389/fnagi.2014.00347

Füllgrabe, C., and Rosen, S. (2016a). Investigating the role of working memory in speech-in-noise identification for listeners with normal hearing. *Adv. Exp. Med. Biol.* 894, 29–36. doi: 10.1007/978-3-319-25474-6_4

Füllgrabe, C., and Rosen, S. (2016b). On the (un)importance of working memory in speech-in-noise processing for listeners with normal hearing thresholds. *Front. Psychol.* 7:1268. doi: 10.3389/fpsyg.2016.01268

Gates, G. A., Cobb, J. L., Linn, R. T., Rees, T., Wolf, P. A., and D'Agostino, R. B. (1996). Central auditory dysfunction, cognitive dysfunction, and dementia in older people. *Arch. Otolaryngol. Head. Neck Surg.* 122, 161–167. doi: 10.1001/archotol.1996.01890140047010

Gittings, N. S., and Fozard, J. L. (1986). Age related changes in visual acuity. *Exp. Gerontol.* 21, 423–433. doi: 10.1016/0531-5565(86)90047-1

Glasberg, B. R., and Moore, B. C. J. (2000). Frequency selectivity as a function of level and frequency measured with uniformly exciting notched noise. *J. Acoust. Soc. Am.* 108, 2318–2328. doi: 10.1121/1.1315291

Göthberg, H., Rosenhall, U., Tengstrand, T., Sterner, T. R., Wetterberg, H., Zettergren, A., et al. (2019). Cross-sectional assessment of hearing acuity of an unscreened 85-year-old cohort – Including a 10-year longitudinal study of a sub-sample. *Hear. Res.* 382:107797. doi: 10.1016/j.heares.2019.107797

Grégoire, J., and Van der Linden, M. (1997). Effect of age on forward and backward digit spans. *Aging Neuropsychol. Cogn.* 4, 140–149. doi: 10.1080/13825589708256642

Heinrich, A., and Schneider, B. A. (2011). Elucidating the effects of ageing on remembering perceptually distorted word pairs. *Q. J. Exp. Psychol.* 64, 186–205. doi: 10.1080/17470218.2010.492621

Heinrich, A., Schneider, B. A., and Craik, F. I. (2008). Investigating the influence of continuous babble on auditory short-term memory performance. *Q. J. Exp. Psychol.* 61, 735–751. doi: 10.1080/17470210701402372

Heyl, V., and Wahl, H.-W. (2012). Managing daily life with age-related sensory loss: cognitive resources gain in importance. *Psychol. Aging* 27, 510–521. doi: 10.1037/a0025471

Howell, D. C. (2002). *Statistical Methods for Psychology, 4th Edn*. Belmont, CA: Duxbury.

Humes, L. E., Watson, B. U., Christensen, L. A., Cokely, C. G., Halling, D. C., and Lee, L. (1994). Factors associated with individual differences in clinical measures of speech recognition among the elderly. *J. Speech Hear. Res.* 37, 465–474. doi: 10.1044/jshr.3702.465

Johannesen, P. T., Perez-Gonzalez, P., Kalluri, S., Blanco, J. L., and Lopez-Poveda, E. A. (2016). The influence of cochlear mechanical dysfunction, temporal processing deficits, and age on the intelligibility of audible speech in noise for hearing-impaired listeners. *Trends Hear.* 20:2331216516641055. doi: 10.1177/2331216516641055

Jorgensen, L. E., Palmer, C. V., Pratt, S., Erickson, K. I., and Moncrieff, D. (2016). The effect of decreased audibility on MMSE performance: a measure commonly used for diagnosing dementia. *J. Am. Acad. Audiol.* 27, 311–323. doi: 10.3766/jaaa.15006

Kahneman, D. (1973). *Attention and Effort*. New Jersey: Prentice-Hall.

Klein, R., Klein, B. E. K., Linton, K. L. P., and De Mets, D. L. (1991). The Beaver Dam eye study: visual acuity. *Ophthalmology* 98, 1310–1315. doi: 10.1016/S0161-6420(91)32137-7

Lin, V. Y. W., Chung, J. W., Callahan, B. L., Smith, L., Gritters, N., Chen, J. M., et al. (2017). Development of cognitive screening test for the severely hearing impaired: hearing-impaired MoCA. *Laryngoscope* 127, S4–S11. doi: 10.1002/lary.26590

Lindenberger, U., Scherer, H., and Baltes, P. B. (2001). The strong connection between sensory and cognitive performance in old age: not due to sensory acuity reductions operating during cognitive assessment. *Psychol. Aging* 16, 196–205. doi: 10.1037/0882-7974.16.2.196

Lorenzi, C., Gilbert, G., Carn, H., Garnier, S., and Moore, B. C. J. (2006). Speech perception problems of the hearing impaired reflect inability to use temporal fine structure. *Proc. Natl. Acad. Sci. U. S. A.* 103, 18866–18869. doi: 10.1073/pnas.0607364103

MacLeod, C. M. (1991). Half a century of research on the stroop effect: an integrative review. *Psychol. Bull.* 109, 163–203. doi: 10.1037/0033-2909.109.2.163

McCoy, S. L., Tun, P. A., Cox, L. C., Colangelo, M., Stewart, R. A., and Wingfield, A. (2005). Hearing loss and perceptual effort: downstream effects on older adults' memory for speech. *Q. J. Exp. Psychol.* 58A, 22–33. doi: 10.1080/02724980443000151

Moore, B. C. J. (2008). The choice of compression speed in hearing aids: theoretical and practical considerations, and the role of individual differences. *Trends Amplif.* 12, 103–112. doi: 10.1177/1084713808317819

Moore, B. C. J., and Glasberg, B. R. (1993). Simulation of the effects of loudness recruitment and threshold elevation on the intelligibility of speech in quiet and in a background of speech. *J. Acoust. Soc. Am.* 94, 2050–2062. doi: 10.1121/1.407478

Myerson, J., Emery, L., White, D. A., and Hale, S. (2003). Effects of age, domain, and processing demands on memory span: evidence for differential decline. *Aging Neuropsychol. Cogn.* 10, 20–27. doi: 10.1076/anec.10.1.20.13454

Nasreddine, Z. S., Phillips, N. A., Bédirian, V., Charbonneau, S., Whitehead, V., Collin, I., et al. (2005). The Montreal Cognitive Assessment, MoCA: a brief screening tool for mild cognitive impairment. *J. Am. Geriatr. Soc.* 53, 695–699. doi: 10.1111/j.1532-5415.2005.53221.x

Nejime, Y., and Moore, B. C. J. (1997). Simulation of the effect of threshold elevation and loudness recruitment combined with reduced frequency selectivity on the intelligibility of speech in noise. *J. Acoust. Soc. Am.* 102, 603–615. doi: 10.1121/1.419733

Pichora-Fuller, M. K., Kramer, S. E., Eckert, M. A., Edwards, B., Hornsby, B. W., Humes, L. E., et al. (2016). Hearing impairment and cognitive energy: the framework for understanding effortful listening (FUEL). *Ear Hear.* 37, 5S–27S. doi: 10.1097/AUD.0000000000000312

Rabbitt, P. (1991). Mild hearing loss can cause apparent memory failures which increase with age and reduce with IQ. *Acta Oto Laryngol.* 111, 167–176. doi: 10.3109/00016489109127274

Rabbitt, P. M. A. (1968). Channel-capacity, intelligibility and immediate memory. *Q. J. Exp. Psychol.* 20, 241–248. doi: 10.1080/14640746808400158

Rönnberg, J., Arlinger, S., Lyxell, B., and Kinnefors, C. (1989). Visual evoked potentials: relation to adult speechreading and cognitive function. *J. Speech Hear. Res.* 32, 725–735. doi: 10.1044/jshr.3204.725

Ruggles, D., Bharadwaj, H., and Shinn-Cunningham, B. G. (2012). Why middle-aged listeners have trouble hearing in everyday settings. *Curr. Biol.* 22, 1417–1422. doi: 10.1016/j.cub.2012.05.025

Salthouse, T. A. (2004). What and when of cognitive aging. *Curr. Dir. Psychol. Sci.* 13, 140–144. doi: 10.1111/j.0963-7214.2004.00293.x

Salthouse, T. A., and Babcock, R. L. (1991). Decomposing adult age differences in working memory. *Dev. Psychol.* 27, 763–776. doi: 10.1037/0012-1649.27.5.763

Saunders, G. H., Odgear, I., Cosgrove, A., and Frederick, M. T. (2018). Impact of hearing loss and amplification on performance on a cognitive screening test. *J. Am. Acad. Audiol.* 29, 648–655. doi: 10.3766/jaaa.17044

Schneider, B. A., and Pichora-Fuller, M. K. (2000). "Implications of perceptual deterioration for cognitive aging research," in *The Handbook of Aging and Cognition*, eds. F. I. M. Craik and T. A. M. Salthouse (Mahwah, NJ: Erlbaum), 155–219.

Semel, E., Wiig, E. H., and Secord, W. A. (2003). *Clinical Evaluation of Language Fundamentals - Fourth Edition (CELF-4)*. San Antonio, TX: The Psychological Corporation.

Shen, J., Anderson, M. C., Arehart, K. H., and Souza, P. E. (2016). Using cognitive screening tests in audiology. *Am. J. Audiol.* 25, 319–331. doi: 10.1044/2016_AJA-16-0032

Shen, J., Sherman, M., and Souza, P. E. (2020). Test administration methods and cognitive test scores in older adults with hearing loss. *Gerontology* 66, 24–32. doi: 10.1159/000500777

Smith, S. L., and Pichora-Fuller, M. K. (2015). Associations between speech understanding and auditory and visual tests of verbal working memory: effects of linguistic complexity, task, age, and hearing loss. *Front. Psychol.* 6:1394. doi: 10.3389/fpsyg.2015.01394

Smits, C., Kapteyn, T. S., and Houtgast, T. (2004). Development and validation of an automatic speech-in-noise screening test by telephone. *Int. J. Audiol.* 43, 15–28. doi: 10.1080/14992020400050004

Smits, C., Merkus, P., and Houtgast, T. (2006). How we do it: the dutch functional hearing - screening tests by telephone and internet. *Clin. Otolaryngol.* 31, 436–440. doi: 10.1111/j.1749-4486.2006.01195.x

van Boxtel, M. P. J., van Beijsterveldt, C. E. M., Houx, P. J., Anteunis, L. J. C., Metsemakers, J. F. M., and Jolles, J. (2000). Mild hearing impairment can reduce verbal memory performance in a healthy adult population. *J. Clin. Exp. Neuropsychol.* 22, 147–154. doi: 10.1076/1380-3395(200002)22:1;1-8;FT147

Wayne, R. V., and Johnsrude, I. S. (2015). A review of causal mechanisms underlying the link between age-related hearing loss and cognitive decline. *Ageing Res. Rev.* 23, 154–166. doi: 10.1016/j.arr.2015.06.002

Wechsler, D. (1997). *Wechsler Adult Intelligence Scale - Third UK Edition (WAIS-III UK)*. Oxford: Harcourt Assessment. doi: 10.1037/t49755-000

Wechsler, D. (2008). *Wechsler Adult Intelligence Scale - Fourth Edition (WAIS-IV)*. San Antonio, TX: Pearson. doi: 10.1037/t15169-000

Wechsler, D. (2009). *Wechsler Memory Scale - Fourth Edition (WMS-IV): Technical and Interpretive Manual*. San Antonio, TX: Pearson.

Willott, J. F. (1996). Anatomic and physiologic aging: a behavioral neuroscience perspective. *J. Am. Acad. Audiol.* 7, 141–151.

Wingfield, A., Stine, E. A. L., Lahar, C. J., and Aberdeen, J. S. (1988). Does the capacity of working memory change with age? *Exp. Aging Res.* 14, 103–107. doi: 10.1080/03610738808259731

Wingfield, A., Tun, P. A., and McCoy, S. L. (2005). Hearing loss in older adulthood - what it is and how it interacts with cognitive performance. *Curr. Dir. Psychol. Sci.* 14, 144–148. doi: 10.1111/j.0963-7214.2005.00356.x

World Health Organization (2019). *Deafness and Hearing Loss*. Available online at: https://www.who.int/news-room/fact-sheets/detail/deafness-and-hearing-loss (accessed January 18, 2020).

Permissions

The contributors of this book come from diverse backgrounds, making this book a truly international effort. This book will bring forth new frontiers with its revolutionizing research information and detailed analysis of the nascent developments around the world.

We would like to thank all the contributing authors for lending their expertise to make the book truly unique. They have played a crucial role in the development of this book. Without their invaluable contributions this book wouldn't have been possible. They have made vital efforts to compile up to date information on the varied aspects of this subject to make this book a valuable addition to the collection of many professionals and students.

This book was conceptualized with the vision of imparting up-to-date information and advanced data in this field. To ensure the same, a matchless editorial board was set up. Every individual on the board went through rigorous rounds of assessment to prove their worth. After which they invested a large part of their time researching and compiling the most relevant data for our readers.

The editorial board has been involved in producing this book since its inception. They have spent rigorous hours researching and exploring the diverse topics which have resulted in the successful publishing of this book. They have passed on their knowledge of decades through this book. To expedite this challenging task, the publisher supported the team at every step. A small team of assistant editors was also appointed to further simplify the editing procedure and attain best results for the readers.

Apart from the editorial board, the designing team has also invested a significant amount of their time in understanding the subject and creating the most relevant covers. They scrutinized every image to scout for the most suitable representation of the subject and create an appropriate cover for the book.

The publishing team has been an ardent support to the editorial, designing and production team. Their endless efforts to recruit the best for this project, has resulted in the accomplishment of this book. They are a veteran in the field of academics and their pool of knowledge is as vast as their experience in printing. Their expertise and guidance has proved useful at every step. Their uncompromising quality standards have made this book an exceptional effort. Their encouragement from time to time has been an inspiration for everyone.

The publisher and the editorial board hope that this book will prove to be a valuable piece of knowledge for researchers, students, practitioners and scholars across the globe.

List of Contributors

Daoli Xie, Tong Zhao, Lihong Kui, Qin Wang, Yuancheng Wu, Tihua Zheng, Ruishuang Geng, Ying Yang and Bo Li
Hearing and Speech Rehabilitation Institute, College of Special Education, Binzhou Medical University, Yantai, China

Xiaolin Zhang
Department of Otolaryngology-Head and Neck Surgery, Binzhou Medical University Hospital, Binzhou, China

Peng Ma
Department of Genetics, School of Pharmacy, Binzhou Medical University, Yantai, China

Yan Zhang
Department of Otolaryngology, Head and Neck Surgery, Second Affiliated Hospital, Xi'an Jiaotong University School of Medicine, Xi'an, China

Helen Molteni
Department of Otolaryngology, Head and Neck Surgery, Case Western Reserve University, Cleveland, OH, United States

Qing Yin Zheng
Department of Otolaryngology, Head and Neck Surgery, Case Western Reserve University, Cleveland, OH, United States

Guanyun Wei, Chengyun Cai, Jiajing Sheng, Mengting Xu, Cheng Wang, Qiuxiang Gu, Chao Guo, Dong Liu and Fuping Qian
Key Laboratory of Neuroregeneration of MOE, Nantong Laboratory of Development and Diseases, School of Life Sciences, Co-innovation Center of Neuroregeneration, Nantong University, Nantong, China

Xu Zhang
Key Laboratory of Neuroregeneration of MOE, Nantong Laboratory of Development and Diseases, School of Life Sciences, Co-innovation Center of Neuroregeneration, Nantong University, Nantong, China
Translational Medical Research Cente Wuxi No. 2 People's Hospital, Affiliated Wuxi Clinical College of Nantong University, Wuxi, China

Fangyi Chen
Department of Biomedical Engineering, Southern University of Science and Technology, Shenzhen, China

Department of Biology, Brain Research Center, Southern University of Science and Technology, Shenzhen, China

Yitong Lu, Na Zuo, Renchun Yan, Cheng Wu, Jun Ma, Shaofeng Liu and Chuanxi Wang
Department of Otolaryngology-Head and Neck Surgery, Yijishan Hospital of Wannan Medical College, Wuhu, China

Dongmei Tang, Yingzi He and Zhiwei Zheng
State Key Laboratory of Medical Neurobiology and MOE Frontiers Center for Brain Science, ENT Institute and Department of Otorhinolaryngology, Eye and ENT Hospital, Fudan University, Shanghai, China
NHC Key Laboratory of Hearing Medicine, Fudan University, Shanghai, China

Xin Wang and Dong Liu
Nantong Laboratory of Development and Diseases, School of Life Sciences, Co-innovation Center of Neuroregeneration, Key Laboratory of Neuroregeneration of Jiangsu and MOE, Nantong University, Nantong, China

Hongfei Xu
Department of Forensic Medicine, Soochow University, Suzhou, China

Bieke Dobbels, Griet Mertens, Annick Gilles, Paul Van de Heyning, Olivier Vanderveken, Vincent Van Rompaey and Annes Claes
Faculty of Medicine and Health Sciences, University of Antwerp, Antwerp, Belgium
Department of Otorhinolaryngology and Head and Neck Surgery, Antwerp University Hospital, Edegem, Belgium

Julie Moyaert
Department of Otorhinolaryngology and Head and Neck Surgery, Antwerp University Hospital, Edegem, Belgium

Raymond van de Berg
Division of Balance Disorders, Department of Otorhinolaryngology and Head and Neck Surgery, Maastricht University Medical Center, Maastricht, Netherlands
Faculty of Physics, Tomsk State University, Tomsk, Russia

Li Zhang and Sen Chen
Department of Otorhinolaryngology, Union Hospital, Tongji Medical College, Huazhong University of Science and Technology, Wuhan, China

Yu Sun
Department of Otorhinolaryngology, Union Hospital, Tongji Medical College, Huazhong University of Science and Technology, Wuhan, China
Institute of Otorhinolaryngology, Tongji Medical College, Huazhong University of Science and Technology, Wuhan, China

Milan Jilek, Vaclav Vencovsky and Josef Syka
Department of Auditory Neuroscience, Institute of Experimental Medicine of the Czech Academy of Sciences, Prague, Czechia

Oliver Profant
Department of Auditory Neuroscience, Institute of Experimental Medicine of the Czech Academy of Sciences, Prague, Czechia
Department of Otorhinolaryngology of Faculty Hospital Královské Vinohrady and 3rd Faculty of Medicine, Charles University, Prague, Czechia

Zbynek Bures
Department of Auditory Neuroscience, Institute of Experimental Medicine of the Czech Academy of Sciences, Prague, Czechia
Department of Technical Studies, College of Polytechnics, Jihlava, Czechia

Diana Kucharova and Veronika Svobodova
Department of Auditory Neuroscience, Institute of Experimental Medicine of the Czech Academy of Sciences, Prague, Czechia
Department of Otorhinolaryngology and Head and Neck Surgery, 1st Faculty of Medicine, Charles University in Prague, University Hospital Motol, Prague, Czechia

Jiri Korynta
Eye Clinic Liberec, Liberec, Czechia

Amanda J. Barnier, Celia B. Harris and Paul Strutt
Australian Research Council Centre of Excellence in Cognition and Its Disorders, Macquarie University, Sydney, NSW, Australia
Department of Cognitive Science, Macquarie University, Sydney, NSW, Australia

Thomas Morris
Australian Research Council Centre of Excellence in Cognition and Its Disorders, Macquarie University, Sydney, NSW, Australia
Dementia Centre, HammondCare, Greenwich, NSW, Australia

Greg Savage
Australian Research Council Centre of Excellence in Cognition and Its Disorders, Macquarie University, Sydney, NSW, Australia
Department of Psychology, Macquarie University, Sydney, NSW, Australia

Ming Li, Yurong Mu, Hua Cai, Han Wu and Yanyan Ding
Department of Otorhinolaryngology, Union Hospital, Tongji Medical College, Huazhong University of Science and Technology, Wuhan, China

Natalia Smith-Cortinez, Rana Yadak, Dyan Ramekers, Robert J. Stokroos, Huib Versnel and Louise V. Straatman
Department of Otorhinolaryngology and Head & Neck Surgery, University Medical Center Utrecht, Utrecht, Netherlands
UMC Utrecht Brain Center, University Medical Center Utrecht, Utrecht University, Utrecht, Netherlands

Ferry G. J. Hendriksen and Eefje Sanders
Department of Otorhinolaryngology and Head & Neck Surgery, University Medical Center Utrecht, Utrecht, Netherlands

Dan Li
School of Biology, Food and Environment, Hefei University, Hefei, China Co-innovation Center of Neuroregeneration, Nantong University, Nantong, China
School of Life Sciences and Technology, Southeast University, Nanjing, China

Yangnan Hu, Wei Chen, Yun Liu, Xiaoqian Yan, Menghui Liao and Renjie Chai
Co-innovation Center of Neuroregeneration, Nantong University, Nantong, China
School of Life Sciences and Technology, Southeast University, Nanjing, China

Mingliang Tang
Co-innovation Center of Neuroregeneration, Nantong University, Nantong, China
Department of Cardiovascular Surgery of the First Affiliated Hospital and Institute for Cardiovascular Science, Medical College, Soochow University, Suzhou, China

Lanlai Yuan and Yu Sun
Department of Otorhinolaryngology, Union Hospital, Tongji Medical College, Huazhong University of Science and Technology, Wuhan, China

Dankang Li and Yaohua Tian
Department of Maternal and Child Health, School of Public Health, Tongji Medical College, Huazhong University of Science and Technology, Wuhan, China Ministry of Education Key Laboratory of Environment and Health, State Key Laboratory of Environmental Health (Incubating), School of Public Health, Tongji Medical College, Huazhong University of Science and Technology, Wuhan, China

Fuxin Ren, Wei Zong, Guangbin Wang, Fei Gao and Bin Zhao
Shandong Medical Imaging Research Institute, Shandong University, Jinan, China

Wen Ma
Department of Otolaryngology, Jinan Central Hospital, Shandong University, Jinan, China

Muwei Li
Vanderbilt University Institute of Imaging Science, Vanderbilt University, Nashville, TN, United States

Huaiqiang Sun
Huaxi MR Research Center, Department of Radiology, West China Hospital of Sichuan University, Chengdu, China

Qian Xin
Central Laboratory, The Second Hospital of Shandong University, Jinan, China

Weibo Chen
Philips Healthcare, Shanghai, China

J. Riley DeBacker
VA RR&D National Center for Rehabilitative Auditory Research, VA Portland Healthcare System, Portland, OR, United States
Oregon Hearing Research Center, Oregon Health and Science University, Portland, OR, United States

Breanna Langenek and Eric C. Bielefeld
Department of Speech and Hearing Science, The Ohio State University, Columbus, OH, United States

Yin Chen, Xia Gao, He Li and Ling Lu
Jiangsu Provincial Key Medical Discipline (Laboratory), Department of Otolaryngology Head and Neck Surgery, Drum Tower Hospital Clinical College of Nanjing Medical University, Nanjing, China

Ruiying Qiang, Yuan Zhang, Leilei Wu, Pei Jiang, Jingru Ai, Xiangyu Ma, Shasha Zhang and Ying Dong
State Key Laboratory of Bioelectronics, Jiangsu Province High-Tech Key Laboratory for Bio-Medical Research, School of Life Sciences and Technology, Southeast University, Nanjing, China

Wei Cao
Department of Otorhinolaryngology, Head and Neck Surgery, The Second Hospital of Anhui Medical University, Hefei, China

Renjie Chai
State Key Laboratory of Bioelectronics, Jiangsu Province High-Tech Key Laboratory for Bio-Medical Research, School of Life Sciences and Technology, Southeast University, Nanjing, China
Co-innovation Center of Neuroregeneration, Nantong University, Nantong, China
Institute for Stem Cell and Regeneration, Chinese Academy of Sciences, Beijing, China
Beijing Key Laboratory of Neural Regeneration and Repair, Capital Medical University, Beijing, China

Lindsey Roque, Sandra Gordon-Salant and Samira Anderson
Department of Hearing and Speech Sciences, University of Maryland, College Park, College Park, MD, United States

Hanin Karawani
Department of Hearing and Speech Sciences, University of Maryland, College Park, College Park, MD, United States
Department of Communication Sciences and Disorders, University of Haifa, Haifa, Israel

Jia-Wei Chen, Peng-Wei Ma, Hao Yuan, Wei-Long Wang, Pei-Heng Lu, Xue-Rui Ding, Yu-Qiang Lun and Lian-Jun Lu
Department of Otolaryngology Head and Neck Surgery, Tangdu Hospital, Fourth Military Medical University, Xi'an, China

Qian Yang
Department of Experimental Surgery, Tangdu Hospital, Fourth Military Medical University, Xi'an, China

Lianhua Sun, Dekun Gao, Junmin Che, Shule Hou, Yue Li, Yuyu Huang, Jianyong Chen and Jun Yang
Department of Otorhinolaryngology-Head and Neck Surgery, Xinhua Hospital, Shanghai Jiaotong University School of Medicine, Shanghai, China
Ear Institute, Shanghai Jiaotong University School of Medicine, Shanghai, China
Shanghai Key Laboratory of Translational Medicine on Ear and Nose Diseases, Shanghai, China

Fabio Mammano
Department of Physics and Astronomy "G. Galilei", University of Padua, Padua, Italy
Department of Biomedical Sciences, Institute of Biochemistry and Cell Biology, Italian National Research Council, Monterotondo, Italy

Mary Rudner, Henrik Danielsson and Jerker Rönnberg
Linnaeus Centre HEAD, Swedish Institute for Disability Research, Department of Behavioural Sciences and Learning, Linköping University, Linköping, Sweden

Björn Lyxell
Linnaeus Centre HEAD, Swedish Institute for Disability Research, Department of Behavioural Sciences and Learning, Linköping University, Linköping, Sweden
Department of Special Needs Education, University of Oslo, Oslo, Norway

Thomas Lunner
Eriksholm Research Centre, Oticon A/S, Snekkersten, Denmark

Rodolfo Sardone, Chiara Griseta and Fabio Castellana
Unit of Epidemiological Research on Aging "Great Age Study," National Institute of Gastroenterology-Research Hospital, IRCCS "S. De Bellis," Bari, Italy

Petronilla Battista and Maria Ruccia
Istituti Clinici Scientifici Maugeri I.R.C.C.S., Institute of Cassano Murge, Bari, Italy

Francesco Panza
Unit of Epidemiological Research on Aging "Great Age Study," National Institute of Gastroenterology-Research Hospital,IRCCS "S. De Bellis," Bari, Italy
Geriatric Unit, Fondazione IRCCS "Casa Sollievo della Sofferenza," Foggia, Italy

Madia Lozupone
Geriatric Unit, Fondazione IRCCS "Casa Sollievo della Sofferenza," Foggia, Italy
Department of Basic Medical Sciences, Neuroscience, and Sense Organs, University of Bari Aldo Moro, Bari, Italy

Rosa Capozzo
Department of Clinical Research in Neurology, Center for Neurodegenerative Diseases and the Aging Brain, University of Bari Aldo Moro, "Pia Fondazione Cardinale G. Panico," Tricase, Italy

Emanuela Resta
Department of Cardiac, Thoracic, and Vascular Science, Institute of Respiratory Disease, University of Bari Aldo Moro, Bari, Italy
Translational Medicine and Management of Health Systems, University of Foggia, Foggia, Italy

Davide Seripa
Geriatric Unit, Fondazione IRCCS "Casa Sollievo della Sofferenza," Foggia, Italy

Giancarlo Logroscino
Department of Basic Medical Sciences, Neuroscience, and Sense Organs, University of Bari Aldo Moro, Bari, Italy
Department of Clinical Research in Neurology, Center for Neurodegenerative Diseases and the Aging Brain, University of Bari Aldo Moro, "Pia Fondazione Cardinale G. Panico," Tricase, Italy

Nicola Quaranta
Otolaryngology Unit, Department of Basic Medicine, Neuroscience, and Sense Organs, University of Bari Aldo Moro, Bari, Italy

Jesper Edvardsson Rasmussen, Patrik Lundström, Per Olof Eriksson, Helge Rask-Andersen, Wei Liu and Göran Laurell
Otorhinolaryngology and Head and Neck Surgery, Department of Surgical Sciences, Uppsala University, Uppsala, Sweden

Christian Füllgrabe
School of Sport, Exercise and Health Sciences, Loughborough University, Loughborough, United Kingdom

Index